MW01195912

Essentials of Veterinary Ophthalmology

Essentials of Veterinary Ophthalmology

KIRK N. GELATT, VMD

Distinguished Professor of Comparative
Ophthalmology
Department of Small Animal Clinical Sciences
University of Florida
College of Veterinary Medicine
Gainesville, Florida, USA

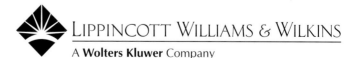

LIPPINCOTT WILLIAMS & WILKINS
A **Wolters Kluwer** Company

Philadelphia · Baltimore · New York · London
Buenos Aires · Hong Kong · Sydney · Tokyo

Editor: Susan Katz
Managing Editor: Dana Battaglia
Marketing Manager: Anne Smith
Production Editor: Paula C. Williams

351 West Camden Street
Baltimore, Maryland 21201-2436 USA

530 Walnut Street
Philadelphia, Pennsylvania 19106-3621 USA

Printed in the United States of America

Library of Congress Cataloging-in-Publication Data

Gelatt, Kirk N.
    Essentials of veterinary ophthalmology / Kirk N. Gelatt.
       p. cm.
    Includes bibliographical references (p.)
    ISBN 0-683-30077-6
    1. Veterinary ophthalmology.   I. Title.

   SF891 .G46 2000
   636.089'77—dc21   00-025601

The publishers have made every effort to trace the copyright holders for borrowed material. If they have inadvertently overlooked any, they will be pleased to make the necessary arrangements at the first opportunity.

To purchase additional copies of this book call our customer service department at **(800) 638-3030** or fax orders to **(301) 824-7390**. International customers should call **(301) 714-2324.**

Visit Lippincott Williams & Wilkins on the Internet: http://www.lww.com.
Lippincott Williams & Wilkins customer service representatives are available from 8:30 am to 6:00 pm, EST, Monday through Friday, for telephone access.

01 02
2 3 4 5 6 7 8 9 10

*To those who teach and those who learn
Veterinary Ophthalmology.*

Preface

The third edition of *Veterinary Ophthalmology*, which was released in January 1999, serves as the eminent clinical and visual science textbook and reference in the field, and it has already been referred as the "gold standard." The previous two editions, which were published in 1981 and 1991, had blue covers and were often referred to as the "blue bibles of veterinary ophthalmology." So the legacy for quality and comprehensiveness continues for this text.

The initial base of essential information for a veterinary medical student is addressed in this clinical pocket reference, which presents the most frequently encountered eye diseases of domestic animals and their treatment. This convenient book also provides critical information for a busy general practitioner or small animal practitioner seeking rapid advice concerning a patient waiting in the examination room. When there is more time, and if the reader seeks additional information on an ophthalmic disorder, the comprehensive third edition can be consulted as well.

This *Essentials of Veterinary Ophthalmology* was conceived while the third edition was being planned (1997). We recognized both the need for and the interest in a small, pocket book that could be carried and used in veterinary medical teaching hospitals and in veterinary clinics and that would provide the basics (or essentials) about the common eye diseases that confront us daily. The primary objectives were to cover the diagnosis and clinical management of the most common eye diseases. Additional details regarding the pathogenesis, pathology, and other aspects of these diseases are available in the third edition; often, the respective page numbers are indicated to assist with this consultation.

Only the clinically relevant chapters from the third edition have been distilled into this "essentials" publication. A few details regarding anatomy and physiology have been incorporated in each chapter to assist in the diagnosis, medical therapy and surgery, and clinical management of these patients. As ophthalmic diseases can be photographed easily and are very educational, most of the illustrations in this pocket reference are in color, facilitating transfer of this information to the clinical patient. Algorithms also have been included when possible to speed the clinical problem-solving process. Because this is a clinical companion text designed for quick consultations, the reader should consult the third edition for a complete list of references concerning any subject.

Therapeutic agents, recommended dosages, and possible side effects are contained in convenient appendices at the end of this book. Tables describing inherited eye conditions in the dog, cat, horse, and food animals are also included in the appendices. Ophthalmology has a unique vocabulary, and this often impedes the teaching of veterinary ophthalmology. As a result, a brief glossary summarizing those ophthalmic words used most frequently in veterinary ophthalmology, often with some adaptation to animals, is included as well.

There are many different ways to "package" information, and I continue to learn new methods to facilitate the instruction of veterinary ophthalmology to students. This "essentials" publication is designed for those students just starting their ophthalmic "exposure" as well as for those veterinarians already in practice who want to refresh their memory. The complete benefits of this book will be achieved when it is carried and used in the clinical environment—either in the clinical service, the hospital, or the practice vehicle. This book is meant to "get dirty," and I encourage you to write in its margins.

If you have suggestions regarding how to improve the "essentials," then by all means, please feel free to contact me with your comments. Because learning is a life- and career-long process, this publication may be your first contact with veterinary ophthalmology. I hope you benefit from and build on this "essential" foundation of clinical veterinary ophthalmology.

Kirk N. Gelatt
25 October 1999

Acknowledgments

Selected chapters from the third edition of *Veterinary Ophthalmology* were used in the preparation of this "essentials" publication. These chapters and their authors include:

Chapter 8: Clinical Pharmacology and Therapeutics (Gorg A. Mathis, Alain Regnier, and Daniel A. Ward)

Chapter 10: Ophthalmic Examination and Diagnostic Procedures (D. Todd Strubbe and Kirk N. Gelatt)

Chapter 11: Ocular Imaging (Dennis E. Brooks)

Chapter 12: Electrodiagnostic Evaluation of Vision (Michael H. Sims)

Chapter 13: Diseases of the Canine Orbit (Bernard M. Spiess and Nils Wallin-Håkanson)

Chapter 14: Diseases and Surgery of the Canine Eyelid (Peter G.C. Bedford)

Chapter 15: Diseases and Surgery of the Canine Nasolacrimal System (Bruce H. Grahn)

Chapter 16: Diseases and Surgery of the Lacrimal Secretory System (Cecil P. Moore)

Chapter 17: Diseases and Surgery of the Canine Nictitating Membrane (Daniel A. Ward and Diane V.H. Hendrix)

Chapter 18: Diseases and Surgery of the Canine Conjunctiva (Diane V.H. Hendrix)

Chapter 19: Diseases of the Canine Cornea and Sclera (R. David Whitley and Brian C. Gilger)

Chapter 20: Surgery of the Cornea and Sclera (Brian C. Gilger and R. David Whitley)

Chapter 21: The Canine Glaucomas (Kirk N. Gelatt and Dennis E. Brooks)

Chapter 22: Diseases and Surgery of the Canine Anterior Uvea (B. Keith Collins and Cecil P. Moore)

Chapter 23: Diseases of the Lens and Cataract Formation (Michael G. Davidson and Susan R. Nelms)

Chapter 24: Surgery of the Lens (Mark P. Nasisse and Michael G. Davidson)

Chapter 25: Diseases and Surgery of the Canine Vitreous (Michael H. Boevé and Frans C. Stades)

Contents

Ophthalmic Examination and Diagnostic Procedures

Because the eye can often be visualized to the level of the posterior segment and the orbit is partially exposed, a complete ophthalmic examination can help to establish a rapid and accurate diagnosis for many ophthalmic and systemic diseases. Furthermore, the eye lends itself to numerous simple and efficient diagnostic procedures, many of which can be performed during a routine examination. This chapter describes the examination techniques, diagnostic procedures, and modalities available to veterinarians, and it differentiates those for a basic eye examination from those that would be performed by a veterinary ophthalmologist. Most of these procedures are noninvasive, and a thorough understanding of these techniques can facilitate the identification and diagnosis of many ocular disorders.

GENERAL AND OPHTHALMIC MEDICAL HISTORY

A thorough medical history can be important in establishing a clinical diagnosis, and it also may help to determine an appropriate therapeutic plan. Though it does not need to be exhaustive, the history should include signalment, primary complaint, current treatment, concurrent disease, and any additional medications being used. Further information may be required depending on the specific complaint. Key questions should not "lead" the animal's owner; if informative answers are obtained, additional questions may focus on more specific eye diseases. Two groups of fundamental questions are necessary:

1. Those that analyze the animal's general condition (Box 1-1), and
2. Those that concentrate on the animal's vision and presenting ophthalmic signs (Box 1-2).

1

BOX 1-1

General Health Core Questions for Ophthalmic Patients

General vaccination and medical history

Other animals in the home

Any recent change in weight, eating habits, personality, and so on

Past and current systemic and topical medications

BOX 1-2

Questions that Focus on Patients with Ophthalmic Diseases and Visual Problems

Vision during dark and light illuminations:

Visual problems at night (i.e., nyctalopia) may indicate rod involvement of the retina

Day-time visual problems (i.e., hemeralopia) may signal cone photoreceptor disease

Vision with moving and stationary objects:

Diseases of the central retina may produce loss of central vision (stationary objects)

Diseases of the peripheral retina may cause loss of peripheral vision (moving objects)

Client's impressions of overt ophthalmic clinical abnormality (duration, sequence and type of signs, and so on)

Does the patient sleep a lot?

Can the animal negotiate stairs?

Current topical medications

GENERAL EXAMINATION

Because patients with a primary ophthalmic complaint are most often presented to their local veterinarian, a complete general examination should precede the eye examination. At this time, the overall condition and temperament of the animal can be ascertained as well.

RESTRAINT

Restraint of most small animal patients is not usually a problem. With aggressive and unruly patients, however, additional manual, mechanical, and chemical aids may be required. Some of these procedures may affect the resting pupil size, light pupillary reflexes, tear measurements, and intraocular pressure. The systemic health of the animal, the extent and duration of the ophthalmic examination, and the needs of the client must be considered before a method of restraint is chosen, and the client should be informed of any potential risk (however unlikely).

Most animals require only manual restraint; however, if chemical restraint is necessary, there are often several drug and dosage selections from which to choose (Box 1-3). Most dogs and cats require only manual restraint for ophthalmic examinations. Muzzles can be employed with aggressive or fearful dogs, and fractious cats can be restrained within towels or cat bags. Horses should be restrained in stocks if possible. A twitch may be used in conjunction with chemical restraint during the examination. Dairy cattle can usually be adequately restrained in a stanchion, with the head pulled laterally by an assistant using a nose lead. Beef cattle may be more difficult to restrain, and squeeze chutes with special head restraints may be necessary. Sheep and goats can usually be restrained manually with the help of an assistant. Goats are examined while standing, and sheep can be examined while seated on their rumps to avoid excessive movements. Rodents, rabbits, birds, and small exotics can usually be restrained manually, and difficult rabbits may be restrained in special box devices if necessary. Nonhuman primates can be similarly restrained in

---

BOX 1-3

Recommended Drugs and Dosages for Sedation of Ophthalmic Patients

Cats: Ketamine, 1–5 mg/kg IV, and Valium, 0.22–0.44 mg/kg IV.

Dogs: Ketamine, 5.5 mg/kg IV, and Valium, 0.28 mg/kg IV; or tiletamine/zolazepam, 6.6–9.9 mg/kg; or acepromazine, 0.025–0.200 mg/kg IV, IM, or SC, and torbugesic, 0.2–0.4 mg/kg IV, IM, or SC, for prolonged sedation. Acepromazine causes nictitans protrusion, and torbugesic induces miosis.

Horse: Xylazine, 0.3–0.4 mg/kg IV, is usually adequate for most examinations. For more invasive diagnostic tests, use a higher dose (1.1 mg/kg IV) or even detomidine, 0.02–0.04 mg/kg IV or IM. Torbugesic, 0.01–0.02 mg/kg IV, may be added for painful procedures such as corneal scrapings or conjunctival biopsies.

Rabbits: Xylazine, 2–5 mg/kg IM.

Nonhuman primates: Ketamine, 5–40 mg/kg IM.

special devices, and sedatives as well as general anesthetics may be used to provide additional restraint.

AKINESIA OF THE EYELIDS

The orbicularis oculi muscle may close the eyelids during the eye examination, especially in large animals. As a result, akinesia of this muscle is routine in the horse, is occasionally required in the cow, but is only rarely performed in small animals. **Eyelid akinesia is performed by infiltrating a local anesthetic around the auriculopalpebral branch or the palpebral branch of the facial nerve, which innervates the orbicularis oculi muscle.** Lidocaine is most often employed for this procedure because of its rapid onset and reasonably long duration; however, procaine, bupivacaine, and mepivacaine can be used as well. With effective akinesia, ptosis, narrowing of the palpebral fissure, and occasionally, lower-lid ectropion result; these effects typically last from 45 minutes to 1 hour. Eye movements, however, are not affected. (For additional details, the reader should consult the third edition, pp. 429–431.)

In the restrained horse, local anesthetic may be injected into the depression just caudal to the ramus of the mandible, at the ventral edge of the temporal portion of the zygomatic arch. The needle is directed dorsally, and 2 to 5 mL of anesthetic are injected subfascially in a fanlike manner. The rostral auricular artery and vein should be avoided. Alternatively, the auriculopalpebral nerve can be blocked just lateral to the highest point of the caudal zygomatic arch, where the nerve may be palpated or "strummed" through the skin by running a finger over the dorsal border of the bone (Fig. 1-1). Anesthetic is injected

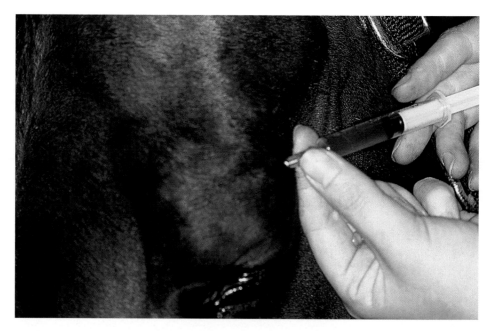

FIGURE 1-1. *The auriculopalpebral nerve block in the horse. This nerve block provides only eyelid akinesia.*

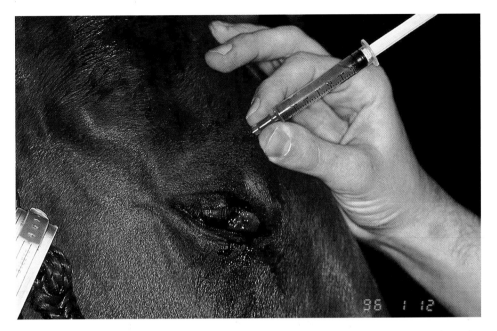

FIGURE 1-2. *The site for the supraorbital nerve block in the horse is the supraorbital foramen within the supraorbital process of the frontal bone. This nerve block provides partial upper eyelid akinesia and anesthesia.*

directly over this nerve (1–2 mL are usually sufficient, but as much as 5 mL may be used).

In the cow, the auriculopalpebral nerve can sometimes be palpated as it passes over a palpable notch in the zygomatic arch at the level of the temporomandibular joint. If the nerve cannot be palpated, anesthetic may be injected subcutaneously along the zygomatic arch, starting at the supraorbital process and continuing for approximately 3 to 4 cm caudally. The needle is directed caudally, dorsally, and medially. When it contacts the zygomatic arch, the needle is then advanced over the dorsal border of the zygomatic arch, and the area is infiltrated with 5 to 10 mL of anesthetic.

REGIONAL ANESTHESIA/ANALGESIA

In the horse, cow, and dog, the frontal nerve innervates most of the central upper lid, the lacrimal nerve innervates the lateral upper lid, the zygomatic nerve innervates most of the lateral lower lid, and the infratrochlear nerve innervates the medial canthus. In the horse, regional injections of local anesthetics are occasionally necessary to perform eyelid and conjunctival biopsies and subpalpebral lavage.

In the horse, the frontal nerve can be blocked as it passes through the supraorbital foramen (Fig 1-2). This foramen can be palpated by grasping the cranial and the caudal borders of the supraorbital process with the thumb and the middle finger, respectively. The digits are then moved medially until the process widens, and the index finger is used to palpate the foramen as it lies midway between the thumb and the middle finger. A 25-gauge hypodermic needle is inserted into or over the foramen, and 2 to 3 mL of anesthetic are infused. (For other nerve blocks in other species, the reader should consult the third edition, pp. 430–431.)

OPHTHALMIC EXAMINATION

The ophthalmic examination begins at a distance from the patient's head. The animal's attitude, overall symmetry and body condition, and ability to navigate in an unfamiliar environment are carefully evaluated as the animal enters the examination area. As mentioned, a general physical examination is performed, and then a thorough ophthalmic examination follows. The ophthalmic examination must be organized and performed at a comfortable rate. Prolonged eye examinations often tax both the patient's and the examiner's patience, but the basic or minimum eye examination should include several procedures (Box 1-4). Additional diagnostic procedures may be conducted after this basic examination depending on the examiner's expertise, the available instrumentation, and the underlying ophthalmic disease.

The ophthalmic examination begins with an indirect assessment of the animal's vision and comfort. How does the animal navigate in an unfamiliar environment? Does it rub or paw at its eyes? The eyes should be evaluated for any asymmetry. Any strabismus or nystagmus should be noted, as should any squinting, ocular discharge, ptosis, swelling, or muscle atrophy. Evaluation of ocular movements can be achieved by turn-

---

BOX 1-4

Diagnostic Components of the Basic Ophthalmic Examination

1. Pupillary light reflexes (direct and consensual/indirect)

2. Menace reflex

3. Schirmer tear test

4. Topical anesthesia and tonometry

5. Instill mydriatic (1% tropicamide recommended)

6. Examine the orbit, eyelids, conjunctiva, nictitating membrane, cornea, anterior chamber, pupil, and iris with adequate illumination and magnification

7. Fifteen minutes later or after complete mydriasis, examine the lens, vitreous, and ocular fundus

8. Apply fluorescein to the dorsal bulbar conjunctiva to evaluate corneal integrity and nasolacrimal system

ing the animal's head from side to side. Normal saccadic and optokinetic movements are noted as the eyes move back and forth in synchronicity, with the fast phase occurring in the direction of the head movement.

Vision, which requires functioning of both the central and the peripheral ophthalmic systems, may be roughly assessed by using a **menace test**, which evaluates cranial nerves II and VII. It is performed by making a menacing gesture with the hand toward the animal's eye while taking care not to touch the vibrissae or to cause excessive air currents that may induce a false-positive result. If the animal can see, it should blink or move its head away from the stimulus. If a patient does not cooperate, which is a common problem with the cat and very young kitten, and puppy, a cotton ball may be thrown across the animal's line of sight. An animal with vision will usually follow this stimulus.

The **palpebral reflex** should be tested in animals that fail to blink completely. The pupils should be observed for asymmetry in both light and dark settings. The examiner may assess pupil asymmetry more accurately by looking through a direct ophthalmoscope from a distance of 1.0 to 1.5 m. The **pupillary light reflex (PLR)** can then be tested using a focal, bright light source. The PLR is a subcortical reflex that requires functioning of the retina, cranial nerves II and III, midbrain, and iris sphincter muscle, which explains why cortically blind animals can have a normal PLR. Both direct and consensual (i.e., constriction of the contralateral pupil) PLRs should be tested. Because all optic nerve fibers decussate to varying extents at the optic chiasm in nonmammalian vertebrates, these animals are not expected to have a true consensual PLR. A false consensual PLR, however, may be noted in avian species related to direct passage of an intense light through the illuminated eye, across the thin septum dividing the orbits, and onto the contralateral retina.

In animals suspected of blindness, an **obstacle course** or "maze test" may be used to determine clinical vision. Gray foam cylinders or, usually, examination room furniture such as chairs and waste cans will suffice. The test should be performed in both light and dim illuminations, thereby allowing the animal time to adjust to the darkness, and obstacles may be readjusted to avoid memorization.

If routinely employed, the **Schirmer tear test** should be performed at this point in the examination, before excessive manipulation of the eye and orbit prematurely stimulate reflex tearing. The Schirmer tear test has been divided into the Schirmer 1 (i.e., without the eye being anesthetized) and the Schirmer 2 (i.e., with the eye being anesthetized). Typically only the Schirmer's 1 tear test is performed. In most small animals, and with use of minimal restraint, the commercial test strips are bent at a notch located 5 mm from one end of the paper (Fig. 1-3). This is preferably done while the test strip is still in its packaging, because oils from the examiner's skin could interfere with tear absorption. The folded end is then placed in the middle to the lateral third of the lower conjunctival fornix, where it should remain for 1 minute. The amount of wetting is measured in terms of millimeters per minute.

Reported means for the normal Schirmer I tear test are 18.9 to 23.9 mm/min for the dog, 16.9 mm/min for the cat, and 5.30 mm/min in the rabbit. In the dog, values of less than 10 mm/min are suspicious if combined with clinical signs of keratoconjunctivitis sicca, and values of less than 5 mm/min

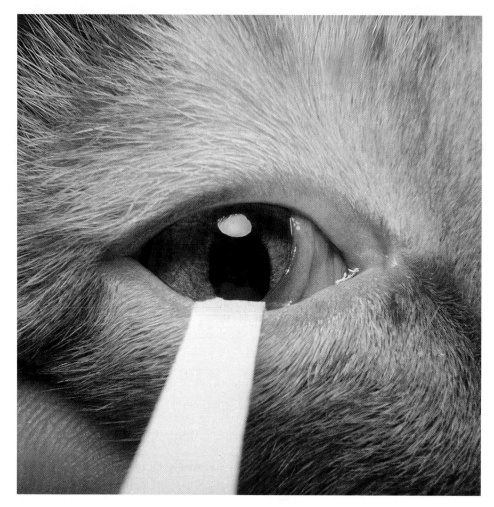

FIGURE 1-3. *To estimate aqueous tear formation, the Schirmer tear test paper strip is inserted into the lower conjunctival fornix of the cat.*

are considered to be diagnostic. Low Schirmer tear test values in the cat must be carefully interpreted in light of the clinical signs, because clinically normal cats can have values as low as 5 mm/min.

The orbit itself is then evaluated by observation, palpation of the bony orbital rim, retropulsion of the globe through a closed eyelid, and manipulation of the mandible. As the coronoid process of the mandible ramus impinges on the lateral orbit, manipulation of the jaw may reveal pain or resistance associated with orbital infections, neoplasia, or trauma. In such instances, the roof of the mouth should be examined for any abnormalities, with particular attention being paid to the soft palate caudal to the last upper molar on the affected side. Additional diagnostic procedures for the orbit include survey radiography, orbital arteriography and venography, special radiographic contrast procedures (i.e., air and radiopaque materials), B-scan ultrasonography, biopsy, and orbitotomy.

Eyelids should be examined for position, movement, and confor-mation using a focal light source and some magnification. Eyelids normally follow the curvature of the cornea, with the meibomian gland openings being exposed and the palpebral conjunctiva being unexposed. Eyelids should be manually everted to examine the conjunctival surfaces as well as the external surfaces and eyelid margins for evidence of tumor or infection.

The nasolacrimal drainage apparatus, which consists of the upper and lower lacrimal puncta and canaliculi, nasolacrimal sac, and nasolacrimal duct, is first evaluated by examining the dorsal and ventral lacrimal puncta, which are located 2- to 5-mm lateral of the nasal canthus and 1- to 3-mm bulbar to the eyelid margins in the canine. Box 1-5 lists the diagnostic procedures to evaluate the nasolacrimal drainage apparatus. The fundamental technique is for patency of this apparatus to be tested by placing fluorescein dye in each eye and then observing its passage at the nares. If passage of the dye is delayed or absent, a nasolacrimal flush may be indicated.

Nasolacrimal flush is the injection of normal saline solution or ocular flush either orthograde or retrograde through the nasolacrimal drainage apparatus. In the dog, cat, and cow, nasolacrimal flush is performed orthograde because of the difficulty in identifying the distal opening of the nasolacrimal duct. For most species, only manual restraint is necessary. After one or more instillations of topical anesthetic, the upper and lower lacrimal puncta are identified near the medial canthus, 1- to 2-mm bulbar to the eyelid margins (Fig. 1-4). The lacrimal puncta are oval in the dog, cow, and horse, but they are round in the cat. In some animals, a small amount of pigment along the margins of the lacrimal puncta facilitates identification. With the upper lid everted to expose the upper lacrimal punctum, a cannula or blunt-tipped hypodermic needle (in the cow, 20–21 gauge; in the dog, 22–23 gauge; in the cat, 24–25 gauge) is gently inserted in a medial direction. Sterile saline is then slowly injected until it flows from the lower lacrimal punctum. This establishes patency of the upper and lower lacrimal puncta, upper and lower canaliculi, and lacrimal sac. If the lower lacrimal punctum is imperforate, a small bleb rises under the conjunctiva in that area. Pressure is then applied to occlude the lower punctum, and 2 to 10 mL

BOX 1-5

Methods to Analyze the Nasolacrimal Drainage Apparatus

Fluorescein passage

Nasolacrimal flush

Nasolacrimal probing

Nasolacrimal catheterization

Dacryocystorhinography

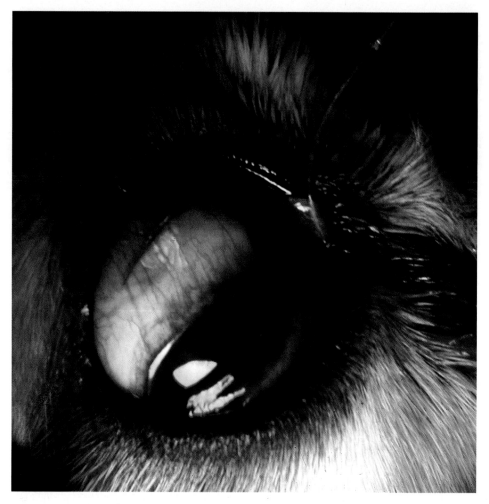

FIGURE 1-4. *To perform a nasolacrimal flush in the dog, the upper lacrimal punctum is cannulated with a gold nasolacrimal needle.*

of sterile saline or ocular flush are injected through the nasolacrimal duct. Any resistance to passage (or failure of passage) is noted, and any debris exiting the duct may be collected for cytology and possible culture. Care must be taken to hold the muzzle down during this procedure; otherwise, the flush may drain caudally into the nasopharynx. In the standing horse, a retrograde nasolacrimal flush is usually performed though the distal opening of the nasolacrimal duct, which is generally visible at the ventral muco-cutaneous junction of the external nares. Approximately 10 to 15 mL of sterile saline are injected, and fluid should be observed to drain from the upper and lower lacrimal puncta. In animals with infection, obstruction, or both, debris may be collected for culture and cytology.

The palpebral, bulbar, and nictitans conjunctiva should be examined for evidence of inflammation, trauma, foreign bodies, petechiae, and lymphoid follicles. With chronic conjunctivitis, the bulbar surface of the nictitans in particular should be examined for lymphoid follicles or trapped foreign bodies. Topical tetracaine or proparacaine is instilled, and the third eyelid is protracted with Van Graefe's forceps (Fig. 1-5). The third eyelid can be everted relatively easily by retropulsing the globe through the upper lid, thereby allowing identification of any cartilaginous, glandular, or other abnormalities. Additional tests for conjunctival diseases include culture, cytology, special stains (Table 1-1), biopsy, immunofluorescent antibody tests, and polymerase chain reaction tests (to detect feline herpesvirus).

Culture and sensitivity tests provide useful information for establishing the diagnosis and determining the appropriate antimicrobial therapy in many corneal and conjunctival diseases. To obtain samples for culture, the eyelids are gently retracted, and a Dacron-tipped applicator is rubbed or rolled over the area to be cultured (Fig. 1-6). The applicator should be moistened with broth or sterile saline before making contact with the cornea or conjunctiva, and care should be taken not to contaminate the sample by inadvertently touching the eyelid margins. The swab is then

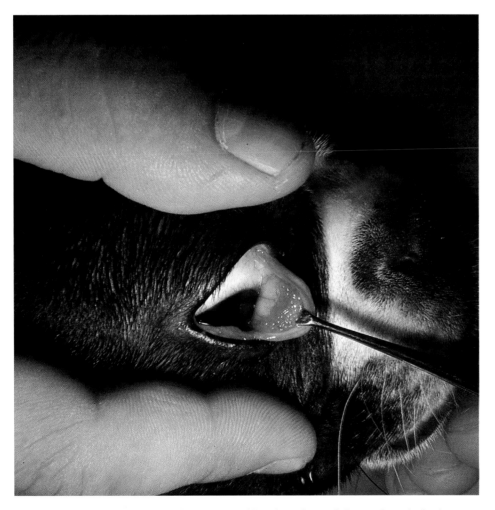

FIGURE 1-5. *Examination of the bulbar (deep) surface of the canine nictitating membrane with thumb forceps and topical anesthesia.*

placed in transport broth for shipping, or it is inoculated either directly onto or into the appropriate culture medium and then incubated.

Cytology is used either alone or in combination with culture techniques to provide rapid results that may influence the immediate course of therapy. Instruments for collecting cytologic samples include cotton or Dacron swabs, cytobrushes, spatulas, and even the blunt end of a scalpel blade. Impression cytology may also be used. Samples should be gently rolled onto glass slides to avoid cell damage. After collection, slides can be fixed with heat, acetone, special cytologic fixative sprays, or some combination of these techniques. The staining methods most commonly used include the Gram stain and various Romanowsky-type stains (e.g., Dif-Quick, Wright-Giemsa).

The cornea is examined next by using a focal beam of light and magnification. The presence of blood vessels, pigment, or other opacities indicates the presence of disease. Corneal integrity is most readily evaluated with fluorescein dye (Table 1-1). When fluorescein is retained, the epithelium is missing, thereby exposing the corneal stroma (i.e., a corneal ulcer); the dye will not bind to Descemet's membrane. Additional tests for corneal disease include culture, cytology, Schirmer tear test, rose Bengal stain, and slit-lamp biomicroscopy.

The anterior chamber and its aqueous humor are examined with a slit beam (as may be found on many direct ophthalmoscopes), pen light, otoscope with the speculum removed, and by the specialist with a slit-lamp biomicroscope. The clarity of the aqueous humor and the depth of the anterior chamber are determined. Increased turbidity of the aqueous humor is determined by using a slit- or tiny circular-beam, which is focused on the cornea and viewed from an angle perpendicular to the beam (normal aqueous, 10–50 mg of protein per 1 dL; with inflammation, the protein content

---

TABLE 1-1

TOPICAL STAINS FOR VETERINARY OPHTHALMOLOGY

Stain	Effect	Indications
Fluorescein	Intercellular spaces	Corneal ulcers and nasolacrimal patency
Rose Bengal	Mucin covering cells Mucus	Keratoconjunctivitis sicca and degenerating corneal and conjunctival cells
Alcian blue	Mucus	Keratoconjunctivitis sicca and conjunctivitis
Trypan blue	Mucus Dead and degenerating cells	Keratoconjunctivitis sicca and conjunctivitis
Methylene blue	Mucus Dead and degenerating cells	

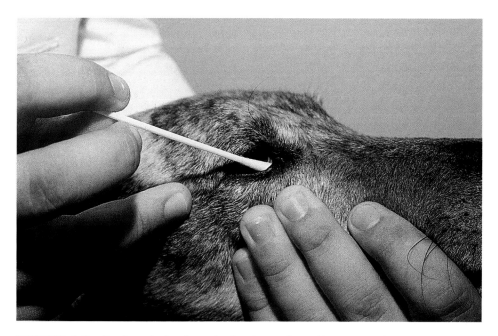

FIGURE 1-6. *Conjunctival culture in the dog using a Dacron swab.*

can elevate to 5–7 g/dL). Under these conditions, both protein and cells suspended in the aqueous humor reflect the focused beam, thus creating the Tyndall effect. Other, more difficult diagnostic tests for the anterior chamber include gonioscopy, B-scan ultrasonography, ultrasonic biomicroscopy using probes from 40- to 60-MHZ, and aqueous humor paracentesis.

The iris is evaluated for color, consistency, pupil size, and pupil shape by using a light beam and some magnification. Some lightly pigmented breeds have blue irides, whereas albino animals have pink to white irides. Iris darkening or thickening (or both) may occur with chronic inflammation and neoplasia. Hypoplastic and atrophic irides are thin and usually transilluminate, and focal holes may be present, especially near the pupil margin. The relative size and shape of the pupil are evaluated as well. Abnormalities of pupil shape may occur with lens luxations, posterior synechiae, iris neoplasia, trauma, or iris atrophy. Most ungulate species have nodular extensions of the posterior pigmented epithelium of the iris (i.e., granula iridica or corpora nigra), which protrude along the dorsal and the ventral pupillary margins. Similar structures are not typically seen in small animals. Further diagnostic procedures include transillumination, retroillumination, gonioscopy, B-scan ultrasonography, slit-lamp biomicroscopy, brush cytology, and biopsy.

Estimation of the intraocular pressure (IOP) is recommended for all ophthalmic patients, even though this may be difficult. Eyes with IOP elevations to between 25 and 40 mm Hg may not demonstrate overt signs of glaucoma. **IOP may be measured with the Schiotz tonometer or, preferably, the TonoPen.** Tonometry, which is the indirect measurement of IOP via digital palpation, indentation, and applanation techniques, is an essential diagnostic procedure during all eye examinations in animals (Table 1-2). A simple and noninvasive procedure, tonometry allows the examiner to

TABLE 1-2

RANGE OF INTRAOCULAR PRESSURES IN ANIMALS

Species	Tonometer	Intraocular Pressure (mm Hg)[a]
Dog	Mackay-Marg	15.7 ± 4.2
	TonoPen	16.7 ± 4.0
	Mackay-Marg	17.8 ± 0.9 (PM)
		21.5 ± 0.8 (AM)
Cat	Mackay-Marg	22.6 ± 4.0
	TonoPen	19.7 ± 5.6
Rabbit	Pneumatonograph	19.5 ± 1.84
		17.9 ± 2.11
Horse	Mackay-Marg	25.5 ± 4.0
	Mackay-Marg	28.6 ± 4.8
	TonoPen	29.6 ± 6.2
	Mackay-Marg	17.1 ± 3.9 (left eye)
		18.4 ± 2.2 (right eye)
	Mackay-Marg	23.5 ± 6.1
	TonoPen	23.3 ± 6.9
	Mackay-Marg	23.5 ± 4.5
	Mackay-Marg	20.6 ± 4.7
Cow	Mackay-Marg	29.5 ± 5.0
		23.4 ± 5.9
Raptors		
Hawks	TonoPen	20.6 ± 3.4
Eagle		21.5 ± 3.0
Owl		10.8 ± 3.6

[a]Mean ± standard deviation.

evaluate intraocular hypertension or hypotension and to intermittently monitor glaucomatous and inflamed eyes for progression or response to therapy. Digital tonometry requires considerable practice, but it may be necessary when indentation and applanation tonometers are unavailable and considerable corneal pathology is present. The index and middle fingers are placed against the patient's closed upper eyelid. One finger applies slight pressure, and the other finger stabilizes the globe (Fig. 1-7). Estimates of IOP do not usually approach the accuracy of results obtained using indentation and applanation tonometers.

The various models of the Schiotz tonometer are the primary indentation tonometers in use today. They consist of a convex corneal footplate; a 3-mm-diameter, jewel-mounted plunger; a holding bracket; a recording scale; and 5.5-, 7.5-, and 10.0-g weight options. The footplate approximates the curvature of the human cornea, and the low-friction plunger protrudes slightly from its concave surface. Depending on the rigidity of the cornea, the plunger is variably depressed so that each 0.05 mm of depression moves the stylet by one scale unit. Scale readings are converted to mm Hg via the instrument's calibration or conversion table. The Schiotz tonometer can provide a reasonable estimation of IOP, but these measurements are still not as accurate as those obtained using applanation tonometers.

The patient is restrained with the head and eyes directed upward, and the eyelids are held open against the orbital rim. After one or more instillations of topical anesthetic, the footplate of the instrument is placed so that it rests on the central cornea. With the instrument being held vertically, the scale readings are then recorded (Fig. 1-8). Three separate readings are taken in this fashion, and the closest two results are averaged. Results of comparative tonometric studies using the Schiotz instrument with the 5.5- and 7.5-g weights and the Mackay-Marg or TonoPen applanation tonometers are suggestive that reasonable correlations are possible.

Applanation tonometers estimate IOP by measuring the force that is required to flatten (or to applanate) a constant area of the corneal surface or by measuring the surface area that is flattened by a predetermined force. Of the different applanation tonometers, the TonoPen is an 18- $\times$ 2-cm, handheld, battery-operated instrument, and it is also the most popular (Fig. 1-9). Although used by all veterinary ophthalmologists, this instrument is sometimes available in larger, small animal practices as well. The footplate is 3.22 mm in diameter, with a central ceramic plunger 1.02 mm in diameter. Recoil of the ceramic plunger after corneal contact produces a signal that is amplified, digitized, and passed through a single-chip

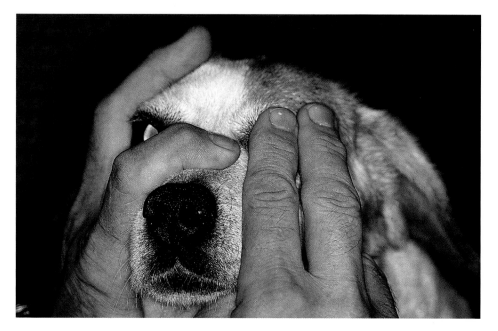

FIGURE 1-7. *To perform digital tonometry in the dog, the first two fingers are used to estimate the intraocular pressure through the closed upper eyelid.*

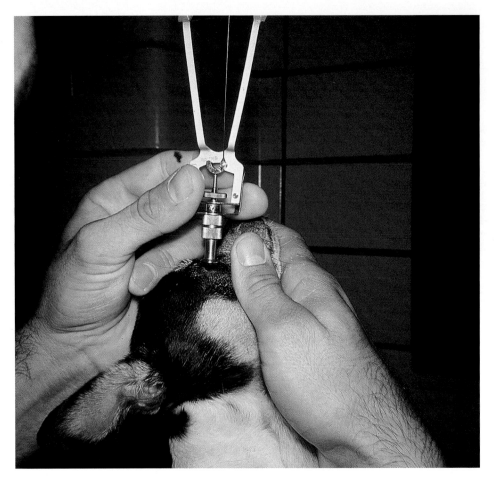

FIGURE 1-8. *To perform Schiotz tonometry in the dog, the instrument is held vertically and placed on the center of the cornea.*

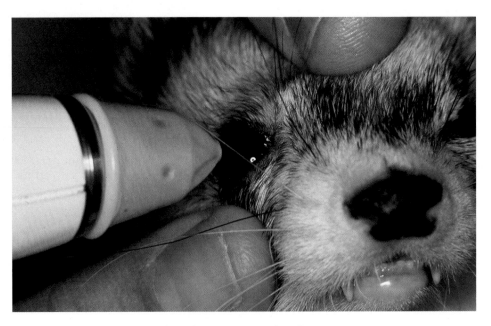

FIGURE 1-9. *TonoPen applanation tonometry in a ferret.*

microprocessor. IOP measurements are then displayed on a liquid-crystal screen. For TonoPen tonometry, topical anesthetic is first instilled, and the eyelids are retracted. The probe tip then gently and repeatedly contacts the central cornea. Brief clicks indicate when individual readings have been recorded, and a sustained tone indicates when the mean IOP has been calculated. The mean IOP is then displayed along with the coefficient of variance (i.e., 5%, 10%, 20%, or >20%). The TonoPen has been used to measure IOP in the dog, cat, cow, horse, American alligator, ferret, raptor, and rat. (For additional information on applanation tonometers, the reader should consult the third edition, pp. 459–462.)

In animals without glaucoma, pupils are chemically dilated to permit complete examination of the lens and the posterior segment (i.e., vitreous, retina–choroid, and optic nerve head). Tropicamide (1%) is preferred in most mammals because of its rapid onset (10–20 minutes) and relatively short duration (6–8 hours). Atropine (1%) is preferred in the rat, and tubocurare derivatives such as vecuronium (0.5% in the raptor) must be used in nonmammalian vertebrates because of the striated muscle fibers in the pupillary sphincter muscle. Inflamed irides usually resist mydriasis and often require multiple mydriatic doses.

The lens is evaluated using both direct illumination and retroillumination. A slit beam is often useful for characterizing cataracts. While directing the beam onto the lens and looking from an oblique angle, the examiner observes a cross-section of the lens. Any opacities of its capsules, cortex, and nucleus should be differentiated. Nuclear sclerosis (i.e., an aging change that leads to a hazy, gray-blue appearance in the center of the lens) must be distinguished from a senile cataract. Other methods of lens evaluation include slit-lamp biomicroscopy, both A- and B-scan ultrasonography, and magnetic resonance (MR) imaging.

The vitreous humor is normally a clear gel that fills the space between the posterior axial lens capsule, posterior chamber, and ocular fundus. In prenatal animals, the hyaloid artery extends from the center of the optic disc to the posterior lens capsule. In very young animals, and especially in ruminants, a persistent hyaloid artery may be visible postnatally for several weeks. **Abnormalities of the anterior vitreous may be observed with direct illumination and some magnification, whereas those in the posterior vitreous require either direct or indirect ophthalmoscopy or the more difficult slit-lamp biomicroscopy using the Hruby and Goldmann lenses, ultrasonography, and vitreous paracentesis (i.e., hyalocentesis).**

With direct and indirect ophthalmoscopy, the ocular fundus is examined. Structures or areas to be evaluated include the optic nerve head (i.e., optic disc or optic papilla), retinal vasculature, tapetal fundus (in species with a tapetum), and nontapetal fundus. Successful examination of the ocular fundus requires intimate knowledge of the normal variations within each species. More difficult diagnostic procedures include slit-lamp biomicroscopy with the Hruby lens, fluorescein angiography, electroretinography (flash and pattern), ultrasonography, biopsy, scanning laser tomography, and optical coherence tomography. Direct and indirect ophthalmoscopy are the primary means to visualize and evaluate the ocular fundus in clinical practice. (For additional information, the reader should consult the third edition, pp. 440–452.)

The modern direct ophthalmoscope consists of an AC or a DC power source and a halogen coaxial optical system. Light is directed via a mirror or prism into the patient's eye, and reflected light is focused through a viewport onto the examiner's fundus (Fig. 1-10). A circular dial holds a series of concave and convex lenses, which can be rotated through the viewing aperture. Green or black numbers on the circular dial represent convex or converging lenses; red numbers represent concave or diverging lenses. A separate dial or switch adjusts the size, shape, and color of the light beam (Table 1-3).

Distances between the normal retina and the surface of such abnormalities can be estimated by changing the dioptric power of the ophthalmoscope. The intensity of the illuminating light is controlled by a rheostat and is generally adjusted to the "comfort zone" of both the patient and the examiner. The resultant image is real, erect, and magnified several times depending on the species being evaluated (Table 1-4). Available monocular direct ophthalmoscopes include the Heine, Keeler, Propper, Reichert, and Welch-Allyn models.

FIGURE 1-10. *Optics for direct ophthalmoscopy.* ***a.*** *Light source.* ***b.*** *Mirror or prism.* ***c.*** *Patient's eye.* ***d.*** *Image.*

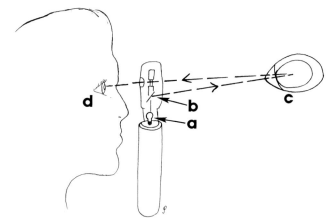

TABLE 1-3	
LIGHT BEAM SELECTIONS FOR DIRECT OPHTHALMOSCOPY	
Small spot	Use with pin-point pupil
Medium spot	Use with pupil in a darkened room
Large spot	Use in a pupil dilated by mydriatics
Red-free light	Use to evaluate retinal vessels and the nerve fiber layer
Graticule	Grid (often of 16 squares) to estimate the size of fundic lesions
Slit beam	Use to estimate fundic elevations/depressions

TABLE 1-4

FUNDUS MAGNIFICATION WITH DIRECT OPHTHALMOSCOPY IN ANIMALS

Animal	Fundus Magnification	Equivalent per Diopter Change (mm)[a]
Cat	19.5	0.22
Dog	17.2	0.28
Cow	10.6	0.74
Horse	7.9	1.33
Sheep	13.9	0.43
Rabbit	25.3	0.13

Modified with permission from Murphy CJ, Howland HC. The optics of comparative ophthalmology. Vis Res 1987;27:599–607.

[a]Change in millimeters with a 1-diopter change in focus with direct ophthalmoscopy.

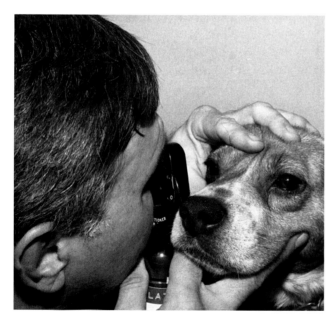

FIGURE 1-11. *Direct ophthalmoscopy in the dog. After locating the fundic reflect, the scope should be advanced as close to the cornea as possible.*

To perform direct ophthalmoscopy, the pupils are first dilated, and the lights of the examination room are dimmed. After adequate mydriasis, the examiner places the direct ophthalmoscope against his or her brow and identifies the patient's fundic reflex from a distance of approximately 0.50 to 0.75 m. Ideally, the examiner's right eye should be used to examine the patient's right eye, and vice versa (Fig. 1-11). In small animals, this minimizes contact between the examiner's nose and the patient's muzzle. Once the fundic reflex is identified, the examiner moves toward the patient, to a point approximately 2 to 3 cm from the eye. If the direct ophthalmoscope is positioned too far from the cornea, the entire fundus cannot be visualized, and even the slightest movement will cause most of the fundic image to be lost.

Indirect ophthalmoscopy, which was first reported in the dog in 1960, is complementary to the direct method (Boxes 1-6 and 1-7). Binocular indirect ophthalmoscopy is the principal method used by veterinary ophthalmologists, but the monocular technique uses only a penlight transilluminator, direct ophthalmoscope, or penlight and a hand-

---

BOX 1-6

Advantages and Limitations of Direct Ophthalmoscopy

Advantages: Greater magnification

  Can be performed through a small pupil

  Availability of options such as the slit and graticule

  Ability to alter the dioptric power of the ophthalmoscope

Limitations: Small field of view

  Short working distance between examiner and patient

  Lack of stereopsis

  Difficulty in examining the peripheral fundus

  Eye movements can be distracting

  Greater distortion when the cornea and lens are not transparent

---

BOX 1-7

Advantages and Limitations of Indirect Ophthalmoscopy

Advantages: Larger (and often safer) working distance from the patient

  Larger field of view

  Stereopsis

  Can be used with some corneal/lens translucency

Limitations: Dilated pupil is necessary

  More difficult to master

  Lower magnification

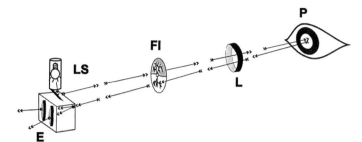

FIGURE 1-12. *Optical principle of the binocular indirect ophthalmoscope. E, examiner's eyes; FI, inverted fundus image; L, handheld corrective lens; LS, light source; P, patient's eye.*

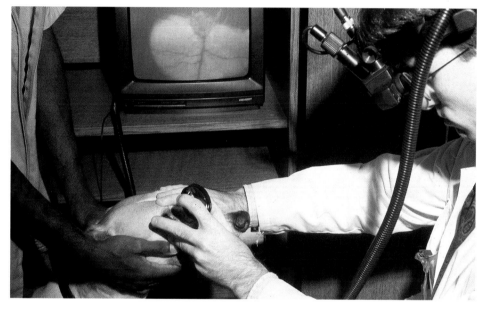

FIGURE 1-13. *Binocular indirect ophthalmoscopy in the dog with a video system attached. The ocular fundus image (seen on the TV screen) is virtual, inverted, and magnified ×2 to ×4. An alternate method is use of the indirect lens (the +20-diopter lens is the most versatile) and a penlight held near the cheek or temple.*

held, converging lens to magnify the reflected image. The light source is placed against the examiner's temple so that both the head and the light source move as a unit. The most common indirect lenses are the 20-, 28-, and 30-diopter powers, which provide a virtual image (i.e., the image is inverted and reversed) of the patient's fundus (Fig 1-12). Fundic magnification varies with the lens and the species but usually ranges from ×2 to ×5. To perform indirect ophthalmoscopy, the examiner grasps the patient's muzzle with one hand to stabilize the head (Fig. 1-13). The other hand holds the eyelids open and positions the lens from 2 to 4 cm in front of the patient's cornea. From a distance of approximately 0.50 to 0.75 m, the examiner then directs the light into the patient's eye and identifies the fundic reflex. The light should be adjusted so that its intensity permits adequate (but not excessive) illumination of the ocular fundus. The indirect lens is moved back and forth until the view of the fundus fills the entire lens. Tilting the lens slightly minimizes any light reflection from the lens surface.

OTHER DIAGNOSTIC PROCEDURES

This chapter presents the basic ophthalmic examination without several of the more difficult diagnostic techniques that veterinary ophthalmologists or veterinarians with considerable ophthalmologic training might employ. Because some patients may require referral for additional diagnostic procedures, however, the indications for several of these techniques are included here.

GONIOSCOPY AND SLIT-LAMP BIOMICROSCOPY

Gonioscopy and slit-lamp biomicroscopy are important but specialized diagnostic procedures that veterinary students will encounter in their clinical ophthalmology clerkships. In practice, however, these procedures tend to be used by specialists. Gonioscopy is most often used in the clinical management of canine and feline glaucoma.

In gonioscopy, the anterior chamber angle or the iridocorneal angle and ciliary cleft are evaluated by placing a special contact goniolens on the cornea. Direct goniolenses allow the examiner to look across the anterior chamber to the opposite iridocorneal angle segment. Many direct and indirect goniolenses are available, and choice is often by personal preference. The Koeppe lenses (either plastic or glass) are most often used. Illumination, magnification, and stereopsis are necessary to observe "the angle," and an otoscope with the speculum removed or a portable slit-lamp biomicroscope serves this function. Small animals can usually be examined with use of only topical anesthetic and minimal restraint. A 1.0% to 2.5% methylcellulose solution is placed on the contact surface of the goniolens before the lens is applied to the cornea (Fig. 1-14). Air bubbles should be avoided, because they will distort both light and the angle of visualization for the iridocorneal angle and ciliary cleft. Special attention should be given to their width, the opening of the ciliary cleft, the pectinate ligament conformation, the inner and outer pigment zones, and the uveoscleral trabecular meshwork. If photographs are desired, a handheld fundus camera may be used, but the flash reflection should be positioned away from the main portion of the photographic field.

Slit-lamp biomicroscopy is a fundamental diagnostic procedure for veterinarians interested in ophthalmology, because it enables the identification and localization of even the most subtle lesions of the cornea, anterior chamber, lens, and anterior vitreous. The basic design of the slit-lamp biomicroscope includes a binocular microscope (usually ×10–20) and an external, pivoting, and adjustable light source. The focused light is modified by a series of diaphragms and filters that adjust the light-beam width, length, orientation, and color. The portable handheld biomicroscope (models include the Clement-Clark, Kowa, Nippon, and Zeiss) has proved to be the most useful and popular for veterinarians interested in ophthalmology. Before performing slit-lamp biomicroscopy, the oculars (i.e., the eyepieces) should be adjusted to accommodate the examiner's interpupillary distance and to correct for the refractive error. This is done by focusing on a target rod that attaches to the instrument at a fixed distance

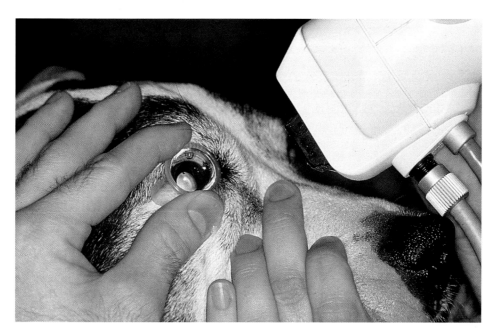

FIGURE 1-14. *The goniolens in position. The iridociliary angle and opening of the ciliary cleft are illuminated and viewed with some magnification. In this patient, the Kowa fundus camera is being used for "angle" photography.*

from the objective (i.e., the focal distance of the slit beam). For biomicroscopy, the animal's head is restrained by an assistant, and the examiner's free hand maintains the eyelids open (Fig. 1-15). The light beam is angled at approximately 20° from the axis of the microscope and usually away from the muzzle to avoid interference. The focal distance of the instrument is 7 to 10 cm, and fine focus is achieved by moving either toward or away from the eye within this range. The most useful light sources are the different sizes of spots and the fine or the medium slit. Several types of illumination techniques are available; those used most frequently are diffuse illumination as well as direct and indirect retroillumination. For both the cornea and lens, the slit beam creates an invaluable parallel-piped or three-dimensional section of these structures. Because of the animal's eye movements, a magnification of ×10 is usually preferred.

IMAGING PROCEDURES

Radiographic examination of the skull is often necessary to completely evaluate the animal patient with ocular or orbital disease. The advantages of plain-film radiographs include their availability at most veterinary medical centers, the relatively basic level of hardware and technical support required, the rapid data acquisition time, and the nominal cost. A Flieringa wire ring placed at the limbus can help to localize the globe and the orbit. Radiographs should be obtained using lateral, ventrodorsal, oblique, and dorsoventral views to differentiate ocular and orbital foreign bodies, tumors, fractures, and the extent of soft tissue or bony lesions.

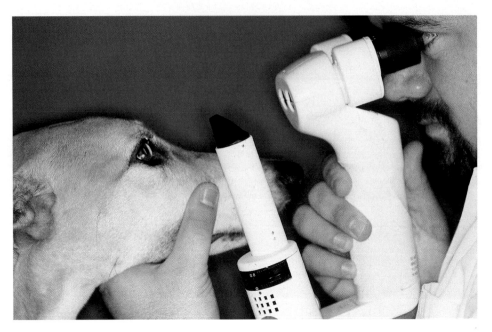

FIGURE 1-15. *Use of the portable Kowa SL-14 slit-lamp biomicroscope in the dog.*

In computed tomography (CT), cross-sectional, two-dimensional slices or scans (i.e., tomograms) of tissue are created by a rotating radiation source that rapidly transmits x-rays from several angles through the tissue in 1° increments. The anatomy of the orbit is an ideal subject for CT, but use of the modality in this area has been somewhat upstaged by MR imaging. Even so, the relatively dense nerves, globe, and extraocular muscles, which are surrounded by lucent orbital fat and are encased in dense bone, provide a tissue of high contrasts on CT scans, which provides anatomic details of orbital bone, soft-tissue, and foreign bodies superior to those of plain-film radiography. CT also provides much better visualization of bony orbital structures than MR imaging. (For additional details, the reader should consult the third edition, pp. 467–471.)

Magnetic resonance images of the globe and orbit are obtained by placing the head within a highly uniform, strong, and static magnetic field. The intraocular structures of the dog and cat visible on proton density–weighted, T1-weighted, and T2–weighted MR images include the cornea, anterior chamber, posterior chamber, iris, lens, ciliary body, choroid, retina, and sclera. The orbital structures of the dog and cat visible on proton density–weighted, T1-weighted, and T2-weighted MR images include the optic nerve and chiasm, extraocular muscles, orbital fat, zygomatic salivary gland, ophthalmic artery and vein, and orbital bones.

Echography (or ultrasonography) is a noninvasive diagnostic procedure that allows qualitative and quantitative evaluation of various orbital and intraocular abnormalities. This technique is particularly useful to examine the posterior aspects of the eye with corneal and lens opacification and for orbital diseases. The resolution of ultrasound measurement depends on the wavelength of the soundwaves, with those of

7.5 to 10.0 MHZ yielding a spatial resolution of approximately 150 mm. The B-scan mode is the most frequently used clinically, because its produces a two-dimensional cross-section of tissue. The ultrasonic transducer (preferably in the sector mode) can be placed in contact with the eyelids via a methylcellulose-coupling agent, directly on the cornea after instillation of a topical anesthetic to evaluate the globe and orbit, or dorsal to the zygomatic arch to scan the orbit.

Dacryocystorhinography evaluates stenosis or obstruction of the nasolacrimal drainage system with the injection of radiopaque material and routine radiography. General anesthesia is required. The upper lacrimal punctum is cannulated with a 22- to 25-gauge silicone catheter containing radiopaque sodium and meglumine diatrizoate contrast material. Radiographic images (lateral and ventrodorsal views) are obtained immediately after injection of the contrast agent.

ELECTRODIAGNOSTIC EVALUATION

Unlike behavioral evaluations of vision, electrodiagnostic assessments are based on objective analyses of changes in electrical potentials among various parts of the visual system. Therefore, no electrodiagnostic procedure should be considered as a measure of vision per se. **The electroretinogram (ERG), for example, remains the most widely reported procedure in the veterinary medical literature. It is often used in establishing the diagnosis of retinal diseases such as progressive retinal atrophy and for evaluating general retinal function before cataract surgery. Other available procedures include the visual-evoked potential, the pattern ERG, and oscillatory potentials.** These procedures have received less attention than the ERG, but they certainly offer additional information concerning retinal function that might otherwise be missing during clinical evaluations. In the dog, the ERG has been useful for the diagnosis or evaluation of retinal function in cataracts, glaucoma, hemeralopia, retinal dysplasia, toxicology screening, degenerative retinopathies, optic nerve hypoplasia, sudden acquired retinal degeneration, and cortical blindness. The ERG can be used in the cat for the diagnosis of retinal diseases such as hereditary retinal degeneration, noninflammatory retinopathy, and central retinal degeneration caused by dietary taurine deficiency. For some retinal diseases, the ERG established the diagnosis much earlier than ophthalmoscopic or behavioral examination, and it even characterizes the function of specific cell types in the retina.

The typical ERG consists of an early, small, corneal negative potential occurring within 10 to 12 msec after a bright light stimulus. The cornea then becomes more intensely positive, only to be followed by a slower, negative trough. After several hundred milliseconds, the cornea again becomes positive. The one negative and the two positive peaks were named the a-, b-, and c-waves, respectively, by Eithoven and Jolly in 1908. The typical canine ERG is recorded using a contact-lens electrode, which is referenced to a needle electrode inserted subcutaneously just posterior to the lateral canthus. The stimulus is usually a white stroboscopic flash delivered to a dog that has been dark-adapted for approximately 5 minutes. The most common effect of general anesthesia on ERGs in the dog is general depression (i.e., reduction in amplitude and increase in implicit times), but these are offset by the elimination of much larger, more consequential artifacts in awake animals.

Some clinical electrodiagnosticians have proposed five ERG responses that should be recorded as a minimum standard protocol:

1. A mixed rod-and-cone response obtained using a high-intensity stimulus in a dark-adapted eye,
2. A rod response obtained using a low-intensity stimulus in a dark-adapted eye,
3. Oscillatory potentials elicited using a high-intensity stimulus in a dark-adapted eye,
4. A cone response obtained using a high-intensity stimulus in the light-adapted eye (or other techniques), and
5. Responses obtained using a rapidly repeated stimulus (i.e., flicker).

Diseases and Surgery of the Canine Orbit

Orbital diseases are not uncommon in the dog. The close vicinity of the oral and nasal cavities, the tooth roots, and the paranasal sinuses render orbital structures susceptible to disease processes extending from any of these cavities through the relatively thin bony wall. Orbital diseases change the orbital volume, impair the function of orbital structures, or both. Orbital diseases may also be associated with reduced ocular motility, strabismus, anisocoria, blindness, congestion of the episcleral vessels, and increased or reduced tear production.

DIFFERENTIAL DIAGNOSIS OF EXOPHTHALMOS AND ENOPHTHALMOS

Orbital diseases are generally divided into those causing exophthalmos (i.e., a more prominent globe) and those causing enophthalmos (i.e., a recessed globe). The most frequent causes of exophthalmia include traumatic proptosis, orbital cellulitis, orbital neoplasia, and myositis of the masticatory muscles, with the latter three conditions occasionally being difficult to distinguish (Table 2-1). The causes of enophthalmia are divided into those disorders with smaller-than-normal globes (e.g., microphthalmia and phthisis bulbus) and those disorders with a normal-size globe that is less prominent within the orbit (Table 2-2).

Dogs with orbital diseases should receive general physical, ophthalmic, and neuro-ophthalmic examinations. Several diagnostic procedures may be indicated as part of the ophthalmic examination for orbital disease (Table 2-3). The orbit, which can be only partially visualized directly, is also imaged by several diagnostic procedures (Table 2-4).

TABLE 2-1

DIFFERENTIAL DIAGNOSIS OF EXOPHTHALMOS IN THE DOG

Clinical Signs/Findings	Cellulitis	Neoplasia	Masticatory Myositis
Local pain	Present	Absent	Variable
Onset	Rapid (few days)	Usually slow (months)	1–2 weeks
Lids	Swollen	Normal	Focal muscle swelling
Conjunctiva	Inflamed	Engorged vessels	Engorged vessels
Nictitating membrane	Inflamed/protruded	Protrusion	Protrusion
Pain on opening mouth	Present	Usually no pain	Present
Globe motility	Impaired	Usually normal	Impaired
Retropulse globe	Difficult	Variable; difficult with large masses	Difficult
Caudal to last molar tooth	Swelling	Possible swelling	No lesion
Complete blood count	Leukocytosis with neurophilia	Usually normal	Eosinophilia

TABLE 2-2

DIFFERENTIAL DIAGNOSIS OF ENOPHTHALMOS IN THE DOG

Globe Size	Clinical Findings/Diagnostic Procedures
Small globe Microphthalmos	Small globe since birth. Small cornea, but usually clear. Often with concurrent ocular abnormalities. More often in certain breeds, and those with the Merling gene. Often bilateral. Impairs development of the orbit (orbital asymmetry). Intraocular pressure usually low normal (±10 mm Hg).
Phthisis bulbus	Usually in adults. History of ocular trauma, intraocular surgery, glaucoma, or intraocular inflammation. Cornea usually not clear, with edema, scarring, and linear Descemet's membrane folds. Cataract formation and retinal detachment concurrent. Intraocular pressure usually less than 5 mm Hg.
Normal globe	Pain secondary to entropion, distichiasis, conjunctivitis, corneal ulceration, anterior uveitis, and so on.
	Horner's syndrome. Look for miosis, ptosis, and nictitans protrusion.
	Loss of orbital tissues (usually adipose tissue).
	Fibrosis of orbital tissues (secondary to proptosis, cellulitis, orbital surgery).
	Dehydration and emaciation.

TABLE 2-3

DIAGNOSTIC PROCEDURES FOR ORBITAL DISEASE

Technique	Indications
Palpation	Orally and caudal of the lateral orbital ligament
Leudde or Hertel exophthalmometer	Measures cornea to lateral ligament distance
Retropulsion of globe	Orbital mass/inflammation may prevent Limited in brachycephalics Oral inspection caudal to last molar tooth Inflammations/neoplasms may protrude
Auscultation of orbit	Arteriovenous fistula/varix

TABLE 2-4

IMAGING PROCEDURES FOR ORBITAL DISEASES

Method	Indications
Plain radiography	Proliferative or destructive osseous lesions and radiodense foreign materials
Pneumo-orbitography	Soft-tissue masses
Orbital arteriography and venography	Vascular abnormalities/deviations
Optic nerve thecography	Intraorbital optic nerve abnormalities
Sialography	Abnormalities of zygomatic salivary gland
Orbital ultrasonography (B-scan)	Soft-tissue abnormalities/foreign bodies
Color Doppler imaging	Orbital and ophthalmic blood flow parameters Guide needle biopsies
Computed tomography	Osseous and soft-tissue diseases, optic nerve, and foreign bodies Intraocular tissues outlined
Magnetic resonance imaging	Most intraocular and orbital soft-tissues outlined

CONGENITAL ANOMALIES OF THE ORBIT AND GLOBE

ANOPHTHALMOS/MICROPHTHALMIA

Complete absence of the eye, or anophthalmos, is very rare. In most cases, some remnants of ocular tissue can be identified histopathologically. **In true microphthalmia, an abnormally small globe is associated with various other ocular anomalies involving the cornea, lens, uvea, vitreous, and retina.** In contrast, a small but otherwise normal globe is called nanophthalmia.

In microphthalmia, vision may be normal, reduced, or absent. Microphthalmia has been described in several breeds, and in some instances, a pattern of inheritance can be established. In the Doberman Pinscher, microphthalmia is associated with anterior segment dysplasia and retinal dysplasia. Congenital cataracts and microphthalmia are recessively inherited in the Miniature Schnauzer. Microphthalmia with multiple ocular anomalies (i.e., equatorial staphylomas, persistent pupillary membranes, cataracts, retinal dysplasia, and retinal detachments) in the Australian Shepherd (Fig. 2-1) is also recessively inherited; these animals are homozygous merles (i.e., excessive white hair coat). Microphthalmia has also been observed in the Beagle, Akita, Chow Chow, Cavalier King Charles Spaniel, and Irish Wolfhound.

VASCULAR ANOMALIES

Orbital varices and arteriovenous fistulas are very rare orbital anomalies; few cases have been reported. Trauma was also suspected in one case of orbital varix in a dog. These dogs are presented with a nonpainful exophthalmos that is either pulsating or intermittent. A systolic or continuous murmur (i.e., a "bruit") may be auscultated over the orbital area. The diagnosis of these vascular anomalies is made on the basis of clinical signs and the results of diagnostic imaging. Treatment has been difficult in the few reported cases, with ligation of the orbital vessels resulting in massive hemorrhage and subsequent enucleation of the globe and ligation of the common carotid artery. Euthanasia was recommended in one of these dogs.

ORBITAL DERMOID CYST

In a young Dachshund, a retrobulbar dermoid cyst produced exophthalmos. The cyst was removed by orbitotomy and contained a yellowish, viscous fluid and long black hair. Histopathologically, the cyst wall consisted of a keratinized squamous epithelium.

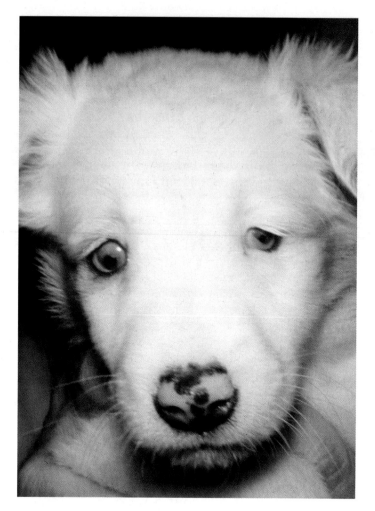

FIGURE 2-1. *Bilateral microphthalmia in an Australian Shepherd puppy. Iridal heterochromia and malformation of the pupil are also present.*

ACQUIRED ORBITAL DISEASES

INFLAMMATORY LESIONS: ORBITAL CELLULITIS/ABSCESS

Orbital inflammatory diseases are rather common in the dog. One reported series involved 13 dogs with a mean age of 4 years. **Typically, the dogs are presented with acute and usually unilateral exophthalmos, protrusion of the nictitating membrane, and conjunctival hyperemia (Fig. 2-2A). There may be serous to mucopurulent ocular discharge. Palpation of the globe and periorbital area as well as opening of the mouth are extremely painful.** The globe itself is usually normal and

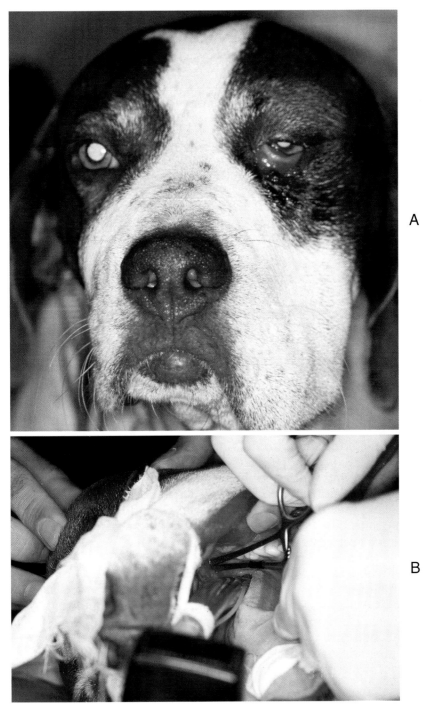

FIGURE 2-2. **A.** *Orbital abscess of 3 days' duration in a Pointer. Note the marked unilateral orbital swelling, exophthalmos, protrusion of the nictitating membrane, edema, and hyperemia of the conjunctiva.* **B.** *Surgical drainage caudal to the last upper molar tooth in the same dog. A hemostat (the jaws are closed) has been inserted through a small incision in the buccal mucosa and into the posterior orbit.*

TABLE 2-5

TREATMENT OF ORBITAL CELLULITIS IN THE DOG

Drainage	Incise the oral mucosa behind the last upper molar tooth. Insert closed hemostat, then slightly open and withdraw. Blood and purulent material may drain from the affected orbit. The area is richly supplied by blood vessels and nerves, but complications are rarely encountered (damage to the optic nerve and ciliary nerves).
Irrigation	Irrigation of the retrobulbar area controversial. Irrigation with crystalline penicillin has been beneficial.
Systemic antibiotics	Use broad-spectrum antibiotics pending culture/sensitivity results. Administer for 5 to 7 days.
Hot packs	Promote healing.
Topical antibiotics	Reduce conjunctival inflammation and lubricate the cornea.

of venous blood flow. In rare and protracted cases, an orbital infection may be accompanied by uveitis. There may be a fluctuating swelling of the oral mucosa behind the last ipsilateral molar tooth as well. Affected dogs are usually febrile and anorectic. White-blood-cell counts may reveal neutrophilia.

Causes of inflammatory lesions may include foreign material, porcupine quills, spread of hematogenous infections, and extension of oral cavity, sinus, and tooth-root infections. In one reported series, *Pasteurella* sp. were cultured from five of 14 orbital abscesses. Infections of the zygomatic gland may present as orbital cellulitis or abscess. Fungal organisms and parasites, however, are rarely identified in dogs with orbital diseases, and the clinical signs are usually pathognomonic for orbital inflammatory diseases. **Treatment of orbital cellulitis is summarized in Table 2-5, and the ventral oral drainage from the orbit is shown in Figure 2-2B.** If the exophthalmos increases temporarily after drainage, a temporary tarsorrhaphy may be necessary. Soft food should be offered until the globe is back to its normal position. The prognosis is usually very good. In most cases, the exophthalmos regresses within 36 to 48 hours, and the general condition of the animal improves markedly. If foreign material is retained in the orbit, however, recurrences are to be expected.

SALIVARY RETENTION CYSTS AND MUCOCELES

Leakage of saliva from the zygomatic gland or its excretory duct causes orbital inflammation and tissue fibrosis. This fluctuating swelling can be dorsolateral or ventromedial, dorsal, ventral in the conjunctiva, or in the oral cavity. Exophthalmos and protrusion of the nictitating membrane are usually present, and pain on opening of the mouth or palpation of the globe is variable but usually minimal. In one case, strabismus and secondary iritis have been observed. A distended excretory duct of the zygomatic gland sometimes can be seen in the oral mucosa as well.

Mucoceles usually result from trauma to the head, both with or without skull fractures. Inflammation and ulceration of the oral mucosa may cause obstruction and retention of salivary outflow, with subsequent cyst formation. The diagnosis is made on the basis of clinical signs and the results of orbital ultrasonography. Aspiration of a yellowish and slightly tenacious fluid with variable amounts of blood is typical, and with nearly complete aspiration of the cyst, the exophthalmos will disappear immediately. Mucoceles are best treated by surgical excision of the cyst and the associated gland, which is performed using a lateral approach dorsal to the zygomatic arch or an approach from the oral cavity.

MYOSITIS

Because of the absence laterally of a bony orbital wall, swelling or atrophy of the masticatory muscles can displace the globe. Inflammatory diseases of the extraocular muscles may also produce exophthalmos.

EXTRAOCULAR POLYMYOSITIS

Polymyositis of the extraocular muscles causing exophthalmos and impaired mobility of the globes has been recently described. Eosinophilic myositis of the masticatory muscles predominantly affects young German Shepherds, Weimaraners, Labrador Retrievers, and Golden Retrievers. Extraocular polymyositis has been diagnosed in Golden Retrievers, a Hovawart, and two Mountain dog crosses. Ultrasonography, computed tomography (CT), or magnetic resonance (MR) imaging will depict swollen extraocular muscles in cases of extraocular polymyositis.

MASTICATORY/EOSINOPHILIC MYOSITIS

Masticatory myositis usually occurs as an acute disease accompanied by fever and anorexia. Jaw movements are limited and painful. Bilateral exophthalmos, protrusion of the nictitating membrane, and congestion of the episcleral vessels are often the presenting signs. In chronic cases, exposure keratitis may ensue. **Swelling of the temporal and pterygoid muscles is responsible for displacing the globe in animals with eosinophilic myositis (Fig. 2-3).** The masseter muscle is also swollen and painful. Without treatment, inflammatory episodes last from 1 to 3 weeks. Acute myositis must be differentiated from orbital cellulitis or abscess, which usually occurs unilaterally. Optic neuritis and subsequent blindness have also been described in association with acute eosinophilic myositis.

With repeated acute attacks, fibrosis of the masticatory muscles eventually result in muscle atrophy and enophthalmos; fibrosis of the extraocular muscles causes mild enophthalmos and strabismus. Severe enophthalmos causes secondary entropion, and enophthalmos and protrusion of the nictitating membrane may impair vision.

Leukocytosis with variable eosinophilia and increased levels of creatine phosphokinase may be present. Biopsy results of affected muscles are usually diagnostic, showing degeneration of muscle fibers and infiltration by neutrophils and eosinophils. Autoantibodies against type 2M myofibers can be identified in frozen sections.

The cause of myositis is not clear, but an immunemediated mechanism is suspected. In one series of dogs with masticatory muscle myositis, 12 had immune complexes limited to type 2M fibers, whereas in another, 13 of 16 sera samples had detectable antibodies against type 2M fibers. Results of immunoblot assays revealed that the antibodies were most often directed against a 185-K protein, myosin heavy chain, and a band that appeared to be myosin light-chain 2-masticatory.

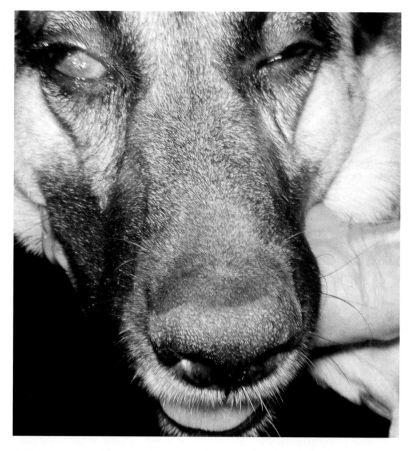

FIGURE 2-3. *Eosinophilic myositis in a German Shepherd. Note the marked swelling of the masticatory muscles and bilateral exophthalmos, which is more marked in the right eye.*

Treatment usually consists of immunosuppressive doses of oral corticosteroids for 3 to 4 weeks. Azathioprine treatment is another possibility. Recurrences are likely, with progressive muscle loss and fibrosis.

ORBITAL NEOPLASMS

Orbital tumors can arise from any orbital tissue, and secondary neoplasms either invade the orbit from adjacent structures or metastasize to the orbit from distant sites. **Orbital neoplasms generally occur in older animals (mean age, 9.5 years). Orbital tumors usually cause slowly progressive, unilateral exophthalmos, with variable displacement of the globe (Figs. 2-4 and 2-5).** Tumors arising within the extraocular muscle cone may produce exophthalmos, whereas those outside the muscle cone usually produce some rotation of the globe. Protrusion of the nictitating membrane is usually evident, though bilateral orbital neoplasms appear to be rare (except for lymphosarcoma).

Orbital neoplasms are not initially painful, and retropulsion of the globe is decreased or impossible. Often, an indentation of the caudal pole of the globe can be seen at ophthalmoscopy and ultrasonography. Even with

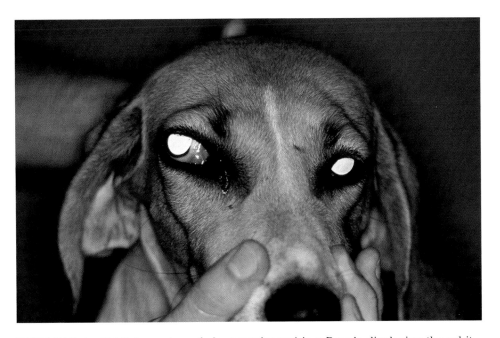

FIGURE 2-4. *Orbital neoplasm (adenocarcinoma) in a Beagle displacing the orbit forward and dorsally. The mass is in the medial and ventral orbit.*

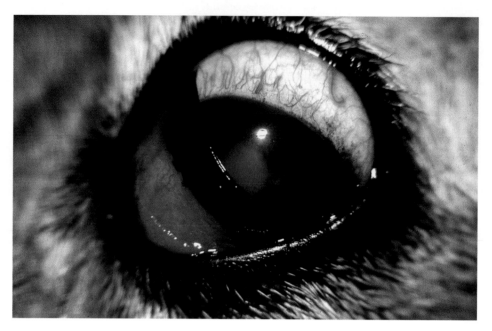

FIGURE 2-5. *Orbital neoplasm in a dog (meningioma) with unilateral exophthalmia, protrusion of the nictitating membrane, and episcleral congestion.*

marked deformation of the globe, the intraocular pressure usually remains within normal range. In most cases, vision is retained; however, tumors arising from the optic nerve or its meninges may cause blindness at an early stage.

Orbital tumors are mostly primary (60–70%) and malignant (80–90%). Fibroma, meningioma, osteosarcoma, and lymphosarcoma were the most common neoplasms diagnosed in one series; osteosarcoma and mastocytoma predominated in another. In a recent series of 24 dogs and six cats, multilobular osteochondrosarcoma was diagnosed most frequently.

Orbital ultrasonography is the most useful and the most available diagnostic procedure to localize the mass. Both CT and MR imaging are even better for this purpose; however, they are not readily available. After localization of the lesion, a fine-needle aspirate is obtained. This usually results in a definite diagnosis. A complete physical examination and chest radiography are usually indicated as well.

Most orbital neoplasms are discovered at an advanced stage, in which euthanasia is the only option. Localized neoplasms without evident distant metastasis may be surgically removed while preserving the globe and, possibly, the animal's vision, but these animals usually have a poor prognosis. If preservation of the globe is not possible, exenteration of the globe or radical orbitectomy may be considered. Surgical management of orbital neoplasia can be combined with radiation therapy, chemotherapy, or both.

TRAUMATIC DISEASES

ORBITAL HEMATOMA

Orbital hematomas, and often subconjunctival hemorrhages, usually result from road accidents. These patients with multiple trauma are presented with marked exophthalmos, lagophthalmos, and secondary xerophthalmia. Contusions of the globe are often associated with lens luxation, vitreal hemorrhage, and retinal detachment. In severe cases, scleral ruptures, usually extending from the lamina cribrosa, may occur. Massive orbital hemorrhage is often associated with proptosis of the globe.

At presentation, the eye must be cleansed immediately and then kept moist. Once the overall condition of the patient is stabilized, plain radiographs of the skull may be obtained and depict fractures, and fractures of the orbital rim and zygomatic arch can often be palpated. Ultrasonography of the globe is indicated when hyphema prevents examination of the posterior segment.

In cases of extensive scleral rupture, enucleation is the only treatment available. Phthisis bulbi is a common sequela of globe contusions. To prevent serious exposure keratitis, a third-eyelid flap or a temporary tarsorrhaphy is indicated. Topical and systemic antibiotic therapy should be instituted as well. Topical application of atropine sulfate is controversial, however, because secondary glaucoma may be a complication of marked hyphema. Corticosteroids should be given systemically and topically if the corneal epithelium is intact. Nonsteroidal anti-inflammatory drugs may increase the risk of further hemorrhages. Hot compresses, however, are beneficial (if they are tolerated by the animal). In cases of severe intraocular hemorrhage, the prognosis for vision is usually grave. As mentioned, phthisis bulbi is a common sequela and often necessitates enucleation at a later date.

ORBITAL EMPHYSEMA

Orbital emphysema is usually a complication of enucleation, but it may also result from fractures of the frontal sinus. Brachycephalic dogs appear to be predisposed, which may result from increased pressure in the nasal cavity during expiration. Air is pressed into the orbit via the nasolacrimal duct. Orbital emphysema resolves spontaneously in most cases, but if an emphysema persists after enucleation, the proximal end of the nasolacrimal duct can be identified and ligated.

PROPTOSIS

Proptosis results from sudden, forward displacement of the globe with simultaneous entrapment by the eyelids behind the equator (Fig. 2-6A). In one series, 50% of the dogs were brachycephalic breeds. In dolichocephalic breeds, greater trauma is necessary to cause proptosis. Proptosis of the globe is a true ophthalmic emergency and requires rapid assessment of the situation as well as immediate medical and surgical therapy. Even if vision cannot be preserved, the globes can often be salvaged for cosmetic purposes by early and correct management.

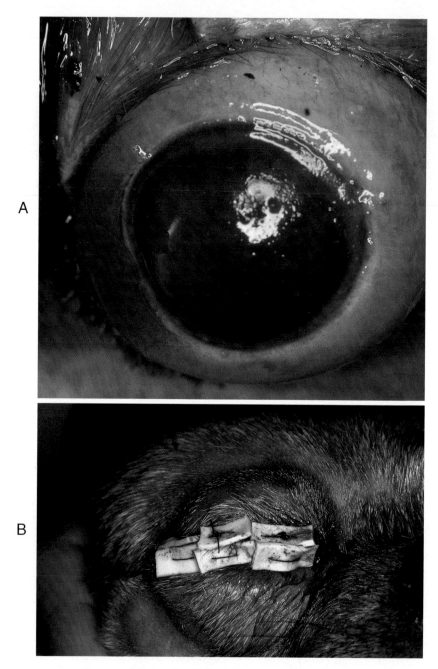

FIGURE 2-6. A. *Proptosis of the left globe in a mixed-breed dog.* **B.** *The same eye immediately after placement of a temporary tarsorrhaphy. Note the marked orbital swelling and pressure under the complete, temporary tarsorrhaphy.*

Determination of the prognosis as well as of the appropriate medical and surgical management for proptosis are summarized in Table 2-6. Only approximately 20% of proptosed globes regain some functional vision. Hence, prognosis refers to the possibility of salvaging the globe for cosmetic purposes as opposed to enucleation. Such a salvaged globe must be free of discomfort to the dog, however, and be cosmetically acceptable to the owner. Keratoconjunctivitis sicca and keratitis resulting from corneal desensitization are common sequelae and may be difficult to manage. Some owners may prefer enucleation rather than a blind eye that requires constant attention for many years. **Treatment for proptosed eyes is summarized in Box 2-1.** Proptosed eyes should be repositioned under general anesthesia as soon as possible (Fig. 2-6B).

The eyelid sutures are removed once a brisk blink reflex returns and the orbital swelling has resolved. It may be best to remove one suture at a time, starting medially, on subsequent visits. Sequelae of proptosis include blindness, strabismus, lagophthalmos, sensory deficit of the cornea, keratoconjunctivitis sicca, exposure keratitis, glaucoma, and phthisis bulbi.

ORBITAL FRACTURES

Fractures of the frontal, the temporal, and the zygomatic bones are not uncommon after head trauma. Clinical signs include exophthalmos or enophthalmos, strabismus, retrobulbar and periocular hemorrhage, pain, lacrimation, and facial asymmetry. Fractures involving the paranasal sinuses may cause orbital or subcutaneous emphysema with crepitus. Plain radiography and ultrasonography should aid in establishing a definitive diagnosis. Animals with orbital fractures should be kept quiet to prevent

---

TABLE 2-6

RECOMMENDED TREATMENTS AND PROGNOSIS FOR TRAUMATIC PROPTOSIS IN THE DOG

Clinical Sign	Possible Prognosis	Treatment
Positive direct pupil reflex	Guarded to good	Replacement of globe
Medial rectus muscle avulsion	Guarded	Monitor/reattach
Two or more rectus muscle avulsions	Poor	Enucleation
Corneal/scleral rupture(s)	Guarded to poor	Repair/enucleation
Massive intraocular hemorrhage	Poor	Repair/possible enucleation later
Optic nerve transection	Poor	Enucleation

BOX 2-1

Treatment Steps for Proptosed Globes

Keep moist with an antibiotic ointment

Cleanse with NaCl solution

Engage eyelids with strabismus hooks, and pull lids over the globe

Lateral canthotomy may be needed to increase the palpebral fissure

Temporary tarsorrhaphy with two or three horizontal mattress sutures with stents (4-0 to 2-0 monofilament nonabsorbable suture). Leave a small opening at medial canthus for medications.

Institute systemic antibiotic and corticosteroid therapy for 7 to 10 days.

Administer topical therapy including atropine sulfate and antibiotic drops.

Apply warm compresses twice daily.

further swelling and hemorrhage, and cold compresses, systemic anti-inflammatory drugs, and local as well as systemic antibiotics should be administered. Small, nondisplaced fractures stabilize spontaneously and do not require surgical reduction and fixation. Large and unstable fractures, however, may require internal fixation.

ORBITAL FOREIGN BODIES/ SHOTGUN INJURIES

Orbital foreign bodies and gunshot injuries often present as acute inflammatory diseases. The point of entry for both foreign bodies and gunshot pellets is not easily identified. Foreign bodies may enter the orbit from the oral cavity or through the conjunctival sac. Most foreign bodies are not recognized on plain radiographs, but gunshot pellets are easily spotted.

MISCELLANEOUS LESIONS

ORBITAL FAT PROLAPSE

Prolapse of orbital fat is rare in the dog. The cause of orbital fat prolapse is unknown, but it involves a rent in the epibulbar fascia. Prolapsed fat presents as nonpainful conjunctival swelling, usually in the dorsolateral quadrant of the eye. The swelling is easily movable and, usually, is nonprogressive. The diagnosis can be made on the basis of fine-needle aspirates of adipose tissue. If necessary, orbital fat prolapse can be treated surgically, by excision of the prolapsed fatty tissue and apposition of any fascial tissue in the defect.

CRANIOMANDIBULAR OSTEOPATHY

Craniomandibular osteopathy is a nonneoplastic, proliferative bone disease that affects primarily Scottish Terriers and West Highland White Terriers from 3 to 6 months of age. The orbit is rarely involved, but exophthalmos has been described in association with this osteopathy. The diagnosis is made on the basis of plain radiographs of the skull that depict typical periosteal lesions of the mandible and the temporal bone. In severe cases, the temporomandibular joint can be damaged. The disease is self-limiting, but damage to the temporomandibular joint may make food intake difficult or even impossible.

SURGERY OF THE GLOBE AND THE ORBIT

ENUCLEATION

Enucleation is the most common orbital surgery and consists of removing the globe. Enucleation is recommended in cases of blind, painful eyes (e.g., uncontrollable glaucoma, endophthalmitis, intraocular neoplasms, and severe ocular trauma with hemorrhage). The most commonly used surgical technique is the subconjunctival approach, which removes the globe, nictitating membrane, and lid margins (Fig. 2-7). Enucleation may also use a lateral approach. After lateral canthotomy to facilitate exposure of the globe and insertion of the lid retractor, the bulbar conjunctiva is incised approximately 5-mm posterior to the limbus, at approximately the 12-o'clock position. The conjunctiva and Tenon's capsule are bluntly dissected from the globe, and the extraocular and retractor bulbi muscles are identified and transected at their scleral insertion. Medial rotation of the globe exposes the optic nerve, which is clamped with curved hemostats and then transected approximately 5-mm behind the globe. Once the globe has been removed, the orbit is packed with gauze sponges to control diffuse hemorrhage, and the nictitating membrane is grasped with forceps and excised at its base (to include the gland of the third eyelid). The lacrimal gland usually is not removed, but 3 to 5 mm of eyelid margin are removed with scissors. After removal of the gauze package, the Tenon's capsule and conjunctiva are sutured with 4-0 absorbable suture material in a continuous pattern. Finally, the eyelids are closed with simple interrupted sutures using 4-0 nonabsorbable monofilament suture material.

In the transpalpebral approach, the eyelids are sutured together in a continuous suture pattern or are held together by Allis forceps. This technique prevents communication between the ocular surface and the orbital contents, and it removes all the conjunctival tissues. Two elliptical incisions approximately 5 mm behind the lid margins are joined near the medial and lateral canthus. Deep dissection allows identification of the bulbar conjunctiva, and forward traction of the eyelids will help with dissection of the conjunctiva until the sclera is encountered at the limbus. Further dissection

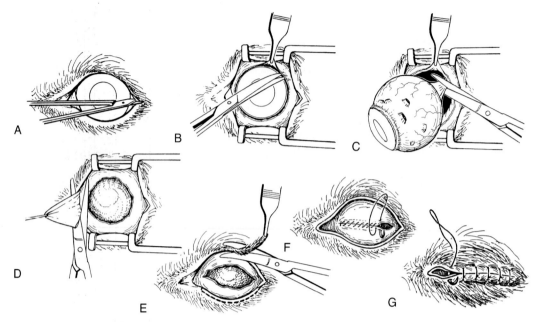

FIGURE 2-7. *Enucleation by the subconjunctival approach.* **A.** *A lateral canthotomy can facilitate exposure of the globe.* **B.** *The bulbar conjunctiva is incised approximately 5-mm posterior to the limbus over the entire circumference of the globe.* **C.** *Sharp and blunt dissection close to the sclera reveals the extra-ocular muscle insertions. Extraocular muscles are severed close to their scleral attachments, and the remaining retractor muscle fibers and optic nerve are clamped with a curved hemostat and then cut with scissors.* **D.** *The orbit is packed with a gauze sponge, and the nictitating membrane is resected.* **E.** *The lid margins are excised approximately 5-mm posterior to the mucocutaneous junction.* **F.** *The conjunctiva is closed with absorbable suture material in a continuous pattern.* **G.** *The lids are closed with simple interrupted sutures.*

and removal of the globe follow the same procedure as that for the subconjunctival approach.

The most common postoperative complication is hemorrhage within the first few hours after surgery, which results in swelling of the surgical site and serous discharge from the suture line. Postoperative care usually involves systemic antibiotics, and lid sutures are removed after 10 to 14 days. Owners should be informed that serosanguinous secretions from the ipsilateral nostril may occur during the first few postoperative days until the nasolacrimal duct is obliterated. Cold compresses, pressure bandages, or both as well as sedation of the patient are usually sufficient to control hemorrhage. Warm compresses applied to the orbit during the days after surgery will help to reduce swelling.

Draining fistulas from the orbit can result from incomplete removal of the caruncle at the medial canthus, incomplete removal of the remaining secretory tissue (e.g., conjunctival goblet cells, third-eyelid gland) within the orbit, or defects in the lid closure.

EXENTERATION

Exenteration involves removal of the conjunctiva, periorbita, extraocular muscles, and the globe. With orbital tumors, exenteration is extended to involve all the orbital contents. A transpalpebral approach is used. The orbital depression is more marked after exenteration than after enucleation, and a prolene or Dacron mesh can be anchored to the orbital rim to avoid this unsightly depression. Alternatively, an orbital prosthesis (i.e., silicone or methyl methacrylate spheres) can be implanted.

ORBITAL PROSTHESIS

As mentioned, to improve the cosmetic appearance after enucleation or exenteration, silicone or methyl methacrylate spheres may be implanted. Silicone spheres are most commonly used. To improve the cosmetic appearance and avoid rotation of the implant, the anterior quarter of the sphere is removed using scalpel blades until a flat, anterior surface with rounded edges is achieved. Possible complications include wound dehiscence, extrusion of the implant, traumatic dislocation and rotation of the implant, orbital seroma, and infection.

EVISCERATION AND IMPLANTATION OF THE INTRASCLERAL PROSTHESIS

Unless they are phthisic or microphthalmic, blind and painful eyes without septic endophthalmitis or intraocular neoplasms may be treated with evisceration and implantation of a silicone prosthesis. Blind eyes with aseptic uveitis and beginning phthisis bulbi can also be fitted with an intrascleral prosthesis to prevent further shrinkage of the globe and secondary adnexal problems. Evisceration involves removing all intraocular contents, leaving only the fibrous tunic, and then filling the cavity with an appropriate-size silicone sphere. The goals of this procedure are to eliminate pain from the inciting disease and to reduce the need for long-term topical and systemic medications.

The size of the silicone sphere should equal the horizontal diameter of the opposite, healthy cornea (or be 1–2 mm larger). Complications include regrowth of unidentified intraocular neoplasms, scleral wound dehiscence, corneal ulceration, and postoperative intrascleral infections. The cosmetic results are usually acceptable and histopathologic examination of the intraocular tissues should be performed (Fig. 2-8).

ORBITOTOMY

Exploratory orbitotomy is indicated to evaluate and biopsy space-occupying lesions. Several approaches to the orbit are possible; the choice depends on localization of the lesion. Removal of localized orbital neoplasms usually requires a more radical approach. A transconjunctival approach provides access to lesions anterior to the equator of the globe. A dorsal, nasal, or temporal approach can be chosen as well. Masses within

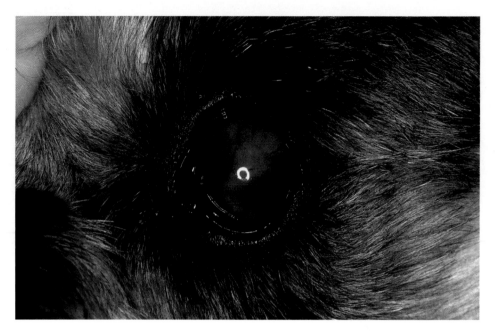

FIGURE 2-8. *Postoperative appearance (at 2 months) of a glaucomatous globe, with some residual corneal scarring, vascularization, and pigmentation, that was treated with an intrascleral prosthesis. The dog is currently free of pain and no longer on any medication.*

the extraocular muscle cone necessitate transsection of the respective rectus and oblique muscles, but even then, visualization is limited with this route. A wider access to the orbit can be gained through a lateral approach, with transsection of the lateral orbital ligament. If deep orbital structures such as the zygomatic salivary gland must be accessed, a portion of the zygomatic arch can be removed with a rongeur (for more details, the reader should consult the third edition, pp. 529–531). Possible complications of lateral orbitotomies include hemorrhage, transient lagophthalmos, postoperative swelling and infection, enophthalmos, and strabismus.

Diseases and Surgery of the Canine Eyelids

Eyelid diseases occur frequently in the dog and are divided clinically into congenital abnormalities, traumatic defects, infections, inflammations, and neoplasms. Breed-related lid conformational anomalies are quite common and may be treated using several surgical therapies. The relationship of the eyelids to the precorneal tear film and cornea is significant in the manifestation and successful treatment of eyelid disease.

The size and shape of the aperture between the eyelids (i.e., the palpebral fissure) dictate the external appearance of the eye. Ideally, the eyelids should rest on the corneal surface, and their contour should be determined by their contact with the globe. During blinking, the eyelids should move smoothly across the corneal surface, maintaining contact with the globe. Complete closure of the palpebral fissure should be easily achieved as well. Eyelid closure of the palpebral fissure physically protects the cornea from threatening trauma and is also involved in the production, distribution, and drainage of the precorneal tear film. Glandular elements within the eyelid's structure directly contribute to the composition of all phases of the tear film, and the blink mechanism is responsible for the constant renewal and distribution of this film across the corneal surface. The eyelids also help to remove foreign bodies from the corneal surface, and their conjunctival surfaces are involved in the exchange of oxygen to the cornea.

Each eyelid is a composite of skin, palpebral conjunctiva, collagen, muscle, and glandular tissue (Fig. 3-1). A central core of collagen, which constitutes the tarsal plate, is poorly defined in the dog. It does, however, provide a surface for muscle attachment, and it contains the meibomian or tarsal glands. The free margins or margo intermarginales of the eyelids, through which the meibomian ducts drain to the outside, meet to seal off the palpebral fissure during the ideal blink. The line of duct openings along the margins is often referred to as the "gray line."

Several muscles are involved in eyelid movement, with most movement that occurs during the blinking process being effected by the

47

FIGURE 3-1. *Cross-section of the normal upper canine eyelid.* ***A.*** *Palpebral conjunctiva.* ***B.*** *Meibomian gland tissue.* ***C.*** *Tarsal plate.* ***D.*** *Levator palpebrae superioris muscle.* ***E.*** *Orbicularis oculi muscle.* ***F.*** *Hair follicles.* ***G.*** *Skin.*

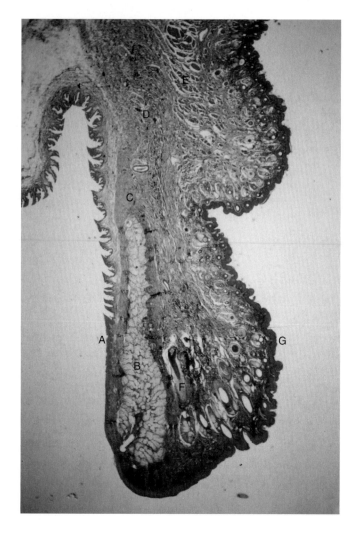

upper eyelid. The levator palpebrae superioris and Müller's muscles maintain the open palpebral fissure. The orbicularis oculi, which is a sphincter muscle completely encircling the palpebral fissure, is responsible for eyelid closure. The orbicularis oculi muscle is innervated by the palpebral branch of the seventh cranial nerve. The levator muscle is innervated by the third cranial nerve, and Müller's muscle is under sympathetic control. Insertions of the frontalis (i.e., upper eyelid) and the malaris (i.e., lower eyelid) muscles, together with the levator anguli oculi medialis muscle, assist in maintaining the open state of the palpebral fissure, and all three muscles are innervated by the facial nerve. The ellipsoidal shape of the palpebral fissure narrows to a horizontal slit during blinking because of the orbicularis oculi muscle anchorage to the orbital tissue, both medially and laterally. At the medial canthus, rigid fixation is achieved by a short, fibrous band (i.e., the medial palpebral ligament) that provides direct attachment to the nasal bones. At the lateral canthus, the retractor anguli oculi muscle anchors the orbicularis oculi to the zygoma. This muscle is innervated by the facial nerve, and its contraction during eyelid closure pulls the lateral canthus laterally. The additional presence of a lateral palpebral ligament in the dog has been recently reported as well, and it has been described as a musculofibrous band attached to the orbital ligament that may contribute to eyelid distortion, particularly in mesaticephalic breeds.

CONGENITAL DEFECTS

The canine palpebral fissure is almost completely sealed at birth, with only a pinhole-size patency at the medial canthus being the earliest indication of the separation that will occur during the subsequent 10- to 15-day period. This period of natural ankyloblepharon is required in the dog because of the relative immaturity of the canine ocular and adnexal tissue, including the eyelid musculature and the lacrimal apparatus, at parturition. **Premature opening of the palpebral fissure is usually accompanied by exposure keratoconjunctivitis and severe corneal ulceration. Globe perforation and uveitis are possible complications as well. In such cases, wetting ointments or gels must be used to protect the ocular surfaces. On occasion, a temporary tarsorrhaphy might also prove to be necessary, particularly if the palpebral fissure opens within the first 3 or 4 postparturient hours.**

ANKYLOBLEPHARON

Delayed or incomplete opening of the eyelids is occasionally encountered in the dog. Most often, this is accompanied by a staphylococcal keratoconjunctivitis, which is usually described as ophthalmia neonatorum. Infection from the dam's genital tract enters the closed conjunctival sac, presumably via the patent medial canthus. **The conjunctival sac often distends with purulent material, and the palpebral fissure should be opened surgically to allow drainage and the use of topical antibiotics.** Otherwise, the lacrimal gland and cornea—and even the whole globe—can be irreversibly damaged. The palpebral fissure is prepared for surgery using a diluted (1:10) povidone-iodine solution, and the line of separation between the two eyelids is cut using scissors. The eye is then examined for corneal damage, and a broad-spectrum topical antibiotic is applied four to six times per day for as long as necessary. Topical corticosteroid therapy should only be used if the corneal epithelium is intact.

EYELID AGENESIS

Congenital absence of part of the palpebral fissure is commonly referred to as a coloboma. Fortunately, such lesions are not as common in the dog as they are in the cat. Absence of eyelid tissue means that the blink mechanism is impaired, and the possible consequence of this is exposure keratitis. Hair adjacent to the defect can cause both corneal and conjunctival irritation, and a lower eyelid defect can result in epiphora. Any part of the palpebral fissure can be affected, and the size of the lesions

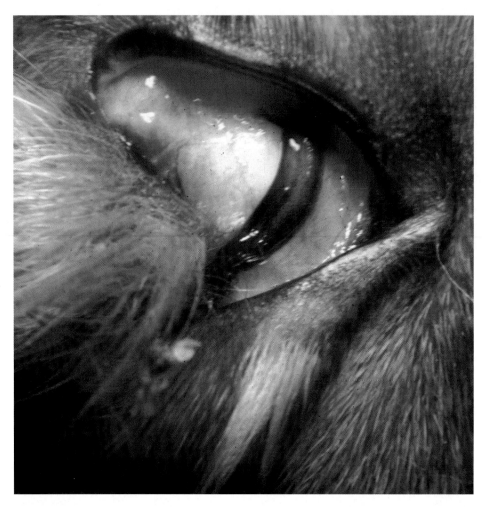

FIGURE 3-2. *Dermoid or choristoma affecting the lateral canthus and lateral lower eyelid in a 6-month-old Golden Retriever.*

varies. Correction is performed similar to that in the cat by using a myocutaneous graft (for more details, the reader should consult the third edition, pp. 537–538 and 999–1000).

DERMOIDS

The dermoid, or choristoma, is an abnormal development of palpebral skin that may involve the conjunctival tissue and the cornea ectopically (Fig. 3-2). Eyelid dermoids may be present unilaterally or bilaterally. Histopathologically, these lesions contain all the elements of normal skin, and the hair they bear is characteristically long. Eyelid dermoids can cause conjunctival and corneal irritation, and the larger lesions may interfere with efficiency of the blink mechanism. Corneal dermoids may affect vision. Genetic predispositions exist in the German Shepherd, Dalmatian, and St.

Bernard, with the latter breed demonstrating a familial relationship between lower eyelid coloboma and dermoid formation.

When the eyelid dermoid is clinically significant, treatment is by resection. Small lesions may be treated by wedge resection. Larger lesions may require excision surgery, which in turn may necessitate repair using sliding skin grafts or other techniques involving the transposition of skin.

DEVELOPMENTAL DEFECTS

Developmental defects are predetermined before birth, but the clinical effects usually are not noted for a period of time. This group of defects includes blepharophimosis (i.e., reduced palpebral fissure), entropion (i.e., lid margin rolled in), ectropion (i.e., eyelid margin rolled outward), distichiasis (i.e., abnormal extra eyelashes or cilia), trichiasis (i.e., hair contacting the eye), and trichomegaly (i.e., abnormally large eyelid lashes).

BLEPHAROPHIMOSIS

An abnormally small or narrowed palpebral fissure, which is referred to as blepharophimosis, blepharostenosis, or micropalpebral fissure, is seen particularly in the Chow Chow, the English Bull Terrier, both Rough and Smooth Collies, and the Shetland Sheepdog (Fig. 3-3). The globe is usually normal in size, but blepharophimosis may accompany microphthalmos. The condition has no clinical significance, unless it

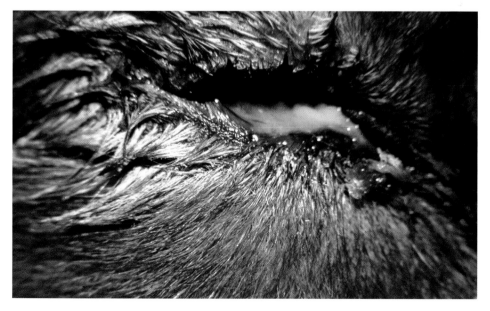

FIGURE 3-3. *Blepharophimosis or a reduced palpebral fissure in a Chow Chow.*

predisposes the animal to entropion and associated ocular surface disease. **Correction is achieved by lateral augmentation canthotomy, which is a lateral canthoplasty that increases the functional length of the palpebral fissure.** A 5- to 10-mm lateral canthotomy is created using tenotomy scissors to release the eyelid tension across the orbit. The palpebral conjunctiva is then lifted to the level of the fornix using blunt dissection and apposed to the edges of the canthotomy wound using 6-0 simple interrupted sutures to prevent its cicatricial closure. In cases with concurrent entropion, additional surgical techniques may be indicated.

EURYBLEPHARON

Euryblepharon, which is also referred to as macroblepharon or macropalpebral fissure, implies an abnormally long eyelid, which may also result in an abnormally large palpebral fissure. In the brachycephalic breeds, euryblepharon results from forward protrusion of the globe through the palpebral fissure. The second type of euryblepharon results from an excess length of eyelid margin, and in these cases, the palpebral fissure is poorly supported by the globe. The shape of the palpebral fissure can be further deformed by lateral canthus instability, small globe size, relative enophthalmos, and heavy facial folds, such as those in the St. Bernard, Bloodhound, and Clumber Spaniel (i.e., "diamond eye" appearance).

Euryblepharon in brachycephalic breeds can be accompanied by lagophthalmos, which involves an inability to complete the blink mechanism and, thus, instability of the precorneal tear film. Pigmentary and ulcerative keratitis can result from early breaking up of the film, and prophylaxis (in terms of supporting the tear film either medically or surgically) becomes essential. Artificial tear medication can be helpful, but surgery to reduce the size of the palpebral fissure, thus allowing lid closure during blinking and sleep, offers a more durable solution. Eyelid length can be reduced using either medial or lateral canthoplasty procedures (Fig. 3-4). Both are possible, but because the ideal goal is to reduce the length of the palpebral fissure by as much as 30%, medial canthoplasty is limited by the complicating presence of the lacrimal puncta and canaliculi. The lateral canthus is more accessible to surgical manipulation, however, and the required amount of shortening can thus be easily achieved.

All canthoplasty techniques to reduce the size of the palpebral fissure involve permanent tarsorrhaphy, in which margo intermarginalis is removed from both the upper and lower eyelids and the resulting wounds are sutured together (for more details, the reader should consult the third edition, pp. 539–542). Variations in technique are designed to reduce the chances of wound breakdown and tissue stretch to ensure an optimal result (Box 3-1). Some surgical overlap of the different tissue layers tends to discourage tissue tension and subsequent atrophy.

ENTROPION

Entropion is the inward rotation of part (or all) of the eyelid margin such that hair-bearing skin can rub against both the conjunctival and the corneal surfaces. It occurs quite commonly in certain breeds. In

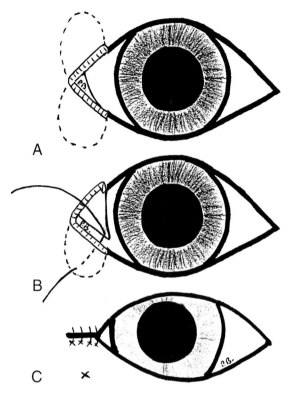

FIGURE 3-4. *Pocket canthoplasty for reducing the length of the palpebral fissure.* ***A.*** *The eyelids are split along the gray line (i.e., openings of the meibomian glands) into the anterior skin and muscle and posterior tarsoconjunctival layers. Two pockets are created by dissecting 10 mm into the split, and the edges of the skin and muscle flaps (upper and lower) are removed.* ***B.*** *A triangular upper tarsoconjunctival flap is created and sutured into the lower eyelid pocket.* ***C.*** *The upper and lower skin and muscle flaps are opposed and sutured.*

BOX 3-1

Surgical Procedures to Reduce the Size of the Palpebral Fissure

Lateral and medial reduction canthoplasty
Roberts-Jensen pocket technique for either the lateral or the medial canthus
Modified Fuchs lateral canthoplasty
Wyman and Kaswan lateral canthoplasty

---

mild entropion, which involves little inversion and loose contact with the ocular surfaces, there may be low-grade discomfort, with possible epiphora or excessive lacrimation. When the trigeminal irritation is severe, however, the patient will be in constant pain, and secondary inflammation of both the conjunctiva and cornea will occur. There can be corneal epithelial erosion because of the trauma, and severe ulceration can also develop. Self-trauma, in an attempt to relieve pain, will contribute to the overall damage as well. Establishing the diagnosis of entropion is usually straightforward, but comprehending the underlying factors is complex.

Entropion is classified as either a developmental defect (i.e., primary) or an acquired lesion associated with another ocular defect or defects (i.e., secondary). Most developmental entropions demonstrate a clear breed predisposition, but the genetic basis is not completely

understood. There may be predisposing conformational factors of the head and eye. Entropion is generally proposed to be inherited as a simple dominant trait, with complete penetrance in some breeds, whereas in others, the incidence is sporadic and the pattern of inheritance difficult to describe. In the gundog breeds, the lateral aspect of the lower eyelid is most commonly involved, whereas in the large or giant breeds, the lateral canthus per se is usually involved. The degree of involvement can vary considerably, however, and the entire palpebral fissure can occasionally be affected. This is a common situation in the Shar Pei, in which a 360° entropion can present as early as 14 or 15 days of age (Fig. 3-5). Undoubtedly, the looseness of the circumorbital skin and the presence of loose facial folds contribute to eyelid distortion in this breed. Of course, in any case of entropion, the primary or anatomical defect causes trigeminal irritation, but the presenting clinical picture may be compounded by considerable spasticity. Medial lower eyelid entropion also occurs, being reported most commonly in Toy and Miniature Poodles.

Predisposition occurs in several breeds, including the Chow Chow, Shar Pei, St. Bernard, both the English and American varieties of Cocker Spaniel, English Springer Spaniel, Labrador Retriever, Bull Mastiff, Great Dane, Irish Setter, Elkhound, and both Toy and Miniature Poodles (Fig. 3-6 and see Appendix N). Most cases of primary entropion present before 6 months of age, but occasionally, spontaneous and sometimes unilateral entropion presents after 12 months. Entropion can be associated with the micropalpebral fissure previously described in the Chow Chow, Bull Terrier, Rough and Smooth Collies, and Shetland Sheepdog. In breeds such

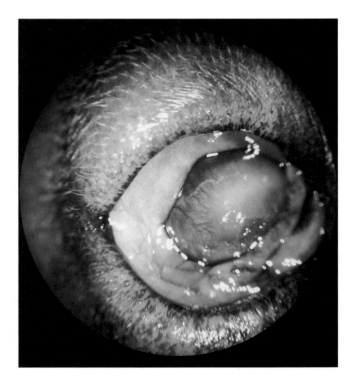

FIGURE 3-5. *Severe corneal disease with granuloma formation and loss of epithelium in a 16-week-old Shar Pei.*

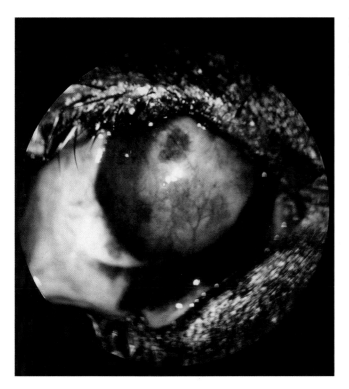

FIGURE 3-6. *Longstanding entropion in an English Cocker Spaniel. The cornea is vascularized, pigmented, and scarred.*

as the St. Bernard, Bloodhound, Newfoundland, Clumber Spaniel, and Neapolitan Mastiff, the euryblepharon or abnormally long lid allows both entropion and concurrent ectropion to occur. The large size and depth of the orbit in the Doberman Pinscher, Bull Mastiff, Great Dane, and Rottweiler contributes to deficient lid support and, in turn, the resulting entropion. For those situations in which the skull and palpebral fissure conformation either predispose or contribute to entropion, simple corrective surgery often proves to be inadequate, and complete therapeutic satisfaction (in terms of restoring normal corneal and conjunctival physiology) may never be achieved.

Acquired entropion can accompany blepharospasm or spasticity, cicatrix formation, or loss of orbicularis oculi tone. Entropion itself can cause blepharospasm, and the amount of lid inversion increases as the result of orbicularis oculi muscle spasticity. This must be considered during surgical correction. It is only necessary to correct the primary or anatomical defect, and inclusion of the spastic component in the surgical correction leads to overcorrection and ectropion formation. Trigeminal pain inducing blepharospasm can also induce a secondary entropion. Fibrosis within palpebral tissue because of trauma or chronic inflammation can lead to lid distortion, and the loss of muscle tone that occurs in old age will allow both lid distortion and inversion to occur. In elderly English Cocker Spaniels, the upper eyelid has a propensity to roll inward laterally, and normal eyelashes are thus directed into a lower conjunctival sac, which is exposed by a developing lower lid ectropion. Normal blink movements then cause irritation.

Assessment for entropion correction includes an evaluation of lid movement, concurrent ocular problems, extent of the primary defect, and amount of the spastic component. This evaluation should be performed before any topical or systemic anesthetic agents are administered. In fact, topical anesthetics may be instilled to differentiate between the structural entropion and the secondary spastic (i.e., pain) entropion. Surgical correction is directed only toward the structural component, thereby reducing the likelihood of overcorrection.

Several nonsurgical techniques have been described, but these are not generally used. Temporary tacking of the eyelids can be effective in very young puppies and is particularly appropriate among Shar Peis, in which the entropion often manifests itself at 14 to 20 days of age (Fig. 3-7). Two or three vertical mattress sutures are positioned in each eyelid such that the inverted lids are everted as the sutures are tied. A 4-0 or 5-0 nonabsorbable suture material is used. The needle enters the skin 1 mm from the margo intermarginalis and eventually emerges such that some 10 to 20 mm of eyelid tissue are encompassed within the suture. The sutures are left in situ for 3 to 4 weeks, by which time many patients will have been permanently corrected.

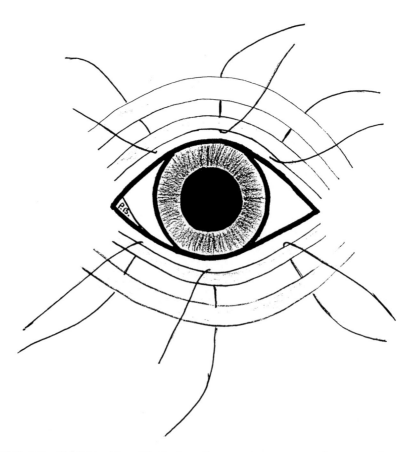

FIGURE 3-7. *Eyelid tacking. Vertical mattress sutures are used to evert the eyelid margins.*

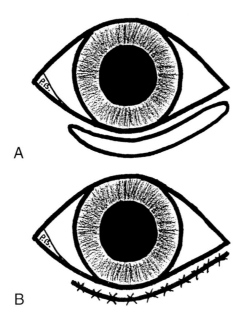

A

B

FIGURE 3-8. *Modified Hotz-Celsus resection for treatment of entropion. **A**. A strip of skin and orbicularis oculi muscle is removed. **B**. The wound is closed with interrupted nonabsorbable sutures.*

BOX 3-2

Key Components of the Hotz-Celsus Procedure for Entropion

Slight undercorrection, because postoperative wound contraction will further evert the eyelid margin.

Initial skin incision parallel to and 1 to 2 mm from the eyelid margin (just enough for sutures).

Section of skin and orbicularis oculi muscle that is excised approximates the entropion defect.

Suture placement starts in the middle of the wound to ensure accurate coaption.

Several surgical treatments have been described for correction of entropion, but the most common approach is the Hotz-Celsus technique (for more details, the reader should consult the third edition, pp. 542–548). In this technique, strips of skin and orbicularis oculi muscle are removed adjacent to the defect, and the wound is closed using sutures through the resected skin and muscle (Fig. 3-8). The technique can be used for the upper eyelid, the lower eyelid, or both, and it can be modified to correct both lateral and medial canthus entropion (Box 3-2).

ECTROPION

Ectropion is the outward rolling of part (or all) of the eyelid such that conjunctival tissue is exposed and lagophthalmos may occur. The lower eyelid is usually involved, but cicatricial eversion of the upper lid may be seen as well. Ectropion may (or may not) be clinically significant, but exposure of the conjunctiva can lead to low-grade conjunctivitis and predispose the animal to epiphora and precorneal tear film deficiency (Fig. 3-9). Ectropion is classified as either developmental (i.e., primary) or acquired (i.e., secondary). Developmental ectropion always involves the lower eyelid and is a characteristic of the St. Bernard, Bloodhound, Great Dane, Newfoundland, Bull Mastiff, and several Spaniel breeds (see Appendix N). Laxity of the palpebral fissure is common in these breeds, and the ectropion may be associated with marked euryblepharon and deficiency of the lateral retractor muscle. Acquired ectropion of either eyelid may result from trauma or cicatrix formation because of chronic inflammation, and loss of orbicularis oculi tone because of senility or palpebral nerve damage can result in lower eyelid eversion.

Ectropion as part of euryblepharon is a breed-standard desired feature in the several breeds just mentioned, and chronic ocular discharge is often accepted as a way of life for these dogs. Surgical correction is always indicated, however, if ongoing conjunctival and progressive corneal pathology cannot be prevented. Fortunately, several surgical procedures are available (Table 3-1). Simple, full-thickness wedge resection more than adequately addresses developmental ectropion in which laxity rather than overlength of the eyelid is the problem. The excision is completed at the lateral canthus to reduce the chances of noticeable notching of the postoperative lid margin, and the amount of tissue removed should account for the additional shortening that results from fibrosis. A triangular wedge is removed using scissors while maintaining tension on the eyelid using forceps. The wound is repaired using a two-layered closure consisting of 6-0 simple interrupted

FIGURE 3-9. *Marked lower eyelid ectropion in an 8-month-old Labrador Retriever.*

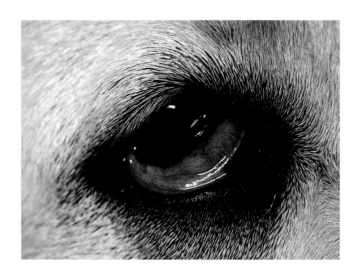

TABLE 3-1

SURGICAL PROCEDURES TO CORRECT ECTROPION

Technique	Effects
Full-thickness wedge resection	Shortens lid
Kuhnt-Hembolt	Shortens lid
Kuhnt-Szymanowski	Shortens lid/stabilizes lateral canthus
Munger and Carter	Shortens lid/stabilizes lateral canthus
Wharton-Jones "V"- to "Y"-plasty	Treats mild cicatricial ectropion

---

absorbable sutures in the tarsoconjunctival tissue and 4-0 to 6-0 simple interrupted nonabsorbable sutures to close the skin and muscle layers. The margo intermarginalis must be accurately reformed, and the first suture should be at this level (through the skin and muscle layer). Alternatively, a figure-of-eight suture can be used to ensure accurate apposition of the eyelid margin.

When eyelid overlength is not excessive, the Kuhnt-Hembolt technique may be used. This resection involves the central part of the eyelid, and it requires an extensive lid split along the gray line to a depth of approximately 10 to 15 mm. A triangular wedge of the central tarsoconjunctival flap is removed, and a similar-size excision of the skin and muscle flap lateral to this central excision is then completed.

Both full-thickness wedge resection and the Kuhnt-Hembolt technique effectively shorten the lower eyelid, but instability at the lateral canthus can lead to recurrence of the ectropion. Thus, techniques addressing laxity of the canthus offer a better prognosis when the ectropion is associated with marked euryblepharon. **Excellent results are routinely obtained using a modified Kuhnt-Szymanowski procedure, in which the length of the lower eyelid is reduced and increased stability at the lateral canthus is achieved (Fig. 3-10).** A triangular flap of skin is raised at the lateral canthus, and the lower eyelid is split along the gray line into anterior skin and muscle and posterior tarsoconjunctival flaps. The length of the split equates to the amount of lid shortening that is required. Using tenotomy scissors, a triangular wedge of the tarsoconjunctival flap is removed, and the defect is closed by apposing its edges with a 6-0 interrupted absorbable suture. The lower eyelid anterior skin and muscle flap is then sutured into the triangular facial skin defect, and any excess facial skin is removed. This lateral translocation of lower eyelid tissue to the canthus lifts the shortened lower eyelid and helps to stabilize the canthus. A further modification of this procedure by Munger and Carter avoids splitting the margo intermarginalis and, thus, damaging the meibomian ducts. The initial skin and muscle incision is placed 3 mm from the eyelid margin and runs parallel to it (starting some 10- to 15-mm lateral to the canthus).

FIGURE 3-10. *Modified Kuhnt-Szymanowski technique for correction of ectropion associated with marked euryblepharon.* **A.** *A triangular flap of eyelid skin and muscle and facial skin is prepared.* **B.** *A triangular wedge of tarsoconjunctival flap is removed to shorten the lower eyelid.* **C.** *The skin flap is lifted into the lateral facial wound and the excess skin removed.*

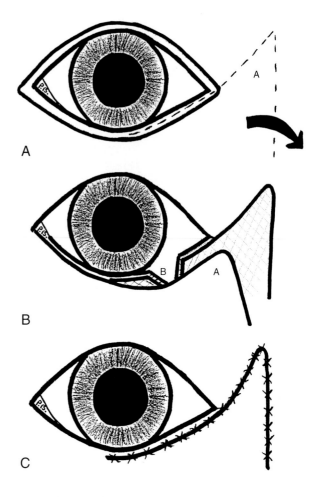

COMBINED ENTROPION–ECTROPION

A combination of both entropion and ectropion is seen in those breeds with a requirement for pronounced euryblepharon. The desired "diamond eye" appearance of the Bloodhound or St. Bernard, for example, is achieved as a variable combination of factors, in which excessive overlength of the palpebral fissure is the most significant (Fig. 3-11). Small globe size and relative enophthalmos both contribute to lack of support for the eyelids. Weakness of the lateral retractor muscle leads to an instability of the lateral canthus, and heavy facial skin folds as well as pendulous pinnae help to pull the palpebral fissure ventrally. The possible presence of a lateral palpebral ligament has been mentioned and may additionally contribute to the overall distortion. As a result of all these factors, the palpebral fissure droops across the orbit, thereby masking the globe and exposing a protruded membrana nictitans and the lower palpebral conjunctiva. Entropion of both the upper and lower eyelids at the lateral canthus as well as ectropion of the central part of the lower eyelid are seen. The effect on the animal's sight is obvious, and the clinical appearance is characterized by impaired tear film drainage and ocular surface disease.

Effective correction requires consideration of two factors: reduction of the eyelid length, and stabilization of the lateral canthus (Box 3-3). The Wyman lateral canthoplasty achieves stabilization by using pedicles of orbicularis oculi muscle to mimic the lateral retractor muscle and attaching the palpebral fissure directly to the zygomatic arch to produce the desired degree of lateral retraction. The orbicularis oculi is approached through a "C"-shaped skin excision at the lateral canthus, with the arms of the "C" extending along the lateral eyelid margins to correct the entropion on closure.

A "Y"- to "V"-plasty is an alternative to the "C"-shaped skin resection. In this technique, the muscle pedicles are based at the canthus and rotated some 180° to allow their fixation by suture to the periosteum of the zygoma. A simplified version of this technique uses a nonabsorbable suture instead of the orbicularis oculi pedicles. More recently, Gutbrod and Tietz have described a technique in which the lower eyelid is shortened and the canthus skin removed to correct the combined entropion–ectropion defect. In addition, Bigelbach has described a combined tarsorrhaphy canthoplasty technique that can also correct lateral entropion.

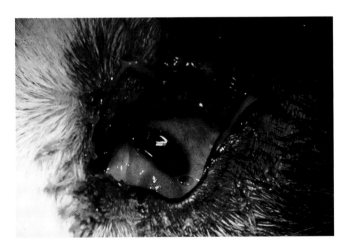

FIGURE 3-11. *"Diamond eye" accompanied by marked conjunctivitis in a 10-month-old St. Bernard. The nictitans is prolapsed.*

BOX 3-3

Surgical Procedures to Treat Combined Entropion–Ectropion

Wyman's lateral canthoplasty

"Y"- to "V"-plasty

Gutbrod and Tietz

Bigelbach

Kuhnt-Szymanowski (modified by Bedford)

"Face lift"

The Kuhnt-Szymanowski lateral canthoplasty, as modified by Bedford, involves the additional splitting and resection of the upper eyelid. This produces a smaller palpebral fissure that is supported at the lateral canthus by the transposed lower eyelid tissue. The modified Kuhnt-Szymanowski technique is completed in the usual manner, but the upper eyelid is split along the gray line to a depth of approximately 10 mm to produce anterior skin and muscle as well as posterior tarsoconjunctival flaps. The length of this split equates to the amount of lid shortening that is required, and the lateral part of the skin and muscle flap is then removed as a triangular resection, with the releasing scissor cut running into the distal end of the original vertical facial incision. The lower eyelid skin and muscle flap is then transposed into this upper eyelid surgical defect overlying the upper tarsoconjunctival flap, and it is tailored to fit the triangular facial skin resection. Some dogs may require subsequent resection of redundant forehead skin to obtain the optimal effect.

A relatively simplistic approach to the problems of euryblepharon is removal of facial and dorsal cervical skin (i.e., a "face lift") to elevate the palpebral fissures to a normal position. This allows exposure of the globe in most patients, and it even reduces the degree of ectropion in some. During rhytidectomy, skin is removed from the dorsal cervical area. During facial skin removal, skin is excised from the midline, running from the medial canthi to the nuchal crest.

DISTICHIASIS

Distichiasis is the presence of adventitious cilia, which usually arise from or, rarely, adjacent to the meibomian duct openings along the margo intermarginales (Fig. 3-12). The cilia originate in the posterior distal tarsal plate adjacent to the subconjunctival tissues approximately 5- or 6-mm below the eyelid margin. Rather than breaking through the conjunctiva, most cilia use the meibomian ducts as the "route of least resistance" for emergence from the eyelid. The meibomian glands are modified hair follicles, and the distichia actually develop from undifferentiated meibomian tissue. The hairs may emerge either singly or in clumps through each duct opening, and several ducts are usually involved. Both lids can be affected, and the condition usually demonstrates a bilateral presence. In most of the affected dogs, the condition may have no clinical significance, with the cilia simply floating on the corneal surface in the precorneal tear film. **Their presence, however, can cause trigeminal irritation, as indicated by excessive lacrimation, blepharospasm, mild conjunctivitis, and superficial keratitis.** Occasionally, corneal ulceration presents with distichiasis, and though the cilia may be directly responsible for any loss of epithelium, self-trauma may also be involved. A secondary entropion may also be present, but distichiasis can be seen accompanying primary entropion as well. Distichiasis has a marked breed predisposition, with American and English Cocker Spaniels and the Miniature Longhaired Dachshund being most commonly affected. In both American and English Cocker Spaniels, the incidence of distichiasis in the United Kingdom is greater than 80%, and it is probably higher for the Miniature Longhaired Dachshund. An appreciable incidence has also been recorded in other

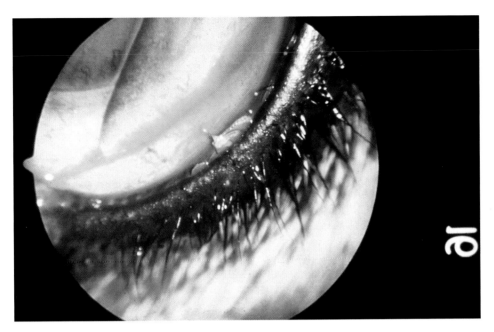

FIGURE 3-12. *Distichiasis of the lower eyelid. Fluorescein stains the mucus that coats the distichia.*

breeds, including the English Bulldog, Pekingese, Yorkshire Terrier, Flat-Coated Retriever, Shetland Sheepdog, and Toy as well as Miniature Poodles. The condition usually makes its presence known in young animals, with clinical signs manifesting at 4 to 6 months of age.

Distichiasis may be diagnosed with the naked eye, particularly when the cilia are long or in clumps, and its presence is often indicated by a disturbance of the precorneal tear film at the eyelid margin. Mucus may accumulate on the cilia, however, and mask their visualization. Focal illumination and magnification assist considerably in establishing the diagnosis, and epilation may be helpful in deciding if the cilia are responsible for the clinical signs observed.

No single technique offers guaranteed resolution, however, and the possibility of recurrence should be stressed to the owner when prognosis is being discussed (Box 3-4). Cryotherapy is the most commonly practiced technique for destruction of the hair follicles in situ. A double freeze–thaw cycle using a nitrous oxide cryounit and specific probes produces a −25°C freeze, which can destroy the follicles but spare the adjacent eyelid tissue. The eyelid is everted, and the cryoprobe is applied to the palpebral conjunctiva directly over the follicles, approximately 4-mm below the margo intermarginalis. A 60-second freeze is followed by a brief thawing period and then an additional, 30-second freeze. The most immediate postoperative effect is considerable swelling of the treated eyelid, so much so that blinking might be impossible. Corticosteroid therapy and corneal lubrication are helpful, however, and the swelling should last no more than 48 hours. Depigmentation of the frozen areas occurs within 72 hours, but repigmentation usually occurs (though it sometimes takes as

---

BOX 3-4

Methods to Treat Distichiasis

Mechanical epilation	For few distichia; regrowth common (~4 weeks)
Hotz-Celsus resection	Produces mild ectropion
Electrolysis	Limited to few distichia
Diathermy/electrocautery	Limited to few distichia
Eyelid splits	More difficult/for few distichia
Partial resection of the distal tarsal plate	More difficult/for few distichia
Transpalpebral conjunctival dissection	More difficult/for few distichia
Cryotherapy	More swelling after freezing; lid margin depigmentation usually temporary

---

long as 6 months to complete). Scarring and distortion are unlikely, but temperatures lower than −30°C will produce necrosis and eyelid distortion. Use of thermocouple needles, however, will ensure that the tissue temperature does not fall to lower than −25°C.

ECTOPIC CILIA

A variant of distichiasis, which is referred to as ectopic cilium, occurs where the cilia emerge through the palpebral conjunctiva and impinge directly on the cornea. The upper eyelid is primarily involved, usually in the 12-o'clock meridian, and single or multiple cilia emerge some 4- to 6-mm below the margo intermarginalis. The condition is accompanied by intense pain, as indicated by blepharospasm and excessive lacrimation. The onset is acute, and rapid corneal erosion and ulceration are not unusual. Clinical signs may be obvious before the actual emergence of the cilia. Ectopic cilia are found in young patients, and though this condition is not breed selective, a predisposition is possibly developing in the Flat-Coated Retriever. Treatment is by scalpel excision of hair and follicles through the palpebral conjunctiva.

TRICHIASIS

Trichiasis is a condition in which normal eyelid hair, arising from normally positioned follicles, deviates to contact the corneal and conjunctival surfaces. It may be a primary condition, but it can also be associated with other eyelid conditions. The irritation produced is indicated by blepharospasm and excessive lacrimation. Conjunctivitis and keratitis can ensue as well. The primary condition, which involves the lateral aspect of the upper eyelid, is most common in the English Cocker Spaniel and brachycephalic breeds. It can be treated by Hotz-Celsus resection, but the Stades technique, in which a section of the upper eyelid skin containing the hair is removed, can also be very effective. In this technique, the skin is incised approximately 1-mm external and parallel to the margo intermarginalis. The incision is started 2- to 4-mm lateral to the medial canthus and extends for 5 to 10 mm beyond the lateral canthus. An ellipsoidal section of skin 15- to 20-mm deep at its widest portion is then removed. The wound may be partially repaired by apposing the upper eyelid skin to the exposed subcutis some 5 mm from the margo intermarginalis using a 4-0 or 5-0 simple interrupted nonabsorbable suture, but this is not necessary. The open wound heals by secondary intention, and the new skin contains no (or few) hair follicles.

Trichiasis may be associated with prominent nasal folds, and it may also accompany entropion, euryblepharon, dermoid formation, and medial canthus hair. Nasal fold trichiasis can be treated by routine use of petroleum jelly to flatten the hair and to break the corneal contact, but a permanent solution lies in surgical removal of the nasal folds, which can be easily achieved by using Mayo scissors and apposing the wound edge with a 4-0 to 5-0 single interrupted nonabsorbable suture. Other instances of trichiasis similarly dictate the method of correction for the cause.

TRICHOMEGALY

Trichomegaly refers to abnormally elongated eyelid cilia and is most commonly observed in American Cocker Spaniels. It has no clinical significance.

ACQUIRED DISEASE

Mechanical injury, infection, inflammation, and neoplastic disease are all relatively common in the dog. An abundance of mast cells within the subcutis ensures a marked response to any disease process with an inflammatory component, including edematous swelling and distention as key features. The therapeutic response to most acquired defects, however, can be rewarding.

TRAUMA

Palpebral tissue usually heals well, and a sufficiency of skin means that even with considerable avulsion, repair can be achieved relatively easily. Most trauma injury is sustained because of fights, but infection is rarely a complicating factor. Abrasions and superficial wounds require little more attention than the necessary lavage and possible debridement. **Full-thickness wounds must be repaired as quickly as possible, however, with the edges being accurately apposed such that normal function**

is restored (i.e., two-layered closure involving tarsoconjunctival tissue as well as the skin and muscle layer). Defects of the margo intermarginalis can lead to lagophthalmos, and abnormal cicatrix formation can lead to eyelid distortion. Whenever possible, the lacrimal puncta and canaliculi should be preserved. The other adnexal structures as well as the globe itself should also be examined to exclude the possibility of less apparent damage.

BLEPHARITIS

Blepharitis refers to several inflammatory conditions of the eyelid, with the primary cause often being masked (to some extent) by possible secondary complications. The inflammation may be focal or diffuse, with variable involvement of all four eyelids. Because the eyelids are highly vascular structures, hyperemia and edema are usually marked. Pain is indicated by blepharospasm and excessive lacrimation, and there may be exudate, evidence of self-trauma, alopecia, erosion, and scaliness. Chronic inflammation can lead to eyelid distortion, with both entropion and ectropion resulting from cicatrix formation.

HORDEOLUM

Hordeolum formation usually results from staphylococcal infection of the eyelid glandular tissue. An external hordeolum (or stye) results from infection of the Zeis or Moll glands, and it manifests either as single or multiple abscess formation and swelling along the eyelid near its margins. It occurs primarily in young animals. Infection of the Meibomian gland is referred to as an internal hordeolum (Fig. 3-13). The infection is contained deeper within the tarsal plate, and swellings are seen distending the palpebral conjunctiva. Treatment of both conditions involves hot compresses, possible manual expression of the lesions under topical analgesia, and both topical and systemic antibiosis.

The term *chalazion* **refers to granuloma formation as the result of retained meibomian secretions within the gland.** Leakage of this material into the surrounding tissues elicits the inflammatory response, which is visible through the palpebral conjunctiva. Treatment is by scalpel incision and curettage, with the incision healing by secondary intention. Postoperative topical antibiotic and corticosteroid therapy is used for a 7-day period.

IMMUNE-MEDIATED BLEPHARITIS

Several autoimmune and immune-mediated phenomena can involve the canine eyelid, either in isolation or in association with other clinical features. **An allergic blepharitis is usually characterized by an acute-onset edema and hyperemia, and it may result from local exposure to a contact allergen or as part of a generalized response.** Swelling of the eyelids and muzzle are seen after insect bites and as a postvaccinal

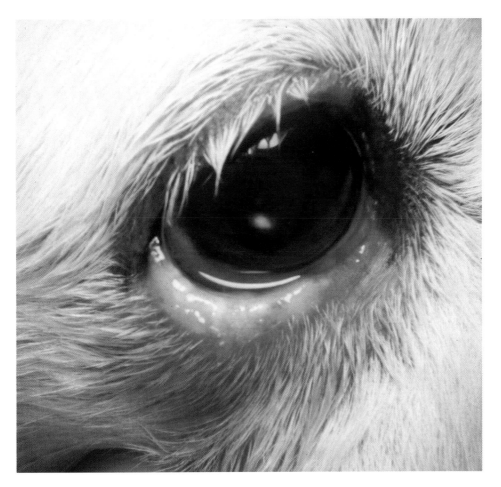

FIGURE 3-13. *Internal hordeolum or infection of the meibomian glands of the lower eyelid in a 3-year-old American Cocker Spaniel.*

reaction. Topically applied drugs may be responsible for contact allergy, with neomycin being the most commonly involved. Seasonal or nonseasonal reaction to environmental allergens is seen with atopy, which involves an inherited predisposition to immunoglobulin E–antibody production. Several breeds are involved, with West Highland White Terriers demonstrating high incidence. Clinical signs manifest in young dogs, usually from the age of 1 year, and periocular hyperemia, facial pruritus, and conjunctivitis are common. Identification of the specific allergen and desensitization are rarely possible; thus, treatment relies on topical and systemic corticosteroids and antihistamines. Food allergies and systemic drug reactions can cause periocular dermatitis and blepharitis, with avoidance of the allergen and cessation of the therapy being the obvious lines of treatment.

The pemphigus group of vesiculobullous epidermal diseases can involve the mucocutaneous junctions, with inflammation and ulceration of the eyelid tissue commonly observed. In both pemphigus foliaceus and pemphigus erythematosus, the facial lesions usually involve the eyelids.

Pemphigus vulgaris is the most severe type of pemphigus. It involves the oral cavity, nail beds, and skin in addition to ulcerative lesions of the eyelids, lips, external nares, and ears. In all types of pemphigus, the lesions result from autoantibody production against the intercellular matrix of the epidermis. In bullous pemphigoid, however, autoantibody production against epidermal basement membrane produces clinical signs that are indistinguishable from those of pemphigus vulgaris. Treatment of this disease complex requires systemic and topical corticosteroid therapy, with additional immune suppression being achieved with cyclophosphamide or azathioprine in refractory cases.

BACTERIAL BLEPHARITIS

In puppies, purulent blepharitis occurs as part of juvenile pyoderma, with meibomianitis being a dominant feature. There is considerable pain, and complicating self-trauma can only be prevented by effective antibiosis and judicious use of an Elizabethan collar. Antibiotic therapy should be determined on the basis of culture and sensitivity results, with trimethoprim-sulfadiazine being used as first-line therapy until the sensitivity results are available. A topical, broad-spectrum antibiotic ointment can be used to help lubricate and protect the cornea, and this may be combined with a corticosteroid in the absence of ulceration.

Staphylococcus and *Streptococcus* sp. **are most commonly involved in bacterial blepharitis among adult patients.** Acute cases are characterized by hyperemia and crusting, whereas ulceration, fibrosis, and alopecia can occur during long-term infection. Abscessation of the meibomian glands may be seen, possibly resulting from an allergic response to the bacterial dermatotoxins. Antibiotic therapy must be determined on the basis of culture and sensitivity results, with expression of exudate from the eyelid margin or the pyogranulomas being necessary to ensure an adequate culture. Acute cases can be treated with topical therapy; chronic blepharitis requires additional systemic antibiosis. Pyogranuloma formation can be treated using intralesional antibiosis. Staphylococcal toxins have a necrotizing effect, but topical corticosteroid medications can help to limit the damage. Autogenous vaccine can be effective in cases of chronic and seemingly resistant staphylococcal infection.

MYCOTIC BLEPHARITIS

Blepharomycosis is uncommon, but infection with *Microsporum* and *Trichophyton* sp. occurs as part of a generalized dermatological problem in young dogs. Expanding alopecia, scaling, and hyperemia are the clinical features, and the diagnosis is confirmed by the results of stained skin scrapings (Gram or Giemsa stain) or by culturing the organisms on Sabouraud's agar. Povidone-iodine scrubs together with topical miconazole nitrate or clotrimazole creams are effective for superficial infection, but corneal contact should be avoided. Persistent and deep-seated infection is most effectively treated by the addition of systemic griseofulvin or, occasionally, oral ketoconazole to the previously mentioned therapy.

PARASITIC BLEPHARITIS

Both demodectic and sarcoptic mange can include the eyelids, with lesions being characterized by hyperemia, alopecia, and pruritus as well as often being complicated by secondary bacterial infection and self-trauma. ***Demodex canis* is considered to be a normal inhabitant of hair follicles, sebaceous glands, and sweat glands, with the associated disease developing only when large numbers of the parasite are present on patients with immunosuppression or possible inherited T-cell deficiency.** In young dogs, the disease tends to be restricted to the face, and eyelid involvement is commonplace. Spontaneous regression is to be expected, but topical rotenone or isoflurophate ophthalmic ointment can be used and, seemingly, is effective. In older dogs, a more generalized disease occurs that often proves to be resistant to treatment. *Sarcoptes scabei* var *canis* infection causes intense pruritus, with several parts of the body being classically involved in addition to the eyelids. Treatment routinely involves use of sulphur dips, whereas amitraz is currently proving to be effective as a potential first-line therapy.

NEOPLASTIC DISEASE

The eyelid is common site of tumor formation in older dogs. A tumor is always of cosmetic concern, but with accompanying trigeminal irritation, lagophthalmos, hemorrhage, or the possibility of malignancy, treatment becomes essential. Fortunately, most eyelid neoplasms in this species are benign clinically, and corneal irritation is the exception rather than the rule. Malignant tumors tend to be locally invasive only, and they rarely metastasize (Table 3-2). In general, however, eyelid

TABLE 3-2

HISTOGENIC CLASSIFICATION AND FREQUENCY OF EYELID TUMORS IN THE DOG

Sebaceous adenoma	28.7–60%
Squamous papilloma	10.6–17.3%
Sebaceous adenocarcinoma	2.0–15.3%
Benign melanoma	12.9–17.6%
Malignant melanoma	2.8–7.9%
Histiocytoma	1.6–3.5%
Mastocytoma	1–2.5%
Basal cell carcinoma	1.2–2.5%
Squamous cell carcinoma	1–2%
All others	1–5%

tumors should be removed before they attain size, and routine histopathologic examination is always advisable, particularly considering the possible recurrence of a malignancy should the surgical excision have been insufficiently radical. Unfortunately, impression smears are rarely helpful in establishing a diagnosis. Excision guarantees the best possible prognosis.

Eyelid neoplasia most commonly involves older dogs. Some surveys indicate a breed predisposition, but surveys also always reflect the popularity of certain breeds within different countries and regions. **The most frequent neoplasia is of glandular origin (i.e., adenoma and adenocarcinoma) (Fig. 3-14).** The **papilloma** also has a high incidence and, in young patients, may accompany oral papillomatosis. Although the lesion has a viral origin, the therapeutic value of autogenous vaccines is doubtful. Papillomas tend to regress over a relatively short time, with their removal being necessary only if accompanying corneal irritation is present. In young dogs, **histiocytoma** also tends to regress spontaneously, but the invasive potential of this tumor is so high that surgical removal is always advocated. Both **basal cell and squamous cell carcinoma** rarely occur as eyelid lesions in the dog.

Pseudotumor formation involving the eyelid tissue is unusual in this species, but when it occurs, it presents as subcutaneous lesions that may cause discomfort and distortion. Such lesions can be difficult to differentiate clinically from neoplasia. Corticosteroid therapy can be helpful, but surgical excision is curative. Microscopic examination of any excised eyelid tissue is recommended.

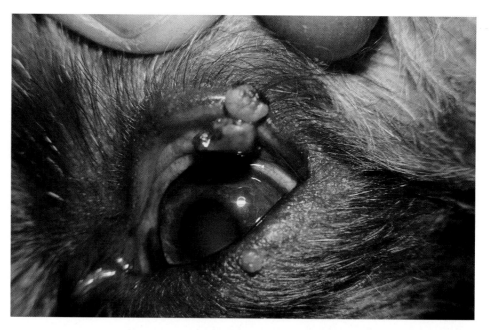

FIGURE 3-14. *Meibomian adenocarcinoma of the upper eyelid of an aged Brittany Spaniel. The tumor is primarily on the palpebral (deep) surface of the eyelid.*

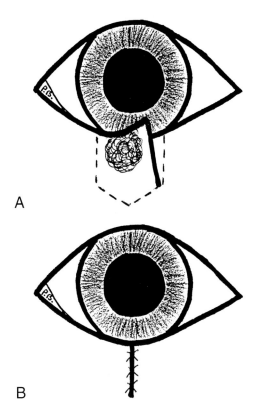

FIGURE 3-15. *Four-sided, full-thickness excision for removal of an eyelid neoplasm. A. A full-thickness wedge of tissue is removed using tenotomy scissors. B. The wound is repaired as a two-layered closure.*

Eyelid tumors generally should be removed and a histopathologic diagnosis sought. The smaller the neoplasm, the easier the reconstruction of the eyelid. Size, however, is not a particular complication, and difficulty may only be experienced if the lacrimal puncta or canaliculi are involved. Electrosurgery generally should not be used, both because of the unnecessary tissue destruction and swelling that it causes and because the repair tends to be associated with excessive scar formation. The decision to use sharp surgery or cryoablation is a personal one, but in cases of larger lesions, the latter technique necessitates use of thermocouples to monitor the extent of freezing. A small tissue sample must be obtained for histopathologic examination before cryoablation; sharp excision of lesions allows the whole neoplasm to be obtained. The size of the lesion dictates the sharp surgical technique to be used, but a sufficiency of eyelid and facial skin allows for whole-lesion excision on all occasions. **For tumors involving one-third of the eyelid margin or less, a full-thickness, "V"-shaped excision can be used. A four-sided full-thickness excision may possibly allow for an easier and stronger repair (Fig. 3-15).** In both techniques, the wound is closed using two layers of sutures, with the tarsoconjunctiva being apposed by a 4-0 to 6-0 simple interrupted absorbable suture and the skin and

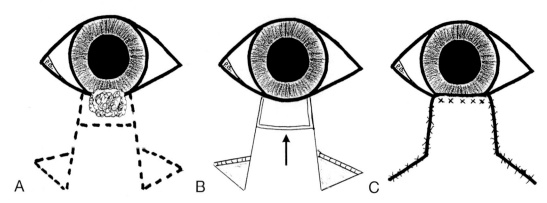

FIGURE 3-16. *Sliding skin graft to repair large eyelid deficits.* **A** *and* **B.** *The neoplasm is removed using full-thickness excision, and the adjacent skin is lifted as a pedicle using two slightly divergent scalpel incisions. Burows triangles are excised to allow the pedicle to be advanced into the surgical defect.* **C.** *Adjacent conjunctiva is mobilized to cover the skin flap, and the pedicle is sutured into the surgical defect with its leading margin edge 1-mm above the adjacent margo intermarginalis to allow for wound contraction and graft shrinkage.*

muscle layer being closed using a 4-0 to 6-0 simple interrupted nonabsorbable suture. Accurate reformation of the margo intermarginalis is the essential feature in preventing postoperative notching. A relief lateral canthotomy may be helpful in reducing the amount of tension on the suture line.

Alternative approaches for larger lid neoplasms include the "Z"-plasty skin flap (i.e., for lateral canthal tumors), local sliding skin grafts (Fig. 3-16), tarsoconjunctival grafts, and the full-thickness Cutler Beard or bucket-handle graft. These same reconstruction blepharoplastic procedures can also be used to repair extensive traumatic lesions and eyelid agenesis as well as to reconstruct the eyelid after dermoid removal (for more details, the reader should consult the third edition, pp. 561–567).

Diseases and Surgery of the Canine Tear and Nasolacrimal Systems

Diseases of the canine tear and nasolacrimal systems are not infrequent, and deficiency of tears (i.e., keratoconjunctivitis sicca [KCS]) is frequently encountered in clinical practice. This chapter presents these interrelated systems with an emphasis on the clinical manifestations of these diseases and their appropriate medical and surgical management.

PREOCULAR/PRECORNEAL FILM DYNAMICS

The preocular tear film is a complex, trilaminar fluid consisting of lipid, aqueous, and mucin components. The thin (0.1 μm), superficial lipid layer is secreted by the tarsal (i.e., meibomian) glands, and it provides a thin, oily covering for the aqueous tear layer, thus retarding evaporation and promoting a stable, even spread of tears across the cornea. The intermediate or aqueous component of canine tears (thickness, ≈ 7 μm or less) is secreted by lacrimal glands of the orbit and the nictitating membrane. Aqueous tears account for most of the total tear volume and consist of water, electrolytes, glucose, urea, surface-active polymers, glycoproteins, and tear proteins, including lactoferrin and some serum proteins. Primary tear proteins include globulins (i.e., secretory immunoglobulin A), albumin, and lysozyme. The deepest tear layer (thickness, ≈ 1.0–2.0 μm) consists of mucin, which is a hydrated glycoprotein produced by conjunctival goblet cells that, in the dog, have their highest density in the conjunctival fornices. Goblet cell–derived preocular mucin fills in any irregularities of the corneal surface, thereby providing an optically smooth ocular surface. Bacteria and foreign particles are trapped

73

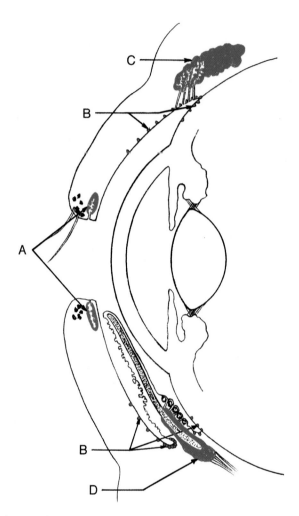

FIGURE 4-1. *Anatomic location of the secretory tissues responsible for production of the tear components.* **A.** *Meibomian glands within the tarsal plate.* **B.** *Conjunctival goblet cells.* **C.** *Orbital lacrimal gland.* **D.** *Nictitans lacrimal gland. (Courtesy of G. Constantinescu.)*

by mucoproteins. Mucin also harbors immunoglobulins (i.e., immuno-globulin A) and lysozyme, and it aids in lubrication and hydration of the conjunctiva and cornea.

The lacrimal glands of the orbit and the nictitating membrane are tubu-loacinar and histopathologically similar. In the dog, three to five ductules from the orbital lacrimal gland open into the dorsolateral conjunctival fornix, whereas the nictitans gland delivers aqueous tears onto the corneal surface through multiple ducts between the lymphoid follicles on the pos-terocentral third eyelid (Fig. 4-1). **The orbital lacrimal gland is the main source of tears in some dogs, whereas the nictitating membrane gland is the main source in others** (for more details, the reader should consult the third edition, pp. 583–586).

DEVELOPMENT AND MORPHOLOGY OF THE NASOLACRIMAL DRAINAGE APPARATUS

The nasolacrimal duct system develops from surface ectoderm within the nasolacrimal groove (i.e., furrow), which separates the lateral nasal fold and the maxillary process. Ectodermal cells grow along this groove, sink into mesenchyme, and are buried. These cells then form a cord in the dog as the maxillary process fuses with the lateral nasal fold between days 23 and 26 of gestation. The upper end of this cord develops two buds, which grow into the upper and lower eyelids near the medial canthus and develop into the superior and inferior canaliculi and puncta. The cord next becomes a duct through a process of canalization and is normally patent at birth.

The superior and inferior lacrimal puncta are oval-to-slitlike openings of approximately 1.0 ± 0.3 mm, with their long axis running parallel to the lid margin (Fig. 4-2). They are located on the palpebral conjunctiva at the edge of the upper and lower eyelids 2 to 5 mm from the medial canthus, or approximately where the tarsal glands end. The puncta are the openings to the superior and inferior canaliculi, which are approximately 4 to 7 mm in length and 0.5 to 1.0 mm in diameter. The canaliculi extend through the orbicularis oculi muscle, and they join together ventral to the medial canthus to form a poorly developed lacrimal sac, which lies within a slight depression (i.e., the lacrimal fossa) in the lacrimal bone. The nasolacrimal duct itself is constricted as it traverses the lacrimal bone, and this narrowing is important in the dog for retention of foreign bodies and development of dacryocystitis. The duct then passes through a canal on the medial surface of the maxillary bone and ends in a nasal punctum. The nasal puncta are usually located in the ventrolateral nasal meatus, which opens approximately 1 cm inside the external nares. In approximately 50% of dogs, the nasolacrimal

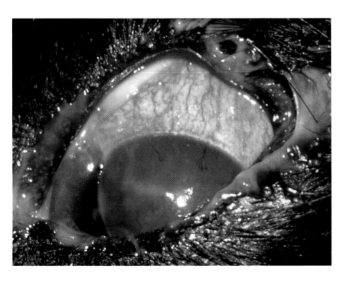

FIGURE 4-2. *Left eye of a dog with keratoconjunctivitis sicca. Note the intense conjunctival hyperemia, thick mucopurulent discharge, and chronic keratitis characteristic of a subacute or chronic aqueous tear deficiency.*

duct also has a second opening in the oral mucosa of the central hard palate, behind the incisors at the level of the canine teeth. The nasolacrimal duct is approximately 1 mm in diameter, but this length varies considerably between brachycephalic, mesocephalic, and dolichocephalic dogs.

The sole purpose of the nasolacrimal duct system is to drain tears from the surface of the eye to the nasal passages. Drainage occurs through multiple forces, and most (60%) of the tear volume is normally drained through the inferior punctum and canaliculus.

PATHOGENESIS OF TEAR FILM DISEASE

Disease states may cause decreased secretion of tear components by affecting the secretory tissues either directly or indirectly (e.g., by compromising the nerve supply to the lacrimal glands). **Keratoconjunctivitis sicca (or dry eye) is the clinical condition associated with lacrimal gland hyposecretion.** Abnormalities or deficiencies of tear components other than aqueous fluid (usually the mucin layer) are considered here to be qualitative disorders.

KERATOCONJUNCTIVITIS SICCA

Keratoconjunctivitis sicca is a common ocular disease in the dog. It is characterized by aqueous tear deficiency, which results in desiccation and inflammation of the conjunctiva and cornea, ocular pain, progressive corneal disease, and reduced vision. The most recently reported incidence of KCS in canine patients is approximately 1% (i.e., 9–12 cases per 1000 admissions).

CAUSES OF AQUEOUS TEAR DEFICIENCY

Absence or reduction of lacrimal secretions may result from a single disease process or a combination of conditions affecting both the orbital lacrimal and the nictitans glands (Box 4-1).

Several breeds are disproportionately affected by acquired KCS, thus suggesting a genetic predisposition. Several breeds are also at greater risk of developing KCS (Box 4-2).

CLINICAL FINDINGS

Clinical signs of KCS vary depending on the time since onset and the extent of dryness. **A very acute, severe form of KCS is sometimes seen in which the eye becomes acutely painful in association with axial corneal ulceration. In such cases, suppurative inflammation may result in progressive corneal disease with stromal malacia, descemetocele**

BOX 4-1

Causes of Keratoconjunctivitis Sicca in the Dog

Immune-mediated dacryoadenitis/dacryoadenopathy

Canine distemper virus

Chronic blepharoconjunctivitis

Congenital acinar hypoplasia (congenital alacrima)

Drug-induced keratoconjunctivitis sicca may occur in the dog after:

Systemic sulfonamide therapy (phenazopyridine, sulfadiazine, sulfasalazine, and trimethoprim-sulfonamide combinations)

Topical atropine

Removal of the nictitans gland

Uncorrected prolapse of the nictitans gland

Traumatic or inflammatory orbital diseases

Loss of parasympathetic innervation to lacrimal glands (cranial nerve VII)

Loss of sensory innervation (sensation) to the ocular surface (cranial nerve V)

Local radiation therapy for head neoplasms

Systemic metabolic diseases (hypothyroidism, diabetes mellitus, and Cushing's disease)

BOX 4-2

Breeds at Highest Risk of Keratoconjunctivitis Sicca

English Bulldogs

West Highland White Terriers

Pugs

Yorkshire Terriers

American Cocker Spaniels

Pekingese

Miniature Schnauzers

English Springer Spaniels

formation with resultant staphyloma, and iris prolapse. In most cases, however, the onset is more gradual, with the severity increasing during a period of several weeks (Fig. 4-3). These eyes initially appear to be red and inflamed, with intermittent mucoid or mucopurulent discharge. As the severity increases, however, the ocular surface becomes lackluster, the conjunctiva appears to be extremely hyperemic, and persistent, tenacious mucopurulent ocular discharge is observed. Progressive keratitis characterized by extensive corneal vascularization and pigmentation, with or without ulceration, also may occur. Severe pigmentary keratitis may be refractory to medical and surgical therapy. Blepharitis and periocular dermatitis often occur with an accumulation of exudates on the eyelid margins and periocular skin. With progressive disease, the level of discomfort intensifies, thus resulting in persistent blepharospasm.

DIAGNOSIS

The diagnosis of KCS is established on the basis of typical clinical signs, positive ocular-staining results using vital stains, and reduced Schirmer tear test (STT) results. Rose Bengal stain will detect devitalized cells, subtle epithelial defects on either the conjunctiva or the corneal surfaces, and adherent mucus tags. Fluorescein stain detects concurrent corneal ulceration and also may be used to evaluate tear film breakup (discussed later). Schirmer tear tests may be done either without (i.e., STT I) or with (i.e., STT II) use of topical anesthetic. The STT I measures the ability of the eye to produce reflex tears in addition to basal secretions and is the one most commonly performed STTs, whereas the STT II estimates only basal tear secretion.

FIGURE 4-3. *Pigmentary keratitis, a common manifestation of canine keratoconjunctivitis sicca, in the left eye of an affected dog. In addition to tear deficiency, predisposing factors for the pigmentary keratitis include an inherently heavily pigmented eye, conformational exophthalmos, and frictional irritation to the cornea (entropion/trichiasis).*

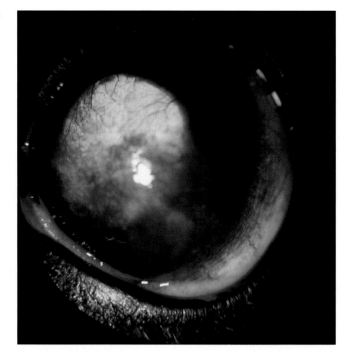

Both STT I and STT II values are significantly different in the normal dog. In the clinical setting, STT I readings are generally interpreted as follows:

15 mm/min = normal production,
11–14 mm/min = early or subclinical KCS,
6–10 mm/min = moderate or mild KCS, and
5 mm/min = severe KCS.

Fluctuations in STT values may occur on a daily and a weekly basis; however, only weekly fluctuations are considered to be biologically significant.

QUALITATIVE ABNORMALITIES

Problematic cases of KCS can occur in which the aqueous tear volume appears to be adequate and other, recognized causes of surface disease (e.g., infection, frictional irritation, ineffectual blinking) have been excluded. In such cases, qualitative tear deficiency from an abnormality of the lipid or the mucin tear components may be a primary (or a contributing) cause of the surface disease.

QUALITATIVE TEAR DEFICIENCIES OF LIPIDS AND MUCIN

Dogs with disturbances of the tarsal or meibomian glands (i.e., the lipid layer of the tear film) and of the conjunctival goblet cells (i.e., the mucin layer of the tear film) may show the clinical signs of KCS but have STT measurements that are usually within the normal range. With diseased meibomian glands, highly polar lipids are produced that disrupt the nonpolar lipid surface of the tear fluid. The resultant loss of the normal oily covering may allow for premature dispersion of the aqueous layer. Insufficient production of preocular mucin also results in the loss of tear film stability, with subsequent corneal desiccation. In the dog, the pathogenesis of spontaneously occurring, mucin-deficient dry eye disease may vary among cases.

CLINICAL FINDINGS

Dogs with acute meibomianitis typically have swollen eyelid margins, with a slight "pointing" of the meibomian openings. Chronic meibomianitis may result in rupture of glandular acini and release of lipid secretions into the periacinar tissues. Formation of lipid granulomas and multiple chalazia may frictionally irritate the eye and, in turn, complicate any tear film abnormality that may be present. In some cases of chronic meibomianitis, superficial keratitis is also present. Clinical findings in this keratopathy may be somewhat subtle, with faint localized or geographic epithelial edema, small and multifocal punctate areas of roughened epithelium that may (or may not) retain fluorescein stain, and fine as well as superficial perilimbal

FIGURE 4-4. *Tear film breakup time test measures the time (in seconds) to the beginning of fluorescein dissipation (or dry spots) within the corneal tear film. After the instillation of fluorescein, the eyelids are held open, and the tear film is observed by biomicroscopy.*

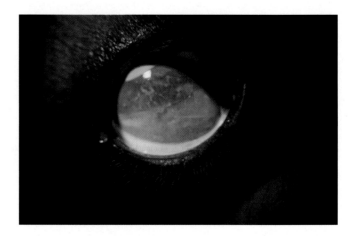

vascular infiltrates. The corneal disease in such cases likely may be attributed to both lipid deficiency with unstable tear film and direct frictional effects from roughened eyelid margins.

Loss of conjunctival goblet cells results in an unstable tear film, as manifested by rapid breakup of the tears over the eye, lackluster appearance of the ocular surface, and corneal desiccation. Clinical features of preocular mucin deficiency in the dog may include chronic keratoconjunctivitis, corneal ulceration, and the absence of appreciable ocular discharge in animals with adequate aqueous tear measurements. In some cases, the conjunctiva may appear to be thickened and inelastic.

DIAGNOSIS

Establishing the diagnosis of lipid tear abnormalities depends on clinical findings from a detailed examination using a focused light and a magnifying source, with particular attention to the appearance of the eyelid margins and the meibomian glands. Swollen, rounded eyelid margins indicate acute or subacute marginal blepharitis. Hyperemia of the mucocutaneous junction with dry, crusty, porphyrin-stained exudates on the lid margins is also indicative of marginal blepharitis. Any elevated, focal, and beige subconjunctival masses typical of chalazia should be noted; when present, chalazia indicates chronic meibomianitis, with periglandular granulomatous inflammation. After administration of a topical anesthetic solution, gentle manipulation of the eyelid margin using blunt-tipped forceps with shallow serrations allows for inspection of secretions expressed from the meibomian glands. Normal meibomian lipid appears to be a clear, viscous oil, which is similar in appearance to vegetable cooking oil. Abnormal meibomian secretions are typically thick, opaque, and may appear to be inspissated, with a cream-cheese consistency. Expression of coiled, semisolid strands of abnormal lipid is not uncommon in cases of chronic meibomian disease.

The clinical diagnosis of canine ocular mucin deficiency may be supported by the results of a tear film breakup time test (Fig. 4-4). The diagnosis may also be confirmed by the results of conjunctival biopsy and quantification of epithelial goblet cells. The tear film breakup time test is performed by instilling one drop of fluorescein stain into the eye and then manually holding the eyelids open. The time is recorded from the last blink to the appearance of the first dry spot, which appears as a dark area in the yellow-green fluorescent film. A cobalt-blue filter should be used when viewing the cornea. A normal breakup time in the dog should be 20 seconds or longer. In the dog with mucin deficiency, however, tear breakup usually occurs in less than 5 seconds.

MEDICAL TREATMENT

Medical therapy is the primary means of treating tear-deficient ocular surface disease. Such therapy should be adjusted for each KCS patient (Box 4-3).

CHOLINERGIC AGENTS

Because of the parasympathetic innervation of the lacrimal glands, cholinergic drugs have historically been used to stimulate tear secretions. **For example, ophthalmic pilocarpine solution has been administered, either topically or orally, as a tear stimulant. Oral administration has consisted of applying 1 to 2% ophthalmic solution to the food. A safe initial oral dosage is one drop twice daily of 2% topical pilocarpine per 10 kg of body weight.** The dose may be increased by one-drop increments at each dosing until signs of systemic reaction develop (i.e., salivation, vomiting, diarrhea, bradycardia). Alternatively, topical dilute pilocarpine has been applied directly to the eyes. Concentrations of either 0.125% or 0.25% have been formulated by adding 1 mL of 2% pilocarpine to 15 mL of artificial tears (0.125% solution) or by adding 2 mL of 2% pilocarpine to 14 mL of artificial tears (0.25% solution). Recent results in normal dogs, however,

---

BOX 4-3

Selected Drugs for the Treatment of Keratoconjunctivitis Sicca in the Dog

Topical antimicrobial agents

Mucinolytics

Anti-inflammatory therapy (avoid in acute keratoconjunctivitis sicca)

Lacrimostimulants:

Immunomodulating: topical cyclosporin A

Cholinergic: oral pilocarpine

have indicated that topically applied pilocarpine may not significantly increase tear production and, therefore, have cast doubt on the efficacy of such therapy.

IMMUNOMODULATING AGENTS

The ability of the immunosuppressive agent cyclosporin A (CsA) to stimulate tear production in the dog is well documented. The mechanism of action for CsA regarding tear production is incompletely understood, but both immunomodulating and tear-stimulating properties appear to produce the dramatic responses observed in many affected dogs after topical application. One important mechanism of action is the inhibition of T-helper lymphocytes. In animal models of immune-mediated lacrimal disease, the balance between T-suppressor and T-helper cells plays an important role in regulation of the lacrimal gland. T-suppressor cells normally predominate, but in immune-mediated KCS, T-helper cells become the prevalent T lymphocytes. Before the commercial availability of CsA for ophthalmic use, 1 to 2% oil-based solutions were compounded from 10% oral CsA solution using a vegetable oil (i.e., olive or corn oil) solvent. Currently, the 0.2% commercial ointment (Optimmune; Schering-Plough) is prescribed. To stimulate tear production, topical CsA is generally recommended for initial application to affected eyes every 12 hours; however, in severe cases, treatments may be initially administered every 8 hours. Several weeks of continuous treatment are usually needed before substantial increases in tear production are observed.

The STT measurements may provide some insight regarding the possible response to therapy with CsA. Dogs with pretreatment STT values of between 0 and 1 mm/min have an approximately 50% chance of responding to topical CsA with increased tear secretion. Dogs with pretreatment STT values of 2 mm/min or greater have a more than 80% chance of improved tear production. In responsive animals, the return of functional secretory tissues has been demonstrated histopathologically after treatment with topical CsA. Most dogs show clinical improvement even without increased tear production, however, including those dogs with pretreatment STT values of 2 mm/min or less.

TEAR SUBSTITUTES (LACRIMOMIMETICS)

Tear substitutes contain ingredients (or combinations of ingredients) to replace deficiencies in one or more of the three primary tear components (i.e., aqueous, mucin, lipid). **Many ophthalmic solutions and ointments are commercially available for tear replacement therapy (see Appendix B).** Aqueous tear replacement agents are initially applied to the affected eyes four to six times daily and are generally used concurrently with other topical therapeutic agents. Viscous lubricants enhance wettability of the ocular surface and have extended contact time with the ocular surface. Linear polymers such as dextran and polyvinylpyrrolidone (povidone) have mucinomimetic properties as well. Patented polymers (e.g., Adsorbobase; Alcon) have been combined with buffered solutions of substituted cellulose esters to form preparations for treating deficiencies of both the aqueous and mucin components of the preocular tear film. Viscoelastic substances with mucinomimetic properties include sodium hyaluronate, chondroitin sulfate, and 1 to 2% methylcellulose preparations. Sodium hyaluronate is a naturally occurring, high-molecular-weight glycosaminoglycan with excellent viscoelastic and lubricating properties. Sodium hyaluronate products have been diluted with artificial tears to make a 0.04% solution (0.2 mL of 1% sodium hyaluronate [Healon, Pharmacia and Upjohn] added to 5 mL of tear substitute) to increase tear viscosity, prolong tear retention, and enhance the lubrication of dry eyes.

ANTIBACTERIALS

Antibiotics with broad-spectrum activity (e.g., triple-antibiotic ointment or solution) are commonly administered to control large bacterial burdens that occur with inadequate cleansing of the ocular surface. Initially, treatment is usually given three to four times daily, is then reduced to twice daily as the mucopurulent discharge decreases, and is eventually discontinued when signs of infection have abated.

MUCINOLYTIC–ANTICOLLAGENASE AGENTS

Good ocular hygiene (i.e., frequent cleansing of discharges) is essential to minimize the accumulation of debris with degradative enzymes that contribute to ocular surface inflammation and ulceration. To facilitate removal of the copious exudates and mucoid debris that may accompany KCS, a 5 to 10% solution of acetylcysteine may be applied topically two to four times daily.

ANTI-INFLAMMATORY THERAPY

Anti-inflammatory therapy may be a valuable adjunct to other medical therapy for the improving clinical signs of KCS. **Topical corticosteroids are commonly administered to minimize conjunctivitis, to alleviate discomfort, and to reduce the corneal opacities associated with chronic keratitis.** Triple-antibiotic ointment in combination with hydrocortisone is beneficial in many KCS patients. Caution must be exercised when administering topical corticosteroids, however, because their use will complicate healing of an ulcerated cornea. In addition to its marked lacrimostimulant effects, topical CsA also has beneficial anti-inflammatory properties (e.g., reducing corneal inflammatory infiltrates). Use of CsA appears to be safe in patients with corneal ulceration, does not alter the ocular surface flora, and may also be beneficial in reducing corneal vascularization in dogs with chronic keratitis from causes other than KCS (for more details, the reader should consult the third edition, pp. 593–599).

   Cases of acute KCS may present with corneal stromal ulceration requiring aggressive medical therapy, surgical therapy, or both. Because opportunistic infections may contribute to the rapid degradation of ulcerated cornea, bacterial culture of the ulcer margins with subsequent sensitivity testing is indicated. When corneal ulceration occurs as a sequela to KCS, local administration of atropine is contraindicated, because surface drying will be exacerbated by such application. In cases of deep stromal ulceration or descemetocele formation, reconstructive corneal surgery (i.e., conjunctival grafting) may be necessary to stabilize the cornea and to stimulate fibrovascular resolution of the ulceration.

SPECIAL CONSIDERATIONS IN QUALITATIVE TEAR DEFICIENCIES

The specific treatment of lipid tear abnormalities depends on the particular meibomian disorder. Bacterial meibomianitis should be treated with both topical and systemic antibiotics. Chronic bacterial meibomianitis is often recurrent and requires intermittent, intensive treatments or continuous, low-level maintenance therapy. In some of these cases, topical application of an antibiotic ointment two to three times daily may be indicated as long-term maintenance therapy. Surgical curettage of chalazia is indicated for granulomas. Warm, moist compresses applied to the eyelids for several minutes two or three times daily may stimulate local vasodilation and result in improved hemodynamics to the affected areas. Another aspect of treating diffuse meibomian diseases is providing lipid substitutes through topical emollients containing petrolatum, mineral oil, liquid lanolin, or some combination of these ingredients.

Treatment for mucin-deficient keratoconjunctivitis consists of topical mucin replacements (i.e., mucinomimetics), symptomatic treatment of corneal ulcers (if present), and topical anti-inflammatory therapy in selected cases. Topical mucinomimetics applied at 4- to 6-hour intervals are the mainstay of therapy. The more viscous lubricants mimic mucin by enhancing wettability of the ocular surface and by providing extended contact time with the epithelial surfaces.

SURGICAL TREATMENT OF TEAR DEFICIENCIES

Surgical procedures indicated for treatment of selected KCS cases are parotid duct transposition (PDT), which provides saliva as a tear substitute, and permanent partial tarsorrhaphy, which reduces exposure and enhances blinking. Nasolacrimal puncta occlusion is used in humans as a tear-conserving procedure by blocking tear drainage, but use of this procedure has not been reported in the dog. Replacement of the nictitans gland (versus removal of the gland) is regarded as a preventative surgical procedure for canine KCS.

PAROTID DUCT TRANSPOSITION

Because of the physiologic similarities between saliva and tear fluids, PDT has been performed successfully in dogs affected with KCS that were nonresponsive to medical therapy. Since the introduction of CsA in 1987, however, the percentage of KCS cases treated by PDT has declined dramatically. Nonetheless, a few dogs with persistent absolute sicca (STT, 0 mm/min) after several weeks of medical treatment remain candidates for PDT.

Preoperative Considerations

In the dog, PDT is delayed until KCS has been unresponsive to at least 8 weeks of conventional medical therapy. Dogs with KCS may occasionally have xerostomia, and these animals are not candidates for PDT. The flow of salivary fluid from the parotid duct is easily tested by administering a bitter substance (e.g., one drop of ophthalmic atropine solution) to the tongue and then observing for salivary flow from the papilla. The teeth should be cleaned before PDT, and when periodontal disease is present, systemic antibiotics should be administered for 7 to 10 days before the operation.

Surgical Procedures

After general anesthesia, the parotid duct is cannulated by placing a monofilament nylon suture into the duct opening. The optimal suture size generally ranges from 0-0 to 2-0 depending on the size of the duct. Either of two approaches (i.e., closed [oral] or open [lateral]) may be used when performing PDT (Fig. 4-5). Both approaches appear to be equally effective; thus, the choice of an open versus a closed PDT procedure is simply one of the surgeon's preference.

The open PDT procedure involves exposing the parotid duct through a facial skin incision directly over the parotid duct. The duct is then carefully dissected from the masseter muscle and retracted using umbilical tape or a muscle hook (to minimize surgical trauma). The duct continues submucosally for 0.5 to 1.0 cm before terminating at the papilla in the buccal mucosa. Therefore, during dissection, the facial vein and the anastomotic branch between the dorsal and ventral buccal nerves must be avoided. The papilla and surrounding mucosa are carefully dissected free using conjunctival scissors, and the papilla, along with the retained suture and duct, are then retracted back into the facial incision. Using small Metzenbaum scissors, a subcutaneous tunnel is established and directed to the ventrolateral conjunctival fornix, where the papilla is attached. The incisions are finally closed in a routine manner.

Complications, Sequelae, and Postoperative Considerations

Twisting, laceration, or trauma to the parotid duct may occur with either the closed or the open PDT procedure. Trauma associated with dissection of the highly vascular and innervated facial tissues, increased postoperative

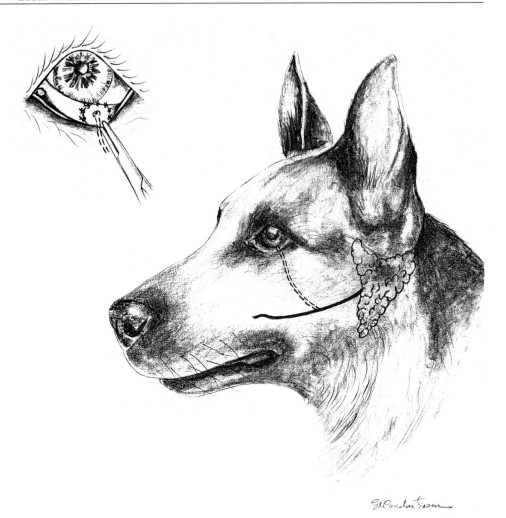

FIGURE 4-5. *Location of the left parotid gland and the duct coursing rostrally through the facial soft tissues to its point of exit into the oral cavity. Dashed lines illustrate the course of the transposed duct resulting from parotid duct transposition.* **Insert.** *Placement of the oral papilla after transposition and attachment of papilla to the ventral conjunctival fornix via interrupted 7-0 polyglactin 910 sutures. (Courtesy of G. Constantinescu.)*

swelling, and potential discomfort from the extensive surgical dissection also may occur soon after surgery. Causes for delayed failure of PDT include retraction of the papilla into the subcutaneous space with fibrous closure of the conjunctival opening, occlusion of the duct by sialoliths, and acute or chronic sialoadenitis. Because of the higher concentration of minerals in saliva compared with tears, owners should be alerted for the development of mineral deposits on the cornea and eyelid margins. Should this occur, a chelating solution containing 1 to 2% ethylenediaminetetraacetic acid (EDTA) in artificial tears may be applied topically two to three times daily to control the mineral precipitates. Continued use of topical CsA also appears to be helpful in reducing irritation from mineral deposits, probably because of its lubricant, mucinogenic, and anti-inflammatory properties. An overabundance of salivary secretions may result in facial wetting and discoloration, which can be objectionable to some owners, especially in light-coated dogs. In rare cases, this overproduction may prompt consideration of duct ligation or even reversal of the surgery itself (for more details, the reader should consult the third edition, pp. 599–605).

OTHER SURGICAL PROCEDURES

A partial permanent tarsorrhaphy may be beneficial in the dog with KCS, especially among brachycephalic breeds, to afford greater corneal protection and to conserve existing tears. Removing a prolapsed nictitans gland or allowing chronic prolapse without treatment may predispose an affected eye to KCS. Repair of a prolapsed nictitans gland using an appropriate replacement procedure, however, reduces (but does not prevent) the onset of KCS.

CYSTS AND NEOPLASMS OF THE LACRIMAL SECRETORY SYSTEM

Cysts involving lacrimal tissue are uncommon, but they have been reported and may originate from either the orbital lacrimal or the nictitans glands. Depending on the site of origin, cysts may distend the conjunctiva and protrude into the palpebral fissure, expand within the orbit and cause displacement of the globe, or both. Surgical excision of cysts is curative. Tear secretion may be compromised depending on how much of lacrimal gland is either involved initially or excised subsequently.

Lacrimal neoplasms are also uncommon in the dog, but when they do occur, they are most often primary adenocarcinomas. These tumors tend to be locally invasive and to have a guarded prognosis. Adenocarcinoma of the nictitans gland constitutes one of the rare indications for complete excision of the nictitans. Orbital exenteration with adjunctive radiation therapy or chemotherapy may be indicated for cases of adenocarcinoma of the orbital lacrimal gland.

CLINICAL MANIFESTATIONS OF NASOLACRIMAL DISEASE

Disorders of the nasolacrimal duct system in the dog are either congenital or acquired, and they are limited to a lack of patency or inflammation. **The clinical manifestations of nasolacrimal system disease include epiphora, mucopurulent punctal and conjunctival discharge, swelling of the ventromedial canthal region, punctal foreign bodies, and draining fistula in the medial canthal region.** The epiphora that develops secondary to obstructed tear flow through the nasolacrimal duct system must be differentiated from the overproduction of tears (i.e., lacrimation) in which the tear volume overwhelms the normal drainage system.

DIAGNOSTIC PROCEDURES

Diagnostic procedures for nasolacrimal drainage diseases include the STT, cytology and microbial culture, fluorescein dye passage test, normograde punctal and canalicular cannulation and lavage, nasal punctal cannulation and retrograde flushing, dacryocystorhinography, ultrasonography, computed tomography (CT), and magnetic resonance (MR) imaging. The normal gross anatomy of the nasolacrimal duct system is illustrated in Figure 4-6. A systematic approach to the diagnosis and

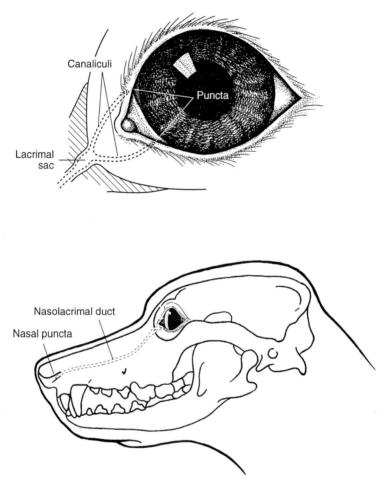

FIGURE 4-6. *Gross anatomy of the canine nasolacrimal duct system. Note the relationship of the eyelids, puncta, canaliculi, lacrimal sac, nasolacrimal duct, and nasal puncta.*

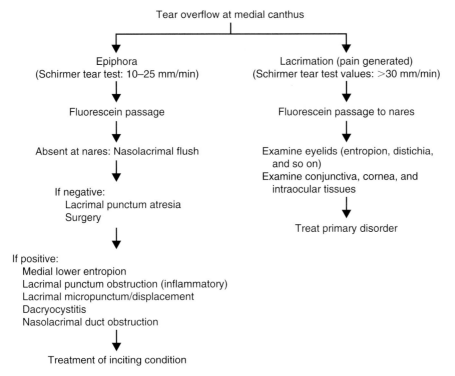

FIGURE 4-7. *Strategy and procedures for the diagnosis and treatment of nasolacrimal (drainage) diseases. (The character of the ocular discharge is mainly serous or seromucus; if the ocular discharge is mucopurulent or purulent, see Chapters 5 and 6.)*

treatment of nasolacrimal system diseases is summarized in Figure 4-7, primarily using the STT, fluorescein passage from the eye to the nares, and the nasolacrimal flush.

Schirmer Tear Test

The STT should be the first diagnostic test during examination of the dog with epiphora. This test estimates the total reflex aqueous tear production; volumes greater than 25 mm/min are consistent with the diagnosis of lacrimation. Lacrimation may overwhelm a functional nasolacrimal duct and result in epiphora.

Fluorescein Dye Passage and Nasolacrimal Flush

Fluorescein dye passage is the primary test of nasolacrimal drainage patency. It involves placing liquid fluorescein dye on the cornea and conjunctiva, and after 3 to 5 minutes have elapsed, both the nasal area and the pharynx are examined with cobalt-filtered or ultraviolet light to confirm dye passage and duct patency. Unfortunately, false-negative results can occur, and a normograde nasolacrimal duct flush is frequently required to confirm patency. A 24-gauge intravenous catheter or nasolacrimal cannula is preplaced on a 3-mL syringe containing a commercial eye wash, and a drop of topical anesthetic is applied to the conjunctiva. The lacrimal punctum and canaliculus are then cannulated, and a small volume of eye wash is injected while observing the contralateral punctum. When fluid passes through the opposite punctum, it is gently occluded using finger pressure. Continued injection into a normal nasolacrimal duct system will produce eye wash at the nostrils or induce swallowing as the solution flows into the pharynx. Retrograde nasolacrimal duct flushing is performed when a normograde flush is not successful. In most dogs, general anesthesia is required before cannulation of the nasal punctum and retrograde flushing can be performed.

Radiographic and Other Imaging Examinations

Lateral and ventrodorsal, open-mouth nasal radiographs are useful for evaluation of the nasal bones along which the nasolacrimal duct passes. This duct is vulnerable to traumatic laceration, erosion, and compression by infectious processes or nasal tumors. Results of dacryocystorhinography will confirm nasolacrimal duct patency. This radiographic contrast study involves the injection of approximately 1 mL of a viscous, radiopaque dye through the cannulated canaliculi. Radiographs are obtained as the dye passes through the nasolacrimal duct system, and perforations or blockages of the nasolacrimal duct are readily detected on these images. Advanced imaging studies (i.e., ultrasonography, CT, MR imaging) are also useful to confirm compression of the nasolacrimal duct system and to determine the extent of primary disease in the nose and the orbit.

CONGENITAL DISEASES

Reported congenital anomalies of the nasolacrimal duct system include punctal aplasia and micropunctum, canalicular and nasal lacrimal duct atresia, misplacement of the punctum and canaliculus, displacement of the punctum secondary to ventromedial ventral entropion, dacryops, and canaliculops.

Lacrimal Punctal Aplasia

Punctal aplasia (or imperforate lacrimal punctum) is the most frequently diagnosed congenital anomaly in the dog. It may affect the superior, inferior, or both puncta, and it may be either unilateral or bilateral. It occurs in numerous breeds and is commonly seen in American Cocker Spaniels, Bedlington Terriers, Golden Retrievers, Miniature and Toy Poodles, and Samoyeds. Superior punctal aplasia is asymptomatic. **The conjunctiva over the canaliculus will bulge during the initial nasolacrimal flush** (for more details, the reader should consult the third edition, pp. 574–575).

Other Anomalies

Incomplete development (i.e., micropunctum) or strictures of the ventral punctum causing epiphora are infrequent, and when they occur, they may be enlarged with a punctal dilator or the "1-2-3 snip" technique and catheterization. Aplasia of the canaliculus, nasolacrimal sac, or duct has not been reported in the dog. Congenital puncta and canaliculi misplacement is often asymptomatic in the dog. When chronic epiphora is present and relates to the position of the ventral punctum, surgical repositioning is indicated; this allows the ophthalmic surgeon to microdissect the punctum and thin-walled canaliculus and then move them through a conjunctival incision to the eyelid margin near the medial canthus.

Inferior puncta and canaliculi are commonly displaced by a subtle, ventromedial entropion. This displacement is integral to the tear-

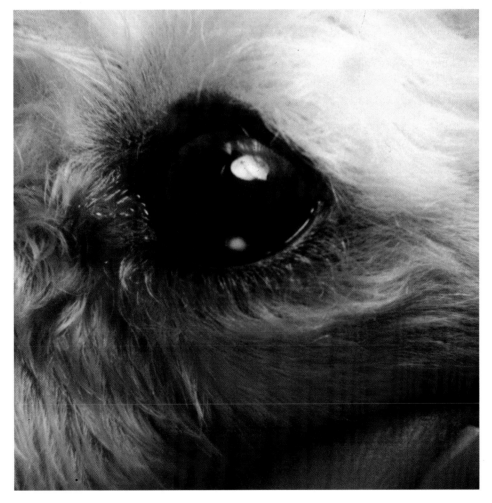

FIGURE 4-8. *Tear-staining syndrome in a 12-month-old Poodle. The clinical manifestation was bilateral tear-staining and epiphora.*

staining syndrome commonly seen among toy and brachycephalic breeds (Fig. 4-8). The results of one study showed that tear staining in the Poodle is related to a prolonged rate of tear excretion. Epiphora and unsightly tear staining in the Poodle and other small breeds develops during the postweaning period. The puncta are usually normal in these dogs, and the clinical signs relate to multiple factors, including displacement of the ventral puncta and compression of the canaliculi by the ventromedial entropion. In addition, tight medial canthal ligaments displace the medial canthus ventrally and, in combination with medial canthal trichiasis and eyelid trichiasis, exacerbate tear spillage in these dogs. Oral tetracyclines and metronidazole have been reported as therapy for Poodle epiphora, but neither has any effect on tear production or excretion. Their success actually relates to reduced staining of the medial canthal region rather than to control of the epiphora; therefore, they are used infrequently as therapy today. Removal of the third-eyelid gland has also been recommended as surgical therapy for epiphora, but this cannot be justified when the tear production is normal. The treatment of choice for this condition is a Hotz-Celsus repair of the ventromedial entropion or a bilateral medial canthal plasty to correct the ventromedial entropion, caruncular trichiasis, and tight medial canthal ligaments.

ACQUIRED DISEASES

Acquired nasolacrimal disorders of the dog include traumatic lacerations, dacryocystitis and obstruction with foreign bodies, and invasion or compression by neoplasms.

Lacerations

Facial trauma may result in lacerations of the puncta, canaliculi, medial canthus, and eyelids. Treatment of lacerated canaliculi involves cannulation of both puncta and injection of air. The resultant bubbling allows the surgeon to detect and cannulate the lacerated canalicular ends with a silastic tube. The lacerated eyelid surfaces are then repaired by apposition of the tissues around the cannulated duct.

Dacryocystitis and Foreign Bodies

Clinical manifestations of dacryocystitis and foreign bodies in the nasolacrimal duct include epiphora, purulent conjunctival discharge, punctal foreign bodies, and draining skin fistulas ventral to the medial canthus (Fig. 4-9). Dacryocystitis in the dog usually develops secondary to foreign bodies that lodge in the nasolacrimal sac; these foreign bodies must be removed for therapy to be effective. The diagnosis of dacryocystitis is confirmed through the results of dacryocystorhinography and cytologic examination of the contents from a nasolacrimal lavage or surgical exploration (i.e., dacryocystotomy). **Foreign bodies may be flushed from the nasolacrimal duct system by retrograde or normograde lavages, or they may be removed via dacryocystotomy. The nasolacrimal duct**

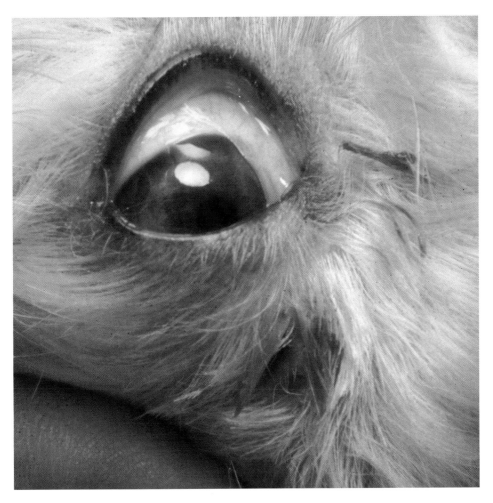

FIGURE 4-9. *Acute dacryocystitis with a ventral draining fistula in a 5-year-old Miniature Poodle.*

system is then cannulated with a silastic tube and treated with topical broad-spectrum antibiotics for approximately 3 weeks.

Neoplasia of the Nasolacrimal Duct

Primary neoplasia of the nasolacrimal duct is rare in the dog. Tumors of the nasal turbinates and maxillary sinus, however, may compress or invade the nasolacrimal ducts and spread into the orbit via the nasolacrimal foramen. In turn, this causes epiphora, mucopurulent or serosanguineous ocular and nasal discharge, masses ventral to the medial canthus, and orbital signs, including prolapse of the third eyelid, enophthalmos, and conjunctival hyperemia. The diagnosis of nasal neoplasia with involvement of the nasolacrimal duct system is established by the results of clinical examination, plain and contrast radiography, or advanced imaging, and it is confirmed by the results of light microscopic evaluation of nasal biopsy specimens.

SURGICAL PROCEDURES TO REPLACE/BYPASS THE NASOLACRIMAL DRAINAGE APPARATUS

Therapeutic options are limited to surgery, and they include conjunctival rhinotomy, conjunctival-maxillary sinusotomy, or conjunctival buccostomy (Fig. 4-10). These procedures create a permanent fistula from the conjunctiva to the nasal turbinates, maxillary sinus, or mouth, respectively (for more details, the reader should consult the third edition, pp. 575–576).

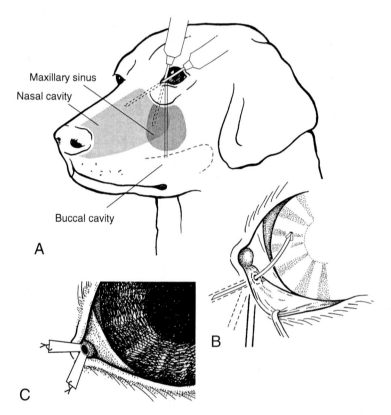

FIGURE 4-10. *Conjunctival rhinotomy.* **A.** *Conjunctival rhinotomy is completed by drilling a hole into the nasal cavity with a Steinmann pin and a Jacob's chuck.* **B.** *Conjunctival maxillary sinusotomy is completed by drilling a hole into the maxillary sinus from the medial canthus.* **C.** *Conjunctival buccostomy is completed by blunt dissection from the medial canthus to the oral cavity. A custom-made cannula is then inserted into the tract and sutured to the medial canthus.*

Diseases and Surgery of the Canine Conjunctiva

The conjunctiva is associated with many adnexal and bulbar diseases because of its exposure and close proximity to both internal and external ocular structures. A thorough physical examination should be performed on all dogs with conjunctival disease, because such disease can be an indication of systemic or blinding disease. The key to clinical management of conjunctival diseases is to determine and, if possible, to eliminate the cause. Fortunately, the cause of a conjunctival disease can often be determined solely on the basis of a patient history and complete ophthalmic examination.

CLINICAL ANATOMY AND PHYSIOLOGY

The conjunctiva plays a role in tear dynamics, immunologic protection of the eye, ocular movement, and corneal healing. As a mucous membrane, the conjunctiva lines the inside of the eyelids (i.e., the palpebral conjunctiva) beginning at the eyelid margin and extending deep toward the orbit to create a fornix (i.e., conjunctival cul-de-sac or fornix), at which point it reverses direction and then extends over the globe to the limbus (i.e., bulbar conjunctiva). The bulbar conjunctiva is freely movable, except near the limbus, which facilitates its use as graft tissue for the cornea. The conjunctiva contains many lymphoid nodules that receive antigen and present it to the circulating mononuclear cells. The lymphatics that drain this area represent the only lymphatic drainage of the eye.

Goblet cells are also present in the epithelial layer of the conjunctiva. These cells produce a gel-like mucin, which forms the deepest of the three layers of the preocular (i.e., the precorneal) tear film. This mucin protects

95

the ocular surface by trapping both debris and bacteria and by providing a medium to which immunoglobulins (i.e., immunoglobulin A) and microbicidal lysozymes adhere.

NORMAL BACTERIAL AND FUNGAL FLORA

Bacteria can be cultured from the conjunctival sac in 70 to 90% of normal dogs. Gram-positive aerobes are the most commonly cultured, with *Staphylococcus* sp., *Bacillus* sp., and *Corynebacterium* sp. predominating. Gram-negative bacteria can be recovered from the conjunctival sac in 7 to 8% of normal dogs. Anaerobes are rarely isolated, and the normal flora appears to vary with the season and the breed. The most commonly isolated fungal flora in the normal conjunctival sac are *Cladosporium oxysporum* and *Curvularia lunata*.

CONJUNCTIVAL CYTOLOGY

Conjunctival cytology may be useful in establishing the cause of conjunctival inflammation. Careful examination may reveal the character of the epithelial cells, the numbers and types of inflammatory cells, amount of mucin, the number (and Gram stain results) for bacteria, any fungi, and even inclusion bodies (i.e., early canine distemper). Table 5-1 provides additional information.

GENERAL RESPONSE TO DISEASE

The conjunctiva responds to acute insults with chemosis (i.e., edema), hyperemia, and cellular exudation. The conjunctiva responds to chronic insults with hyperemia, pigmentation, follicular formation, and exudation. Keratinized epithelial cells may occur secondary to prolonged exposure of the conjunctiva associated with ectropion and lagophthalmos; keratinization may also occur with keratoconjunctivitis sicca (KCS), vitamin A deficiency, and after radiation therapy. Goblet cell proliferation occurs with KCS, chronic conjunctivitis, and vitamin A deficiency.

Ocular redness can result from conjunctival hyperemia and anterior uveal inflammations or from episcleral congestion. Conjunctival hyperemia should be differentiated from episcleral injection, which occurs with glaucoma and anterior uveitis. Generally, conjunctival vessels have a smaller

TABLE 5-1

SUMMARY OF CYTOLOGY RESULTS IN CONJUNCTIVITIS

Cause	Conjunctival Cells	Inflammatory Cells	Mucin	Organisms
Normal	Few nonkeratinized sheets	Few neutrophils	Little	Few bacteria
Bacterial	More nonkeratinized Late: keratinized	Mainly neutrophils	Moderate	Frequent
Viral (distemper)	Early: more nonkeratinized	Mainly lymphocytes	Moderate	Possible inclusion bodies
	Late: more keratinized	Mainly neutrophils	Heavy	Usually no inclusions
Parasitic	More keratinized	Mainly eosinophils and lymphocytes	Moderate	Possible *Thelezia* sp.
Fungal		Mainly neutrophils	Variable	
Allergy	Variable	Mainly eosinophils, plasma cells, and lymphocytes	Little	
Keratoconjunctivitis sicca	Keratinization	Neutrophils ±goblet cells ±pigment cells	Variable	Variable bacteria

diameter and a branching pattern, blanch quickly with administration of topical epinephrine 1 to 2%, and are mobile; episcleral vessels have a larger diameter, do not branch, do not blanch quickly with topical application of 1 to 2% epinephrine, and are not mobile.

INFECTIOUS CONJUNCTIVITIS

Infectious conjunctivitis indicates the association with specific pathogens and is uncommon in the dog. Secondary conjunctivitis is more common, and it is often associated with eyelid abnormalities and KCS.

Examination of the patient with suspected conjunctivitis should include the Schirmer tear test; application of topical fluorescein (and even rose Bengal stain); culture and cytology of severe, medically refractory, and chronic cases; and a complete ophthalmic examination. The character of the conjunctival discharge may also assist in establishing the cause (Fig. 5-1).

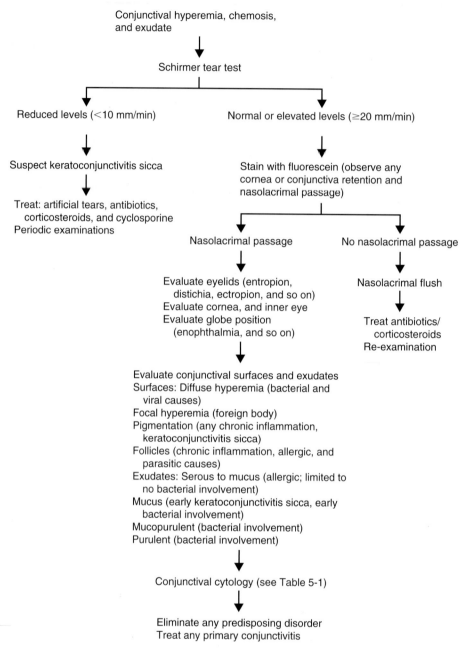

Conjunctival hyperemia, chemosis, and exudate

↓

Schirmer tear test

Reduced levels (<10 mm/min)   Normal or elevated levels (≥20 mm/min)

Suspect keratoconjunctivitis sicca   Stain with fluorescein (observe any cornea or conjunctiva retention and nasolacrimal passage)

Treat: artificial tears, antibiotics, corticosteroids, and cyclosporine Periodic examinations

Nasolacrimal passage   No nasolacrimal passage

Evaluate eyelids (entropion, distichia, ectropion, and so on)   Nasolacrimal flush
Evaluate cornea, and inner eye
Evaluate globe position (enophthalmia, and so on)   Treat antibiotics/ corticosteroids Re-examination

Evaluate conjunctival surfaces and exudates
Surfaces: Diffuse hyperemia (bacterial and viral causes)
Focal hyperemia (foreign body)
Pigmentation (any chronic inflammation, keratoconjunctivitis sicca)
Follicles (chronic inflammation, allergic, and parasitic causes)
Exudates: Serous to mucus (allergic; limited to no bacterial involvement)
Mucus (early keratoconjunctivitis sicca, early bacterial involvement)
Mucopurulent (bacterial involvement)
Purulent (bacterial involvement)

Conjunctival cytology (see Table 5-1)

Eliminate any predisposing disorder
Treat any primary conjunctivitis

FIGURE 5-1. *Clinical strategy for the diagnosis and treatment of conjunctivitis in the dog.*

BACTERIAL CONJUNCTIVITIS

Primary bacterial conjunctivitis is uncommon in the dog. In most cases that do occur, however, bacterial conjunctivitis develops secondary to eyelid abnormalities or KCS. Bacterial conjunctivitis is usually caused by *Staphylococcus* sp. and other Gram-positive organisms. Cytologic examination of conjunctival scrapings from the dog with conjunctivitis can help to confirm the diagnosis. Generally, a complete ophthalmic examination, appropriate ancillary tests (e.g., cytology, culture, and sensitivity), and appropriate treatment (usually broad-spectrum ophthalmic antibiotics in solution or ointment) produce a rapid response.

VIRAL CONJUNCTIVITIS

Canine distemper virus is associated with conjunctivitis, chorioretinitis, KCS, and optic nerve disease (Fig. 5-2). Conjunctivitis generally occurs with the rhinitis and tracheobronchitis that accompanies the initial febrile episode. A mucopurulent discharge is often present as well. Distemper viral antigens can be detected using direct immunofluorescence. After exposure, it takes 6 to 9 days for the virus to reach the epithelial cells, and this appears to occur only in those dogs that fail to develop neutralizing antibody titers (<50%). **Cytoplasmic inclusion bodies may be found in the conjunctival epithelial cells 6 days after infection and are seen more frequently in the cells acquired from the nictitans. In general, however, these inclusion bodies are scarce and infrequently seen.**

FUNGAL CONJUNCTIVITIS

Fungal conjunctivitis is apparently very rare in the dog. Infection with *Blastomyces dermatitidis* can cause nodule formation in the inferior conjunctiva, but treatment with systemic itraconazole may resolve the condition (Fig. 5-3).

RICKETTSIAL CONJUNCTIVITIS

Infection with *Rickettsia rickettsii* is frequently associated with ocular lesions of the conjunctiva, uvea, and retina. Evidence of conjunctivitis usually begins with the onset of fever and includes conjunctival hyperemia, chemosis, petechial hemorrhages, and a mucopurulent to purulent ocular

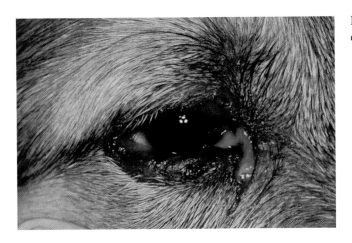

FIGURE 5-2. *Conjunctivitis in a dog with distemper.*

FIGURE 5-3. *Conjunctivitis associated with blastomycosis.*

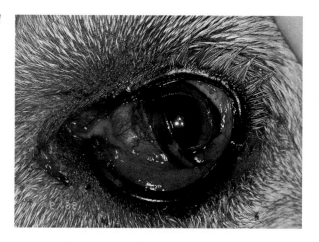

discharge. **Canine ehrlichiosis can cause conjunctival hyperemia, serous ocular discharge, conjunctival hemorrhages, anterior uveitis, and retinal hemorrhages.**

PARASITIC CONJUNCTIVITIS

Ocular thelaziasis occurs in the western United States and is quite prevalent in some provinces of China. **The parasites are found in the conjunctival sac and may cause chronic conjunctivitis. Flushing the conjunctival sac with tetramisole (0.5% solution) is effective in removing the worms.**

NONINFECTIOUS CONJUNCTIVITIS

ALLERGIC CONJUNCTIVITIS

Allergic conjunctivitis occurs frequently in the dog and is often a component of atopic dermatitis. Atopy is classified as a type 1 hypersensitivity reaction. The most common allergens are pollens, dust, and bacterial toxins. The conjunctiva is usually hyperemic and chemotic, and the dog is intensely pruritic and may rub the eyes, thus causing further blepharedema. Serous ocular discharge occurs, and with chronic stimulation, conjunctival follicles develop. Patient history, physical examination, and intradermal skin testing are used to establish the diagnosis of atopy in the dog. Results of cytology and histopathology performed on conjunctival scrapings (Table 5-1) and on biopsy specimens, respectively, can be suggestive regarding the presence of an allergic response.

Avoidance of the offending allergen, hyposensitization, and pharmacologic modification of the clinical signs are the primary forms of treatment. Intermittent use of a topical ophthalmic corticosteroid may be necessary to relieve the clinical signs. Alternate-day treatment with systemic corticosteroids initiated for the skin disease may also relieve the ocular signs.

Intense chemosis and blepharedema may occur as an immediate-type reaction, mediated by histamine and immunoglobulin E, after food absorption, drug administration, spider bites, and bee, wasp, or hornet stings. The chemosis is often bilateral. If caused by an insect, the actual area of trauma is rarely identified, and it may be distant from the eyes. These cases usually respond rapidly to intravenous or intramuscular corticosteroids, and topical corticosteroid ophthalmic ointments administered three to four times daily.

FOLLICULAR CONJUNCTIVITIS

Follicular conjunctivitis is thought to occur secondary to chronic antigenic stimulation, but it does not occur secondary to several viral or bacterial causes. Semitransparent follicles form primarily on the bulbar surface of the nictitans, but they may also form elsewhere on the conjunctiva (Fig. 5-4). Frequently, hyperemia of the conjunctiva and a mucoid ocular discharge are present concurrently. This condition occurs most frequently in dogs younger than 18 months of age.

The diagnosis is established on the basis of characteristic clinical signs. Cytologic results using conjunctival scrapings will confirm the diagnosis by revealing the lymphoid nature of the follicles. **Most dogs respond to treatment with saline irrigation and symptomatic use of ophthalmic corticosteroid ointments. Irrigation appears to play a large role in decreasing the follicular formation, especially in dogs with deep fornices exposed to large amounts of vegetative matter. Nonresponsive dogs can be treated by mechanically debriding the follicles.** After instillation of ophthalmic anesthetic, the follicles are debrided with dry gauze placed over the tip of a cotton-tipped applicator. The follicles should not be excised with a blade or cauterized with copper sulfate crystals, because the lymphoid tissue is critical to the ocular defense system.

Ophthalmic medications can occasionally lead to contact hypersensitivity reactions, which manifest as blepharitis and conjunctivitis. Neomycin, thimerosal, and benzalkonium chloride are the drugs used in

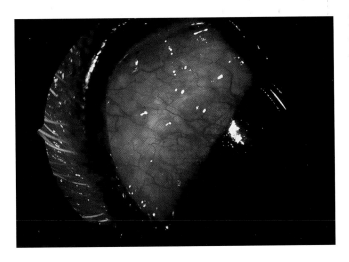

FIGURE 5-4. *Follicular conjunctivitis involving the bulbar conjunctiva.*

canine ophthalmology most likely to cause such reactions. These dogs usually present with a history of conjunctivitis that has been nonresponsive to topical medications. The skin ventral to the medial canthus may eventually become swollen, hyperemic, and then excoriate. Initially, a serous discharge may be present, but this discharge becomes purulent if the conjunctiva is secondarily infected with bacteria. Diagnosis and treatment involve cessation of all medications for 1 week.

CONJUNCTIVITIS ASSOCIATED WITH TEAR DEFICIENCIES

Keratoconjunctivitis sicca is a frequent cause of secondary bacterial conjunctivitis in the dog. Both the Schirmer tear test, which should be performed on all dogs with conjunctivitis, and conjunctival cytology are important diagnostic aids.

LIGNEOUS CONJUNCTIVITIS

Ligneous conjunctivitis has been diagnosed in the Doberman Pinscher. All four affected dogs had thickened, hyperemic, and palpebral conjunctivae with proliferative, opaque membranes. Three of these dogs also had concurrent systemic illnesses. Treatment with azathioprine was used in one dog and appeared to be effective (for more details, the reader should consult the third edition, p. 623).

CONJUNCTIVAL NEOPLASIA

Conjunctival neoplasia occurs infrequently in the dog and includes melanomas, squamous cell carcinomas, angioendotheliomatosis, mast cell tumors, hemangiomas, hemangiosarcomas, angiokeratomas, papillomas, lymphosarcomas, and histiocytomas. Melanomas of the conjunctiva tend to be malignant, and recurrences and metastases are common. Combined excision and cryotherapy appear to be the most effective treatment.

Mast cell tumors of the conjunctiva are both clinically and histopathologically benign. Dogs often present with a several-year history of intermittent conjunctival swelling and redness. The tumors are easily excised, and no recurrence has been noted in the two cases that have been described. Squamous cell carcinoma of the perilimbal area is seen infrequently; these tumors are pink or whitish, elevated, and papillomatous.

Conjunctival hemangiomas tend to occur at the lateral limbus, and they do not adhere to deeper tissue. Resection appears to be curative. Hemangiosarcomas of the conjunctiva are fast-growing and may encroach on the cornea, thereby causing corneal edema and vascularization. Recurrence after excision may be seen, but metastasis has not been confirmed.

Papillomatosis occurs on the palpebral and bulbar conjunctivae as well as on the nictitans. Younger dogs are primarily affected, but excision appears to be curative. Lymphosarcoma may infiltrate around the eye, thus causing conjunctival thickening. Angiokeratomas are rare, benign vascular tumors or telangiectasias of the mucocutaneous tissue or skin and may involve the bulbar conjunctiva and nictitans. Angiokeratomas are generally single, small, and raised red masses, but they may also be black. Excision appears to be curative.

NONNEOPLASTIC CONJUNCTIVAL MASSES

Nonneoplastic conjunctival masses can be inflammatory nodules, displaced orbital fat, or cysts. The conjunctival dermoid is a benign congenital mass of ectodermal and mesodermal origin that usually affects the lateral limbal region but also may involve the cornea, sclera, conjunctiva, eyelid, or nictitans (Fig. 5-5). Frequently, their presence is not appreciated until long, coarse hair extends from the surface and causes irritation. Histopathologically, the tumor resembles normal skin. Complete excision is curative.

MASSES AND INFLAMMATIONS

Nodular granulomatous episclerokeratitis, fibrous histiocytoma, and recurrent proliferative keratoconjunctivitis are thought to represent very similar diseases—or even an identical disease syndrome. Collies appear to be predisposed. This group of nonneoplastic diseases that primarily affect the cornea, limbus, episclera, and nictitans may present as a subconjunctival mass. Histopathologically, the lesions are primarily granulomatous, with lymphocytes, plasma cells, histiocytes, fibroblasts, and reticulin formation. The lesions tend to recur after excision, but

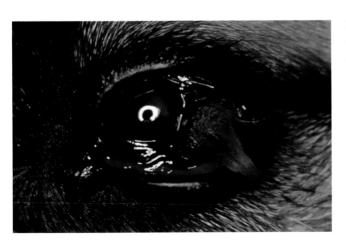

FIGURE 5-5. *Conjunctival dermoid with hair near the lateral aspect of the globe.*

excision with cryotherapy is reported to be a successful mode of therapy. Medically, azathioprine (with or without topical corticosteroids) can be used to induce resolution of these lesions.

Ocular nodular fasciitis, which may be a different disease syndrome, usually causes subconjunctival, scleral, corneal, nictitans, limbal, and eyelid masses. Histopathologically, fibroblasts and abundant reticulin formation are the primary changes, with lesser numbers of lymphocytes, plasma cells, and histiocytes occurring as well. **Excision of these lesions, even when incomplete, appears to be curative.**

SUBCONJUNCTIVAL FAT PROLAPSE

Subconjunctival fat prolapse from the orbit can appear as pink masses at the limbus. Cytologic examination reveals multiple lipid droplets and few mononuclear cells, and surgical removal is curative.

PARASITIC GRANULOMAS

Onchocerciasis can cause masses in the conjunctiva, nictitans, and sclera. This disease has only been reported in the western United States, however, and the parasite is thought to be *Onchocerca lienalis*. Histopathologically, a pyogranulomatous reaction occurs, with degenerate parasites or fibroblasts. When viable parasites are present, the associated inflammation is a mild lymphocytic–plasmocytic reaction. Removal of the parasite is curative.

CYSTS

Conjunctival epithelial inclusion cysts, cystic neoplasms, parasitic cysts, lacrimal cysts (i.e., dacryops), orbital cysts with conjunctival fistula formation, and cysts of the canaliculi occur only rarely in the dog. Lacrimal gland cysts appear as a fluctuant mass within the orbit dorsolateral to the globe. Lacrimal cysts or dacryops present as a subconjunctival cystic swelling in the lateral canthus. In one dog, dissection and histopathology revealed cysts with associated ducts and lacrimal glandular tissue. In another dog, a conjunctival fistula in the lateral canthus developed secondary to what appeared both clinically and histologically to be an orbital cyst originating from the lacrimal gland.

CONJUNCTIVAL DISEASE CAUSED BY TRAUMA

Conjunctival and subconjunctival hemorrhages are common in the dog and most frequently result from trauma. When this condition is caused by trauma, no treatment is necessary if the remaining ophthalmic and physical examinations are normal. If the animal has no history or evidence of trauma, one must consider coagulopathy or vasculitis as the possible cause.

FOREIGN BODIES

Physical irritation caused by foreign bodies lodged within the conjunctiva or the nictitating membrane may cause a severe reaction, including blepharospasm, mucoid discharge, hyperemia, and corneal ulceration. Grass awns and other plant material are the most common culprits. Most foreign bodies can be removed with forceps after use of a topical ophthalmic anesthetic. Chemical exposure can also cause irritation; in one report, conjunctival hyperemia, chemosis, and corneal ulceration occurred in a dog that was sprayed by a walking stick (*Anisomorpha buprestoides*).

ANATOMIC ABNORMALITIES

Conjunctival disease may develop secondary to anatomic defects that cause inadequate tear drainage, chronic exposure, and other changes.

MEDIAL CANTHAL POCKET SYNDROME

Medial canthal pocket syndrome occurs in large and giant breeds, and it is characterized by a chronic conjunctivitis occurring in dogs with enophthalmia, deep orbits, narrow skulls, slight entropion, and inadequate tear drainage. The enophthalmia creates a "pocket" in the ventral conjunctival fornix that collects dust, dirt, and other foreign material. The resulting clinical signs include persistent conjunctival and nictitans hyperemia as well as a slight mucoid discharge. **This syndrome responds poorly to medical therapy.** In certain dogs, and especially in those that are active outdoors, frequent flushing of debris from the ventral fornix with eye wash may help to alleviate the clinical signs.

MEDIAL ABERRANT DERMIS (CARUNCULAR TRICHIASIS)

Aberrant dermis derived from the facial skin may continue past the intermarginal space in the medial canthus and be present on the conjunctiva in some brachycephalic breeds. When this occurs, irritation from the hair, which can grow very long, may cause keratitis, epiphora, or both. Surgical removal of the aberrant dermis using conjunctiva and the medial palpebral ligament for closure has been described. Cryotherapy can also be used to destroy the hair follicles; however, depigmentation of the caruncle can result from this mode of therapy.

CONJUNCTIVAL MANIFESTATIONS OF SYSTEMIC DISEASES

Many systemic diseases cause nonspecific conjunctival manifestations (Box 5-1).

BOX 5-1

Systemic Diseases That May Cause Conjunctival Diseases

Conjunctival hyperemia/conjunctivitis

Leishmaniasis

Generalized *Listeria monocytogenes*

Hepatozoonosis

Tyrosinemia

Multiple myeloma

Systemic histiocytosis

Other conjunctival change

Severe anemia (pallor)

Polycythemia ("brick red" mucous membranes)

Clotting deficiencies (subconjunctival hemorrhages)

Jaundice

EFFECTS OF RADIATION

The conjunctiva is frequently within the field of radiation used during treatment of sinus neoplasia. Mild to severe conjunctivitis is the most frequently occurring, early ocular complication, and this conjunctivitis is usually nonresponsive to medical therapy. The conjunctival disease results from a direct effect of the radiation on the basal epithelial stem cell layer. In addition, KCS can occur as an early or a late complication. Therefore, a Schirmer tear test should be performed on all dogs that develop conjunctivitis as a complication of radiation therapy.

SURGICAL PROCEDURES

The conjunctiva is an invaluable surgical tissue because of its redundancy and rather loose bulbar adhesions. The bulbar conjunctiva can be easily resected and relocated. Conjunctival biopsy specimens can be obtained both easily and quickly, and such biopsies are an effective diagnostic modality in dogs with chronic conjunctivitis or conjunctival masses. Conjunctival grafts that are created by incising the conjunctiva and relocating part of it to the cornea can deliver a focal blood supply to an otherwise avascular cornea in the dog with a progressive infection or deep corneal defects.

CONJUNCTIVAL BIOPSY

Conjunctival biopsy is quite easy to perform and usually involves an awake animal. After several drops of a topical ophthalmic anesthetic have been applied, the conjunctival area in question is elevated with fine-toothed forceps and then excised with tenotomy scissors. The resulting conjunctival defect is allowed to heal by second intention. In addition, an antibiotic ophthalmic solution is instilled for 5 to 7 days. Conjunctival biopsies are indicated for chronic conjunctivitis that is nonresponsive to therapy and for suspected neoplasia.

EXCISION OF SMALL MASSES

Conjunctival neoplasia occurs infrequently, but complete excision of the tumor, either with or without ancillary treatment, is usually the treatment of choice. Most conjunctival neoplasms do not invade the sclera and are dissected rather easily from the underlying tissue. Dermoids can also occur in the conjunctiva and often need to be excised. With small masses, excisional biopsies can be performed in the awake animal. When excising a neoplasm, try to obtain a 2-mm margin. Small defects can be allowed to heal by second intention, but defects larger than 1 cm in diameter should be closed using a simple continuous suture pattern with 5-0 to 7-0 polyglactin 910.

REPAIR OF LACERATIONS

Small lacerations of the conjunctiva (<1 cm) can be allowed to heal by second intention. Large lacerations should be carefully cleansed, but debridement should be kept to a minimum. Any foreign material should be removed. After the area has been cleansed and explored, 5-0 to 7-0 simple interrupted absorbable sutures are used to appose the edges. Most commonly, conjunctival lacerations are associated with a skin laceration of the overlying eyelid (for details on the repair of these lacerations, the reader should consult Chapter 3).

TREATMENT OF SYMBLEPHARON

Symblepharon occurs only rarely in the dog, and then usually secondary to trauma or chemical burns. Surgical correction is difficult, because the healing conjunctiva tends to re-adhere (for more details, the reader should consult the third edition, pp. 626–627).

SURGICAL REPAIR OF CONJUNCTIVAL DEFECTS

Conjunctival defects smaller than 1 cm in diameter can be allowed to heal by second intention or be closed with 5-0 to 7-0 polyglactin 910 suture material in a simple interrupted or simple continuous pattern. Burying the knots decreases postoperative irritation. Repair of defects larger that 1 cm in diameter, however, usually involves autografts from the bulbar conjunctiva of the other eye or from the buccal mucosa.

CONJUNCTIVAL AUTOGRAFTS TO THE CORNEA

Conjunctival autografts are used to treat deep corneal ulcers. Such autografts preserve the corneal and the ocular integrity, replace any lost corneal tissue, and supply vascularization. Many types of grafts have been described. Selection of the conjunctival graft for use in a clinical situation depends on the size, depth, and position of the ulcer, the presence of infection, the surgeon's abilities, and the instrumentation available.

Necessary Instrumentation and Surgical Fundamentals

Specialized ophthalmic instrumentation is necessary to perform conjunctival grafting procedures. A surgical pack containing an eyelid speculum, Steven's tenotomy scissors, Colibri forceps or tying forceps with 1×2 teeth for fixation, and ophthalmic needle holders are the minimal necessary instruments. Generally, 5-0 to 7-0 polyglactin 910 suture is used, with 7-0 being more satisfactory. Magnification with a head loop or an operating microscope is preferable to no magnification during corneal procedures.

Maintenance of the blood supply and prevention of graft retraction are extremely important for the success of these procedures. Grafts must be wide enough to maintain an adequate blood supply, and the base should be wider than the tip. To prevent graft retraction, the Tenon's capsule should be dissected from the substantia propria. The graft should be thin enough that the tips of the scissor blades can be seen through it, and the graft tissue should also be loose enough that it does not retract when positioned over the corneal lesion. This is accomplished by adequate undermining and dissection with tenotomy scissors. In addition, the graft must be larger (<1–2 mm) than necessary to cover the wound to allow for graft contraction. During dissection and removal of the Tenon's capsule, avoid creating holes in the graft, because any holes will tend to expand and cause failure of the graft. If a small hole is created, placing a suture of 7-0 polyglactin 910 across the hole may prevent it from enlarging.

Preparation of the ulcer site is also important for graft retention. Necrotic and "melting" corneal stroma should be debrided using a scalpel blade or cotton swabs. Frequently, a partial-thickness keratectomy is indicated to remove the necrotic tissue, and sutures must be placed in healthy corneal stroma to prevent dehiscence of the graft. Grafts will not adhere to corneal epithelium. Therefore, if corneal epithelium is present at the edge of the wound, it should be excised with a scalpel blade (e.g., Beaver No. 64) if the graft is to cover that specific area.

ISLAND GRAFTS

Island grafts can be created from the bulbar and the palpebral conjunctiva of the upper eyelid and should be 10% larger than the corneal lesion to allow for graft contraction. Grafts are sutured into the prepared ulcer bed using a simple interrupted pattern. To help ensure the success of this type of conjunctival graft, sutures must be placed very close to each other, and the graft must be in perfect apposition to the edges of the corneal wound. Generally, these grafts will remain a blanched white for approximately 10 days, by which time corneal vascularization has usually invaded the graft itself.

PEDICLE GRAFTS

Bulbar Pedicle Graft

The pedicle graft created from the bulbar conjunctiva is the conjunctival graft most frequently used by veterinary ophthalmologists. This type of graft is most easily created from the area lateral and dorsal to the limbus, where the exposure is greatest and incorporation of the third eyelid into the graft can be avoided (Fig. 5-6).

TARSOCONJUNCTIVAL PEDICLE GRAFT

The tarsoconjunctival pedicle graft can be used for deep corneal ulcers. To create this type of graft, a chalazion clamp is placed on the upper eyelid. The pedicle is created with the base toward the eyelid margin, and sharp dissection is used to separate the conjunctiva from the underlying orbicularis oculi muscle. The base of the graft should be wide enough to ensure an adequate blood supply, and the length should be

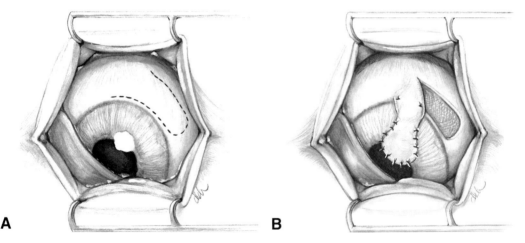

A   **B**

FIGURE 5-6. *Pedicle bulbar conjunctival graft.* **A.** *The pedicle graft is created most easily from the dorsolateral bulbar conjunctiva, because the nictitans can thus be avoided. The tip of the conjunctival pedicle graft should be wider than the base, and the graft should be large enough to allow for contraction. Careful dissection should be used to separate the conjunctiva from the underlying Tenon's capsule.* **B.** *After sufficient dissection has been performed so there is no undue tension on the graft, the graft is sutured to the prepared ulcer bed. The graft can be sutured either to the edge of the ulcer or, if the presence of infection or collagenase activity is uncertain, to healthy cornea that has been debrided of epithelium and that may be distant from the original ulcer. Anchoring sutures may be placed at the limbus. (Courtesy of University of Tennessee College of Veterinary Medicine.)*

constructed to minimize tension and to allow for eyelid mobility. The graft is sutured to the cornea. Disadvantages of this type of graft include the potential for eyelid movement to cause premature retraction of the graft and the greater difficulty of harvesting palpebral conjunctiva compared with bulbar conjunctiva. To minimize the probability of retraction from eyelid movement, a temporary tarsorrhaphy can be performed.

BRIDGE GRAFTS

A bridge graft has a blood supply that feeds the graft from both ends. This type of graft is created by making two parallel incisions in the dorsal bulbar conjunctiva, with the first incision at the limbus. The graft should be at least 10 mm in width to ensure adequate perfusion. Both edges of the graft are sutured to the cornea.

ADVANCEMENT GRAFTS (180° OR HOOD)

Hood grafts, which are also known as advancement or 180° grafts, are most useful for dorsal and lateral paracentral corneal defects and for peripheral corneal defects. This type of graft is created by incising the bulbar conjunctiva near the limbus and then dissecting the conjunctiva from the underlying Tenon's capsule caudally toward the fornix. The graft is sutured to the cornea so that it extends beyond the defect. Supporting sutures are then placed along the remainder of the leading edge of the graft.

COMPLETE BULBAR GRAFTS (360° OR GUNDERSEN)

A 360° bulbar conjunctival graft, which is also known as the Gundersen or a complete bulbar graft, can be used to surgically treat central and paracentral as well as very large-diameter corneal defects. This type of graft has several disadvantages, however, because it covers the entire cornea. Therefore, the patient is blind while the graft is in place, evaluation of the eye is impossible, and penetration of topical drugs is probably impaired. To create the graft, limbal traction is created to rotate the globe ventrally. A 180° incision is then made parallel to, but at sufficient distance from, the limbus so that the graft itself will be wide enough to cover the cornea (Fig. 5-7). After the limbal-based graft is created, a 360° peritomy is made, and the graft is slid into position and sutured either to the inferior and superior limbal cornea, the episclera, or the inferior and superior conjunctival incisions. The graft can be also sutured directly to the corneal defect if corneal rupture is imminent or aqueous humor is leaking.

CORNEOCONJUNCTIVAL TRANSPOSITION

Corneoconjunctival transposition is a modification of the conjunctival graft technique. In this procedure, partial-thickness cornea adjacent

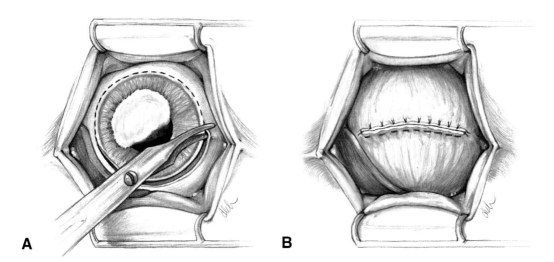

A   **B**

FIGURE 5-7. *The 360° bulbar conjunctival graft. **A**. The 360° conjunctival graft can be created by performing a 360° conjunctival peritomy. Dissection of the bulbar conjunctiva from the underlying Tenon's capsule should be performed caudally, from the limbus, for 360° until enough conjunctiva has been mobilized to cover the entire cornea with minimal tension. **B**. The dorsal and ventral portions of the conjunctiva are sutured together with a horizontal mattress pattern. A temporary tarsorrhaphy may help to decrease tension on the suture line. (Courtesy of University of Tennessee College of Veterinary Medicine.)*

to the defect is mobilized into the defect, with the attached bulbar conjunctiva sliding into the area from which the corneal transplant was harvested. This type of graft is most frequently used with axial corneal lesions, because less scar tissue is associated with transplanted corneal tissue than with a conjunctival pedicle graft. The corneoconjunctival transposition is not recommended, however, for use with an infected cornea, and it is more time-consuming than a bulbar pedicle graft to create. An alternate but even more time-consuming technique, which is known as a corneoscleral transposition, transplants cornea with attached sclera into the defect (for more details, the reader should consult Chapter 7).

GENERAL POSTOPERATIVE CARE AND SUCCESS RATES

Treatment for a corneal ulcer after placement of a conjunctival graft usually includes topical ophthalmic antibiotics and parasympatholytic drugs. Because a blood supply has now been created, systemic antibiotics can reach the corneal ulcer and, therefore, are frequently initiated. Generally, the base of the graft is severed from the limbus after 5 to 8 weeks.

Conjunctival grafts are a highly successful method for treatment of deep and perforated corneal ulcers in the dog. **Studies have noted that corneal quality compatible with useful vision was achieved in 25 of**

35 reported cases, that structural integrity of the cornea was reestablished in 91% of eyes, and that partial or total graft dehiscence occurred in 10 to 32% of eyes. Graft failure has been associated with incorrect corneal graft-bed preparation or suturing, incomplete covering of keratomalacia, aqueous leakage, graft direction of more than 45% from the vertical plane, and excessive stretching of the graft between opposite sutures.

Diseases and Surgery of the Canine Nictitating Membrane

The nictitating membrane (NM), which is also called the membrana nictitans, third eyelid, or haw, is a thin sheet of tissue in the medial canthus of most domestic animal species. It is affected by several primary disorders, shares a number of diseases with the conjunctiva, and can also be used to strategic advantage during corneal surgery as a corneal protectant and graft source. Diseases of the NM occur not infrequently in the dog, and they are characterized by protrusion and changes in structure (Fig. 6-1).

ANATOMY, HISTOPATHOLOGY, AND FUNCTION

The basic shape of the canine NM is defined by a "T"-shaped piece of hyaline cartilage (Fig. 6-2). The arm of the "T" parallels the free margin of the NM, and the shaft runs perpendicular to the free edge. The ventral extent of the shaft originates from the periorbital connective tissue associated with the inferonasal aspect of the globe. The base of the NM is intimately associated with the fasciae of the ocular musculature, and conjunctiva covers both the anterior and the posterior surfaces of the NM. The conjunctiva on the posterior surface is contiguous with the bulbar conjunctiva. The conjunctiva on the anterior surface is contiguous with the palpebral conjunctiva. Numerous lymphoid aggregates populate the posterior subconjunctiva of the NM, and goblet cells are found between the lymphatic nodules and epithelium. In contrast to that of the cat, the canine NM lacks a smooth musculature. The tubuloacinar gland of the NM is invested around the ventral portion of the cartilage shaft, so when the NM is in its normal position, the gland is deeply seated

Protrusion of nictitans

Closely observe for focal abnormalities

Curled outward leading margins—eversion of the nictitans cartilage
   Treat by excision of the curled portion of the cartilage
Pink mass from posterior nictitans in young dog—"cherry eye"
   Treat by repositioning the gland (envelope or anchoring procedure)
Pink mass from behind the nictitans in old dogs—possible adenocarcinoma of the
  nictitans gland
   Treat by total excision of the nictitans
Focal mass(es) on anterior nictitans surface—consider several types of tumors
   Treat by local excision or cryosurgery

Generalized enlargement of the nictitans

Plasma cell infiltration—gradual loss of pigment; German Shepherd is predisposed
   Biopsy and treat with topical corticosteroid/cyclosporin A
Nodular granulomatous epikeratitis—nictitans thickened and inflamed. Mainly in Collies.
   Usually other areas involved including cornea, episclera, and bulbar conjunctiva
   Biopsy and treat with corticosteroids/local excision/systemic azathioprine
Ocular nodular fasciitis—similar to granulomatous epikeratitis. Other breeds.
   Biopsy and treat with local excision and topical corticosteroids
Lymphosarcoma and other systemic neoplasms—bilateral involvement
   Biopsy

Protrusion with few or no abnormalities

Inflamed and medial corneal ulcer—foreign body
   Treat by removing the foreign body and topical antibiotics/mydriatics
Primary condition in large breeds—bilateral
   Generally no treatment
Secondary to pain
   Closely examine the conjunctiva, cornea, and inner eye
Horner's syndrome
   Observe for miosis, ptosis, enophthalmia. Test with topical 1–2% epinephrine or 2.5%
   phenylephrine to determine site of sympathetic denervation
Secondary to orbital diseases—cellulitis, tumors, and masticatory myositis
With systemic diseases—tetanus, rabies, and so on

FIGURE 6-1. *Strategy for the diagnosis and treatment of nictitating membrane protrusion.*

(posterior to the orbital rim) and is not visible. **The NM gland contributes a significant proportion of the aqueous tear film,** and because of its histopathologic similarities with the main lacrimal gland, it is presumed to provide immunologic support to the ocular surface via the production of antibodies and lysozyme. The primary purpose of the NM is physical protection of the cornea, sweeping passively over the cornea from inferonasal to superotemporal when the globe is retracted into the orbit.

ANOMALOUS, CONGENITAL, AND DEVELOPMENTAL DISORDERS

BENT (USUALLY EVERTED) CARTILAGE

Eversion of the shaft of the NM cartilage is much more common than inversion. When the medial and lateral tips of the NM cartilage arm are inverted, keratitis and corneal ulceration may result. Treatment is excision of the bent tips. The everted cartilage appears as an anterior folding of the superior portion of the NM, with exposure of the posterior aspect (Fig. 6-3). Eversion of the NM cartilage most commonly occurs in large breeds, and it may be hereditary. It is thought to result from more rapid growth of the posterior portion of the cartilage compared with that of the anterior portion. The result is chronic conjunctivitis and ocular discharge. **The most frequent treatment is simple excision of the folded portion of the NM cartilage through the bulbar (i.e., deep) conjunctival surface (Fig. 6-4).**

PROLAPSE OF THE GLAND

Prolapse of the NM gland (or "cherry eye") is the most common primary disorder of the NM. Prolapse may result from weakness in the connective tissue attachment between the NM ventrum and the periorbital tissues, and this weakness allows the gland, which normally is located ventrally, to flip up dorsally, where it then becomes enlarged and inflamed by chronic exposure (Fig. 6-5). Prolapse of the NM gland can be either unilateral or bilateral, but it generally occurs before 2 years of age. It appears as a red mass at the medial canthus. Chronic conjunctivitis

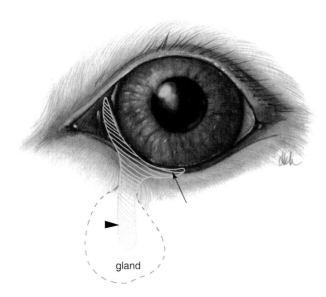

gland

FIGURE 6-2. *Normal canine nictitating membrane. The free edge is parallel to the arm (arrow) and perpendicular to the shaft (arrowhead) of the cartilage. The anterior and posterior surfaces are both covered with conjunctiva, and the ventrum of the shaft is surrounded by the nictitating membrane gland. (Used with permission. ©1997 University of Tennessee College of Veterinary Medicine.)*

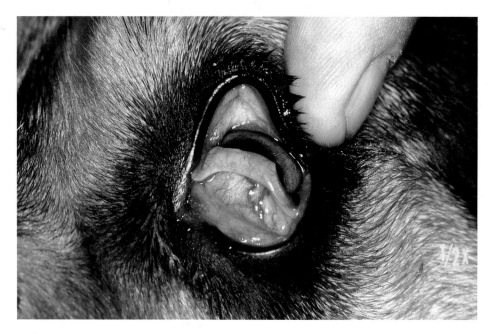

FIGURE 6-3. *Eversion of the nictitating membrane cartilage.*

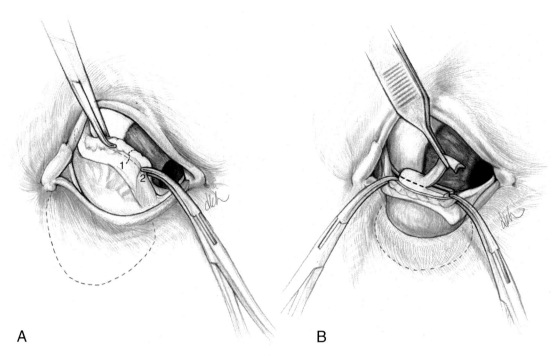

A   B

FIGURE 6-4. *Surgical correction of everted nictitating membrane cartilage. **A.** A conjunctival incision is made over the folded portion of the cartilage. This incision can be either perpendicular (#1) or parallel (#2) to the free edge of the nictitating membrane. **B.** The folded portion is then excised. The conjunctiva does not need to be sutured. (Used with permission. ©1997 University of Tennessee College of Veterinary Medicine).*

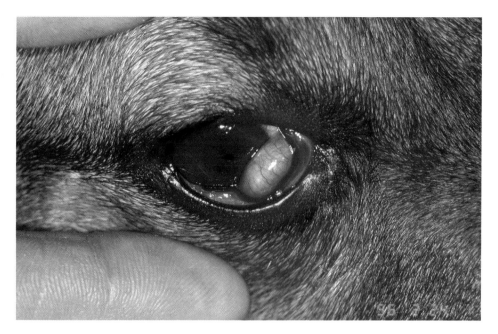

FIGURE 6-5. *Prolapse of the nictitating membrane gland ("cherry eye").*

and ocular discharge are often present, and tear production is affected as well, initially fluctuating to more than normal but then eventually becoming subnormal.

Surgical Repositioning

For several decades, surgical removal of the prolapsed portion of the NM gland was the treatment of choice. As the importance of the NM gland in tear production became apparent, however, surgical repositioning of the gland became widely recommended, and at least eight such repositioning techniques have been published. These techniques are generally divided into anchoring procedures (to the inferior episcleral tissue, inferior episcleral tissue, or periosteum of the ventral orbital rim) and into pocket or envelope methods (Fig. 6-6). The choice of repositioning technique is largely a matter of personal preference. Ease of operation, effects on tear production, likelihood of reprolapse, and cosmesis, however, should all be considered. In my opinion, the pocket techniques are the easiest to learn, but the anchoring techniques, once mastered, are simple and quick to perform. Reprolapse rates of 4% and 0% after the anchoring techniques have been reported. When properly performed, all techniques result in a cosmetically acceptable outcome (for more details, the reader should consult the third edition, pp. 610–614).

PROTRUSION

Primary protrusion of the NM without prolapse of the gland can occur in several large breeds. Although principally a cosmetic problem,

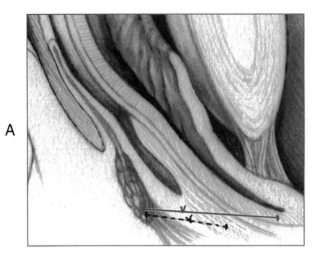

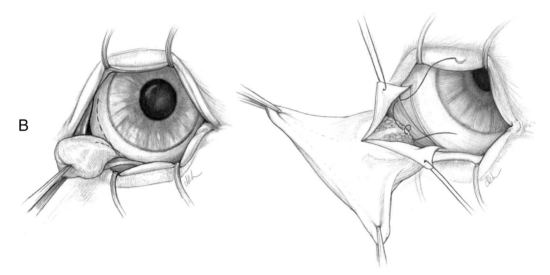

FIGURE 6-6. *Different methods for repositioning the NM gland.* **A.** *The dotted line depicts the suture path of the original anchoring technique of Blogg. Following a posterior conjunctival incision, a suture of 3-0 polyglycolic acid is placed into the deep episcleral tissues on the inferonasal aspect of the globe. The suture is then passed through the ventral aspect of the gland and pulled tight, thus retracting the gland. The solid line depicts the suture path of Gross' modification of Blogg's anchoring technique. This procedure is similar, except the gland is anchored with 5-0 chromic gut to the sclera instead of to the episcleral tissues.* **B.** *Anchoring technique of Albert et al., originally described in the cat. A perilimbal incision is made in the bulbar conjunctiva 4 mm from the inferonasal limbus, and the episcleral tissues are dissected away, thus exposing the inferior oblique muscle. A second conjunctival incision is made perpendicular to the first, thus exposing the gland (left). A 5-0 silk suture is passed through the ventrum of the gland and then through the tendinous origin of the muscle, thus tucking the gland into its natural position (right).*

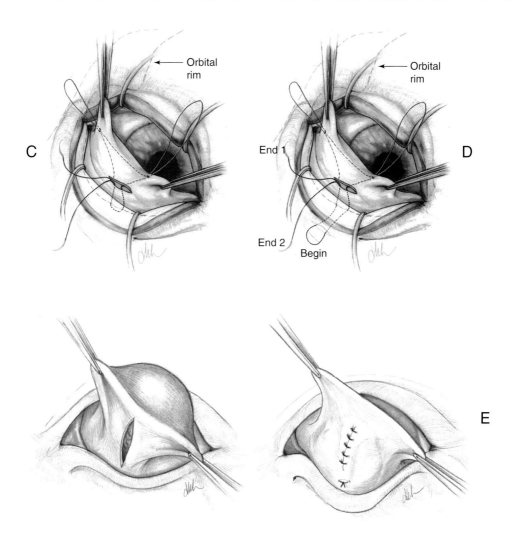

FIGURE 6-6.—*(continued) C. Orbital rim anchoring technique of Kaswan and Martin. An incision parallel to the orbital rim is made in the anterior conjuntiva near the ventrum of the NM, and nonabsorbable, 4-0 monofilament suture material is inserted into the medial extent of the resulting conjunctival pocket and directed toward the orbital rim. A blind bite is taken into the periosteal tissues and directed out of the pocket at its lateral extent; this bite can also be taken from lateral to medial. Adequate purchase into the periosteal tissues should be confirmed by firmly tugging at the suture before proceeding. A pursestring is then placed around the gland by reinserting the suture at each exit point, and the suture is pulled tight, thus anchoring the gland to the orbital rim. The conjunctiva can either be left open or closed with 6-0 polyglactin 910 suture material in a simple continuous pattern. D. In the Stanley and Kaswan modification of the Kaswan and Martin anchoring technique, the approach to the orbital rim is facilitated by an incision into the interior lid near the rim; otherwise, these techniques are similar. E. In the Twitchell technique, an incision is made into the anterior conjunctiva, and a pocket is created by dissection of subconjunctival tissues (left). The gland is then reduced into the pocket and sutured anteriorly with 5-0 absorbable suture material (right).*

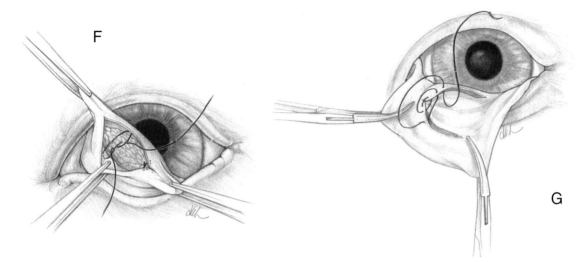

FIGURE 6-6.—*(continued)* *F. Moore described resection of the posterior conjunctiva from over the prolapsed gland and then imbrication of it with two simple interrupted sutures of 7-0 absorbable suture material. A later modification did not involve conjunctival resection (but suggested light scarification) and used a single pursestring suture. **G.** In the Morgan pocket technique, parallel incisions are made into the posterior conjunctiva dorsal and ventral to the prolapsed gland. The gland is reduced into the pocket, and the pocket is closed with a simple continuous suture of 5-0 or 6-0 polyglycolic acid or polyglactin 910 material, securing the knot on the anterior surface. Suturing should begin and end 1 to 2 mm from the ends of the incision to prevent cyst formation because of the entrapment of tears within the pocket. At the end of the suture run, another run using a Cushing pattern may be placed in the opposite direction to conceal the sutures. (Used with permission. ©1997 University of Tennessee College of Veterinary Medicine.)*

protrusion sometimes causes conjunctivitis and epiphora. The NM can be shortened surgically to return it to a more normal position. Secondary protrusion occurs secondary to enophthalmos, microphthalmos, and space-occupying retrobulbar lesions; if the primary problem can be resolved, the NM often returns to its normal position. Protrusion may also occur in animals with Horner's syndrome, dysautonomia, cannabis intoxication, tetanus, and rabies.

NEOPLASMS

Neoplasia of the NM is uncommon in the dog, but melanomas, adenocarcinomas, squamous cell carcinomas, mastocytomas, papillomas, hemangiomas, angiokeratomas, and lymphosarcoma have all been reported. In one study of 47 dogs, eight had local recurrence after resection, and three had confirmed metastasis, with adenocarcinomas and malignant melanomas being the most commonly recurring or metastasizing tumors. Papillomas have papillary, cauliflowerlike surfaces. Excision of the masses along with a margin of normal tissue appears to be curative. **For NM ade-**

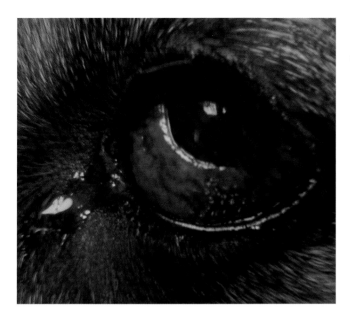

FIGURE 6-7. *Plasma cell infiltration of the nictitating membrane in a German Shepherd.*

nocarcinomas in older dogs, removal of the entire third eyelid is currently the recommended treatment.

INFLAMMATIONS

NODULAR GRANULOMATOUS EPISCLEROKERATITIS

Nodular granulomatous episclerokeratitis is an inflammatory disease that most commonly arises from the temporal corneoscleral junction, but it may involve the NM as well. Collies are predisposed. Clinically, the affected NM is hyperemic, depigmented, and edematous with multiple, smooth, tubular-shaped thickenings involving the palpebral surfaces. At histopathologic examination, these lesions show a chronic granulomatous inflammatory response. The disease process is generally controllable with use of prednisone and azathioprine.

PLASMA CELL INFILTRATION/"PLASMOMA"

Plasma cell infiltration of the NM, or "plasmoma," can cause thickening, depigmentation, and follicle formation. Pannus (i.e., chronic superficial keratitis) is often associated with this condition (Fig. 6-7). German Shepherds appear to be predisposed. Plasmoma has bilateral potential in the Belgian Sheepdog, Borzoi, Doberman Pinscher, English Springer Spaniel, and German Shepherd breeds. At histopathologic examination, the inflammatory infiltrate consists primarily of plasma cells, with fewer lymphocytes. Treatment generally consists of topical, subconjunctival, or systemic corticosteroids. Topical 0.2% cyclosporine ointment and 1.25% to 1.50% cyclosporine drops are also effective.

FOLLICULAR CONJUNCTIVITIS

Follicular conjunctivitis most frequently involves the bulbar aspect of the NM, but the follicles can occur anywhere on the conjunctiva. A small area of lymphoid follicles is normally present on the bulbar side of the NM and closely associated with the NM gland. In animals with follicular conjunctivitis, the follicles are more numerous and larger than normal in size. Conjunctival hyperemia as well as a mucoid discharge commonly are present.

OCULAR NODULAR FASCIITIS

Ocular nodular fasciitis most commonly affects the sclera, episclera, and corneal stroma, but it can also involve the NM. In the one such case described, an irregular nodular thickening involved the anterior aspect of the NM. The mass was excised surgically, and no recurrence has been noted. At histopathologic examination, histiocytes, fibroblasts, capillaries, fibrous connective tissue, and a few inflammatory cells were seen.

TRAUMA, RECONSTRUCTIONS, AND FOREIGN BODIES

Trauma to the medial canthal area may result in lacerations of the NM. Small, partial-thickness tears usually heal spontaneously, but larger, deep or full-thickness lesions should be sutured with 6-0 braided absorbable suture material. Care should be taken not to leave sutures or knots in a position where they could abrade the cornea. If the NM has been removed because of neoplasia or extensive areas lost because of trauma, it may be reconstructed from labial mucosa.

Foreign bodies lodged either within or behind the NM can cause persistent, usually ventromedial corneal ulcerations as well as inflammation of the NM. Other frequently observed clinical signs include epiphora, blepharospasm, protrusion of the NM, and severe discomfort. The foreign bodies (usually grass awns, seeds, or other plant material) generally are loosely embedded and can be removed using thumb forceps after instillation of a topical anesthetic. Topical ophthalmic antibiotics are administered after removal of the foreign body and, if corneal ulceration is present, are definitely indicated.

NICTITATING MEMBRANE SURGERY

The NM can be used as a corneal shield or flap in certain cases of corneal ulceration, iatrogenic ulcers created by lamellar keratectomy in brachycephalic animals, and in particular, refractory indolent ulcers.

NICTITATING MEMBRANE FLAPS

Two types of flaps have been described that temporarily attach the free margin of the NM to the dorsolateral conjunctival fornix or to the dorsolateral episclera. The surgeon must be careful, however, to seat the NM margin as deeply as possible in the superior conjunctival cul-de-sac. If the NM margin is too far from the cul-de-sac, corneal injury from the sutures is more likely to occur (Fig 6-8).

Complications of NM flaps include necrosis of the upper lid if sutures are placed too tightly in the NM-to-superior-lid technique (stents are recommended) as well as inadvertent penetration of the globe in the NM-to-episclera technique. The sutures are generally left in place for 2 to 3 weeks, but with the NM-to-episclera technique, the sutures may pull free prematurely. The suture ends may be left long with the upper lid procedure so that the flap can be released and retied (for more details, the reader should consult the third edition, pp. 616–617).

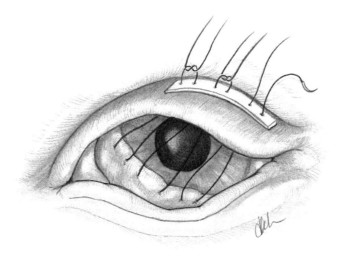

FIGURE 6-8. *Nictitating membrane–to–superior lid flap. Two to three horizontal mattress sutures of 3-0 monofilament nonabsorbable material are placed between the free edge of the nictitating membrane and the lateral aspect of the superior lid. The lid sutures should be placed well within the superior cul-de-sac, and the nictitating membrane sutures should be approximately 2 mm from the free edge, thus incorporating cartilage into the center suture. Alternatively, a single mattress suture can be placed between the superior lid and the midpoint of the cartilage shaft. (Used with permission. ©1997 University of Tennessee College of Veterinary Medicine.)*

7

Diseases and Surgery of the Canine Cornea and Sclera

A unique portion of the outer fibrous tunic of the eye, the cornea is transparent and serves a major refractive function while maintaining a tough, physical, and impermeable barrier between the eye and the environment. The cornea is exposed to environmental hazards, yet it can maintain the smooth outer surface necessary for retinal image formation. This is accomplished by continuously replacing its surface epithelium and by maintaining a preocular tear film on its surface (with the assistance of the lacrimal system and eyelids). Pathologic responses of the cornea are usually associated with a loss of transparency. Fortunately, most corneal diseases are amenable to medical or surgical therapy.

The cornea consists of the outer epithelium and basement membrane, stroma, Descemet's membrane, and the endothelium. Corneal transparency depends on the absence of blood vessels and pigment, its nonkeratinized anterior surface epithelium, the lattice organization of the stroma, and the small diameter of the stromal collagen fibrils. The corneal endothelium uses an active physiologic pump to remove and transport fluid into the anterior chamber. In this way, the corneal endothelium regulates hydration of the corneal stromal collagen matrix, which provides mechanical strength. The endothelial cells normally form a hexagonal, mosaic pattern on the Descemet's membrane (as viewed clinically by specular microscopy). These hexagonally shaped canine endothelial cells tend to enlarge in size but decrease in number with age. In the young dog, the number of endothelial cells averages 2500 to 2800 per mm^2. These findings are suggestive that like the cat and nonhuman primates, the dog has a limited ability for corneal endothelial regeneration (and primarily in young animals). The central corneal thickness in the dog is 0.558 ± 0.076 mm, and the dorsal peripheral cornea is 0.617 ± 0.073 mm.

125

CORNEAL PATHOPHYSIOLOGY

Corneal healing depends on the extent of the initial injury as well as on the size and depth of the defect that requires healing (Table 7-1).

CORNEAL PIGMENTATION

Deposition of corneal pigmentation may occur with chronic inflammation, such as that occurring with chronic superficial keratitis (CSK; i.e., pannus) in the German Shepherd, the "keratitis pigmentosa" syndrome in brachycephalic breeds, keratoconjunctivitis sicca, and chronic ulcerative keratitis. Corneal pigmentation may occur from one or more sources, including migration of melanocytic cells from the limbal and perilimbal tissues, usually with corneal vascularization; melanin pigment within macrophages and fibroblasts, which also may occur in the dog; and anterior synechiae as well as adherence of anterior uveal cysts to the cornea. The pigmented cells may arise from the pigment epithelium of the ciliary body, iridal stroma, and posterior iridal epithelium. In addition, corneal pigmentation may occur because of melanin or melanin-pigmented epithelium phagocytized by the corneal endothelial cells.

TABLE 7-1

DYNAMICS OF CORNEAL HEALING AFTER CORNEAL ULCERATION AND LACERATION

Tissue	Healing Starts	Time to Replace	Clinical Monitoring
Epithelium	1 hour	48–72 hours	Very faint retention of fluorescein (one cell layer)
		14 days	No fluorescein retention (multiple layers)
Corneal epithelial basement membrane		Several weeks	Firm bond; epithelium cannot be dislodged
Corneal stroma	1–2 days	Days to weeks	Stromal replacement requires local fibroblasts; occasional vasculature Occurs under the healing epithelium
Descemet's membrane			Regeneration depends on the endothelium; limited to very young animals
Endothelium			Regeneration in only young animals

CORNEAL EDEMA

After injury, corneal edema or swelling (i.e., corneal overhydration) may result from the imbibition of fluid by the epithelium or stroma. Corneal transparency depends on its physical structure and on the active or cell-based mechanisms that prevent overhydration. The major cellular barriers to edema are the endothelium and the epithelium; when either is damaged, stromal swelling results. The endothelium maintains corneal deturgescence by an energy-dependent, sodium potassium transport pump as well as by a physical barrier. The barrier function of the endothelium results from tight cellular junctions, which are known as zonula occludens and depend on calcium ions. Corneal edema has been regarded simply as an increased corneal water content that, in turn, results in an increased thickness and a decreased transparency as well as in the loss of stromal glycosaminoglycans, collagen lamellae malalignment, and water uptake. Corneal edema in the dog may be associated with a variety of causes, including endothelial dystrophy, endothelial damage occurring with persistent pupillary membranes, mechanical trauma, toxic reactions, anterior uveitis, endotheliitis, glaucoma, neovascularization, and superficial or deep ulceration.

DEVELOPMENTAL ABNORMALITIES AND CONGENITAL DISEASES

Developmental and congenital corneal abnormalities include microcornea (usually with microphthalmia), megalocornea (usually with congenital glaucoma and enlargement of the entire globe), rare corneal dystrophies, pigmentation, and the more frequent dermoids and congenital opacities associated with persistent pupillary membranes.

DERMOIDS

A dermoid is a choristoma, which is a congenital mass of tissue in an abnormal position. Dermoids usually occur at the temporal limbal area, and they generally extend onto the sclera and the cornea (Fig. 7-1). These lesions contain keratinized epithelium, hair, blood vessels, fibrous tissue, fat, nerves, glands, smooth muscle, and even cartilage. Dermoids are present at birth but may not be recognized clinically until the animal is several weeks old. Dermoids are removed by superficial keratectomy and removal of the adjacent, affected conjunctiva.

PERSISTENT PUPILLARY MEMBRANES

Persistent pupillary membranes occur in many breeds, but they appear to be inherited in the Basenji. Persistent pupillary membranes arise from incomplete atrophy of the mesodermal sheet carrying blood vessels that partially fills the anterior chamber during fetal development; this membrane

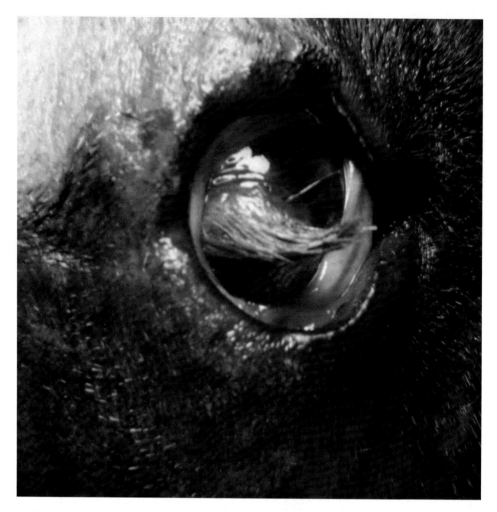

FIGURE 7-1. *Corneal dermoid in a young St Bernard.*

is continuous with the tunica vasculosa lentis that surrounds the developing lens. Atrophy of the pupillary membrane begins during fetal life, but it may not be complete until the dog is 4 to 8 weeks of age (Fig. 7-2). **Persistent pupillary tissue strands arise from the collarette or minor iridal circle region of the iris, and they should be distinguished clinically from posterior synechia formation that is inflammatory in origin.** Pupillary membranes may extend from one section of the iris to another, producing no abnormality; extend from the iris to the cornea, causing focal deep corneal opacity; or extend from the iris to the anterior lens capsule, causing focal capsular and anterior cortical cataract formation. These focal opacities of the cornea may be characterized by thickening and distortion of the Descemet's membrane in the area of the opacity and the endothelium. The endothelium itself may be absent where the Descemet's membrane is altered, with areas of the membrane being replaced by fibroblastic-appearing cells (for more details, the reader should consult the third edition, pp. 639–640).

INFLAMMATORY DISEASES

Corneal inflammations are the most common group of corneal diseases presented to the veterinarian. Fortunately, most can be treated successfully by medical, surgical, or some combination of these therapies.

ULCERATIVE KERATITIS

Corneal ulceration is one of the most common ocular diseases in the dog. Uncomplicated superficial ulcers usually heal readily, however, and with minimal scar formation. Complicated deep ulcers may lead to impaired vision because of corneal scarring or, when corneal perforation occurs, to anterior synechia formation (Fig. 7-3). Severe ulcerative keratitis may lead to loss of the eye because of endophthalmitis, glaucoma, phthisis bulbi, or some combination of these. Fortunately, corneal ulcerations are the most treatable of all vision-threatening ophthalmic disorders. **Corneal ulcers are classified by the depth of the corneal involvement (superficial, deep stromal, and descemetocele; Table 7-2) and by cause.**

Simple/Uncomplicated (Shallow) Corneal Ulcer

Simple/uncomplicated (shallow) corneal ulcers usually occur secondary to minor trauma, self-induced trauma, shampoos, and even eyelash

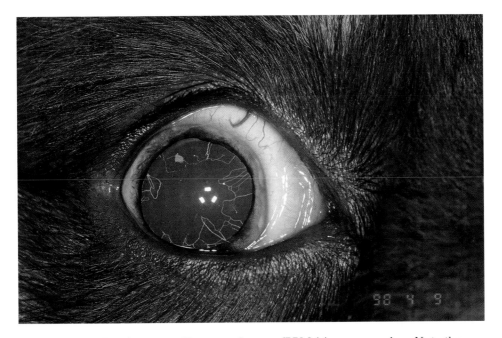

FIGURE 7-2. *Persistent pupillary membranes (PPMs) in a young dog. Note the translucent PPM strands originating from the collarette region of the iris.*

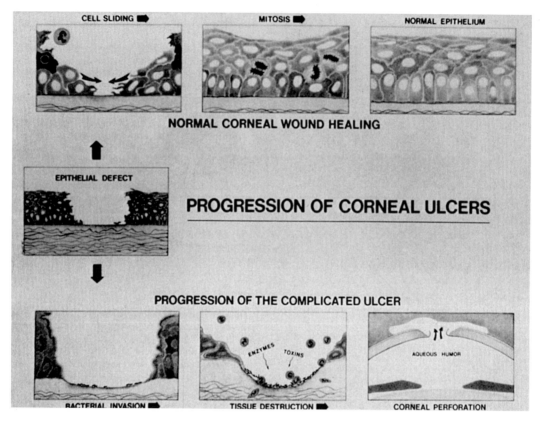

FIGURE 7-3. *Progression of uncomplicated and complicated corneal ulcers. (Reprinted with permission from Nasisse MP. Canine ulcerative keratitis. Comp Cont Educ Pract Vet 1985;7:686–704.)*

abnormalities, eyelid structure and function, and preocular tear film disorders (Fig. 7-4). They usually resolve with topical antibiotic therapy applied three to four times daily to prevent bacterial infection. In addition, 1% atropine is applied to control ciliary muscle spasm and the associated ocular discomfort and to induce mydriasis, thus decreasing the likelihood of synechial formation. Excessive application, however, can decrease tear production. Ophthalmic preparations containing neomycin, bacitracin, and polymyxin B are recommended. The ulcer should resolve in 2 to 6 days; if it does not, the ulcer should be re-evaluated for an undetected, underlying cause or contributing factor.

Refractory Corneal Ulcers

Refractory epithelial erosions, persistent corneal ulcers, recurrent corneal erosion syndrome, recurrent erosion, indolent ulcers, Boxer ulcers, and rodent ulcers are synonyms for superficial corneal ulcers that heal poorly or slowly and that also tend to recur. Refractory superficial corneal ulcers are recognized by their characteristic, encircling lip of undermined epithelium, which is unattached to the corneal

TABLE 7-2

TYPES OF CORNEAL ULCERATIONS IN THE DOG

Clinical Diagnosis	Corneal Layers Lost	Outcome
Superficial ulcer	Epithelium/basement membrane variable	Uncomplicated/progressive
Corneal erosion	Epithelium/basement membrane	Refractory/recurrent
Shallow ulcer	Epithelium/basement membrane/1/4–1/3 stroma	Uncomplicated/progressive
Moderate ulcer	Epithelium/basement membrane/1/2 stroma	Uncomplicated/progressive
Deep	Epithelium/basement membrane/2/3–3/4 stroma	Uncomplicated/progressive
Descemetocele	Epithelium/basement membrane/stroma	Complicated/progressive
Iris prolapse	Epithelium/basement membrane/stroma/ Descemet's membrane/ endothelium	Complicated/progressive

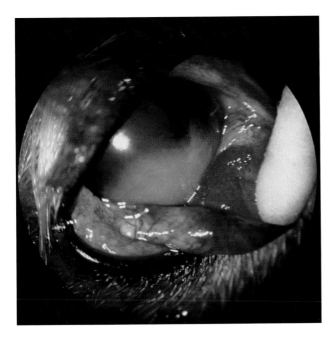

FIGURE 7-4. *Diffuse superficial ulcer in an American Cocker Spaniel caused by a detergent burn.*

stroma or the epithelial basement membrane (Fig. 7-5). The condition was originally described in the Boxer breed, but it may occur in other breeds as well. These refractory or recurrent ulcers are most commonly seen in middle-aged to older dogs.

Pathogenesis

The pathogenesis of refractory corneal ulcers is unknown. Because these ulcers are often breed-related, develop spontaneously, and eventually may affect both eyes, they could represent primary corneal epithelial or superficial stromal dystrophy. Refractory corneal ulcers may represent corneal epithelial dystrophy characterized by basal epithelial cells that produce an abnormal basement membrane and a paucity of hemidesmosomes for attachment. Attachment of the corneal epithelium to the stroma depends on its basement membrane as well as on the associated hemidesmosomes of the basal epithelial cell membrane. These basement membrane complexes are frequently augmented by anchoring fibrils, which add strength to the adhesive bond between cells. Boxers with refractory ulcers have a decreased number of hemidesmosomes and an abnormal epithelial basement membrane (similar to humans with recurrent erosions and epithelial dystrophy).

Diagnosis

Most animals have an acute onset of ocular pain, as evidenced by lacrimation, photophobia, and blepharospasm. The degree of pain is variable, but it decreases with the chronicity of the erosion. These ulcers seem to occur spontaneously and with no history of trauma. **At ophthalmic examination, refractory corneal ulcers are characterized by superficial involvement, with normal-appearing, exposed stroma. Typically, an overlapping lip of nonadherent epithelium is present around the ulcer's edge as well.** Topical fluorescein stain helps to outline the ulcer and delineates the degree

FIGURE 7-5. *Topical fluorescein stain can be used to outline a refractory corneal ulcer. In this case, fluorescein is visible beneath the edge in the nonadherent epithelium (arrows).*

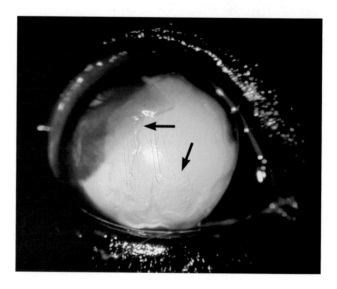

BOX 7-1

Clinical Management of Corneal Erosions in the Dog

Initially:

1. Topical broad-spectrum antibiotics. Some are mildly epitheliotoxic; therefore, administer at low frequency (i.e., two to four times daily).

2. Topical 1% atropine as a cycloplegic for acute ocular pain, usually for 3 to 5 days.

3. Debridement of the nonadherent epithelium, with or without chemical agents. Use dry cotton-tipped applicators, a scalpel blade, a dull spatula (e.g., platinum Kimura spatula, iris spatula), or a fine-toothed forceps. After the cornea has been topically anesthetized, all loose epithelium is removed, usually to a point 1- to 2-mm beyond the margin of fluorescein stain retention. Hence, it is not uncommon to have a large area of abnormal epithelium and to greatly increase the ulcer's size by debridement. Debridement may need to be repeated at 3- to 14-day intervals, but the amount of loose epithelium should decrease with each removal as the ulcer heals. Agents used in chemical debridement include trichloracetic acid, phenol, tincture of iodine, and diluted povidone-iodine. Removal or alteration of the exposed stroma appears to be a necessary part of the healing process.

For Refractory Cases:

1. A second round of treatment with epithelial debridement 3 to 10 days after the initial therapy, topical antibiotics, and limited application of 1% atropine. Surgical therapies to be considered at this time include nictitans flaps, tarsorrhaphy, conjunctival flaps, grid and punctate keratotomies, superficial keratectomy, and keratoepithelioplasty.

2. Corneal contact lenses, collagen shields made from porcine scleral collagen, and cyanoacrylate tissue adhesives.

---

of nonadherent, overhanging epithelium by staining the stroma beneath the loose epithelium. Rose Bengal stain can delineate the nonadherent and degenerating epithelium.

Treatment

Healing of refractory corneal ulcers may span weeks to months, and recurrence is not uncommon. Explaining the progression, expected healing time, possible recurrence, and potential complications to the owner, however, leads to less owner dissatisfaction, greater owner cooperation, and improved results. Less informed clients become frustrated and comply poorly with the recommended therapy. The different treatment strategies are summarized in Box 7-1.

Multiple punctate keratotomy and grid keratotomy are recently introduced procedures for the treatment of refractory ulcers. Multiple punctate keratotomy involves creating multiple anterior stromal punctures into the exposed stroma and 1 to 2 mm of healthy cornea surrounding the ulcer with a 20- to 23-gauge needle (Fig. 7-6). Grid keratotomy involves making scores, cross-hatches, or scratches over the ulcer site with a bent, 25-gauge, disposable hypodermic needle or a diamond knife with a micrometer (Fig. 7-7). With both techniques, the punctures or scores expose normal corneal stroma to which the new epithelium can adhere and allow the formation of normal hemidesmosomes. Both procedures require topical anesthetic and, occasionally, sedation in unruly or nervous patients. Preliminary observations suggest multiple punctate keratotomy and grid keratotomy are very beneficial in healing refractory ulcers.

Other medical therapy for refractory ulcers may include:

1. Topical hyperosmotic agents (e.g., 5% sodium chloride colloidal dextran polysaccharide solutions), which may reduce subepithelial edema and improve epithelial adherence to stroma;
2. Fibronectin, which is a plasma glycoprotein that stimulates cell adhesion, cell migration, and protein synthesis and promotes epithelial attachment and healing in both humans and rabbits;
3. Epidermal growth factor, which is a naturally occurring polypeptide, enhances epithelial regeneration, and promotes mitosis of the corneal epithelium; and
4. Aprotinin, which is an inhibitor of the enzymes plasmin, kallikrein, trypsin, and chymotrypsin.

Excessive plasmin levels may be associated with refractory corneal ulcers. The results of preliminary studies in dogs with refractory ulcers are suggestive that in some cases, topical aprotinin induces rapid healing.

FIGURE 7-6. *A. A hypodermic needle can be used to make multiple punctate keratotomies in the treatment of refractory corneal ulcers. B. A hemostat can be used to grasp the needle tip and so prevent puncturing the cornea too deeply during multiple punctate keratotomies.*

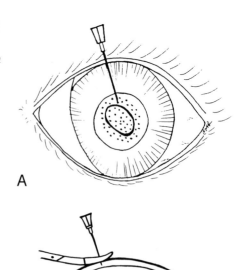

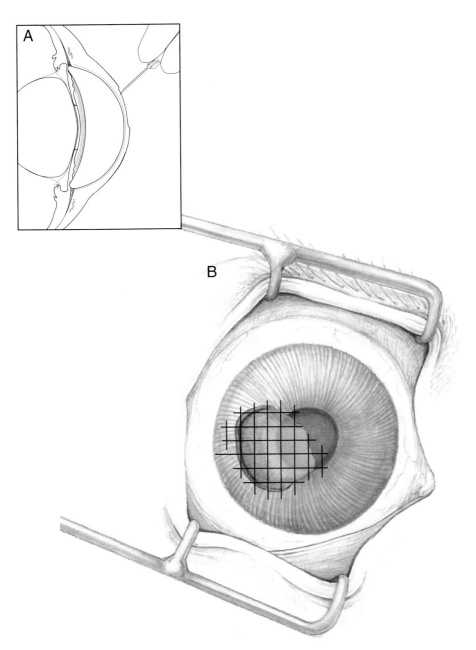

FIGURE 7-7. *Grid keratotomy for an indolent ulcer.* **A.** *After application of a topical anesthetic, a 25-gauge needle is used to lightly scratch the surface of the debrided, indolent ulcer. A diamond knife set at a depth of 0.2 to 0.3 mm can also be used in place of the hypodermic needle.* **B.** *Horizontal and vertical scratches are made, forming a grid pattern and with the scratches extending slightly into the normal epithelium. The scratches should be spaced at approximately 1-mm intervals.*

Stromal Ulcers

Deep (i.e., more than half-thickness) stromal ulcers may be divided into progressive and nonprogressive types. Nonprogressive deep ulcers are managed medically, in the same manner as superficial ulcers but possibly with a conjunctival flap or graft sutured to the ulcer edge as well. Surgical intervention is indicated for progressive stromal ulcers, deep (2/3–3/4 loss of stroma) ulcers, and for descemetoceles. The surgical procedures most commonly used in these cases include conjunctival grafts or flaps. Less frequent procedures include corneoscleral transpositions, corneal tissue adhesives, and corneal transplants, which may also be used as a nonsurgical therapy.

Butylcyanoacrylate tissue adhesive (corneal glue, Tri-Hawk International; Ophthalmic Nexaband, CRX Medical) has been used in the treatment of deep stromal ulcers, descemetoceles, small perforations, and refractory corneal ulcers in the dog. The procedure for applying tissue adhesive involves topical anesthesia (if general anesthesia is not used); debriding the defect (as necessary); drying the site with a cotton-tipped swab, cellulose sponge or a warm-air (i.e., hair) dryer; applying a thin layer of tissue adhesive through a 30-gauge needle; and preventing blinking for 15 to 60 seconds (while the cyanoacrylate solidifies). Care must be taken to apply only a minimal amount of adhesive.

Progressive deep stromal ulcers in the dog are potentially vision- and globe-threatening, and therapy must be aggressive. **Antibiotics are frequently selected on the basis of cytology, cultures, and sensitivity test results.** Topical 1% atropine is administered to minimize the discomfort from ciliary muscle spasm and to prevent synechiae formation. If stromal melting is present, intensive topical antibiotic therapy (every 1–2 hours) is indicated, and the antibiotic spectrum should include Gram-negative rods such as *Pseudomonas* sp. The antibiotics of choice are tobramycin or ciprofloxacin. Topical anticollagenase preparations such as acetylcysteine, serum, disodium ethylenediaminetetraacetic acid (EDTA), and heparin may also be instilled.

A conjunctival graft or flap is indicated for progressive deep ulcers to treat the underlying corneal disease, strengthen the weakened cornea, and prevent the loss of corneal integrity. Several types of conjunctival grafts are available. The conjunctival island or free graft is a segment of conjunctiva completely separated from its blood supply, and from the donor site, before being transplanted to the recipient site in the cornea. The conjunctival flaps, however, are advancement or rotational flaps that retain most of their original blood supply. Corneal grafts using either fresh or cryopreserved corneal tissue also provide support and fill the defect, and they are often covered with a conjunctival graft.

Descemetoceles are very deep ulcers with exposed Descemet's membrane and impending perforation of the globe. Descemetoceles are an ocular emergency and require immediate surgical intervention. Direct suturing has been recommended for small descemetoceles (diameter, ≈3 mm) but produces a high degree of corneal distortion. One limitation of corneal suturing is that the adjacent corneal tissue may be compromised, edematous, and not strong enough to hold the sutures. Large descemetoceles require a conjunctival graft, corneoconjunctival or corneoscleral grafts, or a corneal allograft to provide support and to hasten healing. Of these, the conjunctival grafts or flaps are the most frequently used technique.

Bacterial Corneal Ulcers

Corneal ulcers are frequently traumatic in origin, but they can be rapidly contaminated by bacteria. The diagnosis is established on the basis of cytologic as well as culture and sensitivity results of corneal samples. The most common bacteria isolated from eyes with external disease include *Staphylococcus* sp. (39%), *Streptococcus* sp. (25%), *Pseudomonas* sp. (9.4%), *Escherichia coli* (4.7%), *Corynebacterium* sp. (3.9%), and *Bacillus cereus* (2.4%). In vitro, most *Staphylococcus* sp. are susceptible to bacitracin, gentamicin, and cephalothin. Most *Streptococcus* sp. are susceptible to chloramphenicol, erythromycin, and carbenicillin. *Pseudomonas* sp. are sensitive to gentamicin, tobramycin, and amikacin.

Mycotic Keratitis

Mycotic keratitis is rare in the dog. *Candida albicans* and *Aspergillus* sp. are the most common isolates in cases of fungal keratitis. *Alternaria, Acremonium, Cephalosporium, Curvularia, Pseudallescheria,* and *Scedosporium* sp. have also been associated. Mycotic keratitis may be ulcerative or nonulcerative. The lesions associated with *Candida* sp. are often raised, yellowish-white or grayish-white plaques or ulcerated lesions. Infections with *Aspergillus* sp. are usually ulcerative in nature, with extensive stromal inflammation and melting. A history of long-term topical antibiotic–corticosteroid application and the ocular examination findings are often suggestive of mycotic infection. Results of exfoliative cytologic examination, bacterial and fungal cultures, and histopathologic examination of keratectomy specimens are diagnostic.

Currently available drugs include natamycin, miconazole, nystatin, amphotericin B, ketoconazole, fluconazole, and flucytosine (see Appendix F). Of this group, natamycin (Natacyn; Alcon Laboratories) is the only commercially available preparation that has been approved for ocular use. Commonly, natamycin or miconazole are used initially to treat mycotic keratitis, and appropriate topical broad-spectrum antibiotic therapy is used concurrently. Antifungal drugs are instilled in the conjunctival sac at 1- to 2-hour intervals for the first 2 or 3 days. After this time, the frequency can be reduced to between six and eight times daily for 5 to 10 days, and after that, to four times daily. Therapy should generally be continued for 14 to 21 days or until resolution of the keratitis. Superficial keratectomy to remove fungal corneal plaques and damaged cornea as well as placement of conjunctival grafts are also beneficial in these cases.

Melting Ulcers (Collagenase- and Protease-Associated Ulcers)

Melting ulcers with progressive stromal dissolution are not a specific group. They are a complicating component of corneal ulcers, and they

may occur more frequently in brachycephalic breeds (Fig. 7-8). During normal corneal healing, proteases and collagenases are produced that aid the removal of devitalized cells and debris from the cornea. Corneal epithelial cells, fibroblasts, polymorphonuclear leukocytes, some bacteria, and possibly, some fungi produce proteases and collagenase. *Pseudomonas* sp. most likely produce proteases other than collagenase, however. In some corneal ulcers, these enzymes contribute to the progressive breakdown and rapid "melting" of the corneal stroma.

Acute ulcerative keratitis with progressive melting requires vigorous topical therapy; appropriate broad-spectrum antibiotics and 1% atropine are applied. Initially, the ulcer may be cleansed with povidone–iodine solution (diluted 50:50 with sterile saline or collyrium). Successful management of melting ulcers depends on controlling infection and reducing the impact of collagenase and other proteases on the cornea. The effectiveness of topical collagenase inhibitors in corneal ulcers in the dog is questionable, but compounds attempted to date have included acetylcysteine, cysteine, sodium citrate, sodium ascorbate, tetracycline compounds, thiol-containing peptides, sodium EDTA, calcium EDTA, penicillamine, heparin, and autogenous serum. Acetylcysteine and serum are the main protease inhibitors used clinically. Surgical options include conjunctival flaps or grafts as well as corneal transplantation.

NONULCERATIVE KERATITIS

Pigmentary Keratitis (Superficial Pigmentary Keratitis)

Pigmentary keratitis in the dog usually results from the production of pigment in the corneal epithelium and from the subepithelial stroma

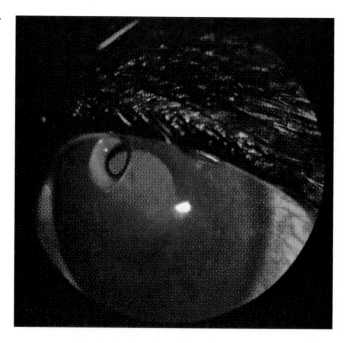

FIGURE 7-8. *Deep corneal ulcer extending to the Descemet's membrane (descemetocele) with coagulase-positive staphylococci being cultured. Note fluorescein staining of the surrounding stromal edges of the ulcer but not of the Descemet's membrane.*

associated with chronic insults. **The most common causes of pigmentary keratitis include chronic irritation from distichiasis, districhiasis, keratoconjunctivitis sicca, and nasal fold trichiasis.** Other causes of chronic irritation include eyelid position abnormalities such as entropion and ectropion, chronic exposure because of prominent eyes with large palpebral fissures (also known as euryblepharon), and congenital euryblepharon, which occurs in many brachycephalic breeds. The pigmentation frequently progresses to cover the central cornea and pupil, thereby interfering with vision. Many owners are not aware of the problem until the animal becomes visually impaired. **Treatment is directed at halting the progression of pigmentation and correcting the inciting cause (e.g., correction of entropion or ectropion, removal of abnormal lashes and aberrant dermis, and possible partial removal of nasal folds).**

If **pigmentary keratitis has resulted in visual impairment, pigmentation can be removed surgically—after the inciting causes have been corrected—by superficial keratectomy or, in some patients, strontium-90 (i.e., beta) radiation therapy. Recurrence of the pigmentation, however, is common.** Great care must be exercised during keratectomy of chronically pigmented corneas, especially in brachycephalic breeds, because the cornea may be thinner than normal. Topical corticosteroids (e.g., dexamethasone) and cyclosporine are frequently used in the treatment of pigmentary keratitis, and these drugs appear to be most useful when the cornea is vascularized.

Chronic Superficial Keratitis (Pannus)

Chronic superficial keratitis is a progressive, inflammatory, and potentially blinding disease of the canine cornea. It is also known as German Shepherd Pannus, Uberreiter's syndrome, and degenerative pannus, and it is a bilateral disease. The German Shepherd is most commonly affected, but CSK can occur in any breed (Table 7-3). Both the incidence and the severity increase at higher altitudes (i.e., >4000 feet). Dogs from lower elevations, such as those in the southeastern United States, tend to respond more favorably and with less intensive topical corticosteroid therapy than dogs from higher elevations, such as those in the Rocky Mountain areas.

Clinically, CSK initially manifests at the temporal or inferior temporal limbus as a red, vascularized, conjunctival lesion that progresses centrally. A white line or small white spots are often seen clinically in the clear corneal stroma 1 to 2 mm in front of the leading edge of the lesion and advancing blood vessels (Fig. 7-9). Eventually, the entire cornea may become vascularized, pigmented, and scarred. Some dogs with CSK also develop concurrent thickening and pigmentation of the palpebral surface of the nictitating membrane.

Both the age of onset and the breed of dog have prognostic value in this condition. In German Shepherds affected at a fairly young age (i.e., 1–5 years), the condition usually is rapidly progressive and severe. In those animals first affected later in life (i.e., 4–6 years), however, the lesions appear to be less severe and to progress more slowly. The Greyhound tends to be affected at younger ages, usually before 2 or 3 years, but exhibits relatively mild lesions.

TABLE 7-3

BREED PREDISPOSITION TO CHRONIC SUPERFICIAL KERATITIS (PANNUS)

Breed	Age of Onset (y)
Airdale Terrier	1–2
Australian Kelpie	
Belgian Sheepdog	2–5
Belgian Tervuren	2–5
Border Collie	
Cattle dogs	
Dachshund	2–4
Dalmation	2–3
English Springer Spaniel	1–3
German Shepherd Dog	1–6
Greyhound	2–5
Miniature Pinscher	7–8
Pointer	2–4
Siberian Husky	1–3

Histopathologic Features and Cause

Histopathologically, CSK appears as a superficial corneal vascularization with infiltration of granulation tissue into the superficial corneal stroma. The invading fibrovascular tissue is accompanied by lymphocytes and plasma cells. The corneal epithelium generally remains intact, but migration of pigment-laden cells (i.e., corneal melanosis) commonly accompanies the fibrovascular inflammatory infiltrate that invades the anterior stroma.

The cause of CSK in the dog has not been established, but this condition may be an immune-mediated disease. The cornea possesses tissue-specific antigens that may be modified by external factors such as ultraviolet light. In fact, CSK is characterized by increased numbers and degranulation of mast cells compared with those in normal dogs or in dogs with other forms of keratitis. Results of immunohistochemical staining of eyes with CSK are indicative that the disease is not an autoimmune reaction against epithelial cell structures. The perilimbal pattern of immunoglobulin deposition is indicative that conjunctival-associated lymphoid tissue, including Langerhans cells, may be involved in the disease process. The predominant cell in the affected cornea is the CD41 lymphocyte, with a high proportion of these secreting interferon-γ. Aberrant major histocompatibility complex class III or IV expression has also been found on epithelial cells in affected areas of dogs with CSK. Circulating autoantibodies to corneal epithelial proteins have been demonstrated in CSK as well (for more details, the reader should consult the third edition, pp. 649–651).

Treatment

Chronic superficial keratitis is a chronic and progressive disease of the cornea. Medical treatment is necessary to control the disease process and to prevent blindness, but once diagnosed, the condition cannot be cured. Owners should be advised of the need for lifelong therapy to control this disease, and that both the severity and the prognosis depend on many factors, including age of onset, altitude, and geographic location. Vision can usually be preserved with medical therapy alone at low to

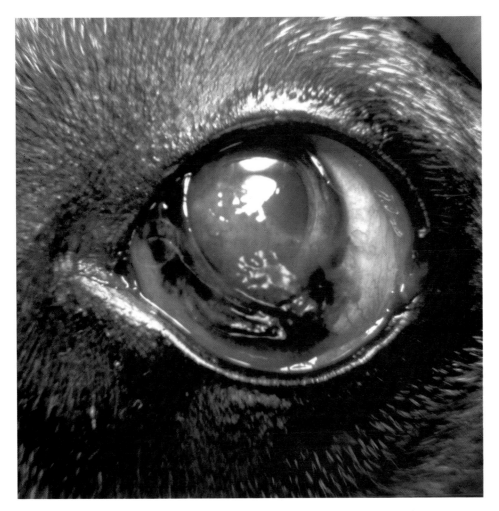

FIGURE 7-9. *Chronic superficial keratitis in a German Shepherd. The superficial cornea is both infiltrated and vascularized.*

medium elevations (i.e., ≤4000 feet) and in cases of mild lesions in middle-aged and older dogs. At higher elevations, however, additional therapy is frequently required.

Initial therapy usually consists of topical corticosteroid ointments or solutions (e.g., 0.1% dexamethasone or 1.0% prednisolone) applied three to four times daily for 3 to 4 weeks, which is followed by a reduced maintenance schedule. Animals on long-term corticosteroid therapy should be monitored by the owner and the veterinarian for ocular infection and corneal ulceration. Topical cyclosporine (0.2–1.0%), with or without concomitant dexamethasone, has been effective in cases of CSK, and 0.2% cyclosporine ophthalmic ointment applied to affected corneas twice daily has been effective in combined treatment with topical dexamethasone at ameliorating clinical signs. Owners should also be advised that improved vision and decreased density of the lesion usually take at least 2 to 4 weeks of therapy to become apparent. The intensity of topical medications can also vary throughout the year. In some cases, however, subconjunctival injection of corticosteroids, in addition to topical therapy, may also be necessary to control the disease.

For eyes with more aggressive CSK, subconjunctival corticosteroids and the application of beta (i.e., strontium-90) radiation therapy may be used. Each area of the keratitis, up to a maximum of six slightly overlapping circles, receives radiation. The area of treatment should overlap the limbus by 1 to 2 mm, and the radiation is applied in one dose of 4500 to 7500 rads per circle. Superficial keratectomy may be required with severe cases, in which blindness has resulted from pigmentation of the central cornea. A maximum of three superficial keratectomies in the dog has been suggested, and every attempt should be made to extend the period between keratectomies by administering intensive medical therapy. Another useful technique in animals with bilateral CSK and blindness is to perform keratectomy in alternate or fellow eyes, thereby allowing vision in one eye and then the other.

NEUROGENIC AND NEUROTROPHIC KERATITIS

Two forms of neurogenic keratitis occur rarely in the dog: neurotrophic keratitis, which is associated with damage to the trigeminal nerve that provides sensory innervation to the cornea; and neuroparalytic (or neurogenic) keratitis, which results from a lack of motor innervation to the orbicularis oculi muscle of the eyelids, with facial paralysis. **Neurotrophic keratitis may follow orbital trauma and usually responds to topical therapy.**

Neuroparalytic keratitis from loss of eyelid movement often results in severe exposure ulcerative keratitis and possible loss of vision. Treatment is often symptomatic. Temporary tarsorrhaphies may prevent corneal trauma and drying. If there is no response in 2 to 3 weeks, a temporary tarsorrhaphy with suturing of the eyelids for up to 6 months or 1 year may be used.

CORNEAL ABSCESSATION

Corneal abscesses are rare in the dog, but when they occur, they consist of an accumulation of inflammatory cell debris in the superficial or the deep stroma. Affected eyes have a distinct, raised, yellow-white corneal stromal opacity. The abscess may be sterile, or it may contain an infectious agent. Therapy consists of topical antimicrobials and atropine as well as curettage or keratectomy followed by placement of a conjunctival graft.

DIFFUSE KERATITIS

Superficial Punctate Keratitis

In superficial punctate keratitis, superficial defects in the corneal epithelium occur that may (or may not) retain fluorescein stain. The affected areas are often multiple, diffusely scattered across the corneal surface, and may give the cornea the pitted appearance of an orange peel. The condition may be induced by multiple insults to the cornea (e.g., chronic exposure), topical anesthetics, and possibly, a virus. **Superficial punctate keratitis may be a form of corneal dystrophy in the Shetland Sheepdog** (for more details, the reader should consult the third edition, pp. 659–660). Superficial punctate keratitis must be differentiated from corneal ulceration, corneal dystrophy or degeneration, corneal edema, and scars. Topical antibiotics, hypertonic sodium chloride, and cyclosporine have been used with variable results.

Florida Keratopathy

Corneal opacities that are apparently unique to tropical and subtropical climates have been described in the dog (and the cat). Multifocal, round, gray to gray-white, fluffy, cottonlike opacities of varying size are commonly seen in the corneal stroma of these species. The opacities occur in both the dog and the cat in warmer climates, and they have been referred to as Florida keratopathy, Florida spots, and Florida fungus. Clinically, this disease is characterized by anterior stromal opacities of variable sizes. The corneal lesion is visible as a large, light-scattering opacity with a dense center and a less dense periphery. These opacities occur at varying levels throughout the corneal stroma; however, most occur in the anterior stroma. The condition appears to be self-limiting and does not seem to respond to treatment with topical corticosteroids and antifungal drugs. The corneas are devoid of any evidence of inflammation, and the eyes usually exhibit no discomfort or irritation. The corneal epithelium is intact, and Schirmer tear test values are within normal limits. The cause (or causes) of "Florida spots" has not been ascertained, but an acid-fast organism within the stromal collagen lamellae or mycobacterial organisms are possibilities.

Endothelial Disease

Endotheliitis (i.e., inflammation of the endothelium) may occur either with or without other ocular signs. The classic example of endothelial involvement occurs with infectious canine hepatitis or postvaccination reaction with canine adenovirus type 1 modified live virus vaccine. The vaccine reaction may produce ocular complications similar to the clinical signs of the natural disease. Ocular manifestations are characterized by delayed development of anterior uveitis that is accompanied by corneal edema, which gives the eye a bluish-white, opaque appearance and is responsible for the characteristic "blue eye" description. The occurrence of uveitis after vaccination for hepatitis with modified live virus is a manifestation of a type III immune complex or Arthus-type reaction rather than a direct effect of viral replication (for more details, the reader should consult the third edition, pp. 653–654).

INJURIES

TRAUMA

Superficial corneal injuries frequently denude the corneal epithelium, thus leaving superficial abrasions that are managed as superficial corneal ulcers. Deep traumatic injuries to the cornea are managed as a deep corneal ulcer. Treatment of corneal lacerations depends on the depth of the laceration. Superficial (i.e., incomplete) lacerations heal readily as a superficial ulcer. Corneal lacerations deeper than one-half of the corneal thickness with edges that gape are apposed with 7-0 to 10-0 absorbable or nonabsorbable sutures. Full-thickness corneal lacerations should be repaired surgically. The prognosis depends on the initial depth of the laceration and the severity of the wound. Corneal rupture from blunt trauma carries a poorer prognosis than lacerations from sharp objects.

FOREIGN BODIES

Corneal foreign bodies, including plant material, flecks of metal, and chips of paint, can adhere to depressions in the corneal epithelium so that the eyelids cannot dislodge them. Foreign bodies adherent to or embedded in the epithelium are easily removed, however, with a moistened, cotton-tipped applicator or with eyewash, or they can be dislodged with a foreign-body spud, spatula, ophthalmic corneal forceps, or sterile 25- or 26-gauge hypodermic needle. Foreign objects embedded in the anterior corneal stroma may require incision with a No. 65 Beaver blade or a razor blade over the long axis of the object before lifting it from the stroma (Fig. 7-10). If the foreign body has completely penetrated the cornea and is partially in the anterior chamber, it may be retrieved from either the corneal surface or from the anterior chamber (whichever is least traumatic). The anterior chamber approach requires intraocular instrumentation, however, and is more difficult.

After removal of vegetative foreign-body material, topical broad-spectrum antibiotics and atropine are administered to control both infection and ciliary muscle spasm. Complications of corneal foreign bodies include secondary bacterial and fungal infection, severe corneal scars, and corneal perforation from inappropriate attempts at removal.

ALKALI-BURNED CORNEAS

Alkali burns to the cornea are rare in the dog, but the clinical signs include edema, opacity, loss of corneal epithelium, pain, and rapid dissolution of

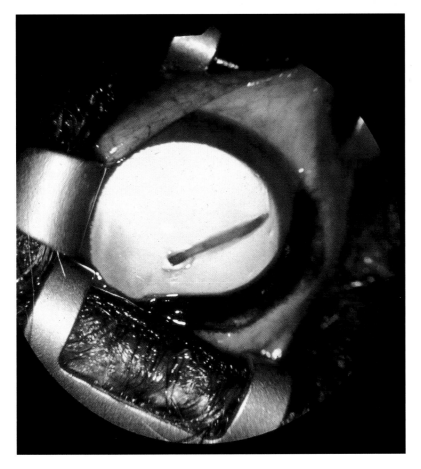

FIGURE 7-10. *A foreign body (thorn) embedded in the corneal stroma.*

the corneal stroma. Later, severe corneal ulceration and anterior uveitis occur. Treating the alkali-burned eye continues to be a major challenge in veterinary ophthalmology (for more details, the reader should consult the third edition, p. 655).

CORNEAL DYSTROPHIES

A corneal dystrophy is any primary, bilateral, and inherited disorder of the cornea that is not accompanied by corneal inflammation or systemic disease. Corneal dystrophy may affect the corneal epithelium (i.e., corneal erosions), stroma, or endothelium, and they are often breed-specific (Box 7-2). Most stromal corneal dystrophies in the dog appear clinically as gray-white or silver and crystalline or metallic opacities in the central or the paracentral cornea (Fig. 7-11). The condition is bilateral and often appears to be nearly symmetric lesions. Variations in both size and density may represent different stages of progression

BOX 7-2

Breeds of Dogs with Corneal Dystrophies

Afghan Hound	Italian Greyhound
Airedale Terrier	Lhasa Apso
Alaskan Malamute	Mastiff
Beagle	Miniature Pinscher
Bearded Collie	Norwich Terrier
Bichon Frise	Pembroke Welsh Corgi
Boston Terrier	Pointer
Chihuahua	Poodle (Miniature)
American Cocker Spaniel	Samoyed
Collie (Rough)	Shetland Sheepdog
Dachshund	Siberian Husky
English Toy Spaniel	Weimaraner
German Shepherd	Whippet
Golden Retriever	Cavalier King Charles Spaniel

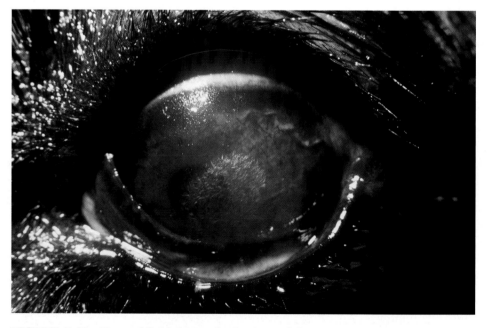

FIGURE 7-11. *Corneal lipid dystrophy in an aged dog.*

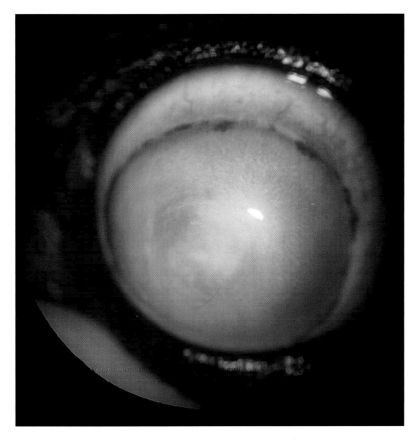

FIGURE 7-12. *Total corneal edema in a 9-year-old Boston Terrier with endothelial dystrophy before corneal transplantation.*

for the dystrophy. With adequate illumination and magnification, a myriad of fine, small particles are often seen throughout the cornea. Frequently, cholesterol crystals and clefts are observed as well.

Corneal dystrophies that occur secondary to endothelial disease manifest with variable edema, usually starting from the center of the cornea. They occur most frequently in the Boston Terrier, Dachshund, and Chihuahua breeds. The disease progresses to complete edema, which is occasionally complicated with recurrent corneal bullae formation, and from visual impairment to blindness (Fig. 7-12). Medical therapy is usually temporary and involves topical osmotic agents as the edema progresses. Treatment includes thermokeratoplasty (i.e., cautery of the superficial corneal stromal) and full-thickness keratoplasty.

TREATMENT

In the breed-associated corneal dystrophies, the diagnosis and elimination of affected dogs as breeding animals may be important. In general, corneal dystrophies do not respond to topical medical treatment, but the lesions often can be removed by keratectomy. Lesions rarely recur after keratectomy; however, faint corneal scarring is often present. Keratectomy also provides corneal tissue samples for light microscopy and ultrastructural studies.

CORNEAL DEGENERATIONS

Corneal degenerations are secondary pathologic changes. Lipids, cholesterol, calcium, or some combination thereof may be deposited secondary to inflammation. Vascularization and pigmentation (i.e., melanosis) may also precede or accompany degeneration. Clinically, corneal degenerations have a highly variable appearance. Lesions may be dense white, grayish-white, and crystalline and have well-demarcated borders. Degenerations may be unilateral or bilateral, and opacities are generally paraxial and inferior to the central axis. Epithelial disruption with vascularization is common, and cholesterol and calcium deposits also occur as the degeneration progresses. Corneal degenerations are not necessarily inherited but are, perhaps, related to other ocular or breed abnormalities (for more details, the reader should consult the third edition, pp. 663–664).

To determine the presence of any concurrent systemic disease, serum chemistry panels may be useful. In addition to cholesterol, high- and low-density lipoprotein, fasting blood glucose, triglycerides, calcium, and phosphorus levels, evaluation of thyroid and adrenal function may be useful. In some cases, lipid electrophoresis is beneficial as well. Calcium degenerations occur secondary to systemic disease, and hypercalcemia, hyperphosphatemia, hyperadrenocorticism, uremia, and hypervitaminosis D may be accompanied by secondary corneal calcification. Other ocular diseases may also produce secondary calcareous degeneration (e.g., corneal scars, uveitis, phthisis bulbi).

Therapy

When degeneration is progressive, interferes with functional vision, or causes discomfort, superficial keratectomy may be effective. In cases of corneal calcification, topical disodium EDTA (0.40–1.38%) in artificial tears is effective. Some ophthalmologists now use 1 to 5% EDTA topically. In cases of corneal cholesterolosis, dietary restriction of cholesterol, dietary additives to reduce cholesterol (e.g., flax seed oil, oat bran, niacin), and cholesterol-lowering drugs may be effective.

CORNEAL MANIFESTATIONS OF SYSTEMIC DISEASES

LIPID KERATOPATHY

Lipid keratopathy in the dog has been associated with systemic lipid abnormalities. It is characterized by both peripheral and central corneal crystalline opacities, and the deposition of lipid in the corneal stroma is more extensive if the cornea is vascularized. Hyperlipoproteinemia occurs in dogs with hypothyroidism, pancreatitis, diabetes mellitus, spontaneous hyperlipo-proteinemia (types I–IV), or postprandial plasma lipid elevations. It has been recommended that all dogs with lipid keratopathy undergo a lipid serum profile and be screened for thyroid function, pancreatitis (i.e., serum lipase and amylase), and diabetes mellitus (i.e., fasting blood glucose). Most serum lipid profiles include serum cholesterol, serum triglycerides, and serum total lipid measurements as well as lipoprotein electrophoresis. In some cases, serum cholesterol ester and phospholipid measurements are useful as well.

HYPERCHOLESTEROLEMIA (LIPID KERATOPATHY)

During hypercholesterolemia, lipid keratopathy may be induced by corneal trauma, ulcers, suture placement, and corneal surgery. Corneal infiltration with cholesterol and various lipids may occur in an otherwise normal cornea or in a pathologic cornea.

CORNEAL LIPIDOSIS (ARCUS LIPOIDES CORNEAE)

Corneal lipidosis has been reported in the German Shepherd. Lipidosis has been associated with hyperlipoproteinemia resulting from hypothyroidism (i.e., thyroid atrophy and lymphocytic thyroiditis), and corneal lipidosis has been reported in a dog with bilateral thyroid carcinoma.

BAND KERATOPATHY

Band keratopathy is a syndrome characterized by a gray-white, superficial corneal opacity oriented in the horizontal interpalpebral fissure. The opacity usually results from subepithelial deposition of calcium. Calcific band keratopathy can usually be attributed to localized corneal inflammation (i.e., "dystrophic" calcification) or systemic hypercalcemia (i.e., "metastatic" calcification). Calcific band keratopathy has also been associated with hyperadrenocorticism.

INFECTIOUS CANINE HEPATITIS

Anterior uveitis and intense corneal edema occur in approximately 20% of dogs recovering from infectious canine hepatitis. An ocular immune reaction to vaccination with modified live canine adenovirus type I may produce anterior uveitis and corneal edema similar to those of the natural disease. The intense corneal edema, which gives the eye a bluish-white, opaque appearance, is responsible for the "blue eye" that characterizes this disease.

SYSTEMIC HISTIOCYTOSIS

Mild to moderate corneal edema and neovascularization may occur with systemic histiocytosis in the dog, and conjunctivitis with ocular discharge is commonly seen before the corneal changes. Systemic histiocytosis is a familial, histiocytic proliferative disorder that occurs most commonly in the Bernese Mountain dog. A sex-linked inheritance has been suggested (for more details, the reader should consult the third edition, p. 665).

Lymphosarcoma

The clinical signs of ocular lymphosarcoma are variable. Canine corneal lesions include keratitis, neovascularization, corneal edema, a centrally migrating white band, and intrastromal corneal hemorrhage. The lesions can be related to direct tumor invasion. The anterior uvea is commonly infiltrated with tumor cells, thereby resulting in moderate to severe uveitis with aqueous flare, keratic precipitates, miosis, and hypopyon. Fibrin and hypopyon in the anterior chamber are common, and occlusion of the pupil with secondary glaucoma may occur as well.

CORNEOSCLERAL MASSES AND NEOPLASMS

Corneal inflammatory masses and neoplasms are infrequent in dogs. Nodular granulomatous episcleritis (NGE), however, appears to be the most frequent of these diseases.

CORNEAL CYSTS

Cyst formation in the canine cornea is rare and usually superficial. Epithelial inclusion cysts occur as benign, raised, solitary, white to pink corneal masses. Inclusion cysts are generally unilateral, and a traumatic origin is suspected. Treatment consists of superficial keratectomy; recurrence is unlikely unless incomplete excision occurs. Histopathologically, the cystic structures are lined by nonkeratinizing squamous epithelium.

FIBROUS HISTIOCYTOMAS

The term *fibrous histiocytoma* has been used to describe infiltrative, raised masses invading the temporal cornea in the dog (Fig. 7-13). The tumorlike mass is observed most frequently in the Collie, but it also occurs in other breeds. Histopathologically, the masses consist primarily of histiocytes, fibrocytes, plasma cells, and lymphocytes. Treatment consists of superficial keratectomy followed by topical and subconjunctival corticosteroids. Azathioprine (Imuran; Burroughs Welcome) at an initial dose of 2 mg/kg is effective for fibrous histiocytomas, but a more benign treatment protocol has been advocated that uses orally administered niacinamide and tetracycline.

NODULAR FASCIITIS

Ophthalmic nodular fasciitis has been described in the dog involving the cornea, limbus, conjunctiva, and eyelids. Histopathologic findings include solid, cellular, infiltrative masses. Fibroblasts are the predominant cell type, with an abundance of reticulin fiber formation. Surgical excision is effective therapy. In the Collie, *nodular granulomatous episclerokeratitis* is the preferred term.

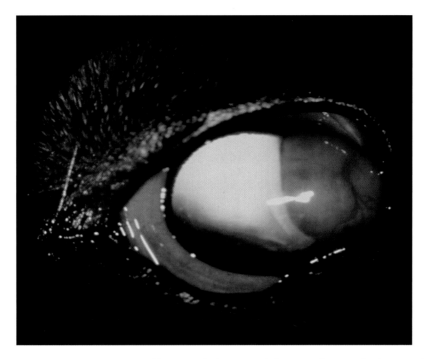

FIGURE 7-13. *Corneal mass (fibrous histiocytoma) in the left eye of a 2-year-old female Blue Tick Hound.*

LIMBAL MELANOMAS

Limbal or epibulbar melanomas may invade the cornea secondarily. These tumors are usually pigmented but may occasionally be non-pigmented (i.e., amelanotic), smooth masses (Fig. 7-14). Canine limbal melanomas occur in two age groups. In the younger group (i.e., 2–4 years), the tumors are invasive and have a history of rapid growth. In the older group (i.e., 8–11 years), the tumors are stationary and are found incidentally during physical examination. **The dorsolateral quadrant is usually the site of origination, and the German Shepherd and Labrador Retriever breeds appear to be predisposed.** An association has also been made between occurrence of melanoma and heavily pigmented dogs.

Primary limbal melanomas must be differentiated from the external extension of intraocular melanomas. In older dogs with nonprogressive limbal masses, periodic surveillance appears to be adequate. Gonioscopy is recommended to rule out intraocular neoplasia. Full-thickness, freehand corneoscleral grafts have been used to maintain a functional eye in younger dogs with progressive limbal melanomas, and grafts of nictitating membrane cartilage with overlying conjunctiva have been used to replace corneal and scleral defects after the removal of limbal melanomas. Surgery with the neodymium:yttrium-aluminum-garnet laser may be an effective means of controlling limbal melanomas in the dog as well, but the diode laser may also be used.

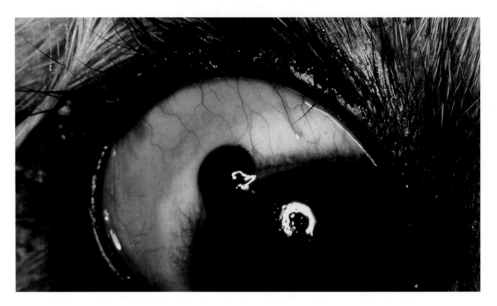

FIGURE 7-14. *Limbal melanoma in the right eye before surgical removal.*

SQUAMOUS CELL CARCINOMA

Primary corneal squamous cell carcinoma occurs rarely in the dog. The neoplastic mass arises directly from the cornea, and it appears as a raised, multilobulated, pink to white mass. Therapy is usually excision by keratectomy, which combined with cryosurgery or beta radiation therapy may decrease the chance for recurrence of the tumor.

PAPILLOMAS

Papillomas (i.e., viral papillomas) appear to be the most common primary corneal tumor in the young dog, and they resemble other papillomatous growths in the mouth and eyelid. Most papillomas respond well to excision by superficial keratectomy. The chance for recurrence may be decreased with cryosurgery using a double freeze–thaw cycle after the mass has been removed by superficial keratectomy or by beta radiation therapy combined with superficial keratectomy.

SCLERAL DISEASES

Several specific inflammatory responses affect the canine episclera and sclera. The common association of episcleritis or scleritis with rheumatoid arthritis in humans, however, has not been established in the dog. Canine episcleritis may be divided into primary and secondary types. The primary form can be further subdivided into simple episcleritis and the more common NGE.

NODULAR GRANULOMATOUS EPISCLERITIS

Several different names have been ascribed to NGE, including nodular fasciitis, fibrous histiocytoma, proliferative keratoconjunctivitis, limbal granuloma, pseudotumor, and Collie granuloma. **Ocular findings in NGE include multiple, elevated, fleshy masses or a single mass arising at the limbus and infiltrating the adjacent corneal stroma. Nictitating membrane involvement is common as well, and the Collie and Shetland Sheepdog breeds are predisposed. The lesions tend to be bilateral and to recur after therapy.** Histopathologic features of NGE are consistent with those of chronic granulomatous inflammation (for more details, the reader should consult the third edition, pp. 668–669).

Generally, NGE tends to be benign, with good response to treatment with oral azathioprine (Imuran; Burroughs Welcome) in conjunction with topical administration of corticosteroids (0.1% dexamethasone suspension [Maxidex; Alcon Laboratories]). **In the past, local surgical excision by lamellar keratectomy, intralesional corticosteroid injections, and beta radiation therapy (7500 rads/surgical site) have been used. Baseline complete blood count and serum biochemical panels are obtained before starting treatment with azathioprine, the toxic effects of which include gastrointestinal toxicosis (i.e., vomiting and bloody diarrhea), hepatotoxicosis, and myelosuppression.** Elevated serum alkaline phosphatase and alanine transaminase activities occur in acute hepatic necrosis.

Azathioprine for NGE is usually administered orally at 1.5 to 2.0 mg/kg once daily for 3 to 10 days, and then at 0.75 to 1.00 mg/kg once daily for 10 to 15 days. Many dogs can be kept in remission with maintenance therapy of 1 to 2 mg/kg once every 3 to 7 days for 1 to 8 months, after which the therapy is discontinued. Cryosurgery for NGE is effective, and a double freeze–thaw technique using nitrous oxide has been described. A more recent treatment protocol for dogs heavier than 10 kg involves oral administration of niacinamide, 500 mg, and tetracycline, 500 mg, three times daily; once improvement occurs, administration is continued at once or twice daily.

SCLERITIS

Inflammatory diseases of the sclera (i.e., scleritis) are rare in the dog but can be divided into nonnecrotizing granulomatous scleritis and necrotizing granulomatous scleritis. Scleritis seems to be most common in the Spaniel breeds, and especially in the American Cocker Spaniel. Dogs with scleritis usually present with pink-tan–colored sector lesions arising near, but posterior to, the limbus. Clinical signs include ocular pain, photophobia, and excessive lacrimation. In some cases, keratitis or anterior uveitis (or both) may be present, because the scleral inflammation extends into these adjacent tissues. Clinical laboratory parameters used to define systemic collagen diseases (e.g., canine rheumatoid factor, anti-DNA-antibody, LE [lupus erythematosus] cell identification) are negative in most cases of scleritis (for more details, the reader should consult the third edition, pp. 668–669).

SURGERY OF THE CORNEA AND SCLERA

Surgery of the cornea and sclera requires magnification, adequate illumination, and a limited number of ophthalmic surgical instruments. This section describes surgical procedures used by the general veterinary practitioner, including the superficial keratectomy, repair of the corneal laceration, and conjunctival grafts. For additional surgical procedures, such as corneal and scleral grafts, the reader should consult the third edition (pp. 675–700).

BASIC SURGICAL INSTRUMENTATION

The basic microsurgical instrument pack should include fine, one-over, two-toothed forceps (e.g., Colibri forceps) as well as corneal section scissors, microsurgical needle holders (e.g., Castroviejo), and microsurgical blade holders (Box 7-3). Acceptable methods of magnification include ×3 to ×5 head loupes or an operating microscope. Depending on the specific procedure, appropriate corneal suture material includes 7-0 to 10-0 nylon, vicryl, or polydioxanone (PDS).

SUPERFICIAL KERATECTOMY

Many superficial corneal lesions are amenable to superficial keratectomy. Such lesions include indolent corneal ulcers, dermoids, corneal neoplasms, sequestra (in the cat), crystalline corneal degeneration, pigmentary keratitis, and others. Superficial keratectomy is also useful in obtaining biopsy material for histopathology of corneal or scleral neoplasms or of inflammatory masses (e.g., nodular granulomatous episclerokeratitis). Determining the depth of the lesion using careful biomicroscopy will help to plan the superficial keratectomy. If the resulting corneal lesion extends from one-half to three-fourths of the corneal thickness, a conjunctival pedicle graft is warranted to protect the cornea, to help prevent perforation, and to promote healing. Because corneal stromal tissue may not regenerate completely, the number of superficial keratectomies that can be performed at the same site is limited to only two or three and depends on the depth of the tissue being removed with each procedure.

Superficial keratectomy can be performed using a standard surgical procedure or using carbon dioxide or excimer laser ablation. **The standard surgical procedure involves removing the corneal epithelium and superficial stroma with a surgical blade (Fig. 7-15).** The initial corneal in-

BOX 7-3

Basic Corneal Microsurgical Instruments

Magnifying loupes (×4 - ×6)

Colibri corneal forceps (0.3-mm teeth with tying platform)

Bishop-Harmon forceps (0.3- or 0.8-mm teeth)

Needleholder

Barraquer

Curved, without lock device

Westcott tenotomy scissors or Stevens tenotomy scissors (curved)

Eyelid speculum

Barraquer

Beaver blade handle

Irrigating cannula (23-gauge)

Other Surgical Supplies:

Suture material

7-0 Vicryl or Dexon

Ophthalmic spatula needle

6-0 Monofilament

Nylon, surgilene, prolene, and so on

Blades

No. 63, 64, and 65 Beaver blades

Irrigating solution

Balanced salt solution (ophthalmic) or lactated Ringer's solution

cision should completely surround the lesion to be removed, and it can be made using a corneal trephine, a diamond knife, or a microsurgical blade. The initial incision can be round, square, or triangular. The edge of the tissue to be removed is then grasped with a forceps, and a corneal dissector (e.g., Martinez corneal dissector, Beaver No. 64 microsurgical blade, iris spatula) is introduced and held parallel to the cornea. The dissector is used to separate the corneal lamella without penetrating any deeper than the original incision. At this point, the cornea is separated until the opposite incision line (or limbus) is reached. Scissors may be needed to connect the

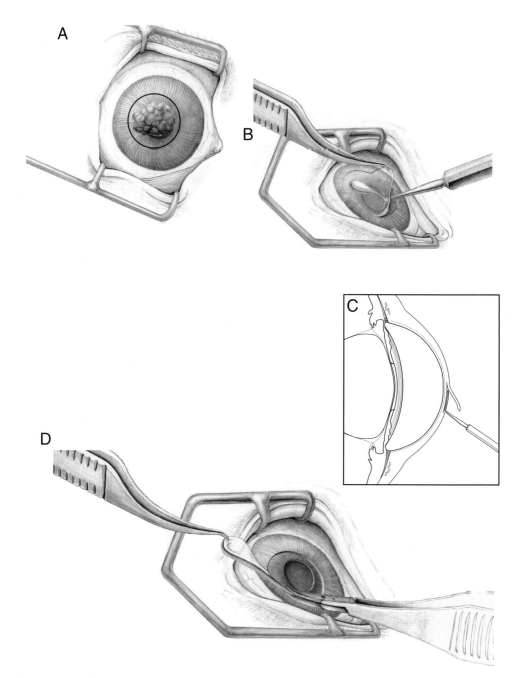

FIGURE 7-15. *Superficial keratectomy.* **A.** *The initial corneal incision, which may be round, square, or triangular, should completely surround the lesion to be removed and can be made using a corneal trephine, a diamond knife, or a microsurgical blade.* **B** *and* **C.** *After the initial incision is made, the edge of the tissue to be removed is grasped using a forceps, and a corneal dissector (e.g., Martinez corneal dissector, Beaver No. 64 microsurgical blade, or iris spatula) is introduced and held parallel to the cornea. The dissector is used to separate the corneal lamella without penetrating deeper than the original incision. The cornea is then separated until the opposite incision line (or limbus) is reached.* **D.** *Scissors may be needed to connect the dissection to the opposite incision or to remove the corneal tissue from the limbus.*

dissection to the opposite incision or to remove the corneal tissue from the limbus.

After keratectomy, the cornea is treated with topical broad-spectrum antibiotics to prevent infection and with topical atropine to decrease both ciliary spasm and discomfort. A potentially devastating complication after keratectomy is corneal perforation, which generally results from infection at the surgical site.

CONJUNCTIVAL GRAFTS OR FLAPS

The most common surgical procedure in the dog for chronic, infected, or progressive corneal ulcers is a conjunctival flap or graft. Conjunctival grafts support the cornea, provide fibrovascular tissue to fill the corneal defects, and bring a blood supply (as well as blood-associated immune components, systemic antibiotics, and natural anticollagenases [e.g., α_2-macroglobulin]) to the lesion. Because partial conjunctival flaps cover only a small area of the normal cornea, the clinician can visualize much of the cornea and the anterior chamber, which in turn allows for continuous examination of these structures and, thus, monitoring for ulcer progression and possible anterior uveitis. Having only a small portion of the cornea covered may also allow the animal to have vision.

All conjunctival grafts consist of thin conjunctival tissue transposed onto the cornea to cover the lesion. The different types of vascularized conjunctival grafts include the total or 360° conjunctival flap, the bridge or bipedicle flap, the hood flap (180°), and the pedicle flap. Conjunctival grafts are generally harvested from the adjacent bulbar conjunctiva; however, the tarsal conjunctiva (i.e., tarsoconjunctival grafts) can also be used. The bulbar conjunctival flap moves with the eye. Thus, no tension is applied to the flap itself. With all conjunctival flaps, the corneal graft bed and the ulcer must be properly prepared. The recipient bed for the conjunctival graft is prepared by debriding the lesion, thereby removing all loose epithelium and devitalized corneal tissue. Great care should be taken to prevent corneal perforation during this debridement.

Total (360°) Conjunctival Grafts

The total (or 360°) conjunctival flap covers the entire cornea and is indicated when most of the cornea is affected by a lesion (see Chapter 5). This graft is not usually preferred by veterinary ophthalmologists because the entire cornea is covered. Because the graft does not need to be sutured directly to the corneal ulcer edges, however, it is used more frequently by the general and the small veterinary practitioner.

Bridge Conjunctival Graft

The bridge or bipedicle flap is a linear graft attached to the conjunctiva at both ends (Fig. 7-16). It is generally indicated in long, linear corneal lesions, such as those corneal lacerations that require conjunctival

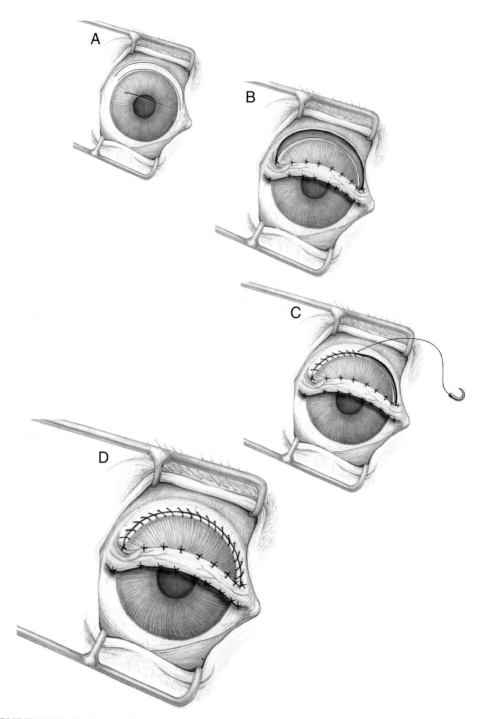

FIGURE 7-16. *Bridge or bipedicle conjunctival graft/flap.* **A.** *The conjunctiva is excised from the limbus for approximately 180° both adjacent and parallel to the linear corneal lesion. This area is extensively undermined, and the underlying fibrous tissue is removed. A second conjunctival incision is then made 5- to 8-mm peripheral and parallel to the original conjunctival incision, thus creating a "bridge" of conjunctiva.* **B** *and* **C.** *The bridge is advanced over the lesion and then sutured, using simple interrupted sutures, into the cornea around the lesion.* **D.** *The original graft-harvesting site is closed by opposing the remaining conjunctiva with a simple continuous suture.*

graft covering after direct suturing. These grafts are started by incising the conjunctiva from the limbus for approximately 180° both adjacent and parallel to the linear corneal lesion. This area is extensively undermined, and the underlying fibrous tissue is removed. A second conjunctival incision is then made 5- to 8-mm peripheral and parallel to the original conjunctival incision, thus creating a "bridge" of conjunctiva. This bridge is advanced over the lesion and then sutured using simple interrupted sutures in the cornea around the lesion. Next, the original graft-harvesting site is closed by apposing the remaining conjunctiva with a simple continuous suture. The advantage of this procedure is that it provides exquisite blood supply to long, linear lesions of the cornea.

Hood (180°) Conjunctival Graft

The hood (or 180°) graft is indicated for peripheral corneal lesions. The conjunctiva adjacent to the lesion is cut from the limbus and undermined. The graft is then advanced to cover the lesion and sutured in place, generally with two or four simple interrupted sutures.

Pedicle Conjunctival Graft

The pedicle or rotational graft is probably the most useful and versatile conjunctival graft and the one usually preferred by veterinary ophthalmologists. The base of the pedicle graft should be directed toward the area of the limbus nearest to the lesion. Once the location of the base is determined, a site 1.0- to 1.5-cm temporal to the base is located; this will be the site where the graft is initiated. A small slit is cut in the conjunctiva perpendicular to the limbus, and through this slit, the entire conjunctival flap site is undermined using blunt dissection. The underlying fibrous tissue (i.e., Tenon's capsule) should be freed from the overlying conjunctiva so that the conjunctiva appears to be transparent. Next, two parallel cuts are made to create a strip of conjunctiva that is rotated to cover the corneal lesion. The flap is then sutured to the cornea with simple interrupted sutures of 7-0 to 9-0 polyglactin 910 or nylon. These sutures are placed first at the distal end of the flap and then at 1.0- to 1.5-mm intervals. To prevent disruption of the blood supply, the sutures are not placed within the pedicle portion of the graft or at the proximal portion of the lesion. The graft-harvest site on the bulbar conjunctiva should be closed using a simple continuous suture of 7-0 to 9-0 polyglactin 910 (see Chapter 5).

Conjunctival grafts adhere to the corneal stroma but not to the adjacent epithelia surrounding the ulcer (Fig. 7-17). Three to 8 weeks after placement of the flaps, the blood supply can be interrupted by cutting the base of the flap at the limbus. This can usually be performed with use of topical anesthesia and Stevens tenotomy scissors. Eliminating the blood supply allows the conjunctival graft to recede and lessens the resulting corneal scar.

Island Conjunctival Graft

A conjunctival free or island graft is a modified conjunctival graft in which the blood supply is severed from the outset. The donor site can

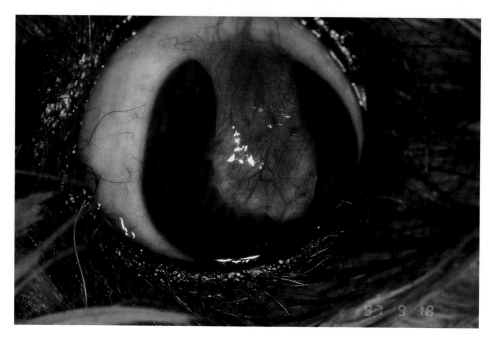

FIGURE 7-17. *A typical conjunctival pedicle graft to treat a deep corneal ulcer in the canine eye.*

be in the tarsal or the bulbar conjunctiva. The conjunctiva is undermined and excised from the donor site, and it is then transposed to cover the corneal lesion. The outer epithelial side must remain external to allow for proper attachment of the graft to the lesion. Simple interrupted sutures, or a combination of simple interrupted and continuous sutures, are used to secure the graft to the cornea. The graft is usually revascularized within 3 to 5 days, depending on the amount of corneal vasculature near the lesion before surgery. Indeed, the success of this surgical procedure may depend on the vascularity of the lesion itself; therefore, lesions without corneal vascularization may heal better with a conjunctival pedicle graft (and an established blood supply). The advantages of free island grafting are that tissue is readily available; a watertight, 360° closure can be made; and the graft does not require trimming after surgery, such as with conjunctival flaps that require excision of their blood supply after surgery (i.e., conjunctival pedicle or bridge flaps).

The most common complication from any conjunctival grafting procedure is dehiscence of the graft from the corneal lesion, which may occur because the corneal lesion is progressing (i.e., worsening) and damaging the cornea where sutures secure the graft. Allowing excessive tension on the graft or a significant portion of the fibrous Tenon's capsule to remain attached to the graft may result in premature dehiscence. Proper placement of sutures in healthy cornea using a thin, conjunctival graft and concurrent, appropriate medical therapy greatly decrease the incidence and severity of complications after conjunctival graft surgery.

CORNEOSCLERAL OR CORNEOCONJUNCTIVAL TRANSPOSITION

Corneoscleral or corneoconjunctival transposition is a type of autogenous corneoscleral graft that uses a sliding pedicle of cornea and attached sclera or conjunctiva to repair corneal defects (Fig. 7-18). These transpositions are more difficult and require more time to perform than conjunctival grafts. They are indicated in central, deep, or perforated corneal lesions with sufficient peripheral healthy cornea that can be used for the grafting procedure. In general, the distance from the peripheral edge of the lesion to the corneal limbus must be at least 1-mm longer than the diameter of the corneal lesion itself. Because "self" tissues are used, corneoscleral transposition eliminates the need for corneal tissue donors, and it also avoids immune-mediated inflammation. This may decrease corneal scarring and allow for a clearer postoperative cornea than that after conjunctival and some other corneal grafts. One disadvantage, however, is that corneoscleral transposition damages normal, healthy corneal tissue.

FULL-THICKNESS CORNEAL LACERATIONS

Surgical repair of most corneal lacerations generally is not overly challenging—provided that proper instrumentation, magnification, and suture materials are used. **A successful visual outcome after traumatic corneal laceration requires a careful, thorough preoperative evaluation and selection of appropriate surgical procedures. The extent of ocular trauma must be determined before repairing the cornea, and in many cases, this can be difficult. Deflation of the anterior chamber, iris prolapse, hyphema, hypopyon, and significant corneal edema may prevent a complete ophthalmic examination from being performed.** A consensual pupillary light response and a dazzle response are positive clinical signs, but these do not ensure a normal posterior segment. Ocular ultrasonography using either a 7.5- or 10.0-MHZ probe can also be used to assess posterior segment damage with corneal lacerations; however, the ultrasound coupling gel should not enter the wound or the anterior chamber. In addition, if ultrasonography of the injured eye is attempted, the animal should be sedated or anesthetized so that movement of the animal does not further damage the eye. A standoff pad (e.g., solid-gel standoff pad or water-filled balloon) should also be used to separate the globe, gel, and eye. If possible, the integrity of the anterior lens capsule should be examined; if a careful examination is not possible before surgery, it should be conducted during the surgical procedure. If the lens capsule is ruptured, significant lens-induced uveitis and cataractogenesis will occur. Phacoemulsification of the lens and implantation of a synthetic intraocular lens during the corneal repair procedure decreases the postoperative inflammatory response and helps to maintain vision.

Full-thickness corneal lacerations may (or may not) have incarcerated uveal tissue. When possible, incarcerated yet viable iris tissue should be repositioned in the anterior chamber; iris tissue that has been prolapsed for longer than 6 to 8 hours should be amputated with electrocautery. When removing a prolapsed iris, gentle traction is placed on the prolapsed portion, and the fresh uveal tissue is cauterized near the cornea. Care must be taken, however, not to cauterize the cornea itself. The anterior chamber is irrigated with balanced salt solution or lactated Ringer's solution, and the lens is carefully inspected (as described earlier). Viscoelastic agents can be used to reinflate the anterior chamber and to keep it formed while the cornea is being sutured, but removal of the viscoelastic agent by irrigation is recommended before placement of the final suture to prevent ocular hypertension from occurring after surgery.

Appropriate suture material for corneal lacerations includes 7-0 to 9-0 polyglactin 910 and 8-0 to 10-0 nylon. The choice of sutures depends largely on the surgeon's preference. Nylon is the easiest to handle and the least reactive in the cornea initially, but in most cases, it needs to be removed after 4 to 6 weeks. Small animal corneas generally require 8-0 to 10-0 suture material. Several suture patterns have been described for corneal wounds, and each has both advantages and disadvantages. Use of simple interrupted, simple continuous or running, shoe lace, and other sutures have been reported. After closure of the cornea, the anterior chamber is reformed with balanced salt solution via a limbal injection using a 27- to 30-gauge needle. After wound closure, sterile fluorescein dye may be applied to the wound to ensure proper closure and to detect leaks (i.e., Seidel test).

KERATOPLASTY PROCEDURES

Keratoplasty procedures can be divided into essentially two types— lamellar keratoplasty, and penetrating keratoplasty—with both types using homologous corneal grafts (i.e., corneal tissue from animals of the same species). Autologous corneal grafts (i.e., graft material from the same animal) were described earlier. Lamellar keratoplasty is the excision

---

FIGURE 7-18. *Corneoscleral transposition. A and B. After debridement of the corneal lesion, a microsurgical blade (Beaver No. 64) is used to create two diverging, linear, one-half to three-fourths corneal thickness incisions extending from the periphery of the lesion to the limbus. The incisions are then extended beyond the limbus and into the conjunctiva and sclera. The width of the graft should be slightly more than that of the corneal defect. C and D. The edge of the lesion at the leading edge of the graft is grasped with a forceps and elevated. E. The cornea is split and undermined both toward and over the limbus and into the sclera or conjunctiva. F. The corneal graft tissue is advanced to cover the lesion and then trimmed to fill the corneal defect. G and H. The graft is sutured to the cornea using simple interrupted sutures of 8-0 to 10-0 polyglactin 910 or nylon. The cornea can be oversewn with a continuous suture. The sclera or conjunctiva (or both) is then sutured to the cornea at the diverging linear incision with a continuous suture pattern using the same type of suture material as that used in the corneal graft.*

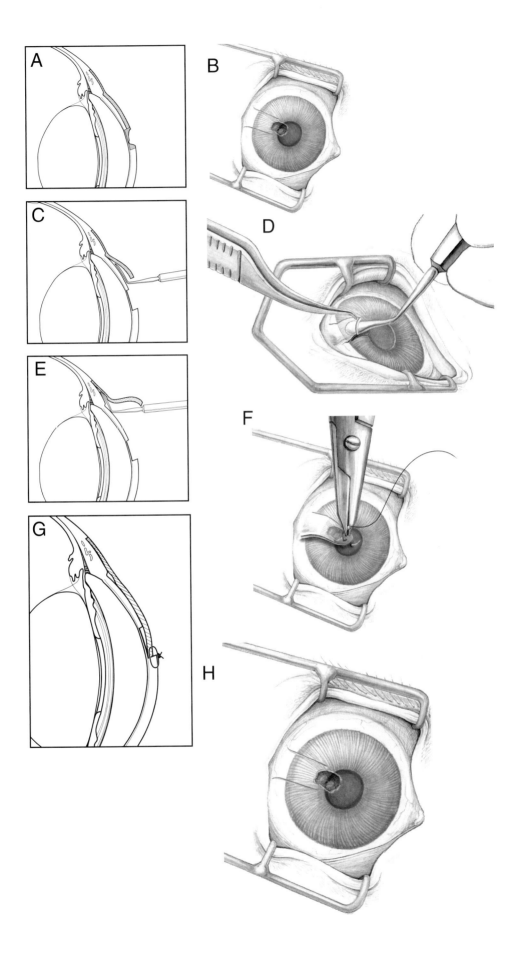

of corneal epithelium and superficial stroma with replacement by graft tissue of equal thickness. With this procedure, the Descemet's membrane remains intact, and the complications of intraocular surgery (e.g., intraocular inflammation) are largely avoided. Indications for lamellar keratoplasty are few but include severe superficial dystrophies, corneal sequestrations (in the cat), and possibly, superficial corneal abscesses. In penetrating keratoplasty, all corneal layers are excised and replaced by a homologous, full-thickness corneal graft. Penetrating keratoplasty is indicated when a central corneal opacity obstructs vision. Generally, the goal is acceptance of this graft and maintenance of a clear cornea; this is achieved by replacing all corneal layers with a graft containing viable endothelial cells. In an eye with glaucoma, keratoconjunctivitis sicca, lid or cilia abnormalities, active infections, or any other inflammatory condition of the anterior segment, however, the likelihood of graft failure is greatly increased. In fact, corneal vascularization of more than two quadrants of the eye is associated with a graft failure rate of 50% in humans. Use of penetrating keratoplasty in veterinary medicine has been rare, but there are several clinical and experimental reports have been published (for more details, the reader should consult the third edition, pp. 692–696).

The Canine Glaucomas

The definition of glaucoma in the dog continues to evolve. At present, **it is best stated as being a group of diseases having the major risk factor of elevated intraocular pressure (IOP) and with an optic neuropathy characterized by the death of retinal ganglion cells (RGCs) and their axons.** Alterations independent of the IOP, such as excitotoxic amino acids, defects in microcirculation of the optic nerve head (ONH), and extracellular matrix abnormalities of the ONH, also may contribute to optic nerve damage in both canine and primate glaucoma.

All glaucomas are diseases of change, and the glaucomas consist of five stages:

1. An initial event or series of events,
2. An obstruction of the aqueous humor outflow system resulting from the initial event or series of events,
3. An increased IOP that is too high for optic nerve axoplasmic flow and blood flow,
4. An RGC dysfunction with resulting optic nerve degeneration and atrophy, and
5. Visual-field loss and blindness.

CLINICAL EFFECTS OF ELEVATED INTRAOCULAR PRESSURE

The clinical effects of elevated IOP are summarized in Table 8-1. For details regarding the pathogenesis of these changes, if known, the reader should consult the third edition, pp. 702–710.

TABLE 8-1

CLINICAL EFFECTS OF ELEVATED INTRAOCULAR PRESSURE IN THE DOG

Ocular Tissue	Changes in Glaucoma
Globe size	Enlargement from stretching of the cornea and sclera; termed *hydrophthalmos, buphthalmia, megaloglobus,* and *macrophthalmia.* Occurs rapidly in puppies.
Cornea	Becomes thicker because of stromal edema. Eventually, corneal endothelial cell death occurs. Focal, linear breaks in Descemet's membrane (i.e., Haab's striae). Exposure keratitis occurs later.
Sclera and lamina cribrosa	Sclera is stretched and becomes thinner. Areas of sclera through which the nerves and blood vessels penetrate may form large staphylomas. Scleral lamina cribrosa is distorted and compressed posteriorly.
Iris	Mydriasis in most types of glaucoma. With time, the iridal stroma becomes thin, and the sphincter muscle becomes atrophied.
Ciliary body	Gradual degeneration with atrophy of the pars plicata and individual ciliary processes.
Anterior chamber angle	Open- and narrow- or closed-angle glaucoma. Secondary changes in the iridocorneal angle and ciliary cleft invariably involve progressive narrowing, and eventual closure, of the iridocorneal angle and collapse of the ciliary cleft.
Choroid and tapetum cellulosum	Depends on the rapidity of onset, duration, and level of the intraocular pressure elevation. Areas of chorioretinal ischemia and degeneration in the ischemic zones. Tapetal changes include degeneration and thinning.
Lens	Cataract formation and changes in the lens position within the patella fossa (from primary zonular disease or secondary to globe enlargement).
Vitreous	Liquefaction and formation of vitreal cortical strands.
Retina and optic nerve head	Progressive degeneration. Large-diameter optic nerve axons appear to be particularly sensitive. The inner retinal layers, especially the retinal ganglion cell and nerve fiber layers, as well as the optic nerve head appear to be very sensitive to intraocular pressure and degenerate. Outer retinal layers may also be impacted, particularly with marked IOP elevations.

DIAGNOSTICS

The three basic procedures in the diagnosis and clinical management of glaucomatous patients are tonometry, gonioscopy, and ophthalmoscopy. Reliable tonometry is essential for the optimal clinical management of canine glaucoma, and of the three available types (i.e., digital, indentation, and applanation), applanation tonometry is the most reliable. Current models include the TonoPen-XL (Mentor O & O) and the pneumatonograph model 30 (Mentor O & O; the former is preferred by veterinary ophthalmologists. When applanation tonometers are not available, the Schiotz tonometer is preferred to digital estimations. With use of only topical anesthesia while the dog is loosely restrained, tonometry can be performed (see Chapter 1). Two or more reproducible readings with consistent IOP measurements should be obtained. Tonometry in the outpatient clinic provides only a "snapshot," however, because diurnal variations in IOP ($\approx$2–4 mm Hg) occur in the normal dog, with higher levels in the early morning and the lowest levels in the early evening. For a glaucomatous patient, instrument tonometry is a critical procedure in both the diagnosis and clinical management.

Gonioscopy is the diagnostic examination of the iridocorneal angle and the opening of the ciliary cleft or the filtration angle (see Chapter 1). Gonioscopy differentiates glaucomas based on the appearance of the iridocorneal angle and the ciliary cleft morphology into the open, narrow, and closed types. Gonioscopy must be performed repeatedly, however, because the angle findings are dynamic and change as the glaucoma and the globe enlargement progress. In most primary or breed-related glaucomas, continual narrowing and eventual closure of these outflow pathways require progressively more aggressive medical and surgical therapy. Gonioscopy is performed with topical anesthesia while the dog is restrained manually (see Chapter 1). Frequent gonioscopic findings in the dog include narrow to closed filtration angles and pectinate ligament dysplasia. Pectinate ligament dysplasia is replacement of the normal, slender, and branching pectinate ligaments that span the opening of the ciliary cleft with broad sheets of pigmented tissues, either with or without "flow holes." Pectinate ligament dysplasia is a developmental disorder of the outflow channels for the aqueous humor and must be distinguished from peripheral anterior synechia, which are inflammatory and often progressive.

A combination of direct (higher magnification) and indirect (larger viewing field) ophthalmoscopy is recommended for the clinical management of canine glaucomatous patients. Both the ONH and the retina are carefully examined for degeneration, when IOP is elevated (i.e., at initial presentation), and after IOP has been medically reduced. Additional diagnostic procedures, such as tonography, A-mode ultrasonography, and pattern as well as flash electroretinography are also available. Other, newer imaging procedures are available to assist with evaluation of canine glaucomatous patients, but these modalities have not yet been used routinely in veterinary ophthalmology (for more details, the reader should consult the third edition, pp. 710–714).

CLASSIFICATION OF GLAUCOMAS

Canine glaucomas are divided on the basis of the possible cause, the gonioscopic appearance of the filtration angle (i.e., iridocorneal angle and ciliary cleft), and the duration or stage of the disease (Box 8-1). Classifications by possible cause include the primary and breed-related glaucomas, secondary glaucomas, and congenital glaucomas. Primary and breed-related as well as the secondary glaucomas constitute the largest clinical groups in the dog.

BOX 8-1

Types of Glaucoma in the Dog

Primary glaucomas

　Open/normal angle (acute/chronic)

　Narrow/closed angle (acute/chronic)

　　Pectinate ligament dysplasia

Secondary glaucomas

　Uveitis

　Lens luxations

　Intumescent cataract

　Phacolytic/phacoclastic uveitis

　Hyphema

　Intraocular neoplasia

　Aphakic

　Malignant/ciliary block

　Melanocytic/pigmentary proliferation

　Giant retinal tears (Schwartz-Matsuno syndrome)

　Anterior chamber silicone oil

　Postoperative ocular hypertension

Congenital glaucomas

　Goniodysgenesis

In the primary glaucomas, the IOP rises without concurrent ocular diseases, is hereditary in some canine breeds, and has a bilateral potential for development. Primary open-angle glaucomas may result from abnormal biochemical metabolism of the trabecular cells of the outflow system. The term *goniodysgenesis* is becoming more frequent in the veterinary literature. In the dog, it usually signals the failure of rarefaction to form pectinate ligaments at gonioscopy, but the status of deeper aqueous humor outflow tissues, especially the trabecular meshwork and the trabecular extracellular matrix, is not known. A more accurate phrase than inclusive goniodysgenesis is pectinate ligament dysplasia. **Pectinate ligament dysplasia has been associated with narrow- and closed-angle primary glaucomas, but narrow- and closed-angle primary glaucomas also occur without pectinate ligament dysplasia.** In our scheme, the persistent mesodermal bands/pectinate ligament dysplasia–associated glaucomas in selected breeds have been classified with the primary glaucomas, because the clinical signs of these glaucomas occur later in life. As the basic pathogenesis for these breed-related glaucomas becomes documented, however, these glaucomas could become classified as secondary types.

In the secondary glaucomas, increased IOP is associated with some known antecedent or concurrent ocular disease that physically obstructs the aqueous humor outflow pathways. These obstructions tend to be unilateral conditions and are not inherited. Some of the conditions that may initiate these forms of glaucoma, however, such as those with cataracts and lens luxation (i.e., dislocation), may be genetically determined in certain breeds. The secondary glaucomas are differentiated by cause as well as by an open or a narrow anterior-chamber angle and ciliary cleft at gonioscopy.

Congenital glaucomas are rare in the dog, and they are usually associated with considerable developmental abnormalities of the aqueous humor outflow pathways. The extent of the angle anomaly may affect the time of onset for the elevated IOP: the more severe the defect, the sooner the elevation occurs.

CLINICAL SIGNS

Clinical signs of the glaucomas depend on the stage of disease and, to some extent, on the type of glaucoma. The stage may be asymmetric in the same dog, with one eye in the advanced stages of the disease and the other apparently normal or at the very early stages (Table 8-2).

The signs of the secondary glaucomas are similar to those of the primary glaucomas, but the cause for the rise in IOP (e.g., an anterior uveitis, an intraocular mass, or a lens luxation) is evident. Congenital glaucomas affect young puppies, usually within the first 3 to 6 months of life. Often, the first clinical sign in these animals is rapid onset of buphthalmia and an inability to completely close the palpebral fissure.

TABLE 8-2	
CLINICAL SIGNS OF GLAUCOMA IN THE DOG	
Stage of Glaucoma	*Clinical Signs*
Early	May be asymptomatic, slight mydriasis, mild transient corneal edema, variable episcleral congestion, normal optic nerve head appearance, intraocular pressures of approximately 20 to 30 mm Hg, visual.
Mild/moderate	Variable mydriasis, episcleral congestion, variable degrees of corneal edema/striae, slight buphthalmia, early lens subluxation, variable retinal and optic disk changes, intraocular pressures of 30–40 mm Hg, vision to visual impairment.
Advanced	Persistent mydriasis, corneal edema with corneal striae, peripheral anterior synechiae and angle closure, buphthalmia, lens displacement from the patella fossa, cortical cataract formation, vitreous degeneration and syneresis, extensive retinal and optic disc degeneration, intraocular pressures of more than 40–50 mm Hg, intermittent visual impairment to total blindness.

PRIMARY BREED-RELATED GLAUCOMAS

INHERITANCE AND BREED PREDISPOSITION

Inherited open- and narrow-angle glaucomas occur bilaterally in purebred dogs. Primary glaucomas are rare in nonpurebred dogs. **Of all the animal species that require veterinary care, the dog exhibits the highest frequency (0.5%) of spontaneous glaucoma, and primary glaucomas have been reported in at least 42 breeds (Table 8-3). Recently identified breeds with primary glaucomas include the Samoyed, Norwegian Elkhound, Bouvier des Flandres, Siberian Husky, Flat-Coated Retriever, Golden Retriever, Great Dane, Welsh Springer Spaniel, Akita, Chow Chow, and Shar Pei.** In only a few breeds has the inheritance for the glaucoma been established. These breeds include the Beagle (autosomal recessive trait), Welsh Springer Spaniel (autosomal dominant with variable expression), and Great Dane (autosomal dominant trait with variable expression).

Breeds having secondary glaucoma associated with luxation of the lens include, most commonly, the Smooth- and Wire-Haired Fox Terriers, Sealyham Terrier, Border Collie, Tibetan Terrier, Cairn Terrier, Welsh Corgi, and Jack Russell Terrier. Other breeds, however, are also affected (Box 8-2). Genetic tests for both primary and lens-related secondary glaucomas have not been reported in the dog.

TABLE 8-3

BREEDS WITH PRIMARY GLAUCOMAS

Breeds Predisposed

Akita	Italian Greyhound
Alaskan Malamute	Lakeland Terrier
Basset Hound	Maltese
Beagle	Miniature Pinscher
Border Collie	Miniature Schnauzer
Boston Terrier	Norfolk Terrier
Bouvier des Flandres	Norwegian Elkhound
Brittany Spaniel	Norwich Terrier
Cairn Terrier	Poodle (Toy/Miniature)
Cardigan Welsh Corgi	Samoyed
Chihuahua	Scottish Terrier
American Cocker Spaniel	Sealyham Terrier
Dachshund	Shih Tzu
Dalmation	Siberian Husky
Dandie Dinmont Terrier	Skye Terrier
English Cocker Spaniel	Smooth Fox Terrier
English Springer Spaniel	Tibetan Terrier
German Shepherd	Welsh Springer Spaniel
Giant Schnauzer	Welsh Terrier
Greyhound	West Highland White Terrier
Irish Setter	Wire Fox Terrier

Types of Glaucomas Reported

Open Angle	Closed Angle
Beagle	Akita[a]
Great Dane[a]	American Cocker Spaniel
Keeshound	Basset Hound[a]
Norwegian Elkhound	English Cocker Spaniel[a]
Poodle (Miniature/Toy)	English Springer Spaniel[a]
Samoyed	Flat Coated Retriever[a]
Siberian Husky[a]	Golden Retriever
	Poodles (Miniature/Toy)
	Samoyed
	Shar Pei[a]
	Welsh Springer Spaniel

[a]Pectinate ligament dysplasia.

BOX 8-2

Inherited and Breed Predisposition to Lens Luxation in the Dog

Inherited	Breed Predisposed
Border Collie	Australian Collie
Cairn Terrier	Basset Hound
Jack Russell Terrier	Beagle
Lakeland Terrier	Chihuahua
Manchester Terrier	German Shepherd
Miniature Bull Terrier	Greyhound
Norfolk Terrier	Miniature Poodle
Norwich Terrier	Miniature Schnauzer
Scottish Terrier	Norwegian Elkhound
Skye Terrier	Spaniel Breeds
Sealyham Terrier	Pembroke Welsh Corgi
Smooth-Haired Fox Terrier	Welsh Terrier
West Highland White Terrier	Toy Poodle
Tibetan Terrier	Toy Terrier
Wirehaired Fox Terrier	

BREED-SPECIFIC PRIMARY GLAUCOMAS

In the dog, the primary glaucomas are divided into open-angle and narrow- or closed-angle glaucomas. The association of abnormalities involving the pectinate ligaments (often termed *goniodysgenesis*) with the narrow- or closed-angle glaucomas appears to be more than coincidental.

Inherited Primary Open-Angle Glaucoma in the Beagle

The elevation in IOP becomes apparent at tonometry in Beagles between 8 and 16 months of age, but the clinical signs of glaucoma are delayed until 2 to 5 years of age. This increase in IOP and decline in facility of outflow, as measured by Schiotz tonography, pneumatonography, and constant-pressure perfusion of the anterior chamber, develop slowly (Fig. 8-1). In affected dogs, pneumatonographic outflow declines from 0.19 ± 0.07 μL/min per mm Hg (age, 3–6 months) to 0.07 ± 0.05 μL/min mm Hg (age, 43–48 months). The mean episcleral venous pressure in both normal and glaucomatous dogs is 10 to 12 mm Hg.

The iridocorneal angle and sclerociliary cleft are initially open and devoid of any abnormalities (fig. 8-2). The IOP in dogs with early stage glaucoma slowly increases from the mean normal IOP of 16 to 18 mm Hg. Animals from 2 to 5 years of age have IOPs in the range of 25 to 40 mm Hg. Diurnal variations (6–10 mm Hg) are greater in affected dogs, with the highest IOP occurring in the morning. Results of serial A-mode ultrasonography indicate that the increased IOP produces enlargement (1–2 mm) of the axial length of the globe, which in turn produces lens subluxation and narrowing of the iridocorneal angle and sclerociliary cleft in dogs between 1 and 4 years of age. Eventual iridocorneal angle and sclerociliary cleft closure result in animals between 4 and 6 years of age. Primary open-angle glaucoma is inherited in Beagles as an autosomal recessive trait and relates to changes in the trabeculae, including compression, disorganization, and the concomitant accumulation of extracellular materials (e.g. glycosaminoglycans).

Retinal and optic nerve changes in affected dogs are currently being studied. Anterior movement of the scleral lamina cribrosa is followed by posterior displacement of the multilayered lamina cribrosa. As the disease progresses, cupping of the canine ONH develops. Such cupping is difficult to use as a clinical guide to glaucoma progression, however, because the rate of cup progression is variable. The retinal blood vessels, and especially the small, peripapillary retinal arterioles and veins, gradually disappear. The optic discs become round with the loss of myelin, depressed, and atrophied (for more details, the reader should consult the third edition, pp. 718–721).

Open-Angle Glaucoma in the Norwegian Elkhound

Primary open-angle glaucoma was originally described among Norwegian Elkhounds in Norway. Affected dogs were mostly males and

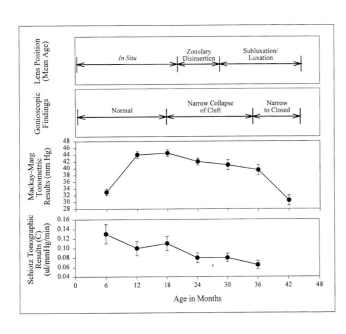

FIGURE 8-1. *Progression of primary open-angle glaucoma in a Beagle with monitoring of the intraocular pressure (applanation tonometry), aqueous humor resistance to outflow (tonography), position of the lens, and appearance of the iridocorneal angle and ciliary cleft (gonioscopy). With globe enlargement (starting at 12 to 18 months), secondary iridocorneal angle and ciliary cleft closure as well as lens luxation with zonular disinsertion occur.*

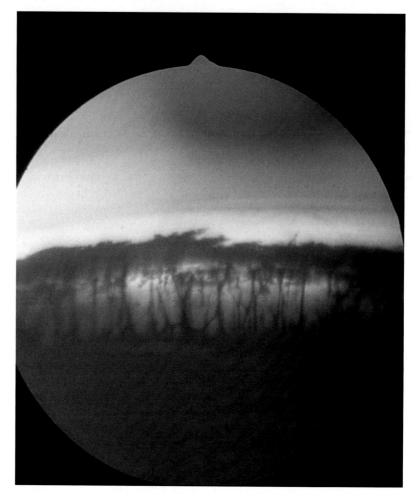

FIGURE 8-2. *Gonioscopic view of the iridocorneal angle and opening of the ciliary cleft in a Beagle with early primary open-angle glaucoma.*

ranged in age from 3.9 to 13.0 years (median age, 6.6 years). The iridocorneal angle and ciliary cleft appeared to be normal in affected dogs at the early stage, with IOPs ranging from the upper twenties to the thirties (mm Hg). Pectinate ligament dysplasia was not observed, but occasional "stout" pectinate fibers were noted, along with some narrowing of the ciliary cleft opening. The ciliary cleft gradually closes as this type of glaucoma advances, and the IOP progressively increases. Synechial closure of the ciliary cleft occurs in advanced cases. Lens subluxation and total lens luxation, buphthalmos and Haab's striae, and ONH atrophy as well as retinal degeneration occur late in the disease, with subsequent loss of vision. Norwegian Elkhounds also exhibit primary glaucoma in the United States, but these dogs have not been studied. Glaucoma with narrow or closed iridocorneal angles and pectinate ligament dysplasia has also been reported in this breed.

Narrow-Angle Glaucoma in the American Cocker Spaniel

Narrow-angle glaucoma in the American Cocker Spaniel (ACS) remains one of the most frequent primary glaucomas. The usual history of narrow-angle glaucoma in the ACS contains few of the classic clinical signs of glaucoma, but occasional histories do include conjunctival hyperemia and even transient corneal edema (Fig. 8-3). Most affected dogs present with either the classic clinical signs of unilateral, acute congestive glaucoma of a few days' duration or with chronic, advanced glaucoma (Table 8-1). Often, the condition becomes bilateral within several months.

Both the history and clinical course are suggestive that this glaucoma may actually be a series of acute IOP attacks, with the subsequent magnitude of the IOP elevation gradually increasing. Tonometry of the acute congestive glaucomas often reveals IOPs as great as 50 to 70 mm Hg, and the corneal edema that parallels the elevation in IOP after approximately 40 mm Hg usually prevents gonioscopy. In the ACS, gonioscopy with ocular hypertension usually reveals a narrow to closed iridocorneal angle and reduced ciliary clefts (Fig. 8-4). As the glaucoma progresses, angle closure and ciliary cleft collapse with peripheral anterior synechial formation are common (Fig. 8-5). More recently, pectinate ligament dysplasia has also been reported in the ACS, but this does not appear to be frequent. With time, the globe becomes enlarged, the lens progressively luxates, and the iridocorneal angle and cleft close (Fig. 8-6).

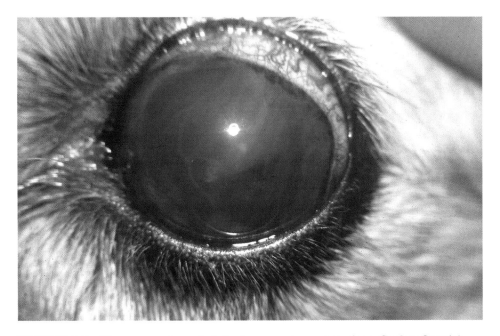

FIGURE 8-3. *Narrow-angle and cleft glaucoma in an American Cocker Spaniel. Both corneal edema and striae are present. The intraocular pressure is 52 mm Hg.*

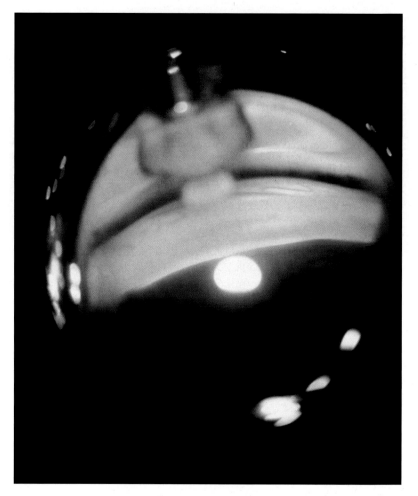

FIGURE 8-4. *Gonioscopic view of iridocorneal angle closure in an American Cocker Spaniel.*

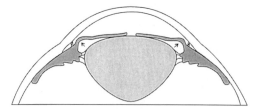

FIGURE 8-5. *One hypothesis for the development of narrow and closed iridocorneal angle glaucoma and ciliary cleft collapse in the American Cocker Spaniel. Tight apposition of the pupillary aspects of the iris increases the pressure slightly within the posterior chamber, which in turn displaces the basal iris forward. Eventually, the basal iris narrows the iridocorneal angle and the opening of the ciliary cleft (arrows). Apposition of the basal iris across the filtration angle causes a potentially reversible angle closure. With continued apposition, peripheral anterior synechiae develop, thereby permanently closing the aqueous outflow pathways.*

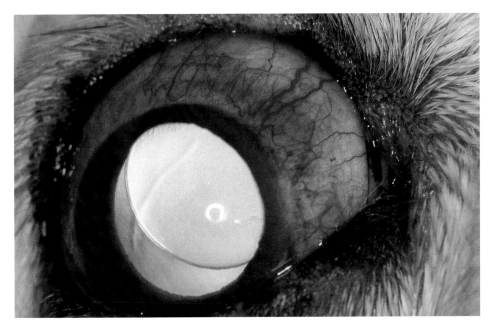

FIGURE 8-6. *Advanced angle closure and cleft closure in an American Cocker Spaniel. The globe is enlarged and the lens subluxated, thereby revealing a large, aphakic crescent.*

Changes of the ocular fundus in the ACS may not correlate with the duration and magnitude of the elevated IOP. An ACS can present with a high IOP (70–80 mm Hg) and a history of the signs of glaucoma being present for less than 1 week, yet after the IOP is lowered to less than 20 mm Hg, the dog loses its vision. Ophthalmoscopically, the ocular fundus cannot be visualized until the IOP is lowered and the corneal edema reduced. The optic nerve and retina initially may appear to be normal, with some vascular attenuation being detected. With the IOP maintained at 20 mm Hg or less, however, progressive retinal and ONH degeneration eventually become apparent within a few weeks (Fig. 8-7). In some of these dogs, the retinal degenerations may affect only limited areas, appearing as radiating or fan-shaped zones from the ONH and representing areas of retinal and choroidal degeneration from ischemia caused by occlusion of the individual short posterior ciliary arteries. Often, ONH degeneration and deterioration of the animal's vision continue despite lowering of the IOP, and this provides classic evidence for the role of non-IOP-related factors in glaucomatous optic neuropathy. Among some animals that have been tested, intravitreal glutamate levels were much higher in the ACS, thereby suggesting that the initial primary optic nerve injury from the elevated IOP induces RGC degeneration and apoptosis, which in turn are caused by, at least in part, glutamate excitotoxicity. The injured, apoptotic RGC then release more glutamate, which predisposes the eye to further, secondary degeneration of the adjacent, healthy RGC and their axons (for more details, the reader should consult the third edition, pp. 722–723).

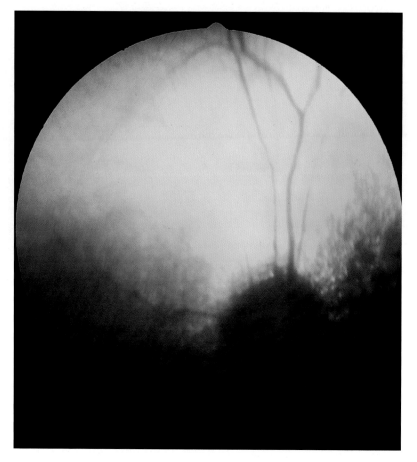

FIGURE 8-7. *Optic nerve and retinal degeneration associated with narrow-angle glaucoma in the American Cocker Spaniel.*

Narrow- and Closed-Angle Glaucoma with Pectinate Ligament Dysplasia in the Basset Hound

Narrow- and closed-angle glaucoma with pectinate ligament dysplasia (i.e., mesodermal dysgenesis) was documented in the Basset Hound during the late 1960s. In one report, 63% of Basset Hounds had some degree of pectinate ligament dysplasia, but fewer than 3% had glaucoma. This form of glaucoma usually presents as a unilateral, acute, congestive, and closed-angle glaucoma or as a chronic, narrow-angle-closure glaucoma with buphthalmia and eventual blindness (Fig. 8-8). Anterior uveitis, along with at least some of the corneal edema that relates to this inflammation, is often present, which is unusual among breed-related canine glaucomas. Whether the uveitis precipitates the glaucoma or the marked elevations in IOP precipitate the uveitis is not known. The inflammation complicates the medical and surgical treatment of this glaucoma.

In the opposite, normotensive eye and in the affected eye, gonioscopy usually reveals a narrow to closed iridocorneal angle, and the opening of the ciliary cleft is spanned by consolidated pectinate ligaments or meso-dermal remnants of varying size and with varying numbers of "flow holes." Normally, the regions of pectinate ligament dysplasia have some gaps, at which the pectinate ligaments appear to be normal and inspection of the trabecular meshwork and the ciliary cleft opening is possible (for more de-tails, the reader should consult the third edition, pp. 723–724).

Narrow-Angle Closure in the Welsh Springer Spaniel

In the Welsh Springer Spaniel, the narrow-angle closure form of primary glaucoma affects females more frequently than males (ratio, 4.2:1). The age of onset ranges from 10 weeks to 10 years (mean age, 2 years and 9 months). Four dogs have been affected before 1 year of age. Time from the onset of glaucoma in the first eye to that in the second eye ranges from 6 days to 3 years. Clinical signs are those of acute congestive glaucoma or those of chronic angle-closure glaucoma. Gonioscopy of affected dogs has revealed eyes with regions of narrow and closed iridocorneal angles and ciliary clefts as well as other eyes with the angles totally closed. This form of glaucoma has been familial, and the mode of inheritance appears to be dominant.

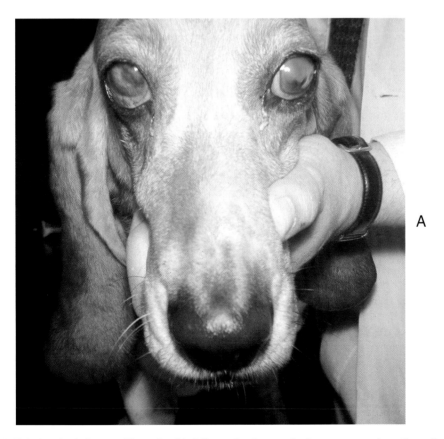

A

FIGURE 8-8. **A.** *A Basset Hound with bilateral advanced glaucoma.*   *(continued)*

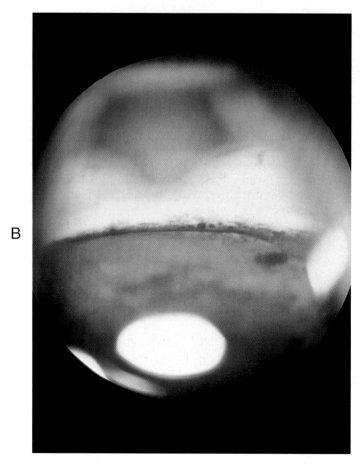

B

FIGURE 8-8—*(continued)* *B. At gonioscopy, large and persistent mesodermal bands rather than the distinct, individual pectinate ligaments are often visible. With extensive involvement, flow holes are present in these dysplastic pectinate ligaments. Because iridocyclitis is often present, these pectinate ligament anomalies must be differentiated from progressive, peripheral anterior synechiation of the aqueous outflow pathways in this type of glaucoma.*

Narrow-Angle Glaucoma in the Samoyed

This form of narrow- or closed-angle glaucoma has been investigated among Samoyeds in Sweden. Ultrasonic measurements of the fellow eyes of unilateral glaucomatous Samoyeds revealed a longer axial length; a shallower anterior chamber; a thicker, more forward-positioned lens; and a longer (anteroposterior) vitreous body. All glaucomatous eyes had closed iridocorneal angles. Eyes with narrow iridocorneal angles had anteriorly positioned lenses and a longer vitreous body.

The classic hypothesis concerning the pathogenesis of narrow-angle glaucoma is a relative block of aqueous humor passage through the pupil, which results from the greater tension applied by the iris against the central lens or, in Samoyeds, by the more anteriorly positioned lens. Increased resistance to the escape of aqueous humor into the pupil from behind the iris results in the more forward displacement of the basal iris, which could be associated with a narrower opening of the ciliary cleft. With time, the outflow pathways become progressively more compromised and, eventually, close.

Narrow-Angle Glaucoma/Pectinate Ligament Dysplasia in the Great Dane

Primary angle-closure glaucoma has occurred in Great Danes from England. Affected dogs have an age range of 1 to 9 years (mean age, 4 years). Most dogs have presented with unilateral acute congestive glaucoma, with 3- to 24-month intervals between binocular involvement. Gonioscopy of the initially affected as well as of the opposite, normotensive eyes has revealed narrow to closed iridocorneal angles with pectinate ligament dysplasia.

Narrow-Angle Glaucoma in the Chow Chow

Primary glaucoma in the Chow Chow has been associated with iridocorneal angle closure and limited pectinate ligament dysplasia. The mean age of affected Chows is 6.2 ± 2.2 years, and two-thirds of these animals have been females. Most animals present with bilateral, acute congestive glaucoma. When possible, gonioscopy reveals narrow to closed iridocorneal angles with short, stout pectinate ligaments. Pectinate ligament dysplasia, which appears as focal areas of solid, pigmented sheets, is usually quite limited (less than one-sixteenth the circumference of the angle). On the basis of clinical observations regarding the extent of pectinate ligament dysplasia, the genesis of this form of primary glaucoma appears to be of the narrow- and closed-angle type. The Chow Chow is another breed with primary glaucoma that often still retains functional vision even late in the disease process despite elevated IOP, buphthalmia, and obvious, extensive ONH degeneration.

Primary Glaucomas in Other Breeds

Primary narrow-angle glaucoma also occurs in Golden Retrievers from England. Angle closure, cleft collapse, and pectinate ligament dysplasia have been observed. Secondary glaucoma associated with anterior uveal cysts and chronic uveitis occurs in this breed as well.

Primary glaucoma also affects Flat-Coated Retrievers from England, but the condition has not been reported among this breed in the United States. Flat-Coated Retrievers with the more extensive forms of pectinate ligament dysplasia are predisposed to glaucoma.

SECONDARY GLAUCOMAS

Secondary glaucomas consist of diseases with increased IOP, open to closed iridocorneal angles and ciliary clefts, and detectably impaired outflow of the aqueous humor. **Clinical management of secondary glaucomas is often more clear-cut than that of primary glaucomas, because the cause of the increased IOP can usually be ascertained (Box 8-3) and the prognosis for development of glaucoma in the nonaffected eye is clear.** Medical or surgical treatment of secondary glaucoma is directed toward removing, if possible, the cause of the elevated IOP. Additional or secondary

---

BOX 8-3

Treatments for the Secondary Glaucomas in the Dog

Anterior uveitis

Peripheral anterior synechiae

Medical: corticosteroids, nonsteroidal anti-inflammatory agents, mydriatics

Pupillary obstruction

Iris bombé

Surgical: coreoplasty, iridencleisis

Lens-associated

Cataract

Surgical: Lens removal

Displacement: anterior luxation, subluxation, posterior luxation

Surgical: lens removal, other

Intraocular neoplasms

Surgical: iridocyclectomy, enucleation

Hyphema

Surgical: aspirate/tissue-plasminogen activator

Melanocytic

Surgical: anterior chamber shunts, enucleation

Aphakic (angle/pupil obstruction)

Surgical: coreoplasty/iridencleisis, anterior vitrectomy

Malignant

Surgical: anterior vitrectomy

Silicone oil

Surgical: aspirate oil/vitreous

changes (e.g., peripheral anterior synechiae) may require application of the standard glaucoma-filtering or cyclodestructive procedures. The most frequent cause of secondary glaucoma in the dog is lens displacement, which manifests as subluxation, anterior luxation, or posterior luxation. Uveitis and intraocular tumors are also associated with secondary glaucoma in the dog.

SUBLUXATED LENSES AND ANTERIOR AND POSTERIOR LENS LUXATIONS

Lens luxations are the most frequent cause of secondary glaucoma in the dog, but they also occur secondary to buphthalmia in the chronic primary glaucomas. Enlargement of the globe causes progressive stretching of the zonules, which eventually breaks the zonules' attachments to the equatorial lens capsule or, infrequently, causes disinsertion of their attachments to the ciliary body. In dogs with bilateral buphthalmia and lens subluxation/luxation, determining if the lens luxations are primary or secondary may be impossible. Even so, the breed, age of onset, and presence or absence of cataract development may aid in making this determination. Total luxation with normal-size globes is more common in the primary luxation syndromes, with subluxations more commonly resulting from the buphthalmia caused by glaucoma.

Lens luxations in Terriers are common (Box 8-3), and these dogs may present with either unilateral or bilateral and acute or chronic secondary glaucoma (Fig. 8-9). The glaucoma may be associated with iridocyclitis from microtrauma between the unstable lens and iris, with resultant increases in the levels of aqueous humor fibrin, proteins, and inflammatory cells, which in turn can interfere with aqueous drainage. The glaucoma also may aid in the formation of preiridal fibropupillary membranes as well as anterior and posterior synechiae, which further compromise drainage of the aqueous humor. Anterior lens movement can mechanically impair the passage of aqueous humor through the pupil, thereby causing increased posterior chamber pressure that, in turn, causes anterior ballooning of the peripheral iris and a reduction in the area of the iridocorneal angle outflow pathways. Such movement of the iris also contributes to the formation of permanent peripheral anterior synechiae and of posterior synechia, which cause a condition known as iris bombé.

The completely luxated lens can remain in the patella fossa, luxate into the anterior chamber, or move posteriorly through the torn anterior vitreal face and into the vitreous. **One recent report claims that glaucoma occurs in 73% of canine eyes with anterior lens luxations, in 43% of those with subluxations, and in 38% of those with posterior lens luxations.** With anterior displacement of the lens from the patella fossa, vitreous that adheres to the posterior lens capsule may occlude the pupil, thereby preventing the pupillary flow of aqueous humor and ballooning the base of the iris, which in turn causes iridocorneal angle and scleociliary cleft closure. This type of iris bombé often masks the basal iridal and filtration-angle changes.

With posterior or vitreal lens luxation, the torn anterior vitreal membrane allows access into the pupil and the anterior chamber of both liquid and formed (i.e., gel) vitreous. Formed vitreous may cause pupillary

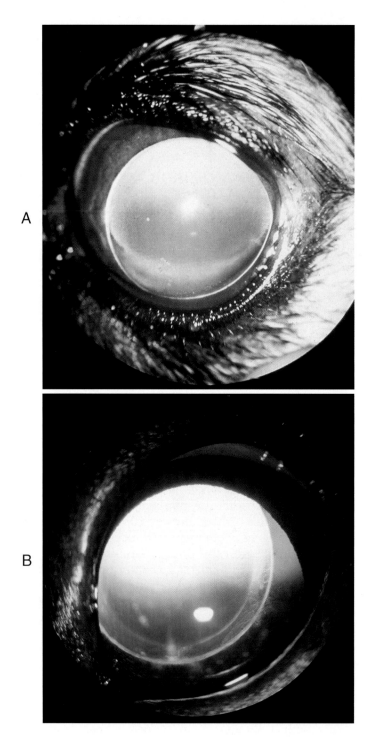

FIGURE 8-9. *Lens luxations in the dog may produce secondary glaucomas, especially in Terriers. Alternatively, lens luxation may develop secondary to globe enlargement. **A.** With anterior lens luxation, the ocular hypertension appears to arise from pupillary obstruction by the cortical vitreous still adherent to the posterior lens capsule, from compression of the iridocorneal angle and ciliary cleft by the basal iris, or from some combination of both. **B.** With lens subluxation, the cause of the ocular hypertension is less obvious. Intermittent pupillary obstructions of aqueous humor passage by the unstable lens and formed anterior vitreous, chronic iridocyclitis, and progressive iridocorneal angle and ciliary cleft closure, however, appear to be important.*

blockage and secondary glaucoma. It can also adhere to the posterior cornea and the iridocorneal angle. Blockage of the iridocorneal angle with formed vitreous in sufficient amounts to increase the IOP is infrequent, but blockage of the pupil from vitreous in sufficient amounts to increase the IOP is more common.

CATARACTOUS VERSUS "CLEAR" LENS

Lens luxation may involve normal as well as cataractous lenses, with the mechanism for the zonular disinsertions possibly differing. In Jack Russell Terriers, Tibetan Terriers, and Border Collies, the zonules appear to possess structural malformations, and bilateral lenticular displacement occurs in dogs of only a few years of age that have clear lenses. In contrast, luxations of hypermature cataractous lenses often occur with inherited cataracts in older dogs of the non-Terrier breeds. The zonular degenerations with cataractous lenses produce subtle to overt degrees of subluxation/luxation, and they appear to relate to the capsular changes associated with cataract hypermaturity and lens-induced uveitis. With focal zonular degenerations, small aphakic crescents develop, and partially liquefied vitreous may protrude through a defect in the anterior hyaloid membrane.

Early removal of displaced lenses, particularly in Terriers, has the highest probability for successful retention of vision and prevention of secondary glaucoma. The primary objective of lens extraction is to prevent secondary glaucoma, diminish inflammation, or treat secondary glaucoma. Delayed medical or surgical treatment of eyes with displaced lenses can result in secondary glaucoma. Surgical removal of subluxated lenses, anterior luxated lenses, and posterior luxated (i.e., intravitreal) lenses is accomplished using the extracapsular, phacoemulsification, or intracapsular techniques.

OTHER FORMS OF LENS-ASSOCIATED GLAUCOMA

The intumescent (i.e., swollen) cataract has been associated with an acute pupillary block, phacomorphic glaucoma in the dog. The enlarged lens displaces the iris forward, thus increasing the posterior chamber pressure and shifting the base of the iris forward, which narrows the iridocorneal angle and the ciliary cleft opening.

Rupture of the lens capsule from ocular trauma or lens-induced uveitis from resorbing hypermature cataracts can cause the phacolytic form of open-angle glaucoma in the dog. If lens-induced uveitis is not carefully monitored and controlled medically, the filtration angle can eventually become obstructed with inflammatory cells, protein-rich aqueous humor, fibrin, and macrophages filled with lenslike material.

With the increasing frequency of extracapsular and phacoemulsification cataract surgery and of the intracapsular lensectomy for luxated lens in the dog, aphakic and pseudophakic glaucomas are becoming more frequent as well. Aphakic glaucomas probably represent multiple causes, with the two most frequent being occlusion of the pupil by inflammatory membranes and closure of the iridocorneal angle and ciliary cleft by formation of preiridal fibrin membranes and peripheral anterior synechia. The aphakic glaucomas that occur secondary to pupillary blockage are usually characterized by a small pupil that has either adhered to itself or been obstructed by a membrane consisting of organized fibrin, inflammatory cells and fibrous tissue, anterior capsule remnants, posterior capsule, the anterior vitreous, or some combination of these. Iris bombé usually occurs as well. The occluded pupil may be depressed and, sometimes, barely visible because of the iris bombé that bulges into the central and the peripheral anterior chamber. As measured by applanation tonometry, the IOP is usually raised, to 30 or 40 mm Hg, with a higher IOP occurring posterior to the iris.

If the pupillary obstruction is acute (<72 hours), intensive medical therapy consisting of 0.1% scopolamine combined with 10% phenylephrine, topical and systemic corticosteroids, topical and systemic nonsteroidal anti-inflammatory agents, and topical or systemic carbonic anhydrase inhibitors (CAIs) can be attempted. Intravenous mannitol can be administered rapidly to reduce the IOP, but its effects may be muted by the increased permeability of the blood–aqueous barrier because of the iridocyclitis. Intracameral tissue-plasminogen activator (TPA; 25–50 mg) can readily assist in resolving fibrin occlusion of the pupil of less than 2 weeks' duration.

If the pupillary flow of aqueous humor is not possible, the occluded pupil can be opened by discission with a sharp blade or hypodermic needle, laser iridotomy, iridectomy, or iridencleisis. (My preference is usually the latter procedure.) Unsuccessful resolution of an occluded pupil and iris bombé results in chronic buphthalmia and blindness. Intraocular hemorrhage should be anticipated during these procedures, because the inflamed canine iris is highly vascular. During iridectomy, a radial (i.e., complete) or basal (i.e., peripheral) section of the iris is excised, and unless these sections are large, the sites will eventually close with iris and inflammatory membranes. The neodymium:yttrium-aluminum-garnet (Nd:YAG) laser may be used to produce full-thickness iris holes (i.e., laser iridotomy); however, and unfortunately, these holes will usually close within a few days.

Malignant (or misdirected aqueous) glaucoma is a variation of pupillary block aphakic glaucoma. It may develop after extracapsular/phacoemulsification, intracapsular cataract, or lens extraction surgery. The pupil is usually of medium size and is obstructed with inflammatory membranes, which are combined with either the posterior lens capsule and the anterior vitreous face (with extracapsular/phacoemulsification) or with the organized anterior vitreal face or membrane. Rather than remaining in the enlarged posterior chamber behind the iris bombé, the aqueous humor is either misdirected or redirected into the vitreous body through a tear in its anterior face as aqueous humor formation continues and the IOP rises. Thus, the organized or formed vitreous is pushed further into the occluded pupil. In this surgical condition, the impermeable pupillary membranes are removed by incisions with iridal scissors, and an anterior vitrectomy is performed. Once these impediments are removed, the pupillary flow of aqueous humor is re-established.

TRAUMATIC GLAUCOMAS

Traumatic glaucomas, which occur secondary to blunt and penetrating trauma, are infrequent in the dog. Complete acute hyphema is usually associated with uveal inflammation and low IOP; chronic or repeated intraocular hemorrhage is more apt to increase IOP. Direct damage to the trabecular meshwork and angle recession, which occurs in humans and results in glaucoma months to years after the traumatic incident, has not been reported in the dog. Canine traumatic glaucomas are usually associated with intense iridocyclitis and are best managed clinically, with aggressive treatment of the inflammation, prevention of peripheral anterior synechia, and control of the IOP (with CAIs). Intracameral TPA may be used to assist in resolving the anterior chamber fibrin after hyphema; however, this may cause more hemorrhage if blood clots dissolve because of the TPA.

UVEITIC GLAUCOMAS

The iridocyclitides are a group of frequent intraocular diseases in the dog, and the development of inflammatory glaucomas is a serious complication of these conditions. Inflammatory glaucomas may develop with either acute, intense iridocyclitis associated with pupillary occlusion and iris bombé; with obstruction of the filtration angle by inflammatory cells, fibrin, and cellular debris; or with chronic iridocyclitis, usually resulting from peripheral anterior synechia but, infrequently, from annular posterior synechia and iris bombé. The iridocyclitides may be associated with localized ocular diseases (e.g., corneal perforation, iris prolapse, iris bombé) and with many systemic infectious diseases. Vogt-Koyanagi-Harada syndrome (i.e., uveodermatologic syndrome) occurs in several Arctic breeds of dogs (Fig. 8-10), and a recently discovered chronic uveitis in the Golden Retriever occurs as chronic intraocular inflammations.

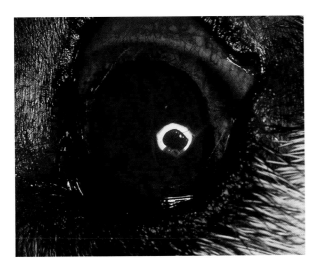

FIGURE 8-10. *Secondary glaucoma from angle closure and formation of extensive peripheral anterior synechiae and preiridal rubeosis in an Akita with uveodermatologic syndrome (Vogt-Koyanagi-Harada syndrome).*

Unfortunately, the serious long-term complications of chronic anterior uveitis are cataract formation and glaucoma.

The clinical signs of uveitic glaucoma are a combination of iridocyclitis and either acute or chronic glaucoma. The pupil may be normal in size, thus manifesting a balance between the iridal inflammation and the IOP. Episcleral venous congestion, which is often present in glaucoma, is partially masked by the conjunctival hyperemia (or the ciliary flush) associated with the anterior segment inflammation. Likewise, corneal edema may represent a combination of the intensity of iridocyclitis and the IOP.

Elevations in the IOP may be acute or gradual (e.g., over several weeks or months). Applanation tonometry is an important diagnostic procedure for uveitis. Most often, iridocyclitis decreases the IOP; however, the onset (within the first hours) of acute iridocyclitis actually produces a transient elevation in the IOP associated with the release of prostaglandins from the iris. The clinical signs of iridocyclitis with the dog with normal IOP may signal the early formation of peripheral anterior synechia. Treatment of uveitic glaucomas occurring secondary to peripheral anterior synechia in phakic eyes is targeted at the underlying uveitis and at controlling the IOP; thus, retinal and ONH damage are minimized. High levels of topical and systemic corticosteroids and nonsteroids are indicated. Neither miosis nor mydriasis is desired; therefore, short-term mydriatics may be used to intermittently move the inflamed iris and pupil and to discourage the formation of posterior synechiae. Topical and systemic antibiotics may also be indicated if an infectious process is present. Topical and systemic CAIs are administered to maintain (hopefully) the IOP within normal limits. Surgical treatments such as laser cyclophotocoagulation and anterior chamber shunts may also be attempted. As in humans, however, success rates in uveitic glaucomas are lower than those in other types of glaucoma in the dog because of the inflammation and the protein-rich aqueous humor.

MELANOCYTIC GLAUCOMA

Melanocytic glaucoma occurs primarily in the Cairn Terrier, and it may affect one or both eyes. Large aggregations of melanocytes occur within the filtration angle, episcleral and subconjunctival tissues, tapetal ocular fundus, and even the meninges around the ONH. What initiates the unchecked proliferations of these melanocytes is unknown, but the condition may represent a diffuse type of benign iris melanoma. Onset of the chronic glaucoma appears to be slow and associated with the accumulation of pigmented cells within the filtration angle and the scleral venous plexus. Medical and surgical treatment have not been successful in the long term, because the proliferating melanocytes eventually obstruct any surgical anterior chamber bypass.

INTRAOCULAR NEOPLASMS AND GLAUCOMA

The primary intraocular neoplasms that occur most frequently in the dog are melanomas and adenomas/adenocarcinomas of the cil-

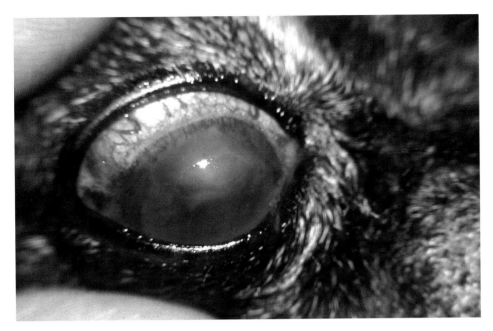

FIGURE 8-11. *Advanced secondary glaucoma associated with an anterior uveal melanoma. With these types of glaucoma, the aqueous humor outflow pathways may be obstructed by tumor, inflammatory debris from iridocyclitis (perhaps secondary to tumor necrosis), hyphema, and preiridal rubeosis.*

iary body and iris. Not infrequently, the presenting clinical sign of these anterior segment tumors is glaucoma, iridocyclitis, hyphema, or some combination of these (Fig. 8-11). Metastatic intraocular neoplasms, which are most often adenocarcinomas, also frequently involve the iris and the ciliary body. Lymphoma/lymphosarcoma may affect the anterior uvea as well. Glaucomas secondary to these neoplasms usually result from direct infiltration of the filtration angle, obstruction of the angle by tumor-associated inflammatory products and peripheral anterior synechiae, or formation of a secondary preiridal membrane. Rapidly growing neoplasms often produce glaucoma, and tumor-related necrosis may produce a secondary iridocyclitis. Most of these tumor-induced glaucomas are treated with enucleation, but local iridocyclectomy (with or without scleral grafts) may successfully remove smaller neoplasms and preserve vision.

GLAUCOMAS SECONDARY TO SILICONE OIL AND RHEGMATOGENOUS RETINAL DETACHMENTS

New glaucomas that have been recently reported or observed in the dog occur secondary to silicone oil in the anterior chamber and to rhegmatogenous retinal detachments.

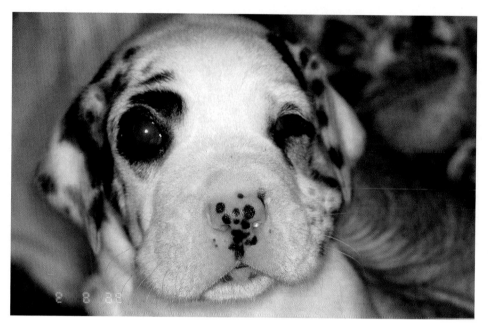

FIGURE 8-12. *Advanced congenital glaucoma in a 10-week-old Dalmatian. The cause was not determined.*

CONGENITAL GLAUCOMAS

Extensive goniodysgenesis/trabecular maldevelopment is rare in the dog. When present, however, it may be unilateral or bilateral and be an isolated defect or occur with other systemic anomalies. Elevations of the IOP occur early in the puppy's life (usually 3–6 months of age), and the primary complaint is one of rapid and often dramatic enlargement of the globe (Fig. 8-12). Histopathologic examination of the few globes with canine congenital glaucomas available for study has revealed multiple anterior segment and aqueous humor outflow abnormalities, including abnormalities of the trabecular meshwork.

MEDICAL AND SURGICAL THERAPY FOR PRIMARY GLAUCOMAS

TARGET, SAFE, AND DIURNAL INTRAOCULAR PRESSURE

The IOP has been firmly established as the primary risk factor, so the establishment of a "target" or "safe" IOP for each canine eye implies a reduction to levels that reduce the loss of RGCs from glaucoma to the normal, age-related levels of loss and thereby achieving an IOP that maintains the threshold number of RGCs necessary for vision. The target range provides a workable framework for therapeutic goals, but it should be re-evaluated periodically by an ophthalmic examination that includes tonometry.

MEDICAL THERAPY FOR THE CONTROL OF INTRAOCULAR PRESSURE

No single treatment regimen for the canine glaucomas is possible because of the many different types that exist (Box 8-4). In secondary glaucomas, the initiating cause is identified and, if possible, either removed or suppressed (Box 8-2). Medical treatment of canine glaucoma is

---

BOX 8-4

Control of Intraocular Pressure

Initial medical control

   IV mannitol (1–2 g/kg IV)

   Miotics (2% pilocarpine BID or TID)

   Adrenergics or β-blockers (SID or BID)

   Prostaglandins (SID -BID)

   Neuroprotective drugs (future)

Short-term control

   Miotics (2% pilocarpine BID or TID)

   Adrenergics or β-blockers (SID or BID)

   Carbonic anhydrase inhibitors (topical dorsolamide or brinzolamide BID or TID; or systemic methazolamide, 1–5 mg/kg per day orally BID in two divided doses)

   Prostaglandins (SID or BID)

   Neuroprotective drugs (future)

   Surgery/laser

Long-term control

   Surgery/laser cyclophotocoagulation

   Supplement with medical control

   Miotics (2% pilocarpine BID or TID)

   Adrenergics or β-blockers (SID or BID)

   Carbonic anhydrase inhibitors (topical dorsolamide or brinzolamide BID or TID; or systemic methazolamide, 1–5 mg/kg orally BID in two divided doses)

   Neuroprotective drugs (future)

a most important aspect, because surgical procedures often still require concurrent medical therapy. Such therapy for narrow- and closed-angle glaucomas is usually short term when employed alone, because eventually, the aqueous outflow becomes so impaired that drug-associated changes in the formation and outflow become inadequate. Results of some clinical studies are suggestive that the earlier in the glaucoma process the surgery is performed, the higher the long-term success rate at controlling IOP and maintaining vision for as long as possible. **Medical therapy for the glaucomas can be quite expensive. Additional information on these drugs can be found in Appendices A (adrenergics), G (CAIs), J (hyperosmotics), and K (miotics).**

Prophylactic treatment of fellow eyes in dogs presenting with unilateral primary glaucoma appears to delay the onset of glaucoma in these eyes for several months or longer (for more details, the reader should consult the third edition, pp. 734–738). Parasympathomimetics or miotics are used in most types of the canine glaucomas (except those associated with severe inflammations of the anterior segment) and are often combined with CAIs and β-adrenergic antagonists. Cholinergic miotics produce pupillary constriction, ciliary musculature contraction, and increased outflow facility of the aqueous humor through the trabecular meshwork. The most frequently used miotics in the dog are pilocarpine and demecarium bromide, though manufacturing of the latter has ceased in some countries.

Adrenergic agents such as epinephrine and dipivalyl epinephrine lower the IOP, but they must be combined with other drugs to achieve the greatest decreases. β-Antagonists or β-blockers (i.e., timolol, betaxolol, and levobunolol) provide inconsistent results in lowering the IOP of normal dogs but are frequently used clinically two times a day in canine glaucoma.

Hyperosmotic agents such as mannitol are used systemically in short-term treatment of acute glaucoma and before surgical procedures for glaucoma. With increased blood osmolarity, water is removed from the aqueous humor and the vitreous body, thus reducing the IOP (and the volume of the vitreous body).

Mannitol is administered intravenously at a dose of 1.0 to 1.5 g/kg. Ocular hypotension becomes evident within 30 minutes and lasts for at least 5 hours.

Systemic (acetazolamide, ethoxyzolamide, methazolamide, and dichlorphenamide) and topical (dorzolamide and brinzolamide) CAIs are useful in the treatment of all canine glaucomas. The CAIs reduce active aqueous humor formation by inhibiting the carbonic anhydrase enzymatic processes within the nonpigmented ciliary body epithelium. No direct effect, however, is exerted on the outflow facility. In the dog, CAIs reduce the IOP by 20 to 30%. The maximal effect usually occurs 4 to 8 hours after oral administration, and the ocular hypotensive effects of these drugs do not depend on diuresis. The CAIs are useful for both short- and long-term management of canine glaucomas.

Certain prostaglandins lower the IOP by increasing unconventional or uveoscleral outflow posteriorly through the ciliary body. Prostaglandin $F_{2\alpha}$ (instilled once or twice daily) lowers the IOP in the dog by approximately 20 to 30%.

Neuroprotection and neuroregeneration of the retina in glaucoma are new concepts, and drugs for this purpose in the dog are still experimental. Nevertheless, drugs will eventually be developed for this function.

SURGICAL TREATMENT FOR PRIMARY GLAUCOMAS

For narrow-angle and angle-closure glaucomas in the dog, surgical treatment is the first choice. Unfortunately, however, surgical treatments of canine primary glaucomas have not been very successful, only lowering the IOP for several months. Medical treatment usually provides a few months of effective IOP control. Anterior chamber shunts (i.e., gonioimplants) and laser cyclophotocoagulation appear to offer longer periods of successful IOP control than the traditional antiglaucoma filtering surgical procedures. Currently, no highly successful glaucoma surgery is available, so additional refinements are imperative.

Historically, the iridencleisis procedure, in which a radial section of iris is permanently positioned through a limbal incision into the subconjunctival spaces beneath the bulbar conjunctiva, is still useful for glaucoma secondary to iris bombé. Two newer treatment modalities, laser transscleral cyclophotocoagulation and anterior chamber shunts (gonioimplants) show promise in the clinical management of canine primary glaucomas. Because of the expense involved, anterior chamber shunts are usually reserved for glaucomatous eyes that are visual or that have the potential for vision. Laser cyclophotocoagulation is less expensive and is used in advanced glaucomatous eyes to reduce or eliminate the need for topical and systemic medications as well as to prevent pain.

The surgery for anterior chamber shunts consists of a fornix-based conjunctival flap and placement of the base of the anterior shunt approximately 10- to 12-mm posterior to the limbus (Fig. 8-13). The shunt's tubing is carefully positioned into the anterior chamber. (For more details, the reader should consult the third edition, pp. 740–746.) The long-term success or failure of the shunts is associated with the fibrosis of the host's capsule that develops around the episcleral base.

Several noninvasive cyclodestructive procedures have also been developed to treat primary glaucomas in small animals by decreasing formation of aqueous humor through partial destruction of the ciliary body processes. Proper positioning of the cryo and the laser probes is critical; these probes must be directly over the ciliary body processes. In the dog, this area is approximately 5 mm from the dorsal limbus.

Transscleral cyclophotocoagulation uses energy developed by different types of lasers to destroy the ciliary body and to reduce the formation of aqueous humor. Both noncontact and contact Nd:YAG and diode lasers have been used in different animal species, and though costly, are promising treatments of canine glaucoma (Fig. 8-14). Current results are suggestive that diode-laser cyclophotocoagulation may effectively lower the IOP for as long as 1 year (<50% of eyes) but is less effective at maintaining vision (22% of eyes).

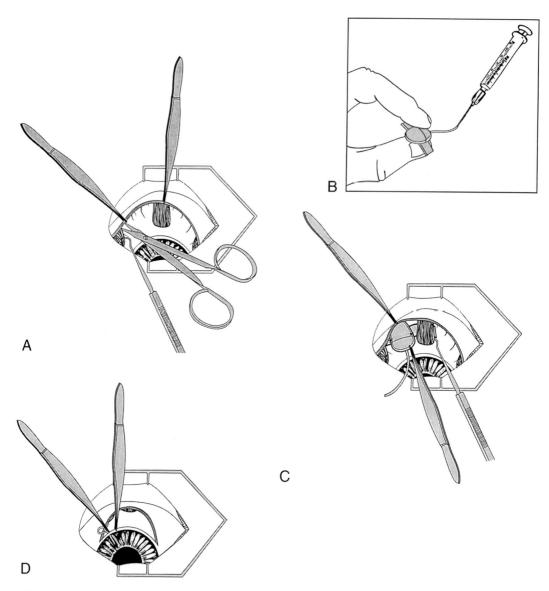

FIGURE 8-13. *Surgical placement is similar for all anterior chamber shunts.* **A.** *The dorso-lateral or dorsomedial quadrant is approached by scissor dissection under a fornix-based conjunctival flap. A space large enough to accommodate the episcleral base of the shunt between the dorsal rectus muscle and either the medial or the lateral rectus muscle is then prepared.* **B.** *The anterior chamber shunt must be primed with balanced salt solution before implantation.* **C.** *The anterior chamber shunt is positioned between the adjacent rectus muscles and, with some implants, under the rectus muscles. It is secured with simple inter-rupted nonabsorbable sutures.* **D.** *After limbal puncture with a 20- to 22-gauge hypodermic needle and creation of the proper length and beveled end for the tube, the silicone tubing is inserted into the anterior chamber. The anterior scleral aspect of this tube should be covered with autogenous or homologous sclera to protect the overlying bulbar conjunctiva.*

(continued)

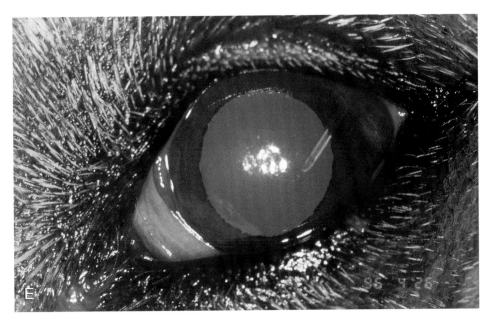

FIGURE 8-13—(continued) *E. Postoperative view showing the proper position of the anterior chamber shunt tubing within the anterior chamber. (Modified from Gelatt KN, Gelatt JP. Surgical procedures for treatment of the glaucomas. In: Handbook of small animal ophthalmic surgery. Vol 2: corneal and intraocular procedures. Oxford: Elsevier Science, 1995:117–161.)*

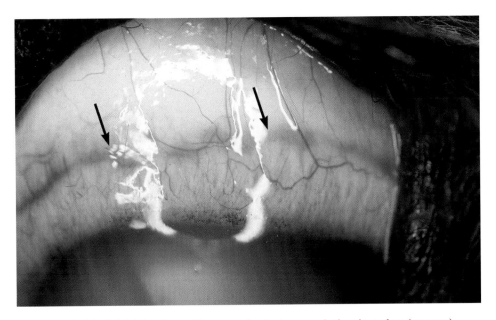

FIGURE 8-14. *Multiple sites of laser cyclophotocoagulation in a dog (arrows). With the contact diode laser, cyclophotocoagulation is performed at 1.2 W per site for 1.2 seconds. Thirty-five sites (20 dorsal and 15 ventral) are treated, for a total of 50 J per eye.*

TREATMENT OF END-STAGE PRIMARY GLAUCOMAS

Salvage procedures to prevent ocular pain, to reduce the enlarged and blind globe to near-normal size, and to provide a cosmetically acceptable eye that no longer requires medications include pharmacologic destruction of the ciliary body with intravitreal injection of gentamicin; intrascleral or intraocular prosthesis, in which a silicone ball is placed in an eviscerated globe; posterior sclerotomy combined with vitrectomy; and enucleation (i.e., surgical removal of the globe).

Pharmacologic destruction of the ciliary body with intravitreal injections of gentamicin is a salvage procedure for advanced-stage and blind canine glaucomatous eyes. Intravitreal gentamicin (25 mg of gentamicin sulfate and 1 mg of dexamethasone) is cytotoxic to the ciliary body epithelium and retina, and such therapy successfully lowers the IOP in 65% of patients undergoing treatment of absolute and blind glaucomatous eyes. Fifty percent of eyes that do not respond to the first injection of gentamicin also do not respond after the second injection, and approximately 10% of eyes will be phthisical after this treatment.

If cost is not a limitation, my preference is for evisceration and intrascleral prosthesis. This procedure treats the pain associated with absolute glaucoma, addresses the corneal exposure, provides a predictable size for the globe, and eliminates the need for antiglaucoma treatments (see Chapter 2; for more details, the reader should consult the third edition, pp. 527–528; and p. 748).

Diseases and Surgery of the Canine Anterior Uvea

The highly vascular and pigmented uveal tract consists of the anterior uvea (i.e., the iris and ciliary body) and the posterior uvea or choroid. Traditional diseases of the uveal tract are divided into anterior uveal disorders and posterior types, though sometimes diseases affect the entire uveal tract. **Anterior uveal diseases, and especially those with an inflammatory origin, are not infrequently seen in veterinary practice.**

IRIS AND CILIARY BODY MORPHOLOGY

The iris is divided histopathologically into the anterior border layer, iridal stroma, sphincter and dilator (i.e., myoepithelial cells) muscles, and posterior epithelium. The iris color depends on melanocytes within the stroma as well as on the pigmented posterior epithelium. The iridal sphincter, which is primarily innervated by parasympathetic fibers from the ciliary ganglion, consists of unstriated muscle fibers that are arranged around the pupil. The iris dilator muscles consist of a single layer of unstriated muscle fibers or highly developed, pigmented myoepithelium innervated primarily by sympathetic fibers. This layer continues to the ciliary body, where it becomes the inner pigmented epithelial layer. The pigmented iris epithelium forms the posterior layer of the iris and then continues posteriorly as the nonpigmented ciliary body epithelium. The iris blood supply is obtained from the long posterior ciliary arteries (located at the 9- and 3-o'clock position) and, within the iris, from the annular major arterial circle (located ≈50% in the base of iris and ≈50% in the anterior ciliary body), the radial arteries from this circle that run toward the pupil, and a variable, minor arterial circle (seen clinically as the collarette area).

The ciliary body is divided macroscopically into the anterior pars plicata (i.e., corona ciliaris) and the posterior pars plana. The anterior, outer part of the ciliary body also forms the ciliary cleft and the filtration angle (see Chapter 8). The anterior pars plicata consists of 70 to 100 ciliary processes, which are highly vascular and pigmented structures covered by the inner, nonpigmented (i.e., the primary source for the active component of aqueous humor production) and the outer, pigmented epithelia, which continues anteriorly with the iridal dilator muscle layer and posteriorly with the retinal pigment epithelial layer. The pars plana is the posterior, smooth portion of the ciliary body that bridges the ciliary processes anteriorly and the peripheral termination of the anterior retina (i.e., ora ciliaris retinae) posteriorly. The width of the pars plana is important clinically and, in the dog, is 7 to 8 mm from the limbus dorsally and laterally but only 4 mm ventrally and medially. Through the pars plana, entry to the vitreous (as with vitreal paracentesis) can be obtained without producing a hole in the retina and, in turn, possible retinal detachment. The main blood supply to the ciliary body is via the long posterior ciliary arteries (for more details, the reader should consult the third edition, pp. 61–79).

Hence, the ciliary body produces the aqueous humor, which nourishes and removes metabolic byproducts from the anterior lens, inner surfaces of the iris, and posterior cornea. It also develops the intraocular pressure (IOP; by the resistance to aqueous humor outflow through the filtration angle) and effects accommodation (via changes in zonular tension to the lens equator and capsules). The anterior uvea is also the site of the blood–aqueous barrier, which normally prevents large, high-molecular-weight proteins from entering the intraocular fluid. Changes in this barrier cause increases in the protein levels, which are seen clinically as "aqueous flare."

The uvea is highly vascular and immunosensitive; therefore, bilateral inflammatory ocular diseases are common and frequently occur as manifestations of systemic diseases. Pupillary light responses, which are critical for assessing cranial nerve functions and gauging the depth of anesthesia, are also altered in patients with anterior uveal disease.

CONGENITAL AND DEVELOPMENTAL DISORDERS

Developmental abnormalities of the canine anterior uvea range from incomplete development (e.g., hypoplasia) and maldevelopment (e.g., polycoria) to incomplete regression of embryonal tissues (e.g., persistent pupillary membranes [PPMs]). Most anterior uveal anomalies in the dog occur sporadically and, except for PPMs, are rare.

COLOR VARIANTS

Because normal ocular embryogenesis depends on the initial development of the pigmented layers of the eye, several congenital defects relate directly to ocular color dilution and, specifically, to the merling gene. Anterior uveal pigmentation in normal dogs exhibits considerable variation, which accounts for the marked differences in eye color both within and among breeds.

HETEROCHROMIA IRIDIS

When multiple colors occur within one iris or between the two irides, the term *heterochromia iridis* (or *irides*) is applicable. In the heterochromic eye, the iris is characterized by at least two distinct and solidly colored areas or by differently colored patches or spots (Fig. 9-1). Owners may use descriptive phrases such as "watch eye" or "china eye" to describe a multicolored iris.

Heterochromia iridis may be the sole manifestation of ocular color dilution in several breeds. These include the Old English Sheep Dog, Siberian Husky, American Fox Hound, American Cocker Spaniel, Malamute, and Shih Tzu. Apart from the variation in appearance, simple heterochromia iridis has no clinical significance.

IRIDAL CHANGES ASSOCIATED WITH THE MERLING GENE

Heterochromia iridis is also a component of ocular merling, and multiple ocular anomalies may be accompanied by iridal anomalies (e.g., iris hypoplasia, PPMs) and, therefore, may result in pupillary abnormalities. Anterior uveal manifestations of the merling gene may include heterochromia irides, thinning of the iris (i.e., iris hypoplasia), a black-rimmed pupil from prominent and exposed iridal pigmented epithelium, and an eccentric pupil (i.e., corectopia). Both typical and atypical iris colobomata and mild to severe PPMs are also common findings in merle dogs. Multiple ocular anomalies, including microphthalmia, cataracts, equatorial staphylomas, retinal dysplasia, and optic nerve hypoplasia, occur as an autosomal recessive trait in merle Australian Shepherds (for more details, the reader should consult the third edition, p. 755–756). Iris anomalies and multiple ocular anomalies also occur in other breeds affected by the merle gene (e.g., Great Danes, Collies, and Dachshunds).

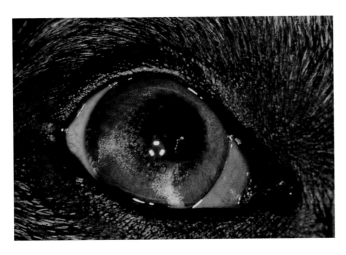

FIGURE 9-1. *Heterochromia iridis. Note the distinct, colored areas of iris.*

PERSISTENT PUPILLARY MEMBRANES

Incomplete resorption of iridal embryonal vasculature and mesenchymal tissues results in retained iris strands, which are termed *persistent pupillary membranes (PPMs)*. These membranes originate at the collarette region of the iris, and they extend to other areas of the iris, the posterior cornea, or the anterior surface of the lens (Fig. 9-2). Persistent pupillary membranes are common findings in the dog. Fortunately, however, most affected animals have only a minor degree of affliction and are not visually impaired. In severely affected eyes, the resultant corneal or lens opacities (or both) may compromise vision. Persistent pupillary membranes may be present either unilaterally or bilaterally. Benign forms include iris-to-iris strands that bridge the iris surface or cross the pupil and remnants with a single iris attachment that occur as small, free-floating

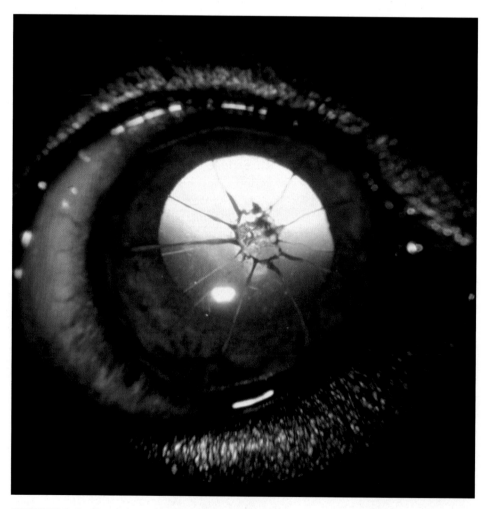

FIGURE 9-2. *Persistent pupillary membranes (PPMs) with confluence over the anterior lens capsule resulting in a cataract at this location. Note attachment of the PPMs to the collarette region of the iris.*

tags. Forms that can produce significant ocular opacification include iris-to-cornea strands and iris-to-lens strands. More than one form of PPM may occur in a single affected eye. Drug-induced mydriasis is not recommended for PPM-associated opacities, however, because pharmacologic dilation may induce tension on the membrane attachments and, thus, aggravate the corneal or lens lesions.

Heritable, clinically significant PPMs occur in the Basenji breed. The incidence of PPMs in these dogs is high, but the severity varies considerably. Familial PPMs occur in the Pembroke Welsh Corgi, Chow Chow, and Mastiff breeds, and use of affected animals for breeding is not recommended. In addition, PPMs have been associated with congenital cataracts in a litter of English Cocker Spaniels and in the Chow Chow.

Surgical alternatives generally are not indicated but include entering the anterior chamber to incise membranes attached to the cornea and extracapsular lentectomy for an extensive anterior capsular or subcapsular cataract. One potential danger of surgical intervention is that some membranes may be vascularized, and if these membranes are incised, intraocular hemorrhage may occur. Use of electrocautery to sever the membranes may minimize hemorrhage, however, and laser surgery offers a noninvasive alternative that also may reduce hemorrhage (for more details, the reader should consult the third edition, pp. 756–758).

UVEAL INFLAMMATIONS

Uveal inflammation (i.e., uveitis) is a component of most intraocular disease processes because of the uvea's highly vascular nature and its proximity to other intraocular structures. Inflammation of the anterior uvea (i.e., the iris and ciliary body) is termed *anterior uveitis* or *iridocyclitis;* inflammation of the posterior uvea (i.e., the choroid) is termed *posterior uveitis* or *choroiditis.* It is often useful to discuss inflammations of the anterior and posterior uvea as separate entities, though anatomically, they are contiguous structures and often simultaneously affected. Inflammation of the entire uveal tract is termed *panuveitis* and may be clinically inapparent but detectable at histopathology. A more advanced condition, which is termed *endophthalmitis,* is inflammation involving the ocular cavities and adjacent structures. Inflammation involving all tunics of the eye is termed *panophthalmitis,* and this may result in the signs of orbital disease as well.

PATHOGENESIS OF UVEITIS

The basic mechanisms in the pathogenesis of the different forms of anterior uveitis are still not completely understood, but as they are elucidated, new therapeutic opportunities are appearing. **A wide variety of exogenous and endogenous causes, both infectious or otherwise, for uveitis exist. Exogenous causes arise external to the eye and most commonly involve trauma (including surgical), corneal ulceration, or perforating** corneal wounds with or without secondary infection. **Endogenous causes arise within the eye or reach the uvea via the bloodstream, account for most cases of uveitis, and include infectious, neoplastic, toxic (which can also be exogenous), metabolic, or autoimmune diseases.** The concept of autoimmune disease has become increasingly important, because various endogenous antigens are now recognized as either initiating or perpetuating uveitis. The exact cause-and-effect relationship is not always apparent, but some endogenous antigens associated with immune phenomena of the eye include the retinal-S antigen, melanin, lens, and corneal proteins. The more commonly recognized causes of uveitis in the dog are listed in Box 9-1.

The pathogenesis of uveitis is extremely complex. It can be divided, however, into general uveal inflammatory responses, chemical mediators of inflammation, and specific immunologic responses (for more details, the reader should consult the third edition, pp. 759–764).

CLINICAL MANIFESTATIONS AND DIAGNOSIS

The diagnosis of uveitis is established on the basis of one or many ocular signs. Because the ocular response to various insults is limited, other primary ocular diseases may appear to be similar to uveitis. **Uveitis may also be an important secondary component of ocular disease, thus requiring therapeutic considerations differing from those of the primary disorder. Bilateral uveitis is often associated with systemic diseases. The clinical signs of uveitis are listed in Table 9-1.**

Excessive lacrimation, blepharospasm, and photophobia are readily ascertained at visual inspection of the animal, and they are suggestive of varying degrees of ocular discomfort not specific to uveitis. The patient history is helpful in establishing both the duration and any episodes of recurrence. **The term** *ciliary flush* **refers to hyperemia of the deep, perilimbal, anterior ciliary vessels (Fig. 9-3) and is more common with deep corneal and intraocular disease (i.e., uveitis).** Ciliary flush may be distinguished from the superficial conjunctival hyperemia that is more common with extraocular disease, but both types of vascular injection are often present in the dog with uveitis. Distinguishing between these vascular patterns may be facilitated by topical application to the eye of a sympathomimetic agent (e.g., 1% epinephrine solution) that will have a greater vasoconstrictive effect on the superficial conjunctival vessels than on the deeper, anterior ciliary vessels. In addition, conjunctival vessels move with the globe, whereas anterior ciliary vessels remain stationary during such movement.

Pupillary constriction (or miosis) is a response to prostaglandins and other inflammatory mediators that act directly on the iris sphincter muscle. Similar actions on the ciliary body musculature cause a painful ciliary body spasm, which in humans with uveitis is often described as "brow ache." Miosis is not present in all cases of uveitis, however. Chronic uveitis may result in adhesions of the iris to the anterior lens surface or posterior synechiae, which in turn results in an immobile or distorted pupil (Fig. 9-4). The pupil may be "fixed" in the constricted or mid-dilated position because of synechiae formation. Clumps of pigment on the

BOX 9-1

Diseases Proved or Suspected of Causing Uveitis in the Dog

Algal

Prototheca sp.

Bacterial

Brucella canis

Borrelia burgdorferi (Lyme disease)

Leptospira sp.

Septicemia of any cause

Fungal

Blastomyces dermatitidis

Coccidioides immitis

Cryptococcus neoformans

Histoplasma capsulatum

Other mycoses

Immune-mediated

Cataracts (lens-induced uveitis)

Immune-mediated thrombocytopenia

Immune-mediated vasculitis

Lens trauma (phacoclastic uveitis)

Uveodermatologic syndrome (similar to Vogt-Koyanagi-Harada in humans)

Metabolic

Diabetes mellitus (particularly diabetic cataract–induced uveitis)

Hyperlipidemia

Systemic hypertension

Miscellaneous

Coagulopathies

Deep necrotizing or nonnecrotizing scleritis

Drug-induced (particularly miotic agents)

Idiopathic

Idiopathic uveitis and exudative retinal detachment

Pigmentary uveitis in the Golden Retriever

continued

BOX 9-1 *(continued)*

Diseases Proved or Suspected of Causing Uveitis in the Dog

Miscellaneous—continued

Radiation therapy

Trauma

Toxemia of many causes (e.g., pyometra)

Ulcerative keratitis (any cause)

Miscellaneous parasitic

Ophthalmomyiasis interna posterior (*Diptera* sp.)

Ocular filariasis *(Dirofilaria immitis)*

Ocular larval migrans (*Toxocara* and *Balisascaris* sp.)

Neoplastic and paraneoplastic disorders

Histiocytic proliferative disease

Hyperviscosity syndrome

Granulomatous meningoencephalitis (formerly reticulosis)

Primary (melanoma) and secondary neoplasms (lymphosarcoma most common)

Protozoan

Leishmania donovani

Toxoplasma gondii

Ehrlichia canis or *platys*

Rickettsia rickettsii

Viral

Adenovirus infection (including postvaccinal "blue-eye")

Distemper virus

Herpes virus

Rabies

anterior lens capsule may indicate previous posterior synechiae and, therefore, uveitis. Lens capsular pigment from uveitis is usually darker than that associated with congenital remnants of the pupillary membrane; in the latter instance, pigment is usually confined to the axial lens surface. The iris commonly is swollen from edema and cellular infiltrates, which together with inflammatory mediators acting on the sphincter muscle impede normal mobility of the pupil. In the eye with uveitis, the pupil often dilates more slowly and incompletely after therapy with short-acting mydriatics (i.e., 1% tropicamide) compared with that in the normal eye, and this observation is itself diagnostic. Conversely, the pupil in the affected eye may respond sluggishly to light or even be nonresponsive because of increased IOP. Inflammatory debris may occlude the uveal trabeculae, thereby resulting in secondary glaucoma, and iris bombé glaucoma may occur, with formation of annular posterior synechiae (Fig. 9-5). Peripheral anterior synechiae in which the basal iris adheres to inner cornea are also possible, occurring either secondary to iris bombé glaucoma or from a chronically swollen iris and dilated pupil.

Increased turbidity of the aqueous humor (i.e., "aqueous flare") occurs as plasma proteins and cellular components accumulate within the anterior chamber after the blood–aqueous barrier has been disrupted. Vitreous flare may occur in a similar manner. Light scattering from particles suspended in the anterior chamber produces a continuous light reflection throughout the chamber. This continuous-beam effect is called the **Tyndall phenomenon,** and it is analogous to shining a flashlight in a smoke-filled room. Observation of the Tyndall phenomenon is indicative of aqueous flare. Varying degrees of aqueous flare are possible, and though this scheme is highly subjective, some clinicians attempt to quantitate flare

TABLE 9-1

CLINICAL SIGNS OF UVEITIS

Anterior Uveitis	*Posterior Uveitis*	*Adverse Sequelae*
Aqueous flare	Choroidal effusion	Cataract
Ciliary flush	Decreased vision	Deep corneal vascularization
Conjunctival hyperemia	Granulomas	
Corneal edema	Optic neuritis	Ectropion uvea
Decreased intraocular pressure	Retinal separation	Endophthalmitis/ panophthalmitis
Decreased vision	Retinal hemorrhage	Iris atrophy
Hyphema	Vitreous opacities	Lens luxation
Hypopyon		Phthisis bulbi
Iris color change (usually darker)		Rubeosis iridis (or preiridal fibrovascular membrane)
Iris swelling		Secluded pupil and iris bombé
Keratic precipitates		Secondary glaucoma
Miosis		
Pain		

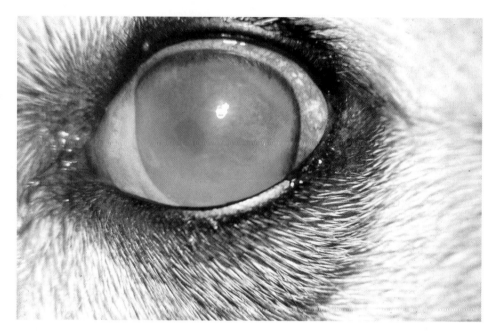

FIGURE 9-3. *Ciliary flush, diffuse conjunctival hyperemia, and miosis in a dog with anterior uveitis.*

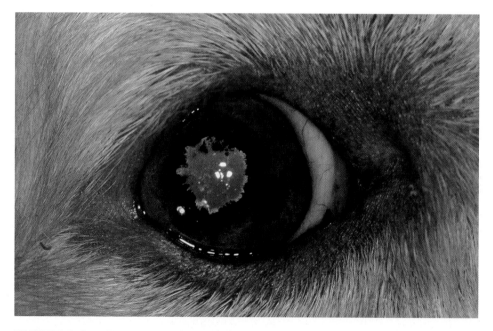

FIGURE 9-4. *Effects of chronic iridocyclitis in the dog: irregular and fixed pupil, numerous posterior synechiae, loss of iridal pigmentation, focal pigmentation proliferation, and foci of iridal tissue adhered to the anterior lens capsule.*

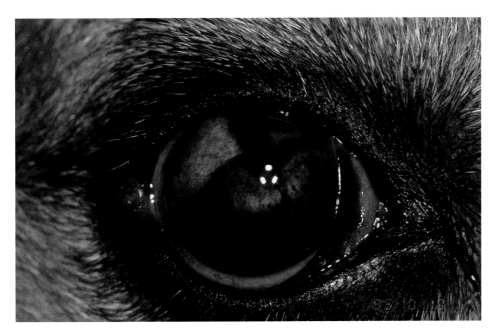

FIGURE 9-5. *Chronic iridocyclitis, annular posterior synechiae, and iris bombé in a dog.*

as "1+" to "4+," with higher numerals indicating increased severity. Slit-lamp biomicroscopy is ideal for the detection of aqueous flare, but other focal light sources (e.g., the small aperture of a direct ophthalmoscope) may be useful as well.

The term *fibrinous* (or *plasmoid*) *aqueous* refers to an increased level of aqueous protein, approximating that of normal plasma. If fibrinous exudation is severe, fibrin clots may form in the anterior chamber. Reported mean values for aqueous protein in noninflamed canine eyes using different assays range from 21 ± 1.2 mg/dL to 37.4 ± 7.9 mg/dL. In sharp contrast, aqueous protein values at various time intervals after the onset of uveitis range from approximately 1200 mg/dL to as high as 6600 mg/dL in experimental and clinical cases, respectively. These values approach those of normal canine plasma, which ranges from 6.0 to 7.5 g/dL.

Visible exudates of red and white blood cells within the anterior chamber are the most marked examples of breakdown in the blood–uveal barrier, and they are termed *hyphema* (Fig. 9-6) and *hypopyon* (Fig. 9-7), respectively. In both instances, cellular components typically gravitate toward the ventral anterior chamber and settle in a homogeneous layer. Keratic precipitates are accumulations of inflammatory cells, fibrin, and pigment that adhere to the corneal endothelium. They are usually deposited in a ventral location on the endothelium because of thermal convection currents.

Cytologic evaluation, bacterial or fungal culture of the aqueous humor, vitreous aspiration, or some combination thereof may be beneficial in determining the cause of uveitis. Aqueous aspiration appears to yield useful and positive results, mainly in eyes with visible exudates or in animals

FIGURE 9-6. *Hyphema associated with iridocyclitis and Rocky Mountain spotted fever in a dog.*

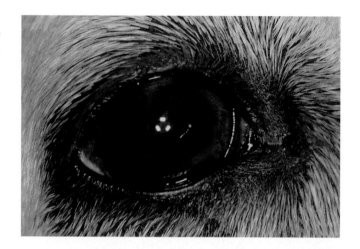

FIGURE 9-7. *Hypopyon and iridocyclitis in a dog with lymphosarcoma. The hypopyon is limited to the lower anterior chamber.*

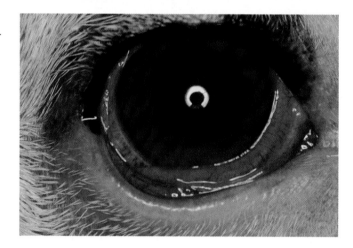

suspected of having lymphosarcoma. The most predictable results of aqueous aspiration are the identification of both nonspecific inflammatory cells and exacerbation of existing uveitis; hence, the procedure is not recommended in most cases.

Decreased IOP is one of the earliest—and most subtle—indications of uveitis. The exact mechanisms for the decreased IOP are undetermined, but proposed mechanisms include decreased aqueous humor production, with breakdown of the blood–aqueous barrier, and increased uveoscleral flow mediated in part by prostaglandins. The IOP will vary depending on the duration or the severity (or both) of uveitis. An absolute IOP determination of less than 10 mm Hg is consistent with the diagnosis of uveitis. Notable differences in IOP (e.g., ≥5 mm Hg) between two eyes, even if the values obtained are in the absolute normal range, should also be considered as significant, and they may suggest that the eye with the lower IOP has uveitis. In acute or subacute uveitis, the IOP is usually decreased because of the previously mentioned reasons; in chronic uveitis, fibrosis or atrophy (or both) of the ciliary body may contribute to decreased secretory function and ocular hypotony. Marked ciliary body dysfunction and hypotony may produce shrinkage of the globe (or phthisis bulbi). If uveitis is intense or persists long enough for inflammatory debris to obstruct the filtration angle or to seclude the pupil, however, secondary glaucoma may occur.

Corneal edema is often present, in varying degrees, with uveitis. Antigen–antibody complexes or inflammatory debris (or both) adhering to the corneal endothelium with disruption of endothelial function is largely responsible for the edema in uveitis.

Systemic Evaluation

After the diagnosis of uveitis is made, the clinician should next attempt to identify the cause. Because of the seemingly unlimited number of potential causes, including immune-mediated disease, a precise etiologic diagnosis may not be possible. **A thorough patient history and general physical examination are indicated in all cases, and a complete blood count, serum biochemistry profile, urinalysis, and thoracic radiography are recommended as minimal screening for uveitis in cases with suspected systemic disease.** Additional diagnostic tests are selected according to one's knowledge of the diseases that are endemic to a given practice area (e.g., coccidioidomycosis in the southwestern United States), any additional physical findings (e.g., coagulation studies if hyphema of undetermined cause or generalized petechiations are present), or simply one's own index of suspicion for a specific disease. (For more details, the reader should consult Chapter 17 and the third edition, pp. 764–768.)

THERAPY FOR UVEITIS

Symptomatic topical anti-inflammatory therapy for uveitis should be instituted immediately after the diagnosis is established—even in those patients with suspected multisystem disease. Failure to institute prompt therapy may result in numerous adverse sequelae of uveitis, including synechiae formation, cataract, glaucoma, endophthalmitis, and phthisis bulbi. **Systemic therapy requires greater discretion, and it may include various combinations of anti-inflammatory, antimicrobial, and additional specific therapy as determined by the specific multisystem disease (Table 9-2). Topical therapy alone may suffice for mild anterior uveitis, but systemic therapy is also indicated for severe anterior uveitis and posterior uveitis. Once a specific cause has been identified, therapy should be modified to treat the underlying disorder** (for more details, the reader should consult the third edition, pp. 768–771).

UVEAL MANIFESTATIONS
OF SELECTED DISEASES

This section summarizes selected diseases that may be presented to the veterinarian. **Unilateral or bilateral uveitis is possible with many multiple system diseases** (for more details, the reader should consult the third edition, pp. 772–774 and 1403–1422).

TABLE 9-2

RECOMMENDED THERAPY FOR ANTERIOR UVEITIS IN THE DOG

Drug	Dose	Effects/Limitations/Comments
Corticosteroids		
Topical		
1% prednisolone or 0.1% dexamethasone	4–6 times daily	Suppress uveal inflammation; decrease aqueous flare.
Systemic (parenteral/oral)		Avoid with the mycosis and corneal ulcers; use caution (or
Prednisolone	0.5–1.0 mg/kg BID	avoid) with diabetes mellitus
Subconjunctival		Avoid in potential surgical
Triamcinolone acetonide, methyl-prednisolone, betamethasone, or dexamethasone	5–10 mg	sites
Nonsteroidal anti-inflammatory drugs		
Topical		
Indomethacin, flur-biprofen, suprofen, or diclofenac	2–4 times daily	
Systemic		
Flunixin meglumine	0.25 mg/kg for up to 5 days, or 0.5 mg/kg for up to 3 days, or 0.25 to 1.00 mg/kg as a single IV dose	May be used either alone or in conjunction with systemic corticosteroids; potential for gastrointestinal complications
Carprofen	2 mg/kg orally BID–TID	Hepatotoxicity has been recognized, particularly in the Labrador Retriever
Immunosuppressives		
Azathioprine	Initial dosage is 2 mg/kg per day for 3–5 days, then taper based on response	Frequent blood and platelet counts as well as liver enzyme determinations because of potential hepatotoxic and myelosuppressive effects of this drug
Antimicrobials		
Topical		
Broad spectrum		Often combined with corticosteroids
Systemic		
Amoxicillin, trimethoprim/sulfadiazine, cephalosporin, and chloramphenicol		Chose based on antibacterial activity and ability to penetrate blood-aqueous barrier

continued

TABLE 9-2

RECOMMENDED THERAPY FOR ANTERIOR UVEITIS IN THE DOG

Drug	Dose	Effects/Limitations/ Comments
Antimicrobials—continued Mydriatics/cycloplegics Atropine (1%)	2–6 times daily	Dilate and provide pupil mobility to decrease posterior synechiae; decrease "ocular" pain; stabilize the blood-aqueous barrier; contraindicated by elevated intraocular pressures; side effects with atropine include decreased tear production
0.3% Scopolamine/ 10% phenylephrine	To effect	Very strong mydriatic combination to break fibrous adhesions and dilate pupils unresponsive to atropine

LENS-INDUCED UVEITIS

Lens-induced uveitis (LIU) is frequently encountered in the dog and is associated with cataract maturity. The degree of LIU varies substantially between individual patients. The results of one recent fluorophotometric study, however, are indicative that all dogs with cataract formation have at least a subclinical uveitis. Recognition and treatment of uveitis are important before cataract surgery is considered, because concurrent LIU increases the likelihood of postoperative complications and decreases the success rate of such surgery. Lens proteins are potentially very antigenic, and it is currently thought that small amounts of lens protein escape the normal lens and induce immunologic tolerance. Exposure to lens proteins after trauma, spontaneous lens resorption, or cataract extraction, however, will produce variable uveitis that depends largely on the degree or persistence of the antigen exposure (or both). The normal, low-dose T-cell tolerance to lens protein is overwhelmed in these latter instances.

At least two distinct types of LIU are currently recognized in the dog, though others may exist. Unfortunately, the terminology used varies among authors. **Phacolytic uveitis occurs in dogs with rapidly developing or hypermature cataracts, in which soluble lens protein leaks through an intact lens capsule.** This type of LIU is characterized by mild lymphocytic–plasmacytic uveitis, not unlike that which occurs with most idiopathic uveitides. This type of uveitis must be treated before cataract surgery and usually responds to conventional therapy.

Another type of uveitis, which is known as granulomatous LIU, may be a more severe manifestation of the nongranulomatous (or phacolytic) uveitis. Granulomatous LIU typically occurs in older dogs with rapidly progressive or long-standing cataracts, and the lens capsule in these dogs is likewise intact. Clinical features include mutton-fat erratic precipitates and a less favorable response to therapy compared with that of the nongranulomatous form. Phacoclastic uveitis is a considerably more intractable form of uveitis that occurs after rupture of the lens capsule. There may be a history of recent ocular trauma, but the eye is often not examined until late in the course of disease, when the cause is not immediately apparent. The results of one study are suggestive that prophylactic lens removal after capsular rupture is associated with a more favorable prognosis compared with that from medical treatment alone. Hence, in the dogs with cataracts, earlier surgical intervention is now recommended (at the onset of cataracts and before blindness) to reduce the adverse effects of LIU.

PIGMENTARY UVEITIS IN THE GOLDEN RETRIEVER

Pigmentary uveitis is a recently recognized, but poorly characterized, disease in the Golden Retriever. It is not associated with any systemic disease. The uveitis may be unilateral at first presentation but will often later become bilateral. Dispersion of pigment in the anterior chamber appears to be important to the disease progression. The iris appears dark and thickened, and clumps of pigment are noted on the anterior lens capsule and, possibly, the corneal endothelium. Pigment cells and aqueous flare are noted in the anterior chamber as well. Sequelae to chronic pigmentary uveitis include posterior synechiae, postinflammatory cataract, and glaucoma.

MYCOSES-ASSOCIATED UVEITIS

Disseminated mycotic infections with ocular involvement are relatively common among dogs in endemic areas. The ocular disease is often the owner's presenting complaint. **Common systemic mycoses include blastomycosis, coccidioidomycosis, histoplasmosis, and cryptococcosis (Table 9-3).** Inhalation is believed to be the primary route of infection for all the major systemic mycoses, with later hematogenous spread to the eye. Direct animal-to-animal or animal-to-human infection, however, is rare. Ocular involvement may be unilateral or bilateral, and infections of the paranasal sinus, orbit, and optic nerve may affect the eye secondarily.

The diagnosis is established on the basis of concurrent clinical signs, identification of organisms in ocular and other tissue aspirates, or the results of fungal culture, histopathologic examination, or various serologic tests. The typical histopathologic pattern for all mycoses is granulomatous or pyogranulomatous inflammation characterized by variable numbers of neutrophils, lymphocytes, plasma cells, histiocytes, and occasionally, epithelioid cells. Histopathologic identification of organisms is facilitated by the use of special stains (e.g., Gomori's methenamine-silver, periodic acid-Schiff, and mucicarmine).

The preferred systemic therapy varies for each type of mycosis (Box 9-2). Current treatment protocols use amphotericin B, itraconazole, ketoconazole, 5-fluorocytosine (i.e., flucytosine), or some combination of these. Eyes that are potentially visual should be treated topically for uveitis, but a painful, blind eye is best enucleated.

TABLE 9-3

DIAGNOSIS AND TREATMENT OF SYSTEMIC MYCOSES AND UVEITIS IN THE DOG

Mycosis	Uvea Affected	Diagnosis	Treatment
Blastomyces dermatitidis	Anterior/ posterior	Vitreous aspirates Serologic tests: agar gel immunodiffusion (specificity, 90%). Cross-reactivity with *H. Capsulatum*.	Itraconazole (5 mg/kg) orally BID for the first 2 weeks, followed by SID administration. Parenteral amphotericin B is somewhat effective, but with potential renal toxicity. Ketoconazole (can also combine with amphotericin) 10 mg/kg per day to 30 mg/kg orally per day.
Coccidioides immitis	Mainly posterior	Serology diagnosis: tube precipitin (immunoglobulin M antibody levels, immunoglobulin M; both appear and disappear early). Complement fixation (immunoglobulin G antibody, which persists longer). Titer of 1:8 or greater is considered to be suspicious; titer of 1:16 or greater is considered to indicate disseminated disease.	Oral ketoconazole, 10 mg/kg orally BID.
Cryptococcus neoformans	Mainly posterior	Identification or culture organism in ocular or cerebrospinal fluid; latex agglutination test.	Systemic amphotericin B and flucytosine (efficacy unknown).
Histoplasma capsulatum	Mainly posterior	Cytologic identification or culture organism. Serology problematic, but complement fixation used.	Amphotericin B and ketoconazole.

UVEODERMATOLOGIC SYNDROME

Uveodermatologic syndrome (UDS) was first reported in 1977, and because of the remarkable similarities with the Vogt-Koyanagi-Harada (VKH) syndrome in humans, the disease has also been called VKH-like in the dog. Uveodermatologic syndrome appears primarily to affect young adult dogs (mean age, 2.8 years). A slightly greater incidence in male dogs has been suggested as well. **An immunogenetic predisposition in the dog is suggested by the more frequent occurrence in the Akita, Samoyed,**

BOX 9-2

Emergency Management of Acute Ocular Trauma

1. Restrain the patient carefully, and if necessary, administer sedatives to examine the eye and associated tissues.

2. Gently irrigate the ocular surface with warm, physiologic saline solution (without preservative) to remove debris or exudates, if present.

3. Determine whether laceration or rupture of the globe has occurred, and if so, attempt to determine the extent. Any globe with hyphema is suspect!

4. If the globe is intact, apply topical anesthetic solution, and inspect the ocular surfaces, including the conjunctival fornices and both sides of the nictitating membrane, for foreign bodies.

5. If the globe is ruptured, determine whether surgical repair is feasible or if enucleation or implantation of an intraocular prosthesis should be advised. This determination is made on the basis of the extent of the intraocular damage, the likelihood of preserving vision, and cosmetic concerns. Ultrasonography may be necessary.

6. Administer systemic antibiotics.

7. Temporary tarsorrhaphy may be used to protect the eye when transport of the animal to a veterinary ophthalmologist is anticipated or the animal's general condition (e.g., concurrent head or chest trauma) necessitates stabilizing the patient.

Siberian Husky, and Shetland Sheepdog breeds. Additional breeds in which UDS is reported include the Golden Retriever, Irish Setter, Old English Sheepdog, Saint Bernard, Australian Shepherd, and Chow Chow. Similar to VKH in humans, viral infection has been postulated to initiate UDS in the dog. **Ocular findings usually precede, or at least are recognized before, dermatologic changes, and they include bilateral anterior uveitis or panuveitis, uveal depigmentation, retinal separation, and blindness (Fig. 9-8). Cataract, extensive posterior synechiae, iris bombé, and secondary glaucoma with buphthalmos are frequent sequelae. Dermatologic findings include vitiligo of the eyelids, nasal planum, lips, scrotum, and footpads. Poliosis may be confined to the facial region or be generalized.** Alopecia occurs inconsistently.

Clinically evident neurologic disease is conspicuously absent in the dog. Analysis of cerebrospinal fluid and postmortem examination of central nervous system tissue have yielded normal results among the limited cases in which these parameters have been examined.

Routine laboratory parameters are normal, and results of immune function tests are usually nondiagnostic. Ocular histopathologic examination reveals primarily granulomatous panuveitis and, often, retinal separation, destruction of the retinal pigment epithelium, and choroidal scarring. Pigment-containing macrophages are a prominent feature as well. Histopathologic examination of the skin reveals interface dermatitis with a primarily lichenoid pattern. Large histiocytic cells, plasma cells, and small mononuclear cells are characteristic.

Variable control of UDS with topical and systemic corticosteroid therapy is possible, but recurrence is common. Uveodermatologic syndrome is difficult to control with steroids alone without causing undesirable weight gain, polyuria, and polydipsia. Subconjunctival injection of a repository steroid is beneficial in controlling inflammation of the anterior segment. **The prognosis for long-term control is less favorable, however, and use of corticosteroids combined with other immunosuppressive drugs may be necessary.** Azathioprine (Imuran) has been used successfully; the starting dose is usually 2 mg/kg per day, with the dosage being reduced after 3 to 5 days.

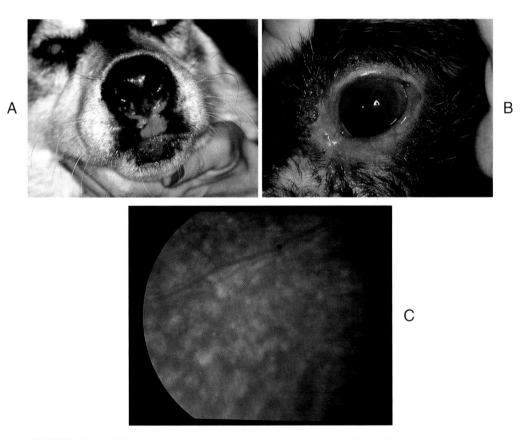

FIGURE 9-8. *Akita with uveodermatologic syndrome.* **A.** *Note the loss of pigmentation or vitiligo of the nasal planum.* **B.** *Chronic iridocyclitis, hyphema, and secondary glaucoma.* **C.** *Funduscopic appearance, with multiple areas of retinal pigment epithelium and choroidal depigmentation.*

DEGENERATIVE DISEASES

SENILE IRIS ATROPHY

Spontaneous progressive thinning of the stroma or pupillary portion of the iris (or both) is a common finding among middle-aged and older dogs (Fig. 9-9). Senile iris atrophy may occur in any breed, but the Toy and Miniature Poodles, Miniature Schnauzer, and Chihuahua are more often affected. Senile iris atrophy may initially manifest as a subtle color change: The natural iris color fades, and foci of hyperpigmentation may be noted as stroma is lost and the pigmented epithelium exposed. As the degeneration progresses, additional thinning may result in the loss of pigmented epithelial layers. With transillumination, affected areas are observed as translucent patches or openings within the iris.

In some cases, the pupillary margin develops a scalloped, moth-eaten appearance. In these dogs, atrophy of the pupillary muscles often results in dyscoria and, eventually, may account for the reduced or absent pupillary light responses and the increased sensitivity to bright illumination. Vision, however, is unaffected by this condition. The cause is unknown, and there is no treatment.

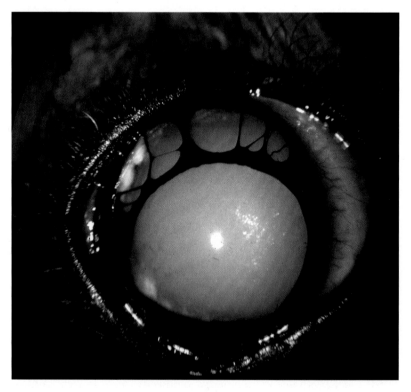

FIGURE 9-9. *Advanced iris atrophy with a hypermature cataract. Note the extensive, diffuse thinning and atrophy of the iridal stroma. Atrophic areas may be mistaken for iris colobomata.*

SECONDARY IRIS ATROPHY

Trauma, chronic uveitis, and glaucoma may cause degenerative changes in the iris resembling those of senile iris atrophy. Signs of pre-existing disease, such as synechiae or pigment dispersion on the anterior lens capsule, may occur as well. Treatment is aimed at controlling the active primary or secondary disease.

UVEAL CYSTS

Cysts of the iris and the ciliary body commonly occur in the dog and may be either congenital or acquired. Because most uveal cysts occur in middle-aged and older dogs, it has been suggested that most are acquired. Trauma and inflammation have been proposed as being causes of acquired cysts, but the cause for most uveal cysts remains unknown.

Most cysts are first noted clinically in adult dogs, and they occur spontaneously, presumably as a degenerative phenomenon. Generally, uveal cysts are benign and occur as incidental findings in the dog. **Iridal or ciliary cysts can be unilateral or bilateral, single or multiple, and spherical, oval, or elongate translucent masses (Fig. 9-10). Iris cysts tend to be black and ciliary body cysts brown, though pale brown or yellow may be seen as well.** Iris cysts are often observed as free-floating structures within the anterior chamber or, less commonly, the posterior chamber. Ciliary body cysts may be evident only with mydriasis or at gonioscopy (or both). Rarely do uveal cysts obstruct vision or cause lens or corneal opacities. Iridociliary cysts in the Golden Retriever have been associated with glaucoma and pigmentary uveitis.

The primary differential diagnosis is a uveal melanocytic neoplasm. Fortunately, clinical differentiation is usually not difficult, because unlike true uveal neoplasms, which are solid masses, most uveal cysts are easily transilluminated. Additional features that distinguish cysts from neoplasms include tremulousness, loculation, multiplicity, and mobility. Ocular ultrasonography may reveal the cystic nature in challenging cases.

Therapy usually is not necessary, and it is not recommended in dogs without symptoms. Techniques to remove uveal cysts include a limbal incision with needle aspiration or electrocautery. The neodymium: yttrium-aluminum-garnet laser is a noninvasive alternative for destroying uveal cysts, but the simplest technique is cyst collapse via anterior chamber paracentesis and fine-needle aspiration using a 25- or 27-gauge needle.

UVEAL TRAUMA

Ocular trauma may result in uveal contusion and intraocular hemorrhage, with or without disruption of the fibrous tunics. Anterior uveal contusion manifests as uveitis, and it may include epibulbar hyperemia, focal corneal edema, iris congestion, miosis, and hypotony. These findings are usually

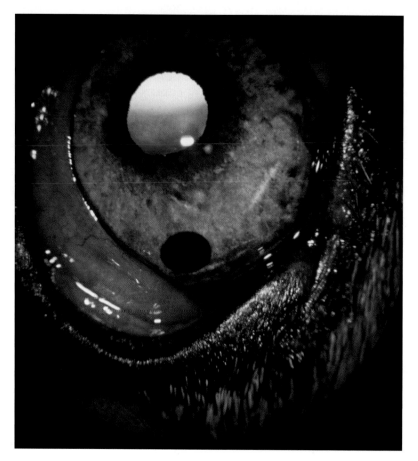

FIGURE 9-10. *A pigmented iris cyst floating within the anterior chamber. The iris cyst is heavily pigmented, but transillumination with an intense, focal light beam is possible.*

accompanied by fibrin and cellular debris within the anterior chamber. Anterior uveal trauma frequently results in vascular damage and subsequent hemorrhage within the anterior chamber, uveal stroma, or around the lens equator. With trauma, the extent of any ocular and periocular damage is established by careful ophthalmologic examination as well as ultrasonic and radiographic imaging.

With penetrating trauma, in which the cornea or the anterior sclera has been ruptured, protrusion of pigmented uveal tissue (i.e., staphyloma) is usually evident. Rupture of the posterior sclera with uveal prolapse, however, generally is not apparent at direct examination. If the cornea is intact and the media is clear enough to permit examination of the intraocular structures, the integrity of the iris, lens, vitreous, and retina may possibly be determined by direct visualization. Corneal edema, miosis, and intraocular hemorrhage, however, may preclude a detailed direct examination and necessitate ultrasonic imaging to assess the extent of intraocular damage. Guidelines for the examination of patients with ocular trauma are summarized in Box 9-2.

TREATMENT OF BLUNT INJURIES

Acute traumatic uveitis from blunt injury is treated in a manner similar to empiric treatment for other causes of anterior uveitis, unless extensive hyphema is a complicating factor (see the discussions of uveal inflammation and hyphema in this chapter). The pressure exerted on the globe during blunt trauma may result in a rebound phenomenon, whereby the vector force reflects off the posterior sclera and is transferred anteriorly, thus causing a "blow out" rupture of the perilimbal cornea or anterior sclera. A ruptured globe resulting from blunt trauma is handled in a manner similar to that for cases of penetrating corneal trauma with uveal prolapse. In cases of blunt ocular trauma with globe rupture, extensive intraocular damage has generally occurred, and severe adverse sequelae (i.e., iris bombé, traumatic cataract, retinal separation, endophthalmitis, phthisis bulbi) may occur. Therefore, the prognosis after severe blunt trauma to an eye may be comparable to that of severe ocular injuries after penetration of the globe. The combination of hyphema, subconjunctival hemorrhages, and retrobulbar hemorrhage often result in phthisis bulbus.

TREATMENT OF PENETRATING INJURIES

Focal "in and out" punctures of the globe may cause minimal damage to the fibrous tunic, and they may seal spontaneously (Fig. 9-11). If the eye is examined within a few hours of the injury, determining whether the cornea or sclera was completely penetrated or the extent of intraocular damage may be difficult. Penetrating corneal injuries that seal spontaneously are treated in a manner similar to nonspecific anterior uveitis. A topical corticosteroid, however, is not applied until the corneal epithelium has healed.

Penetrating injuries of the globe may result in uveal prolapse (or staphyloma), which appears as a protrusion of darkly pigmented tissue through the cornea or sclera. A grayish, fibrinous membrane typically covers the prolapsed uvea. Other associated conditions include a shallow or absent anterior chamber, loss of the pupil, and hyphema. Traumatic staphylomas require surgical repair involving replacement or amputation of the prolapsed uvea; specific steps in the repair of uveal prolapse were discussed in Chapter 7. The prognosis after staphyloma repair varies depending on the time between the injury and treatment, concurrent infection, presence of a pupil opening, patency of the iridocorneal angle, amount of corneal scarring, and the integrity of other intraocular structures (e.g., lens and retina).

MEDICAL TREATMENT OF TRAUMATIC
UVEITIS WITH LENS RUPTURE

Phacoclastic uveitis is a serious sequela of penetrating ocular trauma, and it may precipitate fulminating endophthalmitis. Phacoclastic uveitis occurs when the lens capsule has been ruptured and lens cortex liberated into the anterior or the posterior chamber. **In young puppies, it may occur after penetrating injuries from a cat's claw or, in older dogs, with penetrating buckshot wounds. The results of one study are suggestive that**

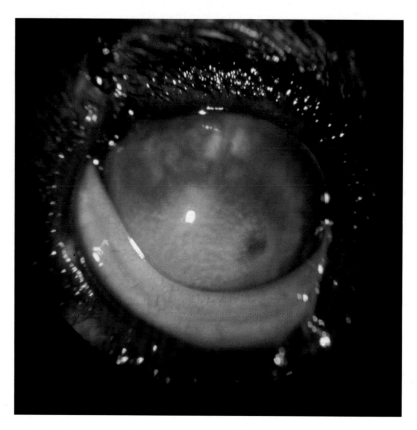

FIGURE 9-11. *Corneal perforation, corneal edema, and iridocyclitis in a dog secondary to buckshot. At ultrasonography, the lens was noted to have been traversed by the buckshot as well.*

early surgical removal of the ruptured lens is associated with a more favorable long-term prognosis. Medical treatment of phacoclastic uveitis is difficult. It requires aggressive and sustained topical as well as systemic corticosteroid therapy, and concurrent with immunosuppressive doses of the systemic corticosteroids, therapeutic doses of oral nonsteroidal anti-inflammatory drugs may be indicated as well. Topical mydriatic therapy with 1% atropine is also recommended. Without removal of the "leaking" lens, intensive medical therapy often results in endophthalmitis or secondary glaucoma. Enucleation or evisceration/prosthesis implantation surgery may be necessary if the affected eye is blind and causes discomfort to the dog.

INTRAOCULAR FOREIGN BODIES

Intraocular foreign bodies may be characterized by a range of clinical signs. This variability in presenting signs results from the type, size, location, and point of entry of the foreign material and from the severity of the initial trauma. Organic foreign bodies most likely to penetrate the globe include wood splinters, thorns, pine needles, cactus needles, and porcupine quills. Inorganic foreign bodies may be subdivided into reactive and nonreactive (i.e., inert) substances. Reactive substances are metals that oxidize within tissues (e.g., iron, steel, copper). Inert materials include lead, silver, gold, stainless steel, glass, and most plastics. **Radiography and ultrasonography are ancillary procedures; their greatest value is in establishing the diagnosis of metallic ocular foreign bodies.** Treatment depends on its nature, size, and location of the foreign body; the extent of any associated tissue damage; and the amount of uveal inflammation.

HYPHEMA

Intraocular hemorrhage occurs when uveal or retinal vessels are torn, disrupted, or anomalously formed, and such hemorrhage often manifests as hyphema (Fig. 9-12). In the dog, intraocular hemorrhage most commonly results from head trauma (e.g., automobile accidents or horse-kick injuries). Traumatic hyphema is frequently accompanied by subconjunctival and orbital hemorrhage; nontraumatic hyphema may result from many different ocular and systemic disorders. The causes of hyphema are summarized in Box 9-3. **Most hyphemas reabsorb without sequelae, but the cause of the intraocular bleed should still be determined and treated.** With spontaneous hyphema, the most informative ancillary diagnostic procedure when evaluating integrity of the globe is ocular ultrasonography. **Medical treatment of traumatic hyphema is similar to that in other forms of uveitis, except that initially, nonsteroidal anti-inflammatory drugs are either not used or are used very cautiously because of their interference with platelet function and the possibility of persistent or recurrent bleeding.** Topical 1% atropine is indicated initially to reduce the possibility of posterior synechiae formation and to stabilize the blood–aqueous barrier. Mydriatics are used judiciously, because an acute increase in the IOP is possible. Topical and systemic corticosteroids are used to both reduce and control intraocular inflammation.

When extensive hyphema has resulted in an elevated IOP or extensive posterior synechiae formation is possible, intracameral injection

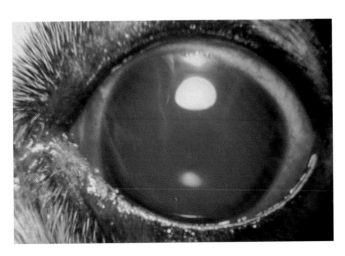

FIGURE 9-12. *Complete and nonclotted hyphema associated with glaucoma and retinal detachment in a Boston Terrier.*

BOX 9-3

Causes of Hyphema in the Dog

Uveitis

Multiple causes

Trauma

Blunt or penetrating

Neoplasia

Primary ocular or systemic

Systemic hypertension

Multiple causes

Coagulation factor abnormalities

Von Willebrand

Dicoumarin toxicity

Liver disease

Disseminated intravascular coagulation

Platelet disorders

Thrombocytopenia

Thrombopathia

Hyperviscosity syndrome

Multiple myeloma

Congenital anomalies

Collie eye anomaly

Vitreoretinal dysplasia

Persistent hyaloid artery

Neovascularization

Iris or retinal

Chronic glaucoma

---

of tissue-plasminogen activator (Activase; Genentech) can result in rapid dissolution of the blood or fibrin (or both). Tissue-plasminogen activator is most effective when injected within 48 hours of clot formation, but it can also be effective in dissolving clots of longer duration. The recommended dosage for intracameral injection is 0.2 to 0.3 mL of a 250-μg/mL solution. It should not be injected if recurrent bleeding is likely.

ANTERIOR UVEAL TUMORS

Intraocular neoplasms are relatively uncommon in the dog, and both primary and secondary anterior uveal neoplasms occur, as in other tissues. The differential diagnosis of intraocular neoplasia should include nonneoplastic uveal proliferations, uveal cysts, granulomatous lesions, extraocular neoplasms with intraocular extension, and perforating wounds of the globe with uveal prolapse. To facilitate the differential diagnosis, consider whether the lesion is single or multiple, focal or diffuse, flat or elevated, unilateral or bilateral, and whether concurrent ocular or systemic disease is present.

BENIGN IRIDAL PROLIFERATIONS

Benign iridal pigmented proliferations may include:

1. *Ectropion uvea*, which refers to a prominence or proliferation (or both) of the pigmented posterior epithelium of the iris, with anterior extension through the pupil;
2. Diffuse iris hyperpigmentation, which often occurs with chronic uveitis;
3. Ocular melaninosis in older Cairn Terriers (sometimes termed *pigmentary glaucoma* in the Cairn Terrier); and
4. Pigment cell clusters, freckles, nevi, and benign melanoma.

Histopathologically benign iridal melanomas resembling the previously described nevi have also been reported in young dogs.

PRIMARY NEOPLASMS

Melanocytic Neoplasms

Melanocytic neoplasms (i.e., melanomas) are the most common primary intraocular neoplasm in the dog, and they occur in the dog more frequently than in other domestic animals. Most canine melanomas arise in the anterior uvea. The incidence of confirmed metastasis for canine anterior uveal melanoma is low (4%). Anterior uveal melanoma is most common in older dogs (age, 8–10 years), but an age range of 2 months to 17 years has been reported in the largest study to date. Inherited iris melanoma has been reported in a family of Labrador Retrievers.

The owner may first observe a peculiar color or structure in the animal's eye, or the eye may become inflamed or enlarged. Nodular growth rather than diffuse infiltration is typical (Fig. 9-13). At clinical presentation, melanoma may be focal and confined to the iris. Alternatively, it may be extensive, either bulging through the pupil, displacing the iris anteriorly, or resulting in dyscoria. Pigmentation is variable, and amelanotic melanomas can occur. Ocular inflammation is a possible sequela with any intraocular neoplasm. Such changes may include keratitis, uveitis, hyphema, secondary glaucoma, buphthalmos, and retinal separation. Anterior uveal melanomas are often locally invasive, and they may extend to

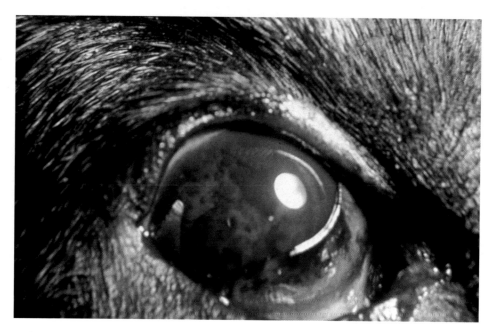

FIGURE 9-13. *Large anterior uveal melanoma arising from the iris periphery and partially occupying the anterior chamber. Note the focal hyphema on the ventral surface of the mass.*

involve the choroid, sclera, filtration angle, and cornea. Lens subluxation may also occur because of displacement by the mass.

Ciliary Body Neoplasms

Ciliary body neoplasms are the second most common primary intraocular tumor in the dog and occur as adenomas and adenocarcinomas. The German Shepherd and, possibly, the American Cocker Spaniel breeds appear to be overrepresented. Ciliary body tumors are more common among middle-aged and older dogs (mean age, 8.0 years). They can arise from pigmented or nonpigmented ciliary body epithelium, but most are nonpigmented. The incidences of adenoma (i.e., benign) and of adenocarcinoma (i.e., potentially malignant) are approximately equal. Distant metastasis of ciliary body adenocarcinoma has been reported but appears to be low. Another ciliary body neoplasm, the medulloepithelioma, arises from undifferentiated cell types (i.e., primitive neuroectoderm) during organogenesis or, possibly, during early neonatal life, but this type of neoplasm is rare.

Secondary Neoplasms

Neoplasms can metastasize hematogenously to the eye from local or from distant sites, or they may invade the eye by local extension from the ocular adnexa, cornea, orbit, paranasal sinuses, or nasal cavity. Hematogenous spread accounts for most secondary neoplasms, and of these, intraocular lymphosarcoma is the most common in the dog (ocular involvement with lymphosarcoma is between 33–37%). Hemangiosarcoma has been suggested as being the second most common metastatic neoplasm to the eye. Additional metastatic neoplasms include cutaneous and oral melanoma, hemangiosarcoma, seminoma, transmissible venereal tumor, transitional cell carcinoma of the urinary bladder as well as urethra, neurogenic sarcoma, rhabdomyosarcoma, anaplastic fibrosarcoma, and pheochromocytoma. Other metastatic neoplasms include adenocarcinoma of the mammary gland, thyroid gland, adrenal gland (presumed), and those of nasal, renal, and pancreatic origin. In contrast to the typical unilateral occurrence of primary ocular neoplasms, bilateral ocular involvement may signal secondary neoplasms. An intraocular mass may (or may not) be readily apparent. Varying degrees of uveitis and all its sequelae, including hyphema and glaucoma, may be the presenting signs.

Treatment of Primary Ocular Neoplasms

Treatment of an intraocular neoplasm is tailored to the individual animal. It may include temporization, local excision, enucleation, orbital exenteration, and possibly, euthanasia if clinical or radiographic evidence of metastatic disease is present. Laser therapy appears to be promising, but current data are limited.

Diseases and Surgery of the Canine Lens

The normal canine crystalline lens is a soft, avascular, transparent, and highly structured tissue that refracts incoming light rays to a point source on the retina. **The canine lens has a volume of approximately 0.5 mL, an anteroposterior thickness of 7 mm, and an equatorial diameter of 10 mm. Its dioptric power is 40 to 41 D. The lens includes a zonular fiber support system, an external capsule comprised of basement membrane, epithelia, and differentiated lens fibers.** Loss of transparency is almost invariably a common denominator in all lens diseases, and because of the prevalence of heritable canine lens disorders, cataracts are among the most common intraocular lesions and a leading cause of vision loss in the dog. Disorders of the lens are classified into those that affect embryologic development, that affect transparency, and that affect correct positioning within the eye.

CONGENITAL AND DEVELOPMENTAL ABNORMALITIES

The lens is an ectodermal structure and, in embryonic life, is surrounded by a vascular envelope. Therefore, anomalous development may occur in the lens cells and capsule or result from abnormalities of the surrounding tissues. Congenital lens abnormalities may result from genetic or exogenous factors. Because proper lens development is crucial in the orchestration of intraocular embryogenesis, eyes with lens anomalies often exhibit multiple ocular defects as well.

RARE LENS ANOMALIES

Congenital absence of the lens is extremely rare in the dog. When it occurs, it usually is associated with multiple ocular defects such as

microphthalmia, deformities of the anterior segment, retinal dysplasia, and staphylomas (as in the St. Bernard). Congenital microphakia, which is an abnormally small lens, may result from optic vesicle derangement that occurs during formation of the neural plate. Microphakia has been associated with multiple ocular defects in the Beagle and the Doberman Pinscher and with congenital cataract and microphthalmia in the Miniature Schnauzer. Lens coloboma is a shortened segment of lens fiber that appears at biomicroscopy as a notch in the equatorial region; it is a rare congenital defect in the dog. Typical lens colobomas (i.e., at the 6-o'clock position) result from an absence of ciliary zonules that are associated in turn with coloboma of the ventral ciliary body. An overt lens zonule defect, however, may not be apparent with atypical colobomas. Congenital deformity of the axial, anterior, or posterior lens surface may result in a circumscribed, conelike (i.e., lenticonus) or spherical (i.e., lentiglobus) protrusion of variable size. Posterior lenticonus involves protrusion of the posterior cortex and capsular regions into the vitreous body, and it is thought to occur at the time of primary lens fiber elongation (i.e., approximately day 25 of gestation). This condition may be unilateral or bilateral, and it is often associated with other ocular anomalies, including congenital cataracts and microphthalmia. Posterior lenticonus has been reported in the Miniature Schnauzer, Cavalier King Charles Spaniel, Old English Sheepdog, Mastiff, and Golden Retriever. Posterior lenticonus occurs in 19% of Miniature Schnauzers with congenital cataracts and microphthalmia. It also occurs in Doberman Pinschers with persistent hyperplastic tunica vasculosa lentis/persistent hyperplastic primary vitreous (PHTVL/PHPV; discussed later and see chapter 11).

EMBYRONIC VASCULAR ABNORMALITIES

The vascular supply of the lens, which is present during prenatal development, consists of the anterior and the posterior tunica vasculosa lentis. The anterior portion is formed by a pupillary membrane extending from the iris; the posterior portion is formed by the intravitreal hyaloid vascular system. Atrophy of the hyaloid vascular system in the dog begins by day 45 of gestation, but the anterior pupillary membrane remains until approximately 14 days after birth. Persistent pupillary membrane is a common congenital ocular anomaly and is seen sporadically in many breeds. The highest frequency occurs in the Basenji and English Cocker Spaniel, thereby suggesting a hereditary predisposition (see Chapter 9).

The most severe lesion associated with abnormal development of the embryonic intraocular vasculature, PHTVL/PHPV is a congenital eye anomaly that leads to cataract formation in most cases (Fig. 10-1). This condition occurs sporadically in many breeds but is perhaps most common in the Doberman Pinscher. The hereditary basis for PHTVL/PHPV among Doberman Pinschers in the Netherlands and Staffordshire Bull Terriers in Great Britain is most likely incomplete autosomal dominant (for more details, the reader should consult the third edition, pp. 799–800 and 861–863). Because of the low success rate in restoring vision, surgery has been advocated only for cases of bilateral PHTVL/PHPV

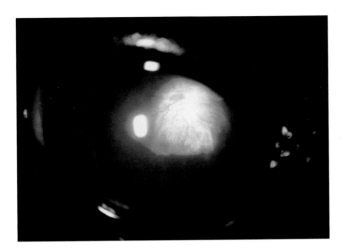

FIGURE 10-1. *Persistent hyaloid artery with posterior capsular and cortical cataract in a mixed-breed dog. Note the patent hyaloid artery system.*

in which vision is lacking. **Intracapsular lens extraction with anterior vitrectomy and cutting of the hyaloid artery has been advocated for dogs with severe PHTVL/PHPV.**

MULTIPLE OCULAR ANOMALIES WITH LENS ABNORMALITIES

Australian Shepherds and other breeds that are homozygous for the merle gene have been reported to develop congenital ocular anomalies. These abnormalities include microphthalmia; microcornea; colobomas of the iris, retina, choroid, sclera, or some combination thereof; and retinal dysplasia, with or without detachment and cataracts. This syndrome is referred to as merle ocular dysgenesis, and it is inherited as an autosomal recessive trait. The cataracts are cortical, and the progression varies among cases.

Congenital cataracts with additional ocular anomalies also occur in the Doberman Pinscher, Chow Chow, English Cocker Spaniel, and Red Cocker Spaniel. Congenital lens abnormalities with hereditary retinal dysplasia occur in the Bedlington Terrier, Sealyham Terrier, Labrador Retriever, and English Springer Spaniel. In the Labrador Retriever, retardation of appendicular skeletal growth, persistent hyaloid remnants, and rhegmatogenous retinal detachment may also be seen. In the Beagle and Old English Sheepdog, cataract, microphthalmia, and retinal dysplasia have been reported. Short-limbed dwarfism is inherited in the Samoyed as an autosomal recessive trait, and anterior as well as posterior cortical cataracts, vitreal liquefaction, hyaloid remnants, and retinal detachment are the associated ocular defects (for more details, the reader should consult the third edition, pp. 797–801).

CONGENITAL CATARACTS

Disruption of lens growth during primary fiber formation results in a fetal nuclear cataract that is generally nonprogressive. With concurrent involvement of the adjacent anterior and posterior cortical regions, however, progression of the opacity may occur. **Congenital cataracts are inherited in the Miniature Schnauzer, Boston Terrier, Old English Sheepdog, Welsh Springer Spaniel, and West Highland White Terrier (Table 10-1).** In ad-

TABLE 10-1

INHERITED CATARACTS IN THE DOG

Breed	Documented Inheritance	Age of Onset	Initial Anatomic Localization
Afghan Hound	Autosomal recessive	6–12 months	Equatorial/posterior cortex
American Cocker Spaniel	Autosomal recessive/ polygenic	>6 months	Posterior/anterior cortex
Boston Terrier	Autosomal recessive	Congenital	Posterior sutures/nuclear
	Autosomal recessive	>3 years	Equatorial/anterior cortex
Chesapeake Bay Retriever	Incomplete dominant	>1 year	Nuclear/cortex
Entelbucher Mountain Dog	Autosomal recessive	1–2 years	Posterior cortex
German Shepherd	Incomplete dominant	>8 weeks	Posterior sutures/cortex
Golden Retriever	Incomplete dominant	>6 months	Posterior subcapsular (triangular)
Labrador Retriever	Incomplete dominant	>6 months	Posterior subcapsular (triangular)
Miniature Schnauzer	Autosomal recessive	Congenital	Nuclear/posterior cortex
	Autosomal recessive	>6 months	Posterior cortex
Norwegian Buhund	Autosomal dominant	Congenital	Fetal nucleus
Old English Sheepdog	Autosomal recessive	Congenital	Nuclear/cortex
Staffordshire Bull Terrier	Autosomal recessive	>6 months	Posterior sutures/cortex
Standard Poodle	Autosomal recessive	>1 year	Equatorial cortex
Welsh Springer Spaniel	Autosomal recessive	Congenital	Nuclear/posterior cortex
West Highland White Terrier	Autosomal recessive	Congenital	Posterior sutures

dition, congenital cataracts may be of maternal origin, resulting from exposure to a toxic or infectious agent in utero.

PATHOPHYSIOLOGIC CHANGES ASSOCIATED WITH CATARACTS

Transparency within the lens is maintained by several complex factors, including a low density of cytoplasm resulting from a lack of intracellular organelles and cell nuclei in lens fibers, small spatial fluctuations in the refractive index of cytoplasm, and a highly organized, lattice arrangement of the fiber cells. Cataract formation is associated with a series of events that relate to changes in the lens protein content, metabolic pumps, ionic concentrations, and antioxidant activity. Cataracts are associated with increased levels of high-molecular-weight, insoluble proteins (i.e., albuminoids), which normally comprise 15% of lens proteins, and with decreased relative amounts of soluble proteins (i.e., crystallins). With congenital cataract in the Miniature Schnauzer, levels of α- and β-light crystallins are increased, and levels of β-heavy and γ-crystallins are decreased. Both hydrolytic and proteolytic enzyme activity increase, and cell membrane rupture is associated with irreversible damage, loss of low-molecular-weight proteins, and increased water content (i.e., the lens gradually becomes white). Further degradation of proteins into amino acids and polypeptides allows small products of proteolysis to diffuse from the lens. Loss of water and nitrogenous material may cause the lens to shrink as well, as with a hypermature cataract.

HISTOPATHOLOGIC CHANGES ASSOCIATED WITH CATARACTS

Specific capsular, epithelial, cortical, and lens nuclear morphologic abnormalities are commonly seen at light microscopy in many types of cataract. Both the anterior and posterior capsules may become thinned with an intumescent lens, and the lens capsule may become wrinkled with an advanced, hypermature cataract. Lens epithelial abnormalities include the formation of "bladder" or Wedl cells, which are balloonlike, swollen lens epithelial cells. Migration of lens epithelial cells past their normal point of termination in the lens bow and along the posterior capsule may occur as well; these cells may have a spindle- or a bladder-cell appearance. Advanced cortical and nuclear cataracts often have a paucity (or even absence) of lens epithelium because of degeneration or necrosis. Lens cortical changes may include particle aggregates within the cytoplasm and increased eosinophilia. Eosinophilic fluid from lytic lens proteins may accumulate in small clefts that form between degenerative fibers, and this fluid may be associated with vacuolization of the lens fibers and pyknotic nuclei. With advanced degradation of the cell wall, larger clefts and pockets of these degenerative proteins may be seen as small eosinophilic aggregates or Morgagni's globules. Hypermature cataracts may be associated with characteristic microscopic features, including advanced liquefaction and loss of cortical and (sometimes) nuclear lens contents, wrinkling of the lens capsule, dystrophic calcification, and formation of multifocal, subcapsular plaques.

CLASSIFICATION OF CANINE CATARACTS

Several classification schemes can be used for canine cataracts. **Common schemes include those associated with cause, age of onset (e.g., congenital-infantile, juvenile, senile), location of incipient stages within the lens (e.g., capsular, subcapsular, zonular, cortical, nuclear, sutural, axial, equatorial), appearance of the cataract itself (e.g., spike- or wedge-shaped, spoke, cuneiform, sunflower, stellate, punctate, purverulent), and stage of progression (e.g., incipient, immature, mature, hypermature).** It is often appropriate to use several classification schemes concurrently to describe a specific type of cataract accurately. Of all classification schemes, the stage of cataract development is perhaps the most useful—and the most widely used—in the dog (Table 10-2). Examples include the incipient cataract (Fig. 10-2), immature cataract (Fig. 10-3), mature cataract (Fig. 10-4), and hypermature cataract (Figs. 10-5 and 10-6).

TABLE 10-2

CLASSIFICATION OF CANINE CATARACTS BASED ON MATURITY

Type	Area Involved	Tapetal Reflection	Vision
Incipient	10–15% involved; cortices and/or sutures	Present	Present
Immature	Normal and opaque areas Intumescent (swollen)	Present	Present
Mature	Entire lens involved Intumescent (swollen)	Obscured	Absent
Hypermature	Reduced overall size Very advanced	Usually obscured Often present	Usually absent Variable

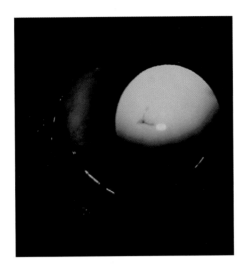

FIGURE 10-2. *Incipient, posterior cortical "Y"-suture–associated cataract as seen with direct retroillumination using the tapetal reflection.*

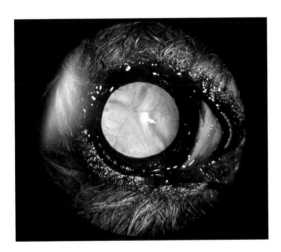

FIGURE 10-3. *Immature cataract as seen with direct retroillumination using the tapetal reflection. Note the prominent cataractous change along the anterior and posterior cortical "Y"-sutures.*

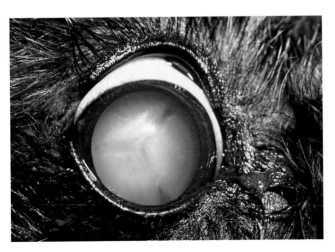

FIGURE 10-4. *Typical appearance of a mature or complete cataract as seen with diffuse illumination. Note the separation of the lens fibers and the formation of a cleft along the anterior "Y"-suture.*

FIGURE 10-5. *Hypermature cataract as seen with diffuse illumination. Note the glistening, refractile appearance of the lens material.*

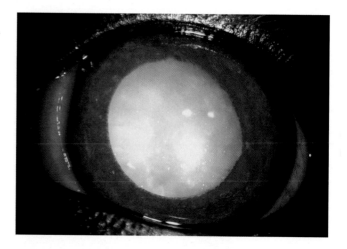

FIGURE 10-6. *Hypermature cataract as seen with direct focal illumination, with the optical section being passed from right to left. Note the increased relucency and glistening refractile property of some lens fibers, with the focal pockets of liquefied lens material appearing as areas of decreased relucency.*

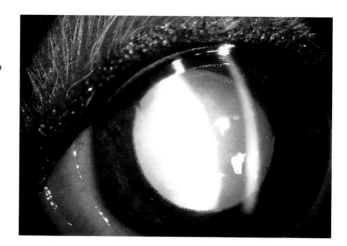

NUCLEAR OR LENTICULAR SCLEROSIS

A consistent finding in dogs older than 7 years, nuclear or lenticular sclerosis is a senescent change in the lens that results from progressive lens fiber formation and internal compression of the older lens fibers, especially those in the lens nucleus. The altered optical properties of the compressed central lens fibers cause light-scattering, thus imparting a clinically apparent, whitish-blue or gray appearance on diffuse illumination of the lens nucleus. With retroillumination, a tapetal or fundic reflection is still visible, and the outline or zone of the lens nucleus may be apparent. Funduscopy is possible through the central lens, but the fine ophthalmoscopic detail may be somewhat obscured.

CLINICAL AND BIOMICROSCOPIC FEATURES OF THE NORMAL AND CATARACTOUS LENS

To examine the entire lens, drug-induced mydriasis is necessary. Adequate illumination and magnification facilitate inspection of the lens, and for veterinary ophthalmologists, the slit-lamp biomicroscope provides both qualities in a convenient diagnostic instrument. The lens is examined using both direct illumination and retroillumination (i.e., indirect illumination using the ocular/tapetal reflection) as well as diffuse illumination and direct focal illumination. With direct focal illumination using a parallelepiped or optical section, the normal canine lens appears at biomicroscopy as a series of opalescent blocks of light. These blocks are produced by the surfaces of the zones of discontinuity from the internal lens architecture (i.e., convex surfaces of the anterior capsule, anterior cortex, anterior adult nucleus, anterior fetal nucleus, and anterior embryonal nucleus; and the similar, concave zones produced by the posterior-situated counterparts of these areas). Both the fetal and the embryonal nucleus is variably visualized, and the zones of discontinuity between the cortex and the adult nucleus become more prominent with age. Sometimes, in fact, they are not even visible in dogs younger than 1 year. "Y"-suture regions are seen as fine, white lines within the light block. These regions may have a central dark zone at high magnification and are visible near the anterior and posterior capsules. On the vitreal aspect of the posterior capsule, Mittendorf's dot (i.e., remnants of the anterior hyaloid artery) and a white, relucent, circular line representing the anterior extent of Cloquet's canal (i.e., arcuate line of Vogt) are generally visible. Depending on their specific structure, cataracts cause reflection, refraction, or dispersion of light. Fluid within the lens, such as that seen with vacuoles, clefts, or Morgagni's globules, appears to be dark or black with focal illumination, because the fluid has a lesser optical density than that of the normal lens fibers. Lens opacities may be localized anatomically by inspecting and estimating their proximity to the adjacent zones of discontinuity. With high-magnification biomicroscopy, minor lens imperfections, which must be differentiated from cataract formation, are commonly detected and include fine particulate opacities or vacuoles in the lens cortex, peripheral capsular opacities, linear "Y"-suture opacities or prominent "Y"-sutures, posterior capsular opacities from hyaloid artery remnants, a distinct zone of separation between the lens cortex and the adult nucleus, minute granules, sheen, and optical discontinuity as well as striations.

HERITABLE OR PRESUMED HERITABLE CATARACTS

Cataracts in young to middle-aged, purebred dogs comprise the largest single type of cataract seen in clinical veterinary medicine. Only in a minority of affected breeds have a heritable basis and mode of transmission been conclusively established (Table 10-1), but many breeds seem to be predisposed (Box 10-1). The frequent and characteristic anatomic localization and appearance of the lens opacity during the initial stages, characteristic age of onset and progression, bilateral nature, and absence of other demonstrable ocular disorders that might cause a cataract, however, are suggestive that in most of the other "suspected" breeds, these cataracts are also likely to have a heritable basis. Most cataracts with an established genetic basis in the dog are inherited as a simple autosomal recessive trait, with the other modes of inheritance (e.g., incompletely dominant) being less common.

BOX 10-1

Breeds Predisposed to Cataracts (Inheritance Suspected)

Affenpinscher	Brittany Spaniel
Alaskan Malamute	Brussels Griffon
American Staffordshire Terrier	Bulldog
American Water Spaniel	Cairn Terrier
Australian Cattle Dog	Cavalier King Charles Spaniel
Australian Shepherd	Chinese Shar Pei
Basenji	Chow Chow
Basset Hound	Clumber Spaniel
Beagle	Collie
Bearded Collie	Curly Coated Retriever
Bedlington Terrier	Dachshund
Belgian Sheepdog	Dalmation
Belgian Tervuren	Doberman Pinscher
Bernese Mountain Dog	English Cocker Spaniel
Bichon Frise	English Springer Spaniel
Black and Tan Coonhound	English Toy Spaniel
Border Collie	Field Spaniel
Borzoi	Flat-Coated Retriever
Boston Terrier	French Bulldog
Bouvier des Flandres	German Shorthaired Pointer
Boxer	

continued

Breeds Predisposed to Cataracts (Inheritance Suspected)— (continued)

German Wirehaired Pointer

Giant Schnauzer

Gordon Setter

Great Dane

Havanese

Ibizan Hound

Irish Setter

Irish Water Spaniel

Irish Wolfhound

Italian Greyhound

Jack Russell Terrier

Japanese Chin

Keeshound

Kerry Blue Terrier

Komodor

Kuvasc

Lakeland Terrier

Lhasa Apso

Lowchen

Manchester Terrier

Mastiff

Miniature Pinscher

Newfoundland

Norbottenspets

Norfolk Terrier

Norwegian Elkhound

Norwich Terrier

Nova Scotia Duck Tolling Retriever

Papillon

Pekingese

Pembroke Welsh Corgi

Pointer

Pomeranian

Poodle (Toy and Miniature)

Portuguese Water Dog

Rhodesian Ridgeback

Rottweiler

Saint Bernard

Samoyed

Schipperke

Scottish Deerhound

Scottish Terrier

Sealyham Terrier

Shetland Sheepdog

Shih Tzu

Siberian Husky

Silky Terrier

Smooth Fox Terrier

Soft-Coated Wheaten Terrier

Standard Schnauzer

Tibetan Spaniel

Tibetan Terrier

Visla

Whippet

Wire Fox Terrier

Yorkshire Terrier

Data from American College of Veterinary Ophthalmologists. Ocular disorders presumed to be inherited in purebred dogs. Purdue University, West Lafayette, IN, 1996; and Rubin LF. Inherited eye disease in purebred dogs. Baltimore; Williams & Wilkins, 1989.

CATARACTS ASSOCIATED WITH SYSTEMIC DISEASE

DIABETES MELLITUS

Diabetes mellitus is commonly associated with rapidly developing, bilaterally symmetric cataract formation in the dog that results from well-described alterations in the lens metabolic pathways (Fig. 10-7). With elevated blood glucose levels, the lens glucose levels increase, and the anaerobic metabolism of glucose by the hexokinase pathways becomes saturated, thus causing a shunting toward an alternate energy pathway involving the enzyme aldose reductase (AR). The AR activity in diabetic cataracts is increased because of increased AR levels rather than because of increased enzyme activation. By using the reduced form of nicotinamide-adenine dinucleotide phosphate, AR reduces the aldehyde form of glucose to sorbitol, which is further oxidized to fructose by nicotinamide-adenine dinucleotide–dependent sorbitol dehydrogenase. Accumulation of sorbitol (i.e., a polyol or sugar alcohol), which does not readily diffuse across the lens capsule, thus results. Water from the aqueous humor is imbibed into the lens through osmotic forces and cause architectural changes in the lens, including fiber swelling and rupture, vacuole formation, and clinically evident cataract. In addition, a series of biochemical changes result in altered electrolyte concentrations; reduced levels of adenosine triphosphate, amino acids, glutathione, and myoinositol; and reduced adenosine triphosphatase activity. The speed of progression as well as the prevalence of cataracts directly relate to the levels of blood sugars, the age of the animal, and a species-dependent concentration of lenticular AR. The activity of AR in the canine lens is similar to that in the human lens (0.39 nm/min per 1 mg of lens protein), is three times less than that in the rat lens, and is much greater than that in the mouse lens, which has almost undetectable levels. Cataracts are one of the most prevalent—and important—complications of canine diabetes mellitus; one retrospective study (involving relatively few animals) cited a prevalence rate of 68%. Canine diabetic cataracts often are so rapidly progressive and osmotically active that intumescence of the

FIGURE 10-7. *Incipient equatorial cataracts in a dog with diabetes mellitus. Note the lens vacuoles, which are characteristic of the early cataractous changes in diabetes.*

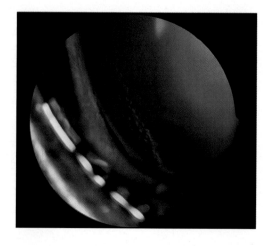

lens as well as leakage of the lens protein (resulting in uveitis) commonly ensues. **Early equatorial vacuole changes may sometimes dissipate after insulin therapy, but substantial cataractous changes with canine diabetes are not reversible through control of hyperglycemia.**

HYPOCALCEMIA

Hypocalcemia, which most commonly results from renal failure or either primary or secondary hypoparathyroidism, may be associated with characteristic cataracts in the dog. These cataracts manifest by multifocal, punctate opacities or coalescing lamellar cortical opacities that are bilaterally symmetric.

HYPERCUPREMIA

A characteristic, sunflower-shaped, anterior subcapsular cataract is associated with elevated serum and aqueous copper levels in humans with Wilson's disease, which is a genetic disorder of copper metabolism, as well as in those with other disorders producing a derangement of copper metabolism. A condition similar to Wilson's disease that is characterized by the excessive accumulation of copper in hepatocytes occurs in the Bedlington Terrier. Cataracts, however, have not been described in these animals.

INBORN ERRORS OF METABOLISM

A single case report of cataracts (and concurrent keratitis) associated with congenital tyrosinemia in a German Shepherd has been published. Bilateral cataract and lens luxation, with the cataract likely occurring secondary to a lens luxation from zonular defects, has been documented in a dog with Ehlers-Danlos syndrome, which is a hereditary disease of the connective tissue.

CATARACTS ASSOCIATED WITH MEDICATIONS OR OTHER TOXIC SUBSTANCES

Several environmental toxins and systemically administered pharmacologic agents produce cataracts in the dog. Initially, toxic cataracts may appear at a variety of locations within the lens, depending on the toxic principle, but they often begin in the anterior and posterior cortical region near the equator (in the area of lens fiber elongation) or in the "Y"-suture regions. They also are often associated with lens vacuole formation (Box 10-2).

The most clinically relevant type of cataract presumed to be toxic in nature is associated with progressive retinal atrophy (PRA) or other

---

BOX 10-2

Drug-Induced Cataracts in the Dog

Diazoxide (an antihypertensive agent)

Phenylpiperazine (an antihypertensive agent)

Hydroxymethylglutaryl–coenzyme A reductase inhibitors (cholesterol-lowering drugs)

Sulfonylurea glimepiride (a hypoglycemic agent)

Pefloxacin (a quinolone)

Dinitrophenol (an anthelmintic agent)

2,6-dichloro-4-mitroaniline (DNCA) (a fungicide)

Progesterone-based oral contraceptives

Ketoconazole

Dimethyl sulfoxide (DMSO)

---

types of retinal degeneration. Cataracts are commonly seen in dogs with moderate to advanced PRA, and these cataracts often obscure the ophthalmoscopic detail of the fundus. The Labrador Retriever, Miniature Poodle, and Toy Poodle are the breeds in which cataractous lens changes have been suggested to be accompanied most frequently by retinal degeneration, though many other breeds have been noted to be affected clinically as well. During the earlier stages, these lens opacities are characterized by the formation of equatorial and posterior cortical vacuoles, "Y"-suture changes, and a diffuse increase in relucency to the posterior subcapsular region. The cataracts are often progressive, eventually involving the entire lens. Because the breeds at risk for PRA also have a high incidence of genetic cataracts, the two disorders may not be interrelated in some dogs; rather, they may reflect two separate, heritable disease states. If these cataracts result from PRA, however, degenerative rod outer segments may release water-soluble dialdehydes from peroxidation of photoreceptor lipid membranes, which may diffuse through the vitreous and be toxic to the cellular membranes of the lens.

DIETARY DEFICIENCIES

A specific syndrome of neonatal cataracts is sporadically seen in puppies fed an oral milk-replacement product. **In mongrel pups that were experimentally fed milk replacements, opacities began during the third week of life, and a brown-colored lamellar zone separating the anterior and posterior nuclear–cortical junctions develops that is visible at biomi-**

croscopy. **This zone progresses to become a dense, white, perinuclear opacity.** Other changes include a feathered appearance to the "Y"-sutures and a transient, extra line of dysjunction in the anterior and posterior cortex. Similar lens changes, especially the nuclear–cortical junction ring, and some vacuolization of the equatorial fibers and "Y"-sutures have been described in naturally occurring cases among puppies and timber wolves. These opacities are often mild, do not threaten vision, and can become less prominent (or even resolve) with age, though more advanced cataractous changes persist into adulthood and may necessitate lentectomy. Arginine deficiency during a critical stage of neonatal lens development has been proposed as a likely cause on the basis of observations of arginine-supplemented wolf pups and of kittens experimentally fed milk supplements. The pathogenesis of these opacities, however, may be more complex than a single amino acid deficiency (e.g., tryptophan, phenylalanine, histidine).

INJURIES TO THE LENS

Mild blunt injury to the globe rarely causes damage to the lens. Moderate blunt injury, however, may result in posterior displacement of the iris, thus causing anterior capsular deposition of pigment from the posterior iris epithelium, sometimes in the shape of the pupillary aperture. Contusion to the lens from blunt injury may produce cataracts because of the resulting contrecoup or ocular compressive forces in turn causing damage to the lens epithelia and, also, the rupture and disruption of the lens fiber membrane spacing in the underlying cortex. Variable degrees of subcapsular cataract formation, which generally occurs adjacent to the site of injury in the anterior superficial cortex, may ensue. Traumatic cataracts sometimes manifest initially along the anterior and posterior lens sutures, thereby producing a stellate shape. With time, a focal traumatic cataract may be displaced to deeper layers of the lens as new lens fibers are formed. Rupture of the lens capsule from blunt trauma without profound globe injury or rupture is rare in the dog but still may occur.

Penetrating ocular injury that perforates the anterior lens capsule invariably causes focal to diffuse cataract formation. Traumatic anterior lens capsule disruption most commonly occurs in young animals from cat-claw wounds or dog bites, though other sources of penetrating injury are possible (Fig. 10-8). Small rents in the lens capsule may spontaneously seal through fibrous metaplasia of the lens epithelia assisted by exudate from the uveal tract, thereby leaving only a focal residual cataract. Rents larger than 1.5 mm often cause progressive opacification of the lens and, in the dog, are generally associated with severe phacoclastic uveitis, which results in vision-threatening sequela. Prophylactic lentectomy has been recommended for lens capsule rents larger than 1.5 mm.

Lens penetration with a metallic foreign body should result in at least a focal cataract and, more commonly, diffuse opacification from substantial disruption of the fiber cells and lens metabolism. Lead shot retained within the globe that does not perforate the lens capsule might not be expected de facto to cause cataract. Gold, silver, glass, and

FIGURE 10-8. *Focal anterior lens capsule perforation associated with a cat-claw wound in a young puppy as seen with direct focal illumination using a parallelepiped being passed from right to left. Note the extrusion of lens material above the capsular surface, cortical cataract, and focal pigment deposition on the capsule.*

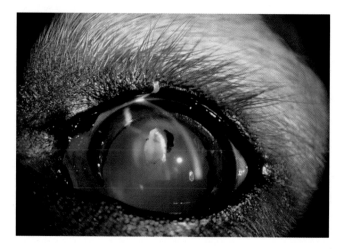

rubber are also relatively inert within the eye. Conversely, copper, zinc, and brass have moderate oxidizing potential, and they often cause panophthalmitis. Iron and steel are the most damaging, causing a severe inflammatory reaction and secondary cataract (i.e., siderosis lentis). Intralenticular iron foreign bodies cause siderotic deposition, thereby resulting in slowly progressive, focal, red-brown or rusty-appearing lens opacities. Iron deposited outside the lens but within the eye may result in siderosis bulbi, with secondary lens epithelial degeneration and necrosis as well as lens cortical degeneration.

Cataracts are a chronic complication from exposure of the eye to ionizing radiation in varying forms. Most commonly, such cataracts are seen clinically after radiation therapy for neoplasms in the head region when the eye is in the radiation field. In two studies, cataracts were reported in 28% of eyes with complications after megavoltage irradiations, in 10.2% of eyes after orthovoltage, and generally 6 to 12 months after therapy. The likelihood of cataracts occurring after radiation therapy relates to the degree of exposure of the eye to the radiation beam and to the radiation dose. The pathogenesis relates to the effect on mitosis and subsequent degenerative changes from the radiation on the equatorial lens epithelium and the formation of newly synthesized lens fibers, thereby resulting in an initial cataract that involves the equatorial, the anterior, and the posterior subcapsular regions. Attempts should be made to protect the globe from the damaging effects of radiation energy during such therapy by using lead shields or other devices, if possible.

AGE-RELATED CATARACTS

Cataracts are commonly seen in aged dogs, and they are often classified as being "senile" or "age-related" if no other antecedent cause is apparent. The age of onset at which a cataract should be considered to be age-related is arbitrary, however, and it relates to the specific breed (in animals >6–10 years of age). The clinical appearance and progression rate of age-related cataracts can vary, but such cataracts often are seen initially as an increase in relu-cency and a punctate to linear opacification in the adult nucleus of the lens, generally occurring concurrently with and after dense nuclear sclerosis. Cor-tical cataractous changes, often in a wedge- or spoke-shaped pattern, also may occur to varying extents, either concurrently with or separate from nu-clear cataracts. The progression of these classic age-related cataracts is often slow; many months to several years may pass for any demonstrable loss of vision is observed. The cause of age-related cataracts in the dog is unknown.

CATARACTS RESULTING FROM INFLAMMATION AND LENS-ASSOCIATED INFLAMMATION

The lens responds in a nonspecific fashion to contiguous inflammation (i.e., uveitis) from any cause by developing a cataract. Formation of synechiae to the anterior lens capsule, with or without any prolifera-tion of fibrovascular membranes onto the lens surface, may result as well. Inflammatory cataracts most commonly form in the anterior sub-capsular or equatorial region and generally result from moderate to severe anterior uveitis.

A common form of lens-associated uveitis that occurs in conjunction with resorbing, typically hypermature cataracts has been termed *phacolytic uveitis*. The prevalence of this generally mild uveitis (i.e., lymphocytic–plasmocytic iridocyclitis) has been reported to be as great as 71% in dogs being screened for cataract surgery. The prevalence of a subclinical dis-ruption in the blood–ocular barrier in dogs with hypermature cataracts may be even higher. A more severe form of phacolytic uveitis, which is also termed *granulomatous lens-induced uveitis,* is sometimes encountered in older dogs with hypermature cataracts.

Phacoclastic uveitis occurs in dogs with traumatic rupture of the lens capsule. Histopathologic changes include varying degrees and types of in-flammation (i.e., suppurative to lymphocytic–plasmocytic), intralenticular neutrophils, and prominent fibroplasia (presumably from the lens epithe-lia). This condition usually responds poorly to anti-inflammatory therapy and often eventually requires enucleation (for more details, the reader should consult the third edition, pp. 816–817).

NONSURGICAL AND CLINICAL CONSIDERATIONS IN CANINE CATARACTS

VISUAL CONSEQUENCES

Clinically evident visual deficits associated with canine cataracts vary greatly, both with the astuteness of the owner and with the individual dog in its level of activity, type of activity, and acuity of the other special senses (e.g., hearing and smell). **Often, clinically apparent changes in behavior that are associated with diminished vision are not detected by the owner until the cataract is 40 to 50% complete–and even then usually not unless both lenses are affected.** An axial cataract generally is associated with earlier, more profound visual deficits. Interestingly, however, some dogs with cataracts appear to have (and are reported by their owners to have) more visual difficulty in daylight as opposed to dim lighting, perhaps because of a larger pupillary diameter with dim lighting. Other owners, however, report the opposite behavior, with dogs having more difficulty in scotopic conditions. Motion detection, such as that manifested in a response to a menacing gesture during an ophthalmologic examination, is often retained until the cataract is nearly complete.

COMPLICATIONS OF UNTREATED CATARACTS

If cataract surgery is not be performed, many canine cataracts will progress, and eventually, they may result in leakage of the lens proteins and subsequent lens-induced uveitis, thereby requiring medical treatment. Spontaneous resorption of cataractous lens material occurs most frequently in dogs younger than 6 years and may be more common in the Toy and Miniature Poodles, Miniature Schnauzer, and American Cocker Spaniel.

The most common complications of lens-induced uveitis include glaucoma and phthisis bulbi. An increased frequency of vitreal degeneration and retinal detachment has also been observed in canine eyes with hypermature cataracts. Long-standing, hypermature cataracts are at risk for subluxation or luxation, which can also produce secondary complications. The lifelong complication rate of untreated cataracts in the dog has not been studied; therefore, definitive statements regarding this subject cannot be made.

CLINICAL TREATMENT OF THE BLIND DOG

Appropriate owner education regarding treatment of the visually impaired or blind dog is an important role for clinicians to undertake. **Most blind dogs develop permanent behavioral changes and are limited functionally, but blind dogs can still cope within their environment and function acceptably as pets.** Common behavioral changes in blind dogs include a tendency to stay closer to the owner and a more cautious approach to the environment. With these changes, a closer relationship between the dog and the owner often forms as well. Many owners also report difficulty recognizing their dog's impairment in a familiar environment because of the compensatory development of other senses. Obvious safety precautions include adequate fencing or containment of the blind dog when outdoors, minimal movement of furniture within the home, and limited access to stairs, decks, or pools.

MEDICAL TREATMENT OF CATARACTS

A variety of therapeutic agents that have been claimed to prevent, delay, or even reverse cataracts are currently available and have been studied in both humans and the dog. **Therapies with topical or systemic selenium–vitamin E, superoxide dismutase, carnosine (a dipeptide antioxidant), or zinc citrate have been advocated for canine cataracts, though none has proved to be efficacious in controlled studies.**

DISLOCATION OF THE CRYSTALLINE LENS

Dislocation of the lens from its normal position within the patellar fossa is termed *subluxation* **(i.e., subtotal dislocation) or** *luxation* **(i.e., total dislocation). Such dislocation relates to a pathologic alteration in the ciliary zonules from abnormal development, degeneration, rupture, tearing, or some combination of these.** Associated clinical findings vary (Box 10-3). These changes in lens position may be associated with additional sequelae as well. **Subluxation or anterior luxation often culminates in secondary glaucoma from several possible mechanisms (Figs. 10-9 and 10-10).** An anterior shift in the lens or vitreal face (or both) may occlude the flow of aqueous humor from the posterior chamber through the pupil, thus diverting the aqueous posterior either to the lens or into the vitreous (i.e., pupillary block or aqueous misdirection glaucoma). Substantial amounts of prolapsed vitreous are often seen in the anterior chamber and the iridocorneal angle; theoretically, this may cause mechanical obstruction of the aqueous outflow. **An anterior luxation into the anterior chamber may result in physical contact between the lens capsule and the corneal endothelium, thereby causing transient or permanent corneal edema.** Secondary uveitis often accompanies lens dislocation, and especially anterior luxation, presumably because of abnormal physical contact by the lens or vitreous with the anterior uveal structures or other, undefined changes in the intraocular spaces.

BOX 10-3

Clinical Findings of Lens Luxation

Increased lens mobility (phacodonesis or tremor of the lens with globe movement)

Iridodonesis (iridal movements resulting from a lack of lens stability)

Asymmetry in the anterior chamber depth (usually resulting from lens tilting)

Appearance of lens equator and ciliary zonules remnants (aphakic crescent)

Degenerative white vitreal strands displaced or prolapsed into the anterior chamber

Lens luxation into the anterior chamber or vitreous

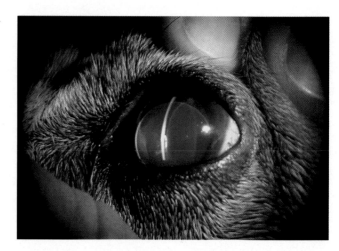

FIGURE 10-9. *Anterior lens luxation in a 4-year-old Jack Russell Terrier as seen with direct focal illumination using a parallelepiped being passed from left to right. Note the asymmetry, decreased anterior chamber depth and the dorsal aphakic crescent.*

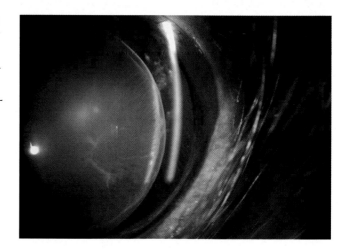

FIGURE 10-10. *Lens subluxation as seen with direct focal illumination using a parallelepiped being passed from right to left. The margin of the lens is visible as an aphakic crescent, and an early cortical cataract formation is present. Vitreal fibers, which have displaced into the anterior chamber, are seen as fine strands with increased relucency.*

Complete posterior luxation of the lens into the vitreous is more innocuous than anterior luxation, and the complications of glaucoma, uveitis, or corneal edema are less prevalent as well. Syneresis or liquefaction is necessary for the lens to fully luxate posteriorly; therefore, mechanical obstruction glaucoma is uncommon. Tractional retinal detachment may occur from changes in the vitreous or from direct contact by the lens capsule with the retinal surface. In addition, because the fully luxated lens often moves freely between the posterior and the anterior segments, surgical removal of the posteriorly luxated lens often continues to be indicated.

Similar to canine cataracts, lens dislocation has been classified using different schemes, though most commonly as being congenital, primary, secondary, or traumatic. Lens dislocations are generally classified as being primary if they occur in an adult dog with no other antecedent ocular disease. There is a strong predilection for a variety of Terrier breeds (most notably the Sealyham, Jack Russell, Wirehaired Fox), Terrier crosses, and in the United Kingdom, the Tibetan Terrier (reportedly not a true Terrier breed), though other breeds that have been reported more sporadically include the Border Collie, German Shepherd, and certain Spaniel breeds. Lens dislocation most commonly manifests bilaterally, but not necessarily with a symmetric clinical presentation. Lens displacement is documented most commonly in 3- to 6-year-old dogs, with the mean age in one study reported to be approximately 4.5, though some variation in this age of onset occurs. In the Tibetan Terrier, primary luxation appears to be an inherited disorder transmitted through an autosomal recessive gene. The disease presumably is heritable in other Terrier breeds, but the mode of inheritance has not been defined.

Evidence is suggestive that the pathogenesis of primary lens displacement relates to an inherited defect in the suspensory apparatus or the ciliary zonules of the lens in certain breeds. Ultrastructurally, an abnormal and haphazard arrangement of zonular material between the major processes of the ciliary body has been found, with these fibers inserting on the posterior aspect of the lens equator. Importantly, no abnormalities were found in the lens zonules arising at the pars plana, the zonular attachments to the lens, and the ultrastructural form, diameter, or periodicity of the individual zonules.

Lens displacement may be associated with glaucoma in a still incompletely defined fashion. **Lens luxation often occurs secondary to chronic glaucoma and enlargement of the globe, and it presumably relates to progressive stretching and rupture of the zonules.** The coexistence of raised intraocular pressure, subluxation of the lens, and an apparently normal-size globe in some dogs at the initial clinical presentation, however, sometimes makes determining the primary or antecedent disease difficult. This has produced speculation that ocular hypertension may precede—and even actually cause—breakdown of the zonules, at least in some cases, through an undefined mechanism unrelated to a change in globe size.

Clinical evaluation of patients with lens luxation should include critical ophthalmic examination for any primary cause. **Because primary or inherited displacement is almost invariably a bilateral disorder, the contralateral eye should be evaluated biomicroscopically after mydriasis for evidence of lens instability or signs that would be compatible with subluxation. Gonioscopy should also be performed, especially if ocular hypertension is documented, in both the affected (if possible) and the unaffected eye to determine any causal relationship. Treatment for dislocated lenses most commonly and appropriately involves surgical removal through an intracapsular lens extraction, with or without sulcus intraocular lens (IOL) placement. If surgical treatment is not possible, subluxated and posteriorly luxated lenses sometimes may be treated conservatively with long-term topical miotic therapy (e.g., phospholine iodide, demecarium bromide).** The rationale for this approach is to maintain the lens in the posterior chamber (or vitreous) to prevent forward migration, in which case complications such as pupillary block glaucoma or corneal edema are more common. Occasionally, anteriorly luxated lens may be manipulated successfully into the posterior chamber by digital pressure on the globe, change in head position, or directing the lens posteriorly with a fine hypodermic needle inserted into the anterior chamber.

SURGERY OF THE LENS

Surgery of the lens is divided into cataract extractions and removal of the lens for lens luxations. These surgeries are the most frequent intraocular procedures performed by veterinary ophthalmologists worldwide. Because of the required training, operating microscope, and microsurgical ophthalmic instruments, cataract and lens removal is not performed by most veterinarians in clinical practice. As a result, patient selection, surgical procedures, expected surgical results, and complications are only summarized here (for more details, the reader should consult the third edition, pp. 827–856).

PATIENT SELECTION

Proper patient selection and preoperative screening are critical to achieving a good surgical outcome. A thorough medical history is obtained, and a general physical examination is performed to rule out any systemic disease that might relate to cataract formation (e.g., diabetes mellitus) or dictate special anesthetic considerations. The owner should be questioned carefully regarding the dog's vision or activities related to vision, and especially regarding any behavior suggesting nyctalopia. Cataract surgery is often very successful in aged dogs; however, owners often attribute specific types of behavior (i.e., decreased mentation and activity level) to a reduction in vision that may, in fact, be associated with other aspects of advanced age. Clarifying the owner's expectations regarding surgical outcome is especially important under these circumstances. The temperament of the dog can also be an important consideration, because postoperative administration of topical medication is challenging with fractious or aggressive patients.

Cataract surgery is generally, but not exclusively, performed in dogs having demonstrably decreased vision associated with the lens opacity. Preoperative evaluation should include critical examination of the eye, and especially the lens. Generally, cataract patients should be referred to be evaluated for cataract surgery at first discovery rather than at the actual onset of blindness. **This earlier surgical intervention attempts to avoid lens-induced uveitis and cataracts of the mature and hypermature types, and it seems to yield the highest surgical success rates.** In addition, the hypermature cataracts often have concurrent or secondary ciliary zonular instability, which might be recognized preoperatively by phacodonesis, spherophakia, an aphakic crescent, or vitreal prolapse into the anterior chamber as well as by the anterior and posterior lens capsular changes. **Funduscopic evaluation is performed when possible to assess the integrity of the retina. Preoperative gonioscopy is recommended in those breeds having both inherited cataracts and the primary glaucomas. Routine electroretinography should be performed in all cases, and especially among dogs in which the fundus is not visible ophthalmoscopically. B-mode ultrasonography should also be performed, with special attention being paid to the vitreous and to the peripheral and dorsal retina (for retinal detachments).** Preoperative keratometry and A-mode ultrasonography (i.e., biometry), which are necessary procedures for calculating the IOL dioptric strength, may be important future considerations as veterinary IOL implantation becomes more sophisticated and IOL formulas are developed for the canine eye.

Whether to perform cataract surgery, and whether to perform it on one or both eyes, are matters of the individual surgeon's preference, and they reflect a balance between the anticipated visual improvement and the risk of substantial postoperative complications. Today, most cataract surgeries involve both eyes. Cataract surgery includes the use of preoperative topical medications, which are often supplemented by the systemic routes. Each veterinary ophthalmologist has a preferred drug selection (e.g., mydriatics, antibiotics, corticosteroids, nonsteroidal agents) and doses. Mydriasis and treatment of any lens-induced uveitis are important considerations as well.

PHACOEMULSIFICATION

After anterior capsulorhexis (i.e., removal of the central portion of the anterior lens capsule), phacoemulsification consisting of a single hand-piece is inserted into the lens capsular "bag" to remove as much of the lens substance as possible (Fig. 10-11). The phaco tip possesses aspiration and power that are piezoelectric in design and produced by an electrical stimulus from a crystal that vibrates at a specific frequency. The phacoemulsification process is completed by meticulous irrigation and aspiration of any residual cortical material.

INTRAOCULAR LENS DESIGN AND IMPLANTATION

A multitude of different prosthetic, veterinary IOLs are available (Fig. 10-12). The 7-mm optic, which is slightly larger than the standard human IOL, represents a balance between minimizing the incision length for insertion and ensuring the proper positioning within the visual axis in the larger canine capsular sac. The IOL is carefully positioned through the capsulorhexis opening, "dialed" (or rotated) into the capsular bag, and then properly centered.

WOUND CLOSURE

The operative wound may be closed with a variety of suture materials and patterns, the choice of which depend on the surgeon's preference. Use of 8-0 to 10-0 suture material with a single or double running pattern and knot burial is common.

ANTICIPATED OUTCOME

The outcome of cataract surgery in the dog has improved since the 1960s because of the now-widespread use of extracapsular cataract extraction techniques. **In separate, retrospective studies of extracapsular cataract extractions, the short-term (6 weeks to 6 months) success rates, with** *success* **being defined in terms of re-establishing functional vision,**

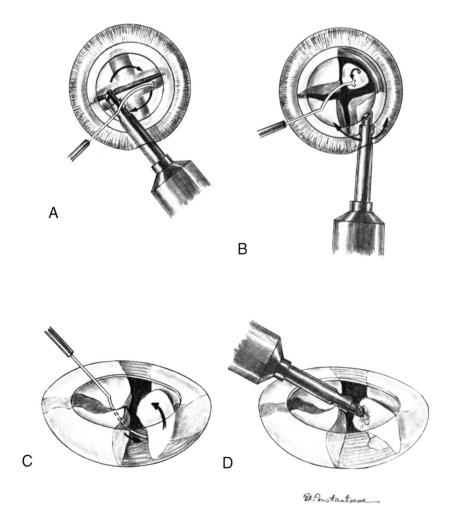

FIGURE 10-11. *A. In the "divide-and-conquer" method, the lens nucleus is rotated 90° after being fractured.* ***B.*** *The lens is fractured again to create four isolated fragments.* ***C*** *and* ***D.*** *The isolated lens fragments are displaced toward the pupil, where they can be easily fragmented and removed.*

were approximately 80%. Bilateral lens removal by phacoemulsification is reported to have a short-term success rate of approximately 95%, but similar to that with extracapsular cataract extraction, a lower success rate is expected with an increased postoperative interval.

DISCISSION/ASPIRATION AND EXTRACAPSULAR CATARACT EXTRACTION

Before the 1960s and the advent of phacoemulsification, discission/aspiration was commonly used to extract both congenital and juvenile cataracts. This procedure is only applicable to the extremely soft lenses of young animals. The anterior lens capsule and body of the cataract are disrupted with a 22- to 25-gauge needle or discission knife inserted through a limbal wound, and the lens material is subsequently aspirated through a large-bore needle, with or without concurrent irrigation through a separate needle. This technique is rarely used at present.

Phacoemulsification is preferred by most veterinary ophthalmic surgeons, but traditional large-incision, extracapsular cataract extraction (i.e., the so-called "open-sky" technique) is still widely used worldwide, especially where the costs or availability of phacoemulsification equipment are prohibitive. The general principles of incision construction, capsulorhexis, lens-loosening techniques, and wound closure are very similar to those previously described for phacoemulsification. The nucleus is expressed from the lens capsule and then is delivered through the incision with a lens loop or an irrigating lens vectis being directed into the dorsal lip of the capsulorhexis. Counterpressure with a blunt instrument (e.g., a muscle hook) at the ventral scleral, just posterior to the limbus, facilitates delivery of the lens. Residual lens cortical material is then removed with a coaxial irrigation/aspiration (I/A) cannula after temporary closure of the wound to 3 mm. At this point, the sutures are removed to allow placement of the IOL. Wound closure is then completed as described for phacoemulsification.

SURGERY FOR LENS INSTABILITY

Lens instability is considered to be primary if attributable to genetic factors (e.g., Terrier breeds) or senile degenerative effects; it is considered to be secondary if associated with primary ocular diseases (e.g., uveitis, glaucoma) that can weaken the ciliary zonules. Lens instability is also a common sequela to hypermature cataract formation and, presumably, occurs secondary to the capsule contracture associated with fibrous metaplasia of lens epithelium, shrinkage in lens volume and stretching of the zonules, or the damaging effects of lens-induced uveitis.

There is considerable diversity of opinion regarding when unstable lenses should be removed. Some avoid surgical intervention for as

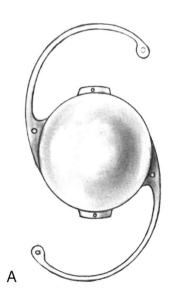

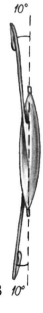

FIGURE 10-12.*Conventional intraocular lens (IOL).* **A.** *Many designs include dialing holes on the optic and suture holes on the haptics.* **B.** *Most lenses are vaulted by 10° to 12°.*

A

B *10°*

long as possible, but recent studies have revealed that the prognosis for vision after intracapsular lens extraction is poor if glaucoma is present at surgery. As a result, unstable lenses should be removed as soon as the instability is detected (for more details, the reader should consult the third edition, pp. 848–853).

INTRACAPSULAR LENS EXTRACTION

Because intracapsular lens extraction requires a 160° to 170° corneal incision, a lateral canthotomy is necessary in most dogs. In the opinion of some veterinary ophthalmologists, unstable lenses can be atraumatically removed only by cryoextraction, for which a 2-mm, nitrous oxide lens probe is the ideal instrument. Regardless of the number of intact zonules, unstable lenses can nearly always be extracted atraumatically if they are very slowly withdrawn from the patellar fossa. As the lens is elevated, the vitreous humor is gently brushed from the posterior capsule with a blunt instrument (e.g., the closed blades of a Westcott tenotomy scissors). In most dogs, the hyaloideocapsular ligament can be left intact, thereby obviating vitrectomy. The incision is then closed with 8-0 vicryl or nylon using a continuous suture pattern, and the anterior chamber is inflated with balanced salt, lactated Ringer's, or saline solution.

Extraction of Subluxated, Hypermature Cataracts

Cataractous lenses that are subluxated because of hypermaturity and capsular fibrosis can often be removed less traumatically if the remaining ciliary zonules are disrupted before the corneal incision is completed.

Suture Fixation of Intraocular Lenses

Currently, suture fixation is the procedure of choice for implanting IOLs in the absence of a lens capsule. The first description of suture fixation for canine IOLs appeared in 1991, and some veterinary ophthalmologists now implant such IOLs routinely.

Perioperative Complications

As with routine cataract surgery, complications may arise from removal of the clear luxated lens or the hypermature cataract with subluxation. The most frequent intra-operative complications include hemorrhage during the extraction and expansion of the vitreous humor. The most common complications postoperatively are retinal detachments and glaucoma.

Prognosis

Less information is available regarding the short- and long-term success rates after intracapsular lens extractions. **Estimates for the success of intracapsular lens extraction without lens implantation of as low as 53% at 1 year after surgery have been reported, and a subsequent study, in which lenses were implanted, revealed a similar success rate (57%) at 32 weeks after surgery. The prognosis after this surgery should improve if the lens is removed early during the course of the disease.**

Diseases and Surgery of the Canine Posterior Segment

The posterior segment includes the vitreous, retina, choroid, and optic nerve head (ONH), which is also called the optic disc and optic papilla. Diseases of these anatomic areas are often shared and, clinically, may appear collectively. **Diseases of the posterior segment are infrequently seen in small animal practice but are more commonly encountered by veterinary ophthalmologists. Diseases of the posterior fundus that impair vision or cause blindness affect large areas of the retina or the optic nerve (or both).**

THE VITREOUS

CLINICAL MORPHOLOGY

The vitreous forms one of the refractive media in the eye, and it provides the necessary pressure to position the neuroretina properly against the retinal pigment epithelium (RPE). Approximately 1% of the vitreous consists of a network of polygonal, hydrated fibrils of hyaluronic acid and collagen (type II); the remaining 99% of the vitreous consists of water. **The outer limits of the vitreous do not consist of membranes. Rather, they are condensations of fibrils that are firmly attached to the ora ciliaris retinae and the pars plana ciliaris. The anterior portion of the vitreous is strongly attached to the posterior lens capsule, which has given rise to the confusing term *hyaloido-capsular ligament* (i.e., Weiger's ligament, Egger's line).** The vitreous is also attached to the region of the ora ciliaris retinae and to the prepapillary area.

253

FIGURE 11-1. *Hyalocentesis. The point of insertion by a 22- to 26-gauge needle (0.70–0.45 mm), 5- to 7-mm posterior to the limbus depending on the ocular quadrant and globe size as determined using calipers or ultrasonography, is of utmost importance.*

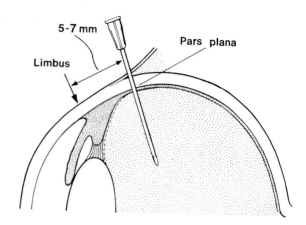

DIAGNOSTIC PROCEDURES

To observe and evaluate the vitreous, the pupil should be dilated using a short-acting mydriatic agent (e.g., 1% tropicamide). **A focal light source and magnification (e.g., the slit-lamp biomicroscope) are used to evaluate the anterior vitreous. Examination of the deeper vitreous requires ophthalmoscopy (direct, indirect, or both) and diagnostic imaging, which usually consists of B-mode ultrasonography (preferably using a 12.5-MHZ probe).** Ultrasonography is particularly useful when direct visual examination of the vitreous is not possible because corneal or lens opacification (or both). Computed tomography and magnetic resonance imaging are other possibilities. Hyalocentesis or vitreal paracentesis involves the aspiration of a small amount of liquid vitreous for analysis, which most often is cytology or microbiologic culture (Fig. 11-1).

THERAPEUTIC PROCEDURES

Medical treatment of posterior segment diseases, including those of the vitreous, requires systemically administered drugs. Topical drugs applied on the corneal surface may affect the anterior vitreous. With breakdown of the blood–aqueous barrier, as occurs during posterior segment inflammations, accessibility to the vitreous by drugs increases. **The most direct way to achieve high drug concentrations in the vitreous is through intraocular injection, but only low doses and volumes are possible.**

Traditional vitrectomies are divided into anterior vitrectomies and posterior vitrectomies. Anterior vitrectomies are usually performed through the pupil, often during cataract or lens removal. Posterior vitrectomies are considerably more difficult, however. They require special instrumentation, and they are used in the treatment of retinal detachments. Anterior vitrectomy can be performed manually using microsurgical cellulose sponges or vitreous forceps, or it can be automated using suction cutters. These cutters can be attached to many of the phacoemulsification units currently being used in cataract surgery.

VITREAL DISEASES

Like corneal and lenticular diseases, vitreal diseases are associated with declines in the transparency and, often, in the consistency of the vitreous.

DEVELOPMENTAL DISORDERS

Vitreal developmental disorders are usually associated with persistent intraocular vasculature or other ocular developmental disorders, such as microphthalmia, anophthalmia, Collie eye anomaly (CEA), and retinal dysplasia.

Persistent Hyaloid Artery

Persistent hyaloid artery (PHA) results from the failure of part (or all) of the hyaloid artery to regress, which produces a small, dense, white string of connective tissue that usually remains adhered to the posterior lens capsule, with variable red or white vascular remnants (Fig. 11-2). The artery may have persisted as a string (and in some cases containing blood) situated in the vitreous space between the optic disc and the lens. Alone, PHA rarely requires surgery. If the associated cataract formation leads to visual impairment, however, surgery may be indicated. In these cases, the risk of complications is slightly higher than that in cases of cataract alone, because in PHA-related cataracts, central fenestration of the posterior lens capsule and anterior vitrectomy are also indicated, which may be especially hazardous when the hyaloid artery is still patent.

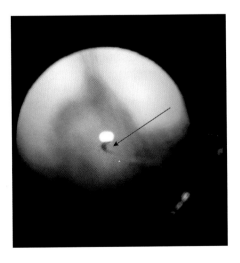

FIGURE 11-2. *Posterior hyaloid artery in a Golden Retriever. The hyaloid artery is visible as a white string (arrow). The optic disc in this patient had the shape of a Bergmeister's papilla.*

Persistent Tunica Vasculosa Lentis

Persistent tunica vasculosa lentis involves fine, white, strandlike deformities (i.e., "spider web") or parts of vascular structures attached to the posterior lens capsule (i.e., persistent tunica vasculosa lentis posterior). These structures generally have no clinical significance, and they are not associated with cataract formation.

Persistent Hyperplastic Tunica Vasculosa Lentis/Persistent Hyperplastic Primary Vitreous

Persistent hyperplastic tunica vasculosa lentis/persistent hyperplastic primary vitreous (PHTVL/PHPV) is a rare and usually unilateral disorder in which parts of the hyaloid system and the primitive vitreous become hyperplastic during early fetal development and persist in this situation postnatally. Its development has been studied extensively in the Doberman Pinscher. The clinical relevance of PHTVL/PHPV centers on its association with cataract formation and, hence, visual impairment. In both the Doberman Pinscher and the Staffordshire Bull Terrier, PHTVL/PHPV generally occurs bilaterally, is inherited (probably because of an incomplete dominant gene in the Doberman), and hence, has a higher prevalence in these breeds than in others. Signs range from very small, retrolentally positioned fibrovascular dots that represent minor remnants of the tunica vasculosa lentis vasculature to severe retrolental and lental malformations (Fig. 11-3). The most severe ocular malformations include intralental or retrolental pigment or hemorrhage, lental coloboma, microphakia, or spherophakia, with or without microphthalmia. Cataract surgery with fenestration of the posterior capsule and transection of the hyaloid artery, if applicable, combined with anterior vitrectomy may be indicated. The prognosis for cataract surgery in cases of severe PHTVL/PHPV is less favorable than that in routine cataract surgery for simple, mature cataracts because of the higher risk for complications (i.e., intra- or postoperative vitreal hemorrhage, formation of traction bands, retinal detachment).

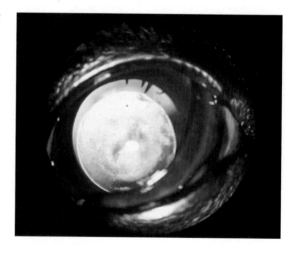

FIGURE 11-3. *Clinical picture of the right eye of a 2-month-old (age approximate) Doberman Pinscher with persistent hyperplastic tunica vasculosa lentis/persistent hyperplastic primary vitreous. Note the elongated ciliary processes at the 12- to 2-o'clock positions, microphakia, and cataract. (Reprinted with permission from Van der Linde-Sipman JS, Stades FC, de Wolff-Rouendaal D. Persistent hyperplastic tunica vasculosa lentis and persistent hyperplastic primary vitreous in the Doberman Pinscher: pathological aspects. J Am Anim Hosp Assoc 1983;19:791–802.)*

TRAUMA

Penetrating trauma, such as that caused by air-rifle or shotgun pellets, may cause floaters of blood in the vitreous. The penetration tunnel is often marked by prolapsed lens material, blood residues, traction bands, and other scars, and the foreign body itself may still be present in the vitreous. Dogs with ophthalmic problems of sudden onset that include signs of trauma such as corneal edema, hyphema, uveitis, and vitreal hemorrhage should also be examined with diagnostic imaging techniques (especially ultrasonography) for the presence of foreign bodies, vitreal changes, and retinal detachment. Survey radiography alone is sufficient for demonstrating metallic foreign bodies. Medical therapy usually consists of topical antimicrobial treatment/prophylaxis, mydriatics/cycloplegics (e.g., 1% atropine), dexamethasone (four to six times daily), and systemic prophylactic antimicrobial as well as extensive anti-inflammatory treatment (e.g., corticosteroids, nonsteroidal anti-inflammatory drugs).

DEGENERATIVE VITREAL DISORDERS AND REACTIONS

Small or large opacities that consist of conglomerates of calcium and lipids, condensations of vitreal fibrils, groups of erythrocytes, or pigment cells (including remnants of the hyaloid system) may persist or develop in the vitreous. Such opacities may move as well and follow the movements of the eye. In older animals, further degeneration of the vitreous can lead to liquefaction (i.e., syneresis), in which case the opacities have a greater tendency to lag behind ocular movements or "whirl up."

Syneresis

Syneresis is a degenerative breakdown of the vitreal gel that separates the liquid from the solid components, thus resulting in liquefaction and development of fluid-filled cavities within the vitreous. This breakdown may result with age, but it can also result from inflammatory reactions or unknown causes. Syneresis may predispose the animal to retinal detachment.

Vitreous Floaters

Vitreous floaters, muscae volitantes, or "flying flies" are larger flakes or streaks in the vitreous that may lag behind ocular movements. If these structures are very moveable, especially against bright light, they can give the impression that something resembling a fly is passing by. Vitreous floaters are uncommon, and they rarely require surgical removal.

Asteroid Hyalosis

Asteroid hyalosis is characterized by many small and, possibly, slightly pigmented particles (i.e., "asteroid bodies") from 0.03 to >0.10 mm in diameter and consisting of calcium or phospholipids in the vitreous of

one or both eyes. These particles move both during and after movements of the globe, but they also return to their initial position (Fig. 11-4). **They generally have no distinct influence on vision.**

Synchysis Scintillans

Synchysis scintillans is characterized by numerous cholesterol particles in a more or less liquefied vitreous. Especially after eye movement, they can resemble a snow flurry behind the lens; against bright light, they may cause dazzling. This abnormality is rare, however, and it seldom causes recognizable problems in the dog.

VITREAL INFLAMMATIONS

Inflammations of the vitreous (i.e., hyalitis, vitreitis) almost always occur secondary to inflammatory reactions of adjacent structures. Floaters of hemorrhagic or other exudate in the vitreous, especially if diffuse or bilateral, often result from exudative uveitis, (chorio)retinitis, or optic neuritis. Therapy should be directed primarily at the underlying cause. The prognosis depends on the underlying cause. Small amounts of blood or exudate may be resorbed, but larger amounts usually cause visual disturbances, even if the inflammatory reaction can be controlled. Vitreal membranes and traction bands may develop as well.

CYSTS

Cysts, most likely originating from the pigmented epithelial layer of the iris or the ciliary body, may extend into the vitreous. These cysts are much less common than anterior chamber cysts, however, and they appear as spherical or oval, translucent bodies that may be stationary or move slowly in liquefied vitreous following movement of the globe. Depending on their size and location, they seldom interfere with vision.

FIGURE 11-4. *Asteroid hyalosis in a dog.*

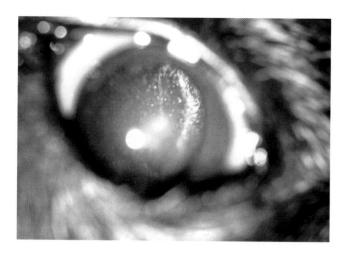

PARASITES

Migrating larvae of *Dirofilaria immitis, Toxocara canis,* the larvae of flies (i.e., ophthalmomyiasis interna), and *Echinococcus* sp. may penetrate the vitreous. Dead or living intraocular parasites may cause local irritation, uveitis, or cyst formation. Killing intraocular dirofilaria using medication (e.g., thiacetarsamide) is sometimes possible, but the intraocular presence of a dead parasite generally induces severe immunogenic uveitis, with possible subsequent endophthalmitis. Therefore, if the parasite can be reached with acceptable risk, surgical removal is preferred.

NEOPLASIA

Intraocular neoplasms generally arise from the uvea. They may occupy part, or almost all, of the vitreous space, and they may cause displacement of the vitreous and lens as well as posterior uveitis and retinal detachment.

THE VITREOUS AND OTHER OPHTHALMIC DISORDERS

LENS LUXATION

The lens may dislocate when its suspension system is compromised by degeneration or rupture of the Zinn's zonular fibers, which are sometimes called the tertiary vitreous. If several zonular fibers have ruptured, vitreous may leak into the anterior chamber along the lental equator and into the pupil; if the fibers have ruptured over a greater area, subluxation of the lens will occur. If the lens becomes completely unattached, it may remain more or less in its normal position, be displaced anterior or posterior, or even topple. Because of its volume and the strong attachment of the posterior lens capsule to the vitreous, a dislocated lens will also dislocate parts of the vitreous. Subsequently, vitreous may prolapse or herniate in the pupil, thus impairing or even blocking drainage of the aqueous between the posterior surface of the lens and the anterior surface of the iris (if the lens has become dislocated into the anterior chamber) or, at the level of the filtration angle, predisposing to secondary glaucoma in all cases. The earliest recognizable sign of a primary lens luxation is slight vitreal protrusions, which are recognizable at slit-lamp microscopy as thin, white clouds in the anterior chamber along the margin of the pupil.

RETINAL DETACHMENTS

A retinal detachment may occupy part, or almost all, of the vitreous space. A small retinal detachment is observed as an indistinctly bordered, grayish-blue "cyst" or fold of the retina. Large detachments look more like grayish-blue to red, parachute-shaped, vascularized bullae positioned either directly behind the posterior lens capsule or deeper in the vitreous. Retinal detachments of a vitreal origin may result from vitreal traction bands (e.g., after perforating trauma or lens luxation), dissolution of the vitreous (i.e., syneresis), or as a complication after vitreal surgery or hyalocentesis.

DISEASES OF THE RETINA AND CHOROID

METHODS OF EXAMINATION

The ocular fundus can be examined using various direct and indirect diagnostic methods. Several are routinely used clinically, whereas others are still evolving and remain more investigative at this time.

Behavioral Testing

After carefully questioning the owner about the animal's vision, the dog's visual performance should be evaluated in an unfamiliar environment using a simple maze, with both daylight and dim light conditions to assess photopic and scotopic vision. Vision may also be assessed through the dog's response to falling objects that do not create noise or air movements (e.g., small cotton balls). Pupillary light reflexes (PLRs) require a functional retina, but they also depend on postretinal transmission of signals. Loss of the PLR is not a confident sign of retinal dysfunction, or even of vision loss. A totally unresponsive pupil might be suggestive of any kind of generalized retinopathy, glaucoma, or lesion involving the reflex pathway. The menace reaction (i.e., the response to a sudden, threatening object coming into the near field of view) may also be used, and this cortical response requires both a functional sensory pathway from the photoreceptors to the visual cortex and an intact motor pathway, including the facial nerve. The normal response is blinking and, possibly, withdrawal of the head.

Ophthalmoscopy

Both direct and indirect ophthalmoscopy are used in veterinary ophthalmology to visualize the fundus. **The ophthalmoscopic examination is performed in a darkened room using short-acting mydriatics, such as 0.5 to 1.0% tropicamide (see Chapter 1).**

Ultrasonography and Fluorescein Angiography

Ultrasonography is a valuable aid in detecting and monitoring pathologic conditions in the canine posterior segment, especially in patients with less-than-clear media (e.g., dense cataracts, intraocular hemorrhage). Fluorescein angiography is a helpful adjunct in establishing the diagnosis of retinal diseases, and it is primarily used to evaluate

disease processes in which the vasculature of the eye is involved (e.g., vascular anomalies, posterior segment neoplasms, hypertension, retinal detachment, inflammatory processes, diabetic retinopathy, degenerative processes). The procedure is performed either in sedated, anesthetized, or awake dogs; the choice depends on the preference and need of the examiner. Fluorescein sodium solution (10%) is given as an intravenous bolus of 10 mg/kg into the cephalic vein. Fundus photography is then performed using a standard fundus camera connected to a powerpack unit to allow for quick recycling of the black-and-white or color film. This test can also be performed with only a direct or indirect ophthalmoscope fitted with the appropriate yellow (light source, Kodak Wratten 15 yellow filter) and blue (viewing area, Wratten blue 47A filter) color filters.

Electrophysiology

When the retina is stimulated by light, a diffuse electrical response is generated by the neuronal and the nonneuronal cells that can be recorded as the electroretinogram (ERG). **The flash ERG is an objective, functional test of the retina and is critically dependent on the function of the photoreceptors (i.e., the rods and cones).** It has a characteristic waveform that varies depending on several factors, though mostly from the type of stimuli used. The ERG is usually recorded in the dog using an active contact-lens electrode as well as reference and ground electrodes. The results displayed on an oscilloscope, ink-writer, or computer screen (for more details, the reader should consult the third edition, pp. 484–494 and 872–873). In clinical veterinary ophthalmology, the flash ERG has two broad applications. The first is to test whether a standard stimulus elicits an ERG response. **This is useful in assessing retinal activity when the fundus is obscured (e.g., before cataract surgery) and in the differential diagnosis of retinal disease when ophthalmoscopic lesions are absent.** The second is to test rod and cone function in conjunction with research into retinal disease processes and in the early diagnosis of hereditary retinal degenerations and dystrophies.

A second type of ERG is the pattern ERG. This type is used experimentally to evaluate the inner retinal layers (mainly the retinal ganglion cells [RGCs]).

Visually Evoked Potentials

The visually evoked cortical potential (VEP), or the visually evoked response, is a gross electrical signal generated at the occipital cortex in response to visual stimulation. These responses are of small amplitude (1–40 μV), and they are extremely sensitive to stimulus changes. Therefore, computer averaging is necessary for their recording, and correct placement of electrodes is necessary to achieve correct and reproducible results. **In veterinary ophthalmology, the VEP is used to test the central visual function, including the optic nerve, higher visual tracts, and visual cortex. It is also useful in blind patients with normal ophthalmic examination results and a normal ERG.**

THE NORMAL OCULAR FUNDUS

The canine ocular fundus is a challenge for the examiner because of the enormous variation in its normal ophthalmoscopic appearance. This great range in normal fundic appearance should, perhaps, be expected when the diversity in the gross appearance of different canine breeds is considered (Fig. 11-5). Certain features of the fundus relate to macroscopic properties (e.g., iris color, coat color).

Proficiency in ophthalmoscopy for canine ophthalmology requires considerable experience. For convenience, the ocular fundus is divided into the tapetal fundus, nontapetal fundus, ONH, and the retinal and optic vasculature.

FIGURE 11-5. *Normal appearance of the fundus in different canine breeds. **A.** A 4-year-old Beagle with a large, mainly yellow tapetal area and a relatively large, round disc at the border of the tapetal and the nontapetal areas. **B.** A 1-year-old Briard with a large, yellow to orange tapetal fundus and a disc at the border of the tapetal and the nontapetal fundus. **C.** A 6-year-old Cavalier King Charles Spaniel with a thin and sparse tapetal fundus. The uneven borders of the optic disc result from pronounced myelination. **D.** A submelanotic right eye in a 1-year-old Papillon. The regular striation of the choroidal vessels is seen against the white sclera, and there are no tapetal cells. The nontapetal fundus is pigmented. The fellow eye had an orange-yellow, "normal" tapetal and a pigmented nontapetal fundus. **E.** A 4-year-old, liver-colored Labrador Retriever with a light brownish coloration of the entire fundus. No tapetal cells are visible. **F.** A 7-week-old Collie pup with an immature, blue-colored fundus.*

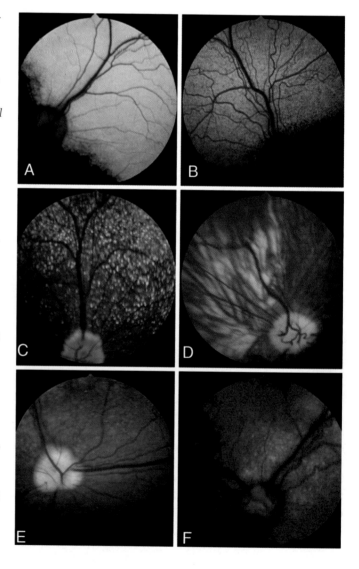

TAPETAL FUNDUS

The combination of the tapetum lucidum and an absence of pigment in the overlying RPE is the anatomic basis for the tapetal fundus, which forms an almost triangular area, with a horizontal base, in the dorsal half of the fundus. This area is usually brightly and beautifully colored and reflective, but the size of the tapetal fundus varies extensively. Usually, the tapetal fundus is large, and it may sometimes surround the ONH in gaze hounds and large breeds. It is often poorly developed, however, in toy breeds (e.g., Papillons). In dogs with a merle coat color (e.g., blue merle Collies, Shetland Sheepdogs, and related breeds), the tapetal fundus may even be absent. Development of the adult tapetal fundus requires approximately 16 weeks in the dog.

NONTAPETAL FUNDUS

The nontapetal fundus comprises the largest area of the canine ocular fundus. The junction between the tapetal and the nontapetal fundus exhibits a continuous variation, from a distinct line of demarcation to a gradual transition with scattered foci of the tapetal cells, which become more and more sparse with increasing distance from the center of the tapetal fundus. The nontapetal fundus has a nonreflective and usually dark or grayish brown to black color. Sometimes, the choroidal vessels will cause a striped or a tigroid appearance when viewed through the ophthalmoscope. In dogs with a subalbinotic fundus, parts of the nontapetal fundus will be unpigmented, thus showing the choroidal vessels overlying the white sclera. Absence of pigment in the entire nontapetal region is common (e.g., in blue merle Collies).

OPTIC NERVE HEAD

The canine ONH (or the optic disc or papilla) also exhibits a wide range of normal variations in ophthalmoscopic appearance. It is located in the center of the fundus, sometimes in the nontapetal fundus and sometimes in the tapetal region. The extent of myelinization affects the size of the ONH. The shape of the ONH may be round, oval, triangular, or polygonal, and the disc edge may sometimes be clearly indented. The color of the ONH varies from pinkish-white to deep pink, depending on the extent of the visible vasculature. The course of these vessels is a useful aid in determining the topography of the ONH. The fundus surrounding the ONH may present as a partial or complete, pigmented ring with focal absence of tapetal tissue.

RETINAL VASCULATURE

The vascular architecture of the canine fundus is classified as being holangiotic. The vasculature consists of arterioles and venules at the surface of the retina. The arterioles (usually 15–20 in number) radiate away from their origin close to the periphery of the ONH. They appear slightly lighter in color compared with those vessels transporting venous blood, and they may be more tortuous than the venules. The main veins (usually 3–4 in number) are obviously larger and darker red in color than the arterioles. They end in the usually incomplete venous circle atop the ONH, but they also may, in part, be covered by the ONH tissue. Several smaller venules coalesce with the major veins, thereby building a branching tree of vessels over the optic fundus. The area centralis–like region has a higher cone density compared with the rest of the retina and is an indistinctly bordered area located slightly superior and temporal to the ONH, which is devoid of blood vessels but is encircled by fine branches.

OPHTHALMOSCOPY OF THE DEVELOPING PUPPY OCULAR FUNDUS

When a puppy's eyelids open at approximately 2 weeks of age and ophthalmoscopic examination can be performed, no difference between the tapetal and the nontapetal fundus can be discerned. Both appear a dull, dark gray in color, the ONH is small, and its anterior surface usually does not protrude over the retinal surface. The retinal blood vessels, however, are easily identifiable and appear relatively large in size. At 3 to 4 weeks of age, the developing tapetal fundus appears paler and the nontapetal region relatively darker. **The tapetal fundus then takes on a lilac to blue coloration, which becomes more intense with increasing age.** At approximately 7 to 8 weeks age, the tapetal fundus becomes more granular in appearance. The bluish, immature tapetal fundus then becomes more brightly colored over time, until the adult structure and coloration are developed at approximately 3 to 4 months of age. These events must be considered during ophthalmoscopy in puppies for congenital and developmental diseases of the ocular fundus.

CHORIORETINAL CONGENITAL AND DEVELOPMENTAL DISEASES

COLLIE EYE ANOMALY

Collie eye anomaly is a congenital ocular syndrome involving defects of the posterior vascular and fibrous tunics of the eye. The pathogenesis of the defect is considered to be an abnormal mesodermal differentiation that results in more or less serious defects, mainly of the sclera, choroid, optic disc, retina, and retinal vasculature. The severity of the disease varies, ranging from no apparent visual deficit to total blindness. It is bilateral, and it has no gender predisposition. There is no difference in frequency related to coat color, coat type, or presence of the merling gene. **The cardinal sign is a geographically defined region of choroidal hypoplasia lateral to the optic disc (Fig. 11-6), which may (or may not) be accompanied by obvious retinal or scleral defects or by colobomas (Fig. 11-7 and Table 11-1). Other anomalies include retinal detachment and intraocular hemorrhage. The CEA anomaly occurs in Collies (i.e., Rough and Smooth Collies), Shetland Sheepdogs, Australian Shep-**

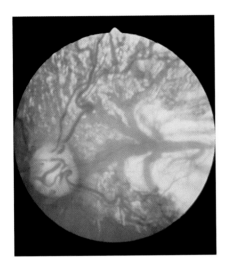

FIGURE 11-6. *Collie eye anomaly with choroidal hypoplasia temporal to the optic disc in a 2-year-old Shetland Sheepdog.*

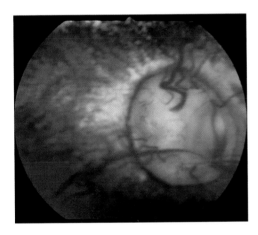

FIGURE 11-7. *Collie eye anomaly with a large, irregularly oval optic nerve head and a pronounced optic nerve coloboma in a Collie. Note the position of the blood vessels as they approach the coloboma.*

herds, and Border Collies, and a simple autosomal recessive inheritance has been postulated.

The prevalence of CEA is extremely high in Rough and Smooth Collies and Shetland Sheepdogs throughout the world. In 1969, the incidence in Collies was between 75 and 97% in the United States, 64% in England, greater than 50% in Sweden, and 41% in Norway. In the Shetland Sheepdog, the prevalence is also high, and the incidence again appears to vary in different countries. The incidence of CEA in Border Collies and Australian Shepherds, however, is low.

Excessive tortuosity of retinal vessels occurs in nearly all eyes affected by CEA. Blood vessel tortuosity can also be found, however, in genetically clear Collies and dogs of other breeds. Therefore, it usually is not regarded as being pathognomonic for CEA, but tortuosity of both arterioles and venules should raise the examiner's index of suspicion for CEA (especially the "Go-Normals" or dogs in which a very small choroidal hypoplastic area becomes pigmented and the dog's fundus appears normal. These dogs, however, breed as affected animals). Vermiform streaks or folds in the neurosensory retina of neonates result from unequal growth of the sclera, the

TABLE 11-1

OPHTHALMOSCOPIC FINDINGS IN COLLIE EYE ANOMALY

Lesion	Appearance
Choroidal hypoplasia	Bilateral, pale to white area lateral (temporal) or dorsolateral (superotemporal) of the optic nerve head, variable size; can be asymmetrical; difficult to detect in merle/subalbinoid dogs. Best to examine puppies at 6–7 weeks of age. Can pigment and later appear normal (Go-Normals).
Posterior colobomas	Involve the optic disc (papillary colobomas) or adjacent area (peripapillary colobomas). Also called "pits" or posterior scleral ectasia. Appear as gray or pink indentations; vary from shallow depressions to more extensive excavations or "holes" ≤30 diopters in depth. May occur in 10–30% of the eyes with choroidal hypoplasia.
Retinal detachment	Partial or complete; unilateral or bilateral; in 5–10% of affected eyes. Appear clinically as nonfixation of the eyes, a tendency toward nystagmus, or even strabismus in affected pups. Affects both pups and adults. Most arise adjacent to the optic disc and extend toward the peripheral fundus, often with subretinal, intraretinal, or preretinal hemorrhages.
Intraocular hyphema	Occurs in ≤5% of affected eyes, often with colobomatous defects and retinal detachments.

choroid, and the retinal layers. They are seen as linear or circular, grayish (in the tapetal area) or white (in the nontapetal area) configurations, usually in the central fundus and most prevalent near the optic disc in the young Collie. As the globe grows, these "streaks" disappear.

The only way to significantly reduce the frequency of CEA from this breed is to avoid using affected animals and their parents (no matter the type or degree of CEA lesions) as breeding stock. The hereditary pattern for CEA is simple autosomal recessive, and the disorder is a congenital defect. The incidence of CEA has remained high throughout the world, however, in the Collie and, to a lesser extent, the Shetland Sheepdog.

RETINAL DYSPLASIA

Retinal dysplasia is an anomalous differentiation of the retina accompanied by a proliferation of one or more of its constituent elements. It is characterized histopathologically by linear folding of the sensory retina and by formation of rosettes, which are composed of variable numbers of neuronal retinal cells around a central lumen. Dysplastic retinal lesions may be associated with systemic abnormalities, or they may occur as a primary ocular defect, either as a single defect or together with other lesions such as microphthalmos or colobomatous defects. Retinal dysplasia involves multiple retinal layers and, occasionally, the vitreous (depending on its severity). It is usually nonprogressive, and it may (or may not) interfere with vision. **Causes of retinal dysplasia include canine herpesvirus, vitamin A deficiency, x-ray radiation, certain drugs, intrauterine trauma, and heredity (the most common cause in the dog). Because of its frequency, retinal dysplasia should be suspected in any blind puppy.**

SPONTANEOUS RETINAL DYSPLASIA

Esotropia, leukocoria, and blindness may be present in those breeds with complete or total retinal dysplasia and retinal detachments. Induced pupillary light responses are variable, and most affected dogs have infundibular (i.e., complete) retinal detachments. Parts of the retina may be attached to the posterior lens capsule. Intraocular hemorrhage may occur as well, and microphthalmia is common. Ophthalmoscopically, the lesions of retinal dysplasia are unilateral or bilateral, and they may be grossly divided into three different types or forms: focal or multifocal, geographic, and complete with retinal detachment (or nonattachment) (Table 11-2).

Multifocal retinal dysplasia does not affect vision, whereas the second and third forms of dysplasia cause severe visual impairment or blindness. In blind puppies with complete retinal dysplasia, leukocoria and a rotary-searching

---

TABLE 11-2

OPHTHALMOSCOPIC FINDINGS IN RETINAL DYSPLASIA

Type	Ophthalmoscopic Findings
Focal or multifocal	Retinal folds and rosettes are seen as areas of reduced tapetal reflectivity, appearing as gray or green dots or linear, "V," or "Y" streaks. Occur anywhere in the tapetal region, but most often central and usually above the optic disc. May appear elevated, distorting the course of the overlying vessels. Retinal folds in the nontapetal fundus appear as gray or white linear or irregular streaks.
Geographic	Appear as an irregular or horseshoe-shaped area, most often in the central tapetal fundus. May include focal retinal thinning and elevation. Usually a hyperreflective area with variable pigmentation.
Complete with detachment	Usually a completely detached neural retina floating in the vitreous, attached around the optic nerve head.

FIGURE 11-8. *Midperipheral tapetal fundus in a 4-year-old Springer Spaniel with severe multifocal retinal dysplasia. The bilateral lesions had progressed since an ophthalmic examination 1 year previously and were now causing visual impairment. Note the hyperreflective central parts of some of the dysplastic lesions, indicating neuroretinal thinning.*

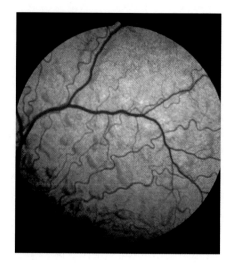

nystagmus sometimes occur. Most lesions of retinal dysplasia do not appear to change significantly with time. Occasional lesions, however, do become less obvious. Some folds may disappear as well, whereas others may become more demarcated, with hyperpigmented spots and streaks and hyperreflective areas in the vicinity of the dysplastic lesions (Fig. 11-8).

Problems of Diagnosis, Interpretation, and Control

Retinal dysplasia includes a diverse group of entities with variable clinical and histopathologic appearances, pathogeneses, and causes. The clinical appearance of retinal dysplasia is often similar, however, regardless of the cause. Among the breeds in which the defect has been recognized as being inherited, certain characteristic features (e.g., the central, mainly tapetal location of the folds and rosettes) are evident, which simplifies establishing the diagnosis (Table 11-3). **Lesions associated with external insults (e.g., intrauterine infection, radiation therapy) may cause problems in establishing the clinical diagnosis.** There are problems in controlling inherited retinal dysplasia among several breeds, especially if blindness does not occur. Though it is certainly suspected by some investigators, whether a genetic relationship exists between the different forms of primary hereditary retinal dysplasia in the various breeds remains unclear.

INHERITED RETINAL AND TAPETAL DYSTROPHIES

The dog exhibits many tapetoretinal dystrophies. Important reasons for this are certainly the establishment of different breeds and the custom of inbreeding dogs, which has favored the emergence and expression of recessive genes that cause a wide spectrum of retinal and tapetal disorders. The

TABLE 11-3

BREEDS OF DOGS AFFECTED WITH RETINAL DYSPLASIA

Breed (Mode of Inheritance)	Type of Retinal Dysplasia	Other Abnormalities
Akita	Complete	Microphthalmia, cataract, posterior lenticonus
American Cocker Spaniel (AR)	Multifocal	None
	Multifocal	Microphthalmia, cataracts, persistent pupillary membranes
Australian Shepherd (AR incomplete penetrance; any breed with homozygous merling)	Complete	Iridal heterochromia, cataracts; staphylomas; retinal detachments
Beagle	Multifocal	Microphthalmia
Bedlington Terrier (AR)	Complete	Microphthalmia, cataracts, retinal detachments
Cavalier King Charles Spaniel	Geographic	Microphthalmia, cataracts, posterior lenticonus
Chow Chow	Complete	Severe ocular defects
Doberman Pinscher (AR)	Complete	Microphthalmia, anterior segment dysplasia, aphakia, hyperplastic primary vitreous
English Springer Spaniel (AR)	Geographic	Microphthalmia, cataracts, retinal detachments
Golden Retriever	Geographic	None
Labrador Retriever	Multifocal	None
	Geographic	None
(AR)	Complete	Microphthalmia, cataracts, intraocular hemorrhage
(AD)	Complete	Cataracts; retarded growth of the radius, ulna, and tibia; separated hypoplastic anconeal and coronoid processes; hip dysplasia; delayed development of the epiphysis
Rottweiler	Multifocal	None
Sealyham Terrier (AR)	Complete	Microphthalmia, cataracts, retinal detachments
Samoyed	Complete	Microphthalmia, cataracts, hyaloid artery persistence, and skeletal defects like those in the Labrador Retriever
Yorkshire Terrier	Multifocal	None

AR, autosomal recessive trait; *AD,* autosomal dominant trait with variable penetrance.

paucity of knowledge concerning the underlying biochemical, physiologic, and morphologic disease mechanisms of humans renders dogs with similar diseases especially important as animal models.

CLASSIFICATION OF CANINE RETINAL DEGENERATIONS

Canine retinal degenerations primarily affect the photoreceptors or RPE (or both). Since the first well-documented report of an inherited retinal degeneration in a Gordon Setter from Sweden, many breeds have been found to be affected by hereditary retinal degenerations. The general term *progressive retinal atrophy (PRA)* has been applied to these conditions, and clinicians have divided PRA into two types, depending on the ophthalmoscopic appearance of the fundus lesions: generalized PRA, and central PRA (CPRA). Generalized PRA involves a generalized hyperreflectivity of the retina at the end stage of the disease, thereby indicating a generalized atrophy of the neural retinal structures and clinical blindness. In CPRA, there are multifocal accumulations of pigment within the retina, with areas of hyperreflectivity encircling these changes at the end stage. **The latter disorder is a primary defect in the RPE but that does not always lead to blindness, hence the recent change to the more appropriate term,** *retinal pigment epithelial dystrophy (RPED).* During the last few decades, PRA has been subdivided even further, into more specific diseases at both the cellular and the molecular levels, and gene symbols are now used to differentiate these disorders.

The classification of hereditary retinal degenerations reflects differing opinions, much discussion, and continued development of new information. **The PRA group is subdivided grossly into developmental and degenerative photoreceptor diseases.** The developmental class represents a large aggregate of genetically distinct disorders that are expressed cytologically during the postnatal period, when the visual cells begin to differentiate. These disorders represent a dysplasia of the rod or cone photoreceptors (or both), and each has its own unique disease course and phenotype as assessed using functional and morphologic criteria. **Typical for the dysplasias is that before the retina becomes adultlike (<10 weeks of age in the dog), it shows rather severe structural alterations of the rod photoreceptor cells. The rate of progression and loss of cones in the disease process, however, varies among these disorders. In contrast, the degenerative diseases represent defects in which photoreceptor cells degenerate after having differentiated normally.** In this latter group, disease occurs more slowly, and it is modified by both temporal and topographic factors. Different alleles have been identified at the same gene locus in dogs affected with progressive rod-cone degeneration (prcd), and these segregate to regulate the rate of photoreceptor degeneration.

CLINICAL SIGNS OF PROGRESSIVE RETINAL ATROPHY

The clinical manifestations of PRA are often remarkably similar, no matter what specific type of disorder is present at the cellular level.

Without exception, PRA is bilateral and leads to blindness. The dog's familiarity with the environment can greatly conceal severe visual deficits. In fact, it is not unusual to obtain animals for diagnosis late in the disease process, when owners have noticed visual problems only after having moved or refurnished their homes. Almost always, the earliest clinical sign is impaired vision in dim light and darkness (i.e., nyctalopia or night blindness). This reduced visual capacity in darkness often may be observed at visual testing, which involves the menace reaction or using falling cotton balls in front of the dog in a dimly lit room. Fundus changes of PRA as observed at ophthalmoscopy are summarized in Table 11-4 and are shown in Fig. 11-9.

Pupillary light reflexes become progressively more sluggish as the disease progresses, and the resting pupillary opening is often wider among affected animals at an advanced stage than among the normal population. Often, however, the PLRs are not lost entirely in PRA, which is a useful feature in the differential diagnosis of blindness. **Secondary cataract is frequently present at advanced stages of disease in several (but not all) breeds with PRA. The initial changes tend to involve the posterior cortex and include vacuolation and opacification.** Irregular radiations are often seen emanating from the posterior pole of the lens and

---

TABLE 11-4

OPHTHALMOSCOPIC CHANGES IN PROGRESSIVE RETINAL ATROPHY

Disease Stage	Ophthalmoscopic Changes
Early	Slight change in tapetal reflectivity or hyporeflectivity is often seen, such as a grayish discoloration, mainly in the peripheral tapetal fundus. Slight vascular attenuation and beading of retinal vessels in the midperipheral and peripheral parts of the tapetal fundus may also be observed.
Moderate	Color changes in the tapetal fundus become more marked and generalized, as does the vascular attenuation. Increased reflectivity or hyperreflectivity of the tapetal fundus, usually most marked in the midperipheral tapetal fundus. Slight decrease in pigmentation of the nontapetal fundus. Optic nerve head changes include early loss of myelin, the disc changing in shape to circular, and reduced number and calipers of blood vessels. Early optic atrophy.
Advanced	Hyperreflectivity progresses to involve the entire tapetal fundus. Continued loss of pigmentation of the nontapetal fundus. Marked decrease in the retinal vasculature, with preservation of only the large and central blood vessels until late in the disease. Ghost vessels peripherally. Optic disk pallor, loss of myelin, and reduction in disc size.

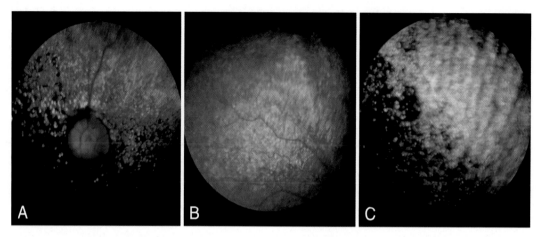

FIGURE 11-9. *Advanced progressive rod-cone degeneration in a 7-year-old Miniature Poodle.* **A.** *The central part of the fundus, with severe vascular attenuation and a grayish tapetal discoloration.* **B.** *The midperipheral fundus, with hyperreflectivity and discoloration in the peripheral part.* **C.** *The periphery of the tapetal fundus, with a marked striation. Note the contours of the choroidal vascular pattern underlying the atrophic neural retina.*

extending to involve the equatorial cortex and, later, the entire lens. Especially in certain breeds, mature cataracts make ERG of utmost importance before surgery to rule out concurrent retinal degeneration.

PHOTORECEPTOR DYSPLASIAS

Breeds with retinal dysplasias are affected clinically during the first year of life, and they include the Irish Setter (rod-cone dysplasia type 1), Collie (rod-cone dyplasia type 2), Norwegian Elkhound (rod dysplasia and early retinal degeneration), Miniature Schnauzer (photoreceptor dysplasia), Belgian Shepherd (photoreceptor dysplasia), and Alaskan Malamute (cone degeneration). The clinical characteristics for these conditions are summarized in Table 11-5.

Rod-cone dysplasia type 1 in Irish Setters is a recessively inherited disease characterized by arrested differentiation of visual cells resulting from abnormal cyclic guanosine 3,5′-monophosphate (cGMP) metabolism. By 10 days of age, deficient cGMP-phosphodiesterase (cGMP-PDE) activity causes the retinal levels of cGMP to rise sharply, achieving concentrations as much as 10-fold higher than normal. These biochemical abnormalities are present, however, before degenerative changes are observed in the photoreceptor cells. The defect in Irish Setters is similar to that in the rd mouse, in which the β-subunit of cGMP-PDE has been identified. Rod-cone dysplasia in the Collie is not influenced by coat color, merling, CEA, or other forms of eye disease, but at times, it may appear simultaneously and coincidentally with them. Rod dysplasia in Norwegian Elkhounds involves no abnormalities in the cyclic nucleotide metabolism, thus distinguishing this disorder from rod-cone dysplasia type 1 in Irish Setters. In addition, matings between the two breeds have failed to produce affected progeny. Early retinal degeneration in the Norwegian Elkhound has been described more recently than rod dysplasia, and abnormalities in retinal cyclic nucleotide metabolism as well as mutations in the *PDEb* gene have been excluded as causes for the early retinal degeneration by the results of breeding and molecular studies.

Photoreceptor dysplasia in Miniature Schnauzers is an unusual PRA, in that it shows a slow clinical progression when assessed using behavioral testing and ophthalmoscopy. When judged using histopathology and ERG, however, it is an early onset disorder. Conclusive and distinct funduscopic changes are not apparent until the very late stages of the disease, and classical PRA lesions are not observed in affected animals until 2 to 5 years of age.

A recessive cone degeneration inherited in Alaskan Malamutes specifically affects the cones and causes congenital hemeralopia or day blindness. It is characterized by specific functional and structural abnormalities limited to the cone photoreceptors; thus, it is unique, being the only model to date for selective cone degeneration in humans. Clinically, behavioral signs in affected dogs are usually apparent at 8 to 10 weeks of age.

TABLE 11-5

CHARACTERISTICS OF RETINAL PHOTORECEPTOR DYSPLASIA IN THE DOG

Breed	Primary Defect	Mode of Inheritance	Diagnosis	
			By Ophthalmoscopy	By ERG and Anatomic Changes
Alaskan Malamute	Cone degeneration	AR	No changes	6 weeks: cone: —; rod: N
Belgian Shepherd	Rod-cone dysplasia	Unknown	11 weeks	4 weeks: cone: —; rod: —
Collie	Rod-cone dysplasia	AR	16 weeks	6 weeks: cone: ↓; rod: —
Irish Setter	Rod-cone dysplasia	AR	16 weeks	6 weeks: cone: ↓; rod: —
Miniature Schnauzer	Rod-cone dysplasia	AR	1.5–5.0 years	6 weeks: cone: ↓; rod: ↓
Norwegian Elkhound	Rod dysplasia	AR	1.0–1.5 years	6 weeks: cone: N/↓; rod: —
Norwegian Elkhound	Early rod degeneration	AR	9 months–1 year	5 weeks: A-wave dominates; cone: ↓; rod: ↓

AR, autosomal recessive trait; *ERG,* electroretinography; *N,* normal.

Hemeralopic dogs show severe loss of vision both in daylight and in high levels of artificial illumination, but such dogs become less insecure when placed in dim lighting. Recovery of vision takes several minutes, though loss of vision on returning to bright light is immediate. The behavioral signs remain unaltered throughout life, and night vision is never abnormal. No funduscopic changes are observed at any stage of this disease, however, and the PLRs are normal in both dim and bright light. **The ERG of affected dogs reveals normal rod function but an absence of cone responses** (for more details, the reader should consult the third edition, pp. 887–894).

LATE-ONSET RETINAL DEGENERATIONS

Late-onset retinal degenerations occur in older or middle-aged dogs, and the basic photoreceptor disorder is usually rod-cone degeneration. Like the photoreceptor dysplasias, these conditions can be diagnosed considerably earlier with electroretinography than with ophthalmoscopy or the onset of visual impairment (Table 11-6). They share the same ophthalmoscopic changes as the photoreceptor dysplasias and affect the Toy and Miniature Poodle, English and American Cocker Spaniel, Portuguese Water Dog, Siberian Husky, Tibetan Terrier and Spaniel, Miniature Longhaired Dachshund, Akita, Papillon, Samoyed, and other breeds.

Of the degenerative group of hereditary retinal diseases recognized in the dog, mutations at the *prcd* gene locus account for several autosomal diseases, but the different mutations responsible for the defined allelic variants among breeds (discussed later) have not yet been identified. To date, however, the peripherin/rds, opsin, and *PDEb* genes have been excluded as being causative. Thus, the term *progressive rod-cone degeneration* today refers to classic PRA as well as to a specific photoreceptor disorder that is a bilateral, late-onset disease of the rods primarily and then of the cones, has typical ERG findings in affected animals, and shows morphologically a typical spatial distribution of disease. **Genetic homology has been found for prcd in the Toy, Miniature, and Standard Poodle, the American and English Cocker Spaniel, the Labrador Retriever, and the Portuguese Water Dog.** More breeds will probably be added to this list in the near future.

During the search for systemic markers in human retinitis pigmentosa and for animal models of this disease, several groups have investigated the level of plasma lipids among affected individuals. In the Miniature Poodle, significantly lower levels of plasma docosahexaenoic acid (22:6n-3) were found in affected dogs compared with normal dogs. The effects of 22:6n-3 supplementation on polyunsaturated fatty acid metabolism were also determined, with the results revealing a defect in 22:6n-3 metabolism among prcd-affected animals. Whether there is any correlation between the reduced renewal rate of photoreceptor outer segments, the lower 22:6n-3 levels, and retinal degeneration in prcd-affected dogs, however, is not yet clear. Results of cross-breeding experiments with prcd-affected Miniature Poodles and retinal-degenerate English and American Cocker Spaniels have shown that the gene mutation in each breed lies at the same (*prcd*) locus. In the English Cocker Spaniel, however, the disease differs phenotypically both in the rate of progression and in the topographic distribution of disease in the retina. Clinically, prcd in the English Cocker Spaniel is phenotypically expressed late in life, with funduscopic alterations that are in-

TABLE 11-6

CHARACTERISTICS OF RETINAL PHOTORECEPTOR DEGENERATION IN THE DOG

| Breed | Primary Defect | Mode of Inheritance | Diagnosis | |
			By Ophthalmoscopy	By ERG and Anatomic Changes
Akita	Not established	AR	1–3 years	1.5–2.0 years: cone: ↓; rod: ↓↓
American Cocker Spaniel	Rod-cone degeneration	AR	2.5–3.0 years	9 months: cone: ↓; rod: ↓↓
English Cocker Spaniel	Rod-cone degeneration	AR	3–8 years	2–3 years: cone: ↓; rod: ↓↓
Labrador Retriever	Rod-cone degeneration	AR	3–6 years	1.5 years: cone: ↓; rod: ↓↓
Miniature Long-haired Dachshund	Unknown	AR	6 months	4 months: cone: ↓; rod: ↓↓
Papillon	Unknown	AR	1.5–5.0 years	9 months–1.5 years: cone: ↓; rod: ↓↓
Portuguese Water Dog	Rod-cone degeneration	AR	3–6 years	1.5 years: cone: ↓; rod: ↓↓
Siberian Husky	Unknown	X-linked	2 years	1 year: cone: ↓; rod: ↓↓
Tibetan Spaniel	Unknown	AR	3–5 years	1.5 years: cone: ↓; rod: ↓↓
Tibetan Terrier	Unknown	AR	1.0–1.5 years	10 months: cone: ↓; rod: ↓↓
Toy and Miniature Poodle	Rod-cone degeneration	AR	3–5 years	9 months: cone: ↓; rod: ↓↓

AR, autosomal recessive trait; *ERG,* electroretinography.

dicative of retinal degeneration usually not becoming prevalent until between the ages of 4 to 8 years. Moreover, appearance of the fundus in affected dogs may be quite variable.

Hereditary retinal degeneration in the Siberian Husky is unusual, in that an excess of male dogs are affected and the disease is transmitted

by an X-linked gene. Furthermore, it is the first canine retinal degeneration that can be assigned to an identified chromosome.

Great variability occurs in the extent and coloration of the visible tapetal fundus in the Papillon, which may confound establishing the diagnosis of PRA in this breed. Some dogs lack visible tapetal fundi, and some have subalbinotic eyes. These variables also often render making the diagnosis difficult, because the retinal blood vessel and optic nerve changes occur later. The ERG is extremely useful in such eyes, but the ERG is also useful in making an early diagnosis of disease in dogs with the more common fundus appearance. (For more details, the reader should consult the third edition, pp. 895–903.)

RETINAL PIGMENT EPITHELIUM (AUTOFLUORESCENT INCLUSION) EPITHELIOPATHY/RETINAL PIGMENT EPITHELIAL DYSTROPHY

The term *central progressive retinal atrophy*, or *CPRA*, has been used for a group of conditions with ophthalmoscopic changes that can be characterized by an accumulation of irregular foci or light-brown pigment spots in the central tapetal fundus (Fig. 11-10). Over time, these foci increase in size and become distributed throughout the tapetal zone. At this stage, visible changes (e.g., hyperreflectivity around the pigment foci) indicate atrophy of the overlying neural retina. The nontapetal fundus shows similar foci, with hyperpigmentation and depigmented areas in between. Originally, CPRA was used to differentiate this condition from generalized PRA. Hence, CPRA affects the RPE primarily, with secondary effects on the neural retina, and differs from the PRA diseases, which primarily affect the photoreceptor layer. **Today, CPRA is referred to as retinal pigment epithelial dystrophy,**

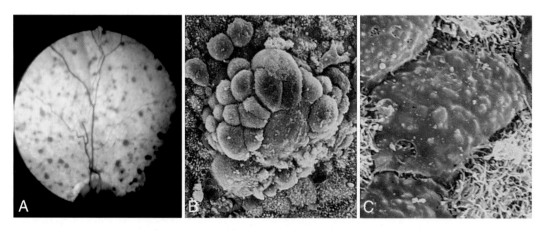

FIGURE 11-10. *A. Retinal pigment epithelial dystrophy in a 5-year-old German Shepherd. Note the generalized pigmented spots, generalized hyperreflectivity, and severe vascular attenuation at this advanced stage. B. Scanning-electron micrograph of the RPE in the same dog. Nests of hypertrophied RPE cells are seen bulging up toward the photoreceptor cells that have been peeled away. (Original magnification, ×480.) C. Scanning-electron micrograph of abnormal RPE cells that have lost their apical microvilli. (Original magnification, ×3000.) (Courtesy of C. Peruccio.)*

or RPED, which has been recognized in many breeds throughout the world but it is, perhaps, most prevalent in England. In particular, cases have been recorded in the Labrador and Golden Retriever, Border Collie, Rough and Smooth Collie, Shetland Sheepdog, English Cocker Spaniel, English Springer Spaniel, Chesapeake Bay Retriever, and others. In the Briard, an unusually high frequency of the disorder has been reported, but recently, the condition is more rarely observed among the various breeds, including the Briard, even in England. A genetic predisposition in an individual breed may possibly be modified by environmental or dietary factors. In this context, that lesions similar to RPED have been produced in dogs fed diets deficient in vitamin E, which is an antioxidant that retards the intracellular accumulation of lipofuscin pigment, is important to consider. Naturally acquired retinopathy resulting from vitamin E deficiency has also been described in the dog. The similarities between RPED and vitamin E deficiency may explain its unique geographic distribution as well. Some affected Briards have been described as being hypercholesterolemic and systemically deficient in vitamin E and taurine. Further investigations into the blood biochemistry of both normal and affected Briards in the United Kingdom have shown a hyperlipidemia characterized by increased plasma cholesterol but normal triglyceride concentrations. No significant difference in plasma cholesterol concentrations between affected and ophthalmoscopically normal dogs were found. This absence of obvious metabolic derangements associated with hypercholesterolemia is suggestive that Briards in the United Kingdom may have a primary abnormality in cholesterol metabolism. That an abnormality of lipid metabolism might play a role in the development of RPED among Briards, however, remains under investigation.

The behavioral signs of RPED are typical. Visual impairment usually is not observed until a moderately advanced stage of the disease. Then, because of the relative sparing of the peripheral as opposed to the central retina, peripheral vision is retained until late in the disease. Vision tends to improve at low light levels and may also appear to be normal for moving and distant objects but impaired for stationary and nearby objects. Not all affected dogs become blind. Secondary cataracts are most often seen at the advanced stage.

HEREDITARY RETINAL DYSTROPHY IN THE BRIARD

A retinal dystrophy has been described among Briards in Sweden that differs from CPRA/RPED. This disease, which was initially described as congenital stationary night blindness, affects Briards from birth. Further clinical and morphologic studies have, indeed, shown a progressive component. Both the neural retina and the RPE are affected by a dystrophy with an extremely slow progression. Both in- and outbreeding as well as backcrossing showed an autosomal recessive pattern of inheritance, but expression of the defect was variable.

Clinically affected dogs were congenitally night blind, whereas daylight vision varied from normal to more or less severely impaired. A rapid, horizontal nystagmus was seen in affected pups. With progression of the disease, a subtle alteration in tapetal sheen could be seen in affected dogs, and in certain individuals, whitish-gray spots could also be seen and were observed most easily in the central and midperipheral nontapetal fundus. It appears that these dogs, which mainly are only night-blind at birth, stay visual in daylight for another 6 to 7 years. The ERGs showed a 40% reduction of dark-adapted b-wave responses in affected pups at 5 weeks of age. This disease has been termed *lipid retinopathy* in the United States, and studies have provided evidence that the Briard retinal dystrophy includes a defect in retinal polyunsaturated fatty acid metabolism (for more details, the reader should consult the third edition, pp. 905–908).

NEURONAL CEROID LIPOFUSCINOSIS

Neuronal ceroid lipofuscinosis, which is a group of inherited and progressive diseases of lipid storage, is characterized by retinal degeneration and fatal encephalopathy. It has been described in several breeds, including the English Setter, Dalmatian, Border Collie, Tibetan Terrier, and others. In the Tibetan Terrier, night blindness occurs in young animals, but the more severe neurologic abnormalities are not observed until later in life. In the Polish Owczarek Nizinny, visual dysfunction and funduscopic alterations occur early in life, often between 1 and 2 years of age. Histopathologic examination has revealed severe inner and outer retinal degeneration and extensive accumulation of fluorescent lipopigment in the central nervous tissue and retina.

MUCOPOLYSACCHARIDE STORAGE DISEASES

In both humans and animals, mucopolysaccharide storage diseases are caused by an inherited deficiency of lysosomal enzymes, and they represent generalized, multisystemic abnormalities of which ocular lesions are but one component. The lysosomal enzymes participate in the degradation of glycosaminoglycans. Results of morphologic studies have shown the accumulation of intracellular inclusions in secondary lysosomes of the enzyme-deficient RPE. In the dog, mucopolysaccharide VII has been described, and within the retinal pigment epithelium, single cytoplasmic inclusions initially are present (during the early postnatal period).

HEREDITARY TAPETAL DEGENERATION

An autosomal, recessively inherited tapetal abnormality of laboratory Beagles has been described. Affected dogs have a light, uniform choroidal pigmentation that precludes visualization of the choroidal vessels. Morphologically, normal numbers of tapetal cells are present at birth. With time, however, progressive degeneration of the tapetal cell layer occurs. Even so, retinal structure and function remain normal.

CHORIORETINAL INFLAMMATIONS AND INFECTIONS

Inflammatory lesions in the ocular fundus are not uncommon in the dog. Retinal involvement, however, is usually secondary to disease processes

extending from the choroid or, sometimes, the vitreous, whereas primary retinal inflammation (i.e., retinitis) is uncommon. The terms *chorioretinitis* (i.e., starting in the choroid) and *retinochoroiditis* (i.e., initially involving the retina) indicate the primary site and direction of spread when both the choroid and the retina are involved. Choroiditis, which is an inflammation strictly confined to the choroid, without involvement of the anterior uvea or retina, appears to be an uncommon condition. Chorioretinitis may have various causes, including several infectious diseases, neoplasia, foreign bodies, and trauma (Box 11-1). Infectious agents may be restricted to the eye, but signs in the ocular fundus may also be part of (or secondary to) a systemic disease. The exact cause of the inflammatory process is usually difficult to establish. Additional tests (e.g., complete blood counts, clinical chemistries, serology, radiology) may aid in determining the cause. The ophthalmoscopic appearance of chorioretinitis is summarized in Table 11-7 and shown in Figures 11-11 and 11-12.

SUDDEN ACQUIRED RETINAL DEGENERATION

Sudden acquired retinal degeneration (SARD) is a retinal disorder of unknown cause that results in sudden and permanent blindness among adult dogs. There is no treatment for this disorder. Clinical signs are characterized by sudden loss of vision (usually within days or 1–2 weeks), pupillary dilatation and unresponsive pupils, absence

---

BOX 11-1

Causes of Chorioretinitis/Retinochoroiditis in the Dog

Virus: Canine distemper morbillivirus, canine herpesvirus, and Mokola virus.

Rickettsia: Canine *Ehrlichia canis* and *Rickettsia rickettsii* (Rocky Mountain spotted fever).

Mycotic Diseases: *Acremonium* sp., *Aspergillus fumigatus*, *Blastomyces dermatitidis*, *Histoplasma capsulatum*, *Cryptococcus neoformans*, *Coccidiodes immitis*, *Geotrichum candidum*, and *Pseudallescheria boydii*.

Algal Disease: Achlorophyllic alga Prototheca.

Protozoal Diseases: *Toxoplasma gondii*, *Neospora caninum*, and *Leishmania donovani*.

Parasitic Diseases: *Toxocara canis*, *Angiostrongylus vasorum*, and order Diptera.

Immune-mediated: Uveodermatologic/Vogt-Koyanagi-Harada syndrome.

TABLE 11-7

OPHTHALMOSCOPIC CHANGES IN CHORIORETINITIS

Stage of Inflammation	Tapetal Changes	Nontapetal Changes
Acute (active) Chronic (inactive)	Indistinct grayish/brownish areas White, perivascular opacities Lesion margins: irregular (fuzzy) Lesion often raised	Grayish to white areas White, perivascular opacities Lesion margins: irregular (fuzzy) Lesion often raised
	Irregular, hyperreflective areas with a distinct (sharp) border May be pigmented Blood vessel attenuation	Distinctly bordered, depigmented areas Blood vessel attenuation Variable pigment proliferation

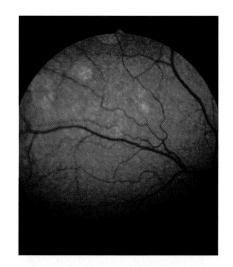

FIGURE 11 11. *Inflammatory changes in the neural retina of the tapetal fundus are often seen as asymmetrical, grayish discolorations, as in this 3-year-old Curly-Coated Retriever.*

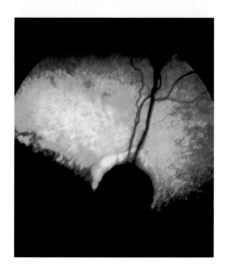

FIGURE 11-12. *An inactive, chronic scar in the tapetal fundus. Note the wide hyperreflective area temporal to the optic disc and the hyperreflective arc around the disc, which is probably unrelated to the scar itself.*

of ophthalmoscopic fundus abnormalities at the early stage, and an extinguished ERG. It appears that all breeds (even cross-breeds) may be affected, often in middle age. After several weeks to months, slight funduscopic alterations may be observed that are indicative of a generalized retinal degenerative process. The end stage is a generalized retinal atrophy, which is indistinguishable from PRA. Affected dogs are usually healthy, but some have a history of weight gain, polyuria, polydipsia, and polyphagia. Some cases have included elevated serum alkaline phosphatase, serum amino transferase, serum cholesterol, or serum bilirubin levels. Frequently, signs suggestive of hyperadrenocorticism occur, and the involvement of faulty fat metabolism in the disorder has been speculated. Implications of an autoimmune mechanism stem from findings that dogs with SARD have circulating antiretinal antibodies; however, attention lately has focused on a possible toxic cause. Morphologically, the initial abnormalities are primarily restricted to the photoreceptor cell layer.

CHORIORETINAL TOXICITIES

Drug-induced retinotoxicity is rarely encountered in clinical practice. Nevertheless, several drugs produce retinal destruction. These include:

1. **Ethambutol**, an antitubercular drug that produces discoloration of the tapetal fundus;
2. **Diphenylthiocarbazone**, a metal-chelating agent that causes a dark-red color and diffuse retinal edema;
3. **Hydroxypyridinethione**, a zinc-chelating drug that causes tapetal necrosis, edema, and retinal detachment;
4. **Quinine**, which produces rapid vasoconstriction of the retinal arterioles and pallor of the optic disc within a few hours of administration and, later, partial or complete destruction of the ganglion cells with subsequent optic atrophy;
5. **Rafoxanide**, which causes optic nerve edema that, in turn, can result in blindness;
6. **Chloroquine**, an antimalarial drug that causes scattered, gray-white specks in the nontapetal fundus;
7. **Azalide**, an antibiotic drug that causes tapetal color changes if administered in high doses; and
8. **Closantel**, an antihelmintic drug that produces generalized atrophy of the retinal and optic disc.

RETINOPATHY INDUCED BY RADIATION

Radiation-induced ocular injury secondary to treatment of nasal cancer occurs in both humans and animals. The immediate changes are usually blepharitis, keratoconjunctivitis, and keratoconjunctivitis sicca. Later (3–6 months posttreatment with 36.0–67.5 Gy in fractionated doses given over 4 weeks using a 6-mV linear accelerator), however, a degenerative angiopathy of the retinal vessels can develop, with multifocal retinal hemorrhages and mild, diffuse retinal degeneration, that first affects the outer retinal layers but then progresses inward.

RETINOPATHIES INDUCED BY NUTRITIONAL AND GENERAL DISEASE PROCESSES

In the dog, systemic diseases causing impaired fat absorption could result in vitamin A deficiency, but this situation is extremely rare. Vitamin E, which is an antioxidant with an important function in maintaining cell membrane stability by preventing lipid peroxidation, may be more important in the dog. A deficiency in vitamin E may result in pathologic changes in the muscle, central nervous system, reproductive tract, and retina. **Experimental vitamin E deficiency in puppies has produced a mottled appearance of the tapetal fundus, particularly centrally, with numerous discrete, yellow-brown foci. With time, the central fundus became hyperreflective, and the retinal vessels attenuate.** Histopathologically, an accumulation of autofluorescent pigment was observed within the RPE cells and, at later stages, within migrating cells at all retinal layers. The obvious similarities between vitamin E deficiency and hereditary RPED are suggestive of some common etiologic factor, and recent reports have substantiated this suggestion. One recent report, for example, is suggestive that low plasma levels of α-tocopherol in RPED-affected dogs resulted, at least in part, from impaired absorption of dietary vitamin E.

CHORIORETINAL VASCULAR DISEASES

The retinal vasculature is well suited to direct, noninvasive examination, and hemorrhages within the retina have distinct shapes (Table 11-8). **Systemic disease as well as local ocular pathology can produce observable changes in both retinal and choroidal vessels (see Chapter 17). Systemic hypertension, hyperviscosity, and hyperlipidemia are the more frequent cases encountered in the dog.** Diabetic retinopathy occurs in the dog, but the extent and severity of these retinal lesions are mild compared with those in humans. The canine ocular lesions include anomalies of the retinal vasculature and cataract formation, however, just as they do in humans.

TABLE 11-8	
OPHTHALMOSCOPIC LOCALIZATION OF VITREAL AND RETINAL HEMORRHAGES	
Ophthalmic Appearance	*Anatomic Site of Hemorrhage*
Discrete, round hemorrhage	Within the retinal layers
Flame-shaped hemorrhage	Within the nerve fiber layer
Indistinct borders; diffuse, dull-red hemorrhage	Subretinal hemorrhage
Keelboat-shaped hemorrhage	Bleeding from the superficial retinal vessels into the space between the inner limiting membrane of the retina and the posterior hyaloid

SECONDARY RETINAL DEGENERATIONS

GLAUCOMA

Histopathologically, loss of RGCs is a consistent finding in canine globes with glaucoma. The degree of changes in the ganglion cell layer has been reported to be more severe (or at least equal) in the nontapetal fundus compared with that in the tapetal area. Eventually all layers of the retina can be affected (see Chapter 8).

RETINAL DETACHMENTS

Various pathologic conditions of the eye can cause focal, multifocal, or total retinal detachment. Usually, the neuroretina is separated from the underlying RPE, which implies a disruption of the intimate and essential (but structurally weak) association between the outer segments of the photoreceptors and the RPE. **A focal retinal detachment affecting a minor area will usually not result in a clinically detectable impairment of vision, whereas detachment of the entire retina is a blinding condition (Fig. 11-13).** Detachments involving large areas of the retina also may result in separation of the peripheral retina from the ora ciliaris retinae or dialysis. The retina will remain attached only at the ONH in dogs with total retinal detachments and dialysis. **Ophthalmoscopy reveals an anterior displacement of the retinal surface and retinal blood vessels.** Large volumes of subretinal fluid can result in segments of the retina ballooning anteriorly or, in extreme cases, even extending

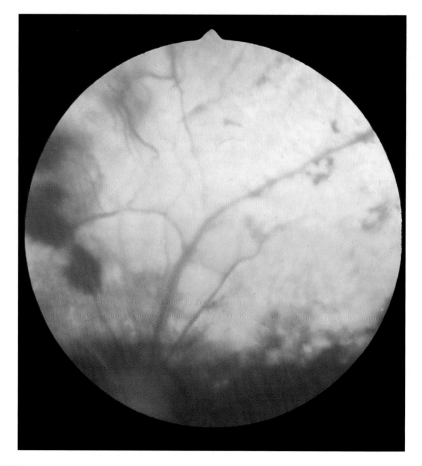

FIGURE 11-13. *Retinal detachment and retinal hemorrhages in the tapetal fundus associated with systemic hypertension.*

to the posterior surface of the lens. If there is a total detachment with dialysis, the retina will hang in folds, resembling a grayish-colored curtain, from the ONH, and the denuded tapetal fundus will appear to be hyperreflective when the light is not absorbed by the retina. Extensive detachments may cause secondary uveitis, and cataract as well as other pathologic changes likely will develop in severely affected eyes. Some vision may be retained during the acute phase of detachments, and residual PLRs will be present at these times.

NEOPLASTIC AND PROLIFERATIVE CONDITIONS

Primary tumors of the retina, choroid, and optic disc are very rare in the dog, and they include the astrocytoma, medulloepithelioma, and choroidal melanoma. Secondary tumors may involve the posterior segment by extension from a primary focus in the anterior segment, optic nerve, or extraocular tissues or by metastasis from a more remote site. Secondary tumors are more common than primary tumors in the dog. Clinical signs usually develop late in the disease, thus delaying both detection and diagnosis, and include intraocular hemorrhage, uveitis, glaucoma, and blindness. Metastatic neoplasms in the choroid and retina are often incidental findings; these neoplasms include mammary gland adenocarcinoma, thyroid adenocarcinoma, renal adenocarcinoma, malignant melanoma, hemangiosarcoma, rhabdomyosarcoma, and neurogenic sarcoma. Malignant lymphoma, which usually affects both eyes, seems to be the most common secondary intraocular tumor (see Chapter 17).

POSTERIOR SEGMENT SURGERY

Posterior segment surgery is receiving renewed attention by veterinary ophthalmologists. Currently, these procedures are performed infrequently because of the expensive instrumentation and the need for specialty training in retinal reattachment surgical techniques. **In addition to the repair of rhegmatogenous retinal detachments (RRDs), posterior vitrectomy may be used in making the diagnosis and in the treatment of severe endophthalmitis, in the treatment of dropped intravitreal lens fragments, or in the surgical treatment of congenital anomalies (e.g., persistent hyperplastic primary vitreous).** Less-invasive posterior segment procedures such as laser retinopexy, pneumatic retinopexy, and scleral buckling may be used to treat some RRDs as well.

The main indication for vitreoretinal surgical procedures is the treatment of retinal detachments. **By definition a retinal detachment is a separation of the neurosensory retina from the RPE. Subretinal fluids then accumulate in the potential space that is the remnant of the optic vesicle. This space is termed the *subretinal space*, though it is truly intraretinal, or the *interphotoreceptor space*.** Nonrhegmatogenous retinal detachments have no retinal tear or break, and in these detachments, the subretinal fluid is usually inflammatory or exudative. In addition, these detachments are often associated with systemic diseases such as hypertension or systemic mycosis. If the underlying condition can be treated, the retina may reattach, and some vision may return.

Nonrhegmatogenous retinal detachments also may result from traction associated with intravitreal hemorrhage or inflammation. If vitreoretinal traction contributes to a retinal detachment, with or without a break, posterior vitrectomy is usually necessary for successful retinal reattachment. RRDs are associated with a break or tear in the retina, which allows liquefied vitreous to enter the subretinal space. It is a surgical condition that requires all retinal breaks or tears be identified, and the edges of those breaks must be sealed against the RPE. Complicated RRDs may have retinal breaks either induced or complicated by vitreoretinal traction. The prognosis for return of vision is usually guarded, but with early and successful surgical intervention, functional vision can be restored.

The incidence of retinal detachment in dogs with CEA varies from 2.4 to 10.0%. Most commonly, it occurs in dogs younger than 1 year of age but can occur at any time in life, and it has been associated with the optic nerve pits or colobomas in CEA. The source of the subretinal fluid

in CEA appears to be the vitreous. Collie eyes with optic disc pits have a direct communication between the optic pit and the vitreous. Photocoagulation with argon and xenon lasers adjacent to the optic nerve and around the optic pit promotes reattachment of the retina in both humans and the Collie; both the diode and the argon laser have been used in dogs with CEA with good results (Fig. 11-14). Treatment should include the peripapillary area adjacent to and a few degrees beyond the retinal detachment borders to minimize damage to the normal retina. In one study, single photocoagulation treatments produced reattachments in 23 of 28 of the eyes with CEA and retinal detachment; additional treatments produced improvement in two more eyes.

Spontaneous RRD may occur in any breed, but it has been reported more frequently in the Shih Tzu. Some cases may represent sequela to trauma or intraocular inflammation. Retinal hole formation as well as vitreous degeneration in association with PRA may also lead to RRD. In the Shih Tzu, vitreous syneresis is a prevalent finding among animals both with and without detachments. In one report, 14 of 16 eyes that underwent retinal reattachment surgery were successfully reattached, and 13 of these regained some degree of clinical vision 2 days to 6 weeks (mean time, 3 weeks) after surgery.

Rhegmatogenous retinal detachment may occur either preoperatively in association with cataracts or postoperatively after cataract surgery. A significant correlation exists between retinal detachment and cataracts, lens luxation, and endophthalmitis. Most detachments associated with cataracts, cataract surgery, or intracapsular lens extraction (ICLE) are presumed to be, or obviously are (i.e., when retinal tears are observed), rhegmatogenous. **The incidence of retinal detachment after cataract surgery in the dog ranges from 1 to 5%.**

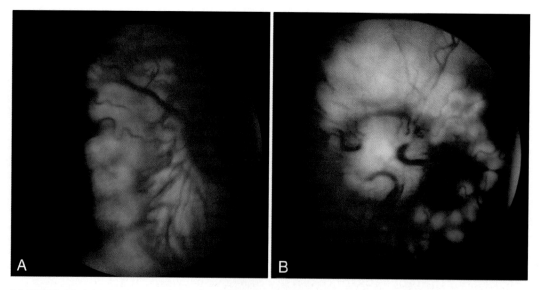

FIGURE 11-14. *Collie eye anomaly with laser burns delivered around the optic nerve. A. The diode laser was used for this treatment. Because of the lack of pigment directly adjacent to the disc, the line of laser burns was made where pigmentation was present. B. The argon laser was used for this treatment. The shorter wavelength is absorbed by hemoglobin; therefore, the peripapillary area can be treated more effectively.*

The basic principles regarding surgical repair of RRDs are to identify all retinal breaks, close all breaks by apposing the retina to the RPE, and then seal the breaks by inducing a chorioretinal adhesion. Apposition of the neural retina to the RPE can be achieved using intraocular tamponade with air, expanding gases, or silicone oil or using extraocular scleral buckling, in which an implant in the orbit is used to indent the sclera so that the RPE contacts the neural retina. Titanium tacks have also been used to maintain retinal attachment while the retinopexy procedures are creating adhesion. Laser or cryoretinopexy is used to create chorioretinal adhesions that seal the retina to the RPE around the break, thus preventing fluid from entering the subretinal space. For successful repair, any vitreous traction on the retina must be relieved. If vitreous traction or proliferative vitreoretinopathy contribute to the retinal tear and detachment, posterior vitrectomy is necessary to relieve the traction and to prevent redetachment. With complicated RRDs, in which vitreal abnormalities including vitreous detachment or proliferative vitreoretinopathy are present, or with RRDs having giant tears, reapposition of the retina to the RPE requires vitrectomy to remove the vitreous exerting traction on the tear edges, tamponade of the retina against the RPE (with gas or oil), and creation of a permanent chorioretinal adhesion with cryotherapy or laser treatment.

DISEASES OF THE OPTIC NERVE

The optic nerve consists of four different regions. The *intraocular* optic nerve contains the RGC layer, nerve fiber layer, ONH or optic disc, and the intralaminar region within the sclera. Posterior to the globe, the retrobulbar optic nerve consists of the *intraorbital* optic nerve, the *intracanalicular* optic nerve (within the optic canal), and the small *intracranial* optic nerve, which merges into the optic chiasm.

CONGENITAL OPTIC NEUROPATHIES

Micropapilla/Optic Nerve Hypoplasia/Optic Nerve Aplasia

The number of RGCs and, thus, the number of optic nerve axons present vary between individual animals. **Small optic discs are associated with small numbers of RGCs and have a range of vision-related clinical signs. If the number of axons is so low that visual and PLR deficits are present, the condition is termed** *optic nerve hypoplasia.* **Micropapilla (i.e., a slightly small optic disc) may result in normal PLR and vision yet, in fact, be a partial optic nerve hypoplasia with subtle visual deficits.** Complete absence of RGCs and the optic nerve is termed *optic nerve aplasia.* Hypoplasia of the optic disc may be unilateral or bilateral, marked or minimal, and associated with either near-normal or reduced visual function. In the dog, this condition may occur alone or accompany other ocular malformations. **The hypoplastic canine optic**

disc is small and gray, with no myelinated fibers on the disc surface (Fig. 11-15). The appearance of the retina and the retinal blood vessels is normal, but they do appear to be large relative to the small size of the optic disc. The PLR is abnormal and the pupil dilated in dogs with optic nerve hypoplasia; in contrast, both the PLR and pupils are normal in dogs with micropapilla.

Micropapilla is found in the Belgian Sheepdog, Belgian Tervuren, Dachshund, Irish Wolfhound, Tibetan Spaniel, Miniature Schnauzer, Norfolk Terrier, Old English Sheepdog, Shih Tzu, Gordon Setter, Great Pyrenees, Irish Setter, Labrador Retriever, Puli, Sheltie, Beagle, Collie, Flat-Coated Retriever, German Shepherd, Miniature Poodle, and Soft-Coated Wheaten Terrier. The heritability of optic nerve hypoplasia is reported to be recessive, dominant, and undefined in the Miniature and the Toy Poodle. Optic nerve hypoplasia has been seen in the Rough Collie, Sheltie, St. Bernard, Beagle, Miniature Schnauzer, American Cocker Spaniel, Dachshund, Irish Setter, German Shepherd, Standard Poodle, Tibetan Spaniel, Soft-Coated Wheaten Terrier, Skye Terrier, Kerry Blue Terrier, Labrador

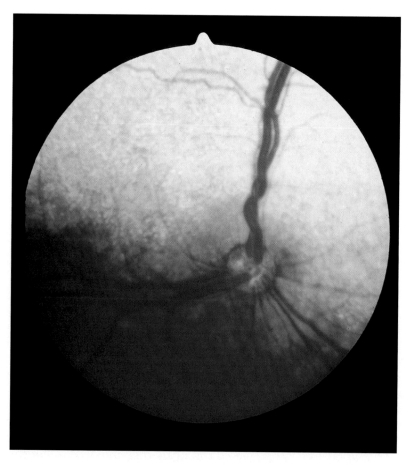

FIGURE 11-15. *Unilateral optic nerve hypoplasia in a Dachshund puppy associated with a fixed, dilated pupil and blindness.*

Retriever, Old English Sheepdog, Pharaoh Hound, Afghan, Borzoi, Collie, English Springer Spaniel, Golden Retriever, Greyhound, Italian Greyhound, Keeshond, and Shih Tzu.

Optic Nerve Colobomas

Optic nerve colobomas are congenital malformations of the ONH and peripapillary retina that enlarge or distort the nerve head circumference. They may appear as enlarged discs containing a deep excavation or as slightly enlarged, irregular discs containing pits within the borders of the nerve head. In the Collie, colobomas of the optic nerve result from faulty closure or fusion (or both) of the embryonic ventral (i.e., fetal) fissure of the optic stalk and cup, and peripapillary colobomas originate from orbital cysts. Optic disc colobomas in the Collie may be small and hard to differentiate from a deep, physiologic cup, or they may be very large in diameter and as great as 30 diopters in depth. They may be "typical," at the 6-o'clock position, or "atypical," at the nasal or the temporal disc margin. Colobomas of the optic disc in this breed result from ectasia of the lamina cribrosa, whereas colobomas of the peripapillary retina are best characterized as foci of ectatic sclera that are lined by attenuated retinal and choroidal tissues (Fig. 11-7). Disc colobomas communicate with the vitreous and subretinal space in the dog, and in the Collie, optic nerve colobomas are always associated with varying degrees of choroidal hypoplasia. Colobomas are also found in the Australian Shepherd, Sheltie, Basenji, American and English Cocker Spaniel, Norfolk Terrier, Siberian Husky, Tibetan Spaniel, Irish Setter, Labrador and Golden Retriever, Whippet, Samoyed, Malamute, Beagle, Bernese Mountain Dog, Flat-Coated Retriever, and German Shepherd.

Pseudopapilledema

Anomalous elevation of the ONH may resemble disc swelling caused by elevated intracranial pressure (i.e., noninflammatory papilledema), and it may be a cause for alarm and result in misdirected diagnostic procedures. In the dog, pseudopapilledema most commonly results from excessive myelination of optic nerve axons beyond the anterior lamina cribrosa. This may occur in isolated regions of the disc, along the retinal blood vessels, or involve most of the ONH. Because the funduscopic appearance is suggestive of papilledema, some patients may receive diagnostic workups or therapy (or both) for intracranial disease. Pseudopapilledema has been reported in the Curly-Coated Retriever, Miniature Poodle, English Springer Spaniel, Labrador Retriever, English Toy Spaniel, German Shepherd, and Golden Retriever.

ACQUIRED OPTIC NERVE DISEASES

Disorders of the prechiasmal visual pathways are a diagnostic challenge. Optic nerve disorders may result from inflammation, cellular infiltration, ischemia, infection, and mechanical compression. In the dog, abrupt onset of vision loss with an ONH having a normal-appearance is highly suggestive of SARD or of retrobulbar optic neuritis. Slowly progressive loss of vision is typical of neoplastic compression or infiltration of the prechiasmal optic nerve.

Differential Diagnosis of the "Swollen Disc"

Active or passive edematous swelling of the optic disc provides nonspecific evidence for distal optic nerve dysfunction. Papilledema (i.e., disc swelling because of increased intracranial pressure) must be differentiated from the "swollen disc" of pseudopapilledema and optic neuritis.

The distinction of congenitally elevated discs (i.e., pseudopapilledema) from papilledema must be made as well. **During the early stage, true papilledema does not affect vision, but optic neuritis is associated with acute loss of vision and diminished PLR.** Disc edema can accompany glaucoma, uveitis, or postoperative hypotony. Both primary and metastatic ONH tumors (e.g., meningioma, glioma) may cause a "swollen disc," and disc tumors may involve hemorrhagic elevation of the disc and peripapillary retina as well as drastic reduction in vision. Orbital mass lesions characteristically produce proptosis, but they also may present as very chronic, unilateral disc edema with insidiously advancing field loss.

Axonal swelling caused by the accumulation of mitochondria and other axoplasmic structures at the lamina cribrosa is primarily responsible for papilledema from elevated intracranial pressure. It also is primarily responsible for disc swelling from orbital tumors, ocular hypotony, and acute glaucoma. Disturbance of both fast and slow axoplasmic transport results in axonal swelling.

Papilledema of Raised Intracranial Pressure

The term *papilledema* is reserved to describe passive, noninflammatory disc swelling associated with increased intracranial pressure. Papilledema is almost always bilateral, and it is not associated with visual deficits, at least during those developmental stages that precede atrophy. **In the dog, brain tumors are associated with papilledema.** The pathogenesis involves a stasis of both fast and slow axoplasmic flow at the lamina cribrosa of the ONH. Papilledema is primarily a mechanical and not a vascular phenomenon. Optic nerve fibers are compressed by elevated cerebrospinal fluid (CSF) pressure in the subarachnoid space of the intraorbital portion of the optic nerve, and the subsequent reduction in axoplasmic flow results in swelling of the axons in the prelaminar region of the optic disc. Venous obstruction and dilation as well as nerve fiber hypoxia are secondary events.

In humans, papilledema may develop within hours of a subarachnoid or an intracerebral hemorrhage. Once the intracranial space is decompressed, venous congestion of the disc will diminish rapidly, but disc swelling, hemorrhages, and exudates will resolve slowly. Early—and even well-developed—papilledema may not be symptomatic. When papilledema has existed for many weeks or months, nerve fiber attrition results in progressive loss of vision and optic nerve atrophy.

In one report, papilledema was associated with brain tumors in 50% of dogs studied, 75% of which had no vision or had PLR deficits. Spindle cell sarcoma, microglioma, oligodendroglioma, astrocytoma, ependymoma, and meningiomas were also reported, and possibly were associated with increased intracranial pressure, in dogs with papilledema. Most dogs in this series were bilaterally affected. Dogs are thought to develop papilledema with increased CSF pressure only rarely, however, because this species does not have a central retinal artery and vein whose flow could be affected by elevated CSF pressure. In the dog, CSF pressure instead is transmitted directly to the retrolaminar tissue space, and a rise in CSF pressure could affect the ONH. If true papilledema has no associated PLR or vision deficits during its early stages, the true incidence of papilledema in dogs with increased CSF pressure simply may not be known. Myelin anterior to the lamina cribrosa in the canine ONH could also provide stability to the axoplasmic flow during conditions of increased intracranial pressure and, thus, minimize the occurrence of papilledema.

Inflammatory Optic Neuropathies

Optic neuritis is more of a clinical syndrome than a single disease. It includes idiopathic, neoplastic, immune-mediated, and infective causes of optic neuritis; inflammatory diseases that contiguously involve the optic nerves of the adjacent paranasal sinuses, retina, brain and meninges, and orbit; and granulomatous as well as neoplastic infiltration syndromes (e.g., reticulosis).

The term *papillitis* refers to the intraocular form of optic neuritis, in which optic disc swelling of varying degrees is observed. Optic neuritis must be distinguished from papilledema and pseudopapilledema, and it is generally idiopathic in the dog.

Optic Neuritis

Inflammation of the canine optic nerve may be either unilateral or bilateral. The optic papilla and retrobulbar optic nerve may be affected as well. Clinical signs of blindness appear suddenly, and the pupils are fixed and dilated. The optic disc itself appears to be swollen and edematous, with blurring of the disc margins (Fig. 11-16). The physiologic cup may be lost, the blood vessels on the disc surface are raised, and hemorrhages may be present. Papillitis is frequently associated with cells in the vitreous. Peripapillary retinal edema and neuroretinitis are commonly seen with optic neuritis in the dog. No ophthalmoscopic signs of disc inflammation may be seen with the retrobulbar form. The ERG is normal with optic neuritis, but VEPs are reduced. **Causes of optic neuritis in the dog include distemper, blastomycosis, cryptococcosis, histoplasmosis, and toxoplasmosis. Idiopathic causes, trauma, toxins, vitamin A deficiency, and reticulosis may also cause optic neuritis in the dog.** Corticosteroids are used systemically in the hope of favorably influencing visual recuperation, but no substantive evidence proves that eventual visual function is affected by therapy. In fact, the prognosis for vision is poor.

FIGURE 11-16. *Optic neuritis caused by reticulosis appears as a swollen, hyperemic disc with indistinct margins. There is no apparent physiologic cup.*

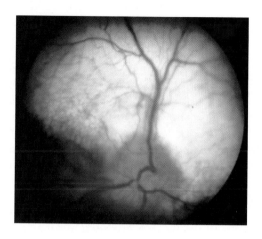

Reticulosis and Granulomatous Meningoencephalitis

Both the inflammatory and the neoplastic form of reticulosis include a continuous spectrum of cellular responses. A variety of mononuclear cells, lymphocytes, plasma cells, monocytes, and macrophages proliferate and accumulate as perivascular aggregates in the central nervous system and cause reticulosis. Granulomatous meningoencephalitis is a more disseminated form of inflammatory reticulosis. **Proliferation of the reticulohistiocytic elements of the central nervous system can cause papillitis, optic neuritis, retinochoroiditis, choroiditis, iridocyclitis, and retinal detachments. Sudden blindness in both eyes with fixed, dilated pupils is a common presentation.** Other neurologic signs may be present as well. The ONH can be hyperemic and swollen, but retrobulbar forms of reticulosis have been noted in the dog. The CSF will have increased protein levels and pleocytosis. **The specific cause is not known, but reticulosis responds to systemically administered corticosteroids during its early stages.**

Contiguous Inflammations

The optic nerve may be secondarily affected by various inflammatory or neoplastic lesions of the adjacent tissues, including the uvea, retina, sclera, orbit, paranasal sinuses, and meninges. Vision defects may result from development of a true optic neuritis or from pressure on the optic nerve because of cellular infiltration or mass compression.

Immune-Mediated Optic Neuritis

Experimental allergic optic neuritis can be produced by immunizing guinea pigs with an isogenic spinal-cord emulsion in complete Freund's adjuvant. These animals develop a retrobulbar neuritis, with infiltration of the optic nerve, chiasm, or brain by mononuclear cells. Focal demyelination of the nerve and neuroretinitis may also occur. This experimental model may be useful in future studies of optic neuritis.

Traumatic Optic Neuropathies

All portions of the optic nerve (i.e., intraocular, intraorbital, intracanalicular, intracranial) are susceptible to injury, and traumatic proptosis and orbital fractures are common in the dog. Taut stretching of the canine optic nerve and posterior tenting of the globe in traumatic proptosis can produce ONH avulsion, globe rupture, optic nerve laceration and shearing, and vascular compromise to the ONH. In avulsion injuries, vision is lost immediately. An afferent pupillary defect is evident as well, and vitreous as well as retinal hemorrhages also may be found. In addition, massive proliferation of glial connective tissue around the ONH occurs after optic nerve avulsion.

Hemorrhage after trauma may disrupt the optic nerve parenchyma or accumulate within the nerve sheaths. Hemorrhage into the optic nerve or interference with its blood supply because of trauma can result in optic neuropathy. Damage to the optic nerve mediated by posttraumatic rupture of the posterior ciliary arteries has been reported in humans. Disturbance of the RPE is indicative of damage to the ciliary vessels.

With damage to the nerve posterior to the entrance of the retinal vessels, the optic disc may initially appear to be normal. Intracanalicular optic nerve trauma can result from direct damage by penetrating foreign bodies, compression, and fractures, or it can result from indirect damage (e.g., a blow to the frontal region). Force applied to the anterior orbit can be transmitted to the optic foramen, with subsequent traction and shearing forces being applied to the optic nerve and the small nutrient vessels. In addition, traumatic optic neuropathy may result from vascular compromise or from shearing of the short posterior ciliary artery vessels, vascular spasm, thrombosis, and subsequent ischemia or contusion necrosis. Several treatment options for traumatic optic neuropathy have been advocated, including osmotic agents, corticosteroids, and surgical decompression of the optic nerve sheath or canal. Spontaneous visual recovery has been reported in humans, and it has also been noted in some traumatic neuropathies in the dog. Aggressive medical treatment is advocated, however, in the absence of optic nerve avulsion.

Glaucoma

The glaucomas are neurodegenerative diseases, because they result in death of the neural cell (i.e., the RGC). Retinal and ONH ischemia as well as neurotropin deprivation from the obstruction of axoplasmic flow to the RGC cause RGC dysfunction and, possibly, Müller cell dysfunction. Excitotoxic amino acids, intra-axonal calcium ion influx, free radicals, nitric oxide, and apoptosis may be common in pathogenesis of the optic neuropathy of glaucoma in the dog (as well as in other species).

OPTIC NERVE TUMORS

Optic nerve tumors in the dog may present with exophthalmos alone or with exophthalmos and a unilateral or a bilateral papilledema and subsequent optic neuritis. Tumor impingement on and infiltration of the optic nerve can reduce the axoplasmic flow. Primary optic nerve tumors that have been reported in the dog include teratoid medulloepithelioma, ganglioglioma, and meningioma. Squamous cell carcinomas, nasal tumors, and orbital tumors may affect the optic nerve.

Feline Ophthalmology

The feline eye exhibits several unique diseases, and in general, its inflammatory responses are more moderate than those of the canine counterpart. **The cat suffers from several infectious conjunctivitides; an acute, recurrent, and chronic viral keratitis; and several viral uveitides. The most frequent form of glaucoma is secondary to anterior uveitis, the chronic forms of which carry increased risks of cataract formation and blindness.** The cat's vertical-slit pupil is less apt to development of obstruction or iris bombé than the canine pupil, however, and inherited ophthalmic disorders are relatively infrequent in the cat compared with the dog. In older cats, the clinical frequency of hypertensive retinopathy has markedly increased during the past several years, which perhaps is indicative of a longer life span for the domestic cat. This chapter discusses the broad scope of ophthalmic conditions in the domestic cat, and it notes the significant differences between the cat and other domestic species.

DISEASES OF THE ORBIT

CONGENITAL AND DEVELOPMENTAL DISORDERS

Multiple abnormalities or colobomas of the eye and associated ophthalmic structures occur infrequently in the domestic cat. Affected breeds include the domestic Shorthair and Persian, and the defect is usually signaled by an upper eyelid agenesis (defect). Other colobomatous defects in single or multiple ocular tissues may affect the iris, optic nerve, and sclera. In addition to heredity, in utero viral causes may be important.

Griseofulvin Teratogenesis

The cat is particularly sensitive to the teratogenic effects of griseofulvin. When given to cats at a weekly dose of 500 to 1000 mg during the first half of gestation, griseofulvin produces ocular defects consisting of cyclopia, anophthalmia, and optic nerve aplasia. Extraocular defects include numerous central nervous system and skeletal abnormalities.

TRAUMATIC PROPTOSIS

Proptosis of the globe is a serious disease in the cat, because it requires considerable trauma to the orbit and head (usually produced by a car) and is associated with concurrent facial fractures (probably most often mandibular symphysis), hyphema, corneal perforation, and ocular desiccation as well as optic nerve damage (Fig. 12-1). The possibility for return of vision is low. Replacement of the globe and temporary tarsorrhaphy combined with medical therapy are the recommended treatments.

ORBITAL INFLAMMATIONS

The feline orbit has a relatively limited space. Therefore, early in the onset of disease, space-occupying orbital inflammations and neoplasms will produce exophthalmos, deviation of the globe (usually exotropia or esotropia), and protrusion of the nictitating membrane. **Orbital cellulitis and abscessation occur infrequently in the cat, but they usually are**

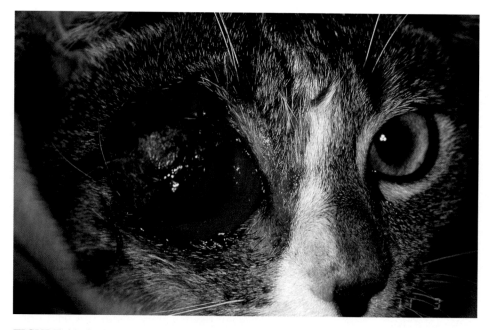

FIGURE 12-1. *Proptosis of the globe and mandibular fracture in a 2-year-old domestic Shorthair after being struck by a car.*

amenable to traditional therapy. The presence of communications to the adjacent paranasal sinuses should be considered.

ORBITAL NEOPLASIA

Approximately 90% of feline orbital neoplasms are malignant, and approximately two-thirds of these neoplasms are epithelial in origin (mostly squamous cell carcinomas). Orbital lymphosarcoma may occur either unilaterally or bilaterally in the cat.

DISEASES OF THE EYELIDS

CONGENITAL AND DEVELOPMENTAL LID DISORDERS

The domestic cat is the main species that develops eyelid colobomas, which tend to be bilateral, to involve the upper lids only, and to occupy primarily the lateral portion of the lid. These colobomas may produce corneal exposure keratitis, vascularization, epithelial hyperplasia, and ulceration attributable to inadequate eyelid function. Other intraocular anomalies (e.g., optic nerve coloboma) are often concurrent and may produce blindness. **Treatment is usually surgical reconstruction of the defective upper eyelid and lid margin using a myocutaneous graft from the lower eyelid that is anchored at the lateral canthus (Fig. 12-2).**

Structural defects of the feline adnexa are uncommon. Occasionally, cats are presented with traumatic eyelid lacerations, which are usually attributable to fighting. Eyelash diseases are rare, though ectopic cilia has been described in a Siamese. **Cicatricial ectropion occurs infrequently, and primary entropion (usually of the lower lid) is the most common acquired structural defect, with a predilection for the Persian and other brachycephalic breeds.** Entropion also may occur secondary to painful ocular diseases that induce chronic blepharospasm. Initially, the entropion might be described as spastic, but the eyelid inversion tends to become permanent with chronicity, thereby suggesting that cicatrices eventually develop. **The modified Hotz-Celsus technique (see Chapter 3) is the procedure of choice for correcting all forms of feline entropion, and it can readily be modified for each patient's individual abnormality.**

FOCAL AND DIFFUSE BLEPHARITIS

Localized demodecosis *(Demodex cati* and an as-yet-unnamed species of *Demodex)* is a rare, parasitic skin disease in the cat. It has a predilection for the eyelids, and the clinical signs include periocular alopecia, erythema, and scaling, with variable pruritus. The diagnosis is established on the basis of identifying the mites in scrapings from the affected skin. **Topical therapy with rotenone (Goodwinol) ointment is effective.**

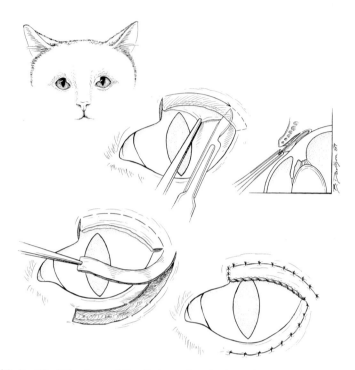

FIGURE 12-2. *Modification of the Roberts' technique for the repair of upper eyelid agenesis in the cat. After separating the conjunctiva from the remaining upper eyelid, a myocutaneous flap is prepared by making parallel incisions 4 to 5 mm from the upper eyelid margin. The lower skin graft is dissected free and then rotated dorsally to become the new upper eyelid. The skin is closed with simple interrupted sutures of 5-0 to 6-0 nylon, and the dorsal conjunctiva is attached to the new eyelid with 6-0 to 7-0 vicryl sutures in a continuous pattern. Alternatively, conjunctiva from the lower fornix may be transposed to the upper eyelid in a fashion similar to that with the skin flap. (Reprinted with permission from Nasisse MP. Feline ophthalmology. In: Gelatt KN, ed. Veterinary Ophthalmology. 2nd ed. Philadelphia: Lea & Febiger, 1991:529–575.)*

Feline scabies is a highly contagious and pruritic disease caused by *Notoedres cati*. Lesions begin on the pinna of the ear, but they quickly progress to involve the eyelids, face, and neck. The lesions are partly alopecic, and excoriation because of self-inflicted trauma is common. The diagnosis is established on the basis of identifying the mite in skin scrapings. Treatment involves dipping the cat in an effective parasiticide, such as lime-sulphur (Lym Dyp; Bermatologics for Veterinary Medicine) or malathion (Flea Off Dip; Adams). Other parasiticides are extremely toxic to the cat, however, and should be avoided. Amitraz (Mitaban; Upjohn) and ivermectin (Ivomec; MSD AgVet) are also effective.

Feline dermatophytosis, which most commonly results from *Microsporum canis* and, to a lesser extent, *M. gypseum* and *Trichophyton mentagrophytes*, may involve the eyelids. The lesions are circular, oval, or irregularly shaped, and they are typically accompanied by folliculitis. The diagnosis is established on the basis of fungal culture and microscopic evaluation (potassium hydroxide preparations) of hairs from the lesion. **Treatment**

of localized dermatophytosis involves topical application of an appropriate antifungal agent, such as miconazole (Conofite; Pitman-Moore), clotrimazole (Veltrim; Haver), or thiabendazole (Tresaderm; MsD AgVet), or systemic therapy with griseofulvin (Fulvicin; Schering) or ketoconazole (Nizoral; Janssen) in the generalized form. The globe must be protected from irritating dermatologic compounds, however, by first applying a protective coating of petrolatum-based ophthalmic ointment.

Myiasis is the intradermal and subdermal migration of fly larva. In the cat, *Cuterebra* sp. cause eyelid myiasis. The condition is easily recognized by the presence of a fistulous opening, and treatment is by careful extraction of the larva after enlarging the opening.

Blepharitis may also be associated with autoimmune diseases, including pemphigus vulgaris, pemphigus erythematosus, and systemic lupus erythematosus. Viral agents that cause dermatologic infections with the theoretic potential of eyelid involvement include catpox and feline herpesvirus (FHV)-1. Blepharitis resulting from inflammation of the marginal eyelid glands (e.g., meibomianitis, chalazion, hordeolum) or tuberculosis, however, occurs only rarely in the cat.

LID NEOPLASIA

Eyelid neoplasms are infrequent in the cat. They also usually are malignant and locally invasive. Ophthalmic neoplasms account for approximately 2% of all feline neoplasms (Table 12-1). The prevalence of eyelid neoplasia increases with advancing age. Squamous cell carcinoma is the most frequent type, and it appears as a slightly raised or depressed, ulcerative lesion either on or adjacent to the eyelid margin. There is a conspicuous predilection for white cats (Fig. 12-3). Metastasis does not occur until late in the disease, but local invasion can be extensive. Regional lymph nodes eventually are involved as well. **Squamous cell carcinomas are amenable to most forms of therapy, including surgical excision with some type of grafting procedure, teletherapy or brachytherapy, cryosurgery, and hyperthermia (for superficial lesions).**

Basal cell carcinoma (i.e., basal cell epithelioma) is a common dermal neoplasm in the cat. Though it has no particular site predilection, it can affect the eyelids. These carcinomas are usually round and well circumscribed, but their tendency to ulcerate allows their appearance to be confused with that of squamous cell carcinoma. Basal cell tumors generally are benign clinically and treated using surgical excision and cryotherapy.

Mast cell tumors also are common dermal neoplasms in the cat. Though demonstrating no site predilection, they do occasionally affect the eyelids. These tumors appear as single or multiple dermal masses. Treatment is by excision or systemic corticosteroid therapy.

Fibrosarcomas are common in the cat and may involve the eyelids. They generally appear as focal, nodular neoplasms that are dermal and subcutaneously situated, often with an ulcerated surface. **Recommended therapy is wide surgical excision, and the prognosis correlates with the mitotic index. In younger cats, multicentric fibrosarcomas result from the feline sarcoma virus (FeSV), which is a mutant strain of the feline leukemia virus (FeLV).** Cats with FeSV-induced fibrosarcomas test positive for FeLV, thus indicating a grave prognosis regardless of therapy.

TABLE 12-1

REPORTED EYELID NEOPLASMS IN THE CAT

Tumor Type	Veterinary Medical Data (%)	Purdue Comparative Oncology (%)
Squamous cell carcinoma	65	36.1
Fibrosarcoma	5	8.3
Lymphosarcoma		11.1
Undetermined	5	
Adenocarcinoma	3.5	
Adenoma/sebaceous adenoma/ cystadenoma	3.5	8.3
Mastocytoma	3.5	11 1
Basal cell carcinoma	2.3	5.6
Carcinoma (unspecified)	2.3	
Fibroma	2.3	
Hemangiosarcoma	2.3	
Melanoma	2.3	8.4
Hemangioma	1	
Neurofibroma	1	
Trichoepithelioma	1	
Squamous papilloma		8.3
Histocytoma		2.8
Total	100	100

Modified from McLaughlin SA, Whitley RD, Gilger BG, Wright JC, Lindley DM. Eyelid neoplasm in cats: a review of demographic data (1979–1990). J Am Anim Assoc 1993;29:63–67.

NASOLACRIMAL AND TEAR DISEASES

Nasolacrimal and tear diseases are infrequent in domestic cats. Epiphora is occasionally seen, most often as an idiopathic condition (particularly in the Persian and Himalayan) or secondary to symblepharon formation and resultant punctal occlusion. This is strictly a cosmetic problem, however, and successful correction can be achieved by conjunctivorhinostomy. Congenitally imperforate lacrimal puncta are uncommon in the cat and can be surgically opened in the same manner as that described for other animals (see Chapter 4). Dacryocystitis likewise is rare in the cat, presumably because the relatively short nasolacrimal duct provides less opportunity for obstruction.

Though uncommon, keratoconjunctivitis sicca (KCS) is the most important lacrimal disease in the cat. The actual causes, however, have been poorly defined. **Most cases of feline KCS occur secondary to chronic blepharoconjunctivitis, at least some of which, in turn, appears to be secondary to recurrent or chronic FHV-1 infection.** Experimentally, transient KCS has been observed in cats with chronic FHV infection.

The diagnosis of feline KCS is established on the basis of compatible clinical signs in conjunction with decreased Schirmer tear test values. As in the dog, less than 5 mm/min of wetting is considered to be diagnostic (mean normal feline wetting, 17 mm/min), though in many cats, no clinical signs will be associated with such low values. Feline KCS is characterized by conjunctival hyperemia, mild and diffuse corneal opacification resulting from epithelial hyperplasia, and rarely, corneal vascularization and pigmentation as well as conjunctival discharges. In acute cases, epithelial ulceration is also seen.

Treatment of feline KCS differs little from that of canine KCS. The foremost consideration is to correct, if possible, any underlying cause. Palliative relief is achieved by application of artificial tears as needed (four times a day to hourly) and use of topical antibiotics to prevent bacterial infection. Pilocarpine may be used (one or two drops of 0.25–0.50% solution mixed in the food), but the patient should be monitored for any adverse systemic cholinergic effects. Cyclosporin A ophthalmic solution is the current

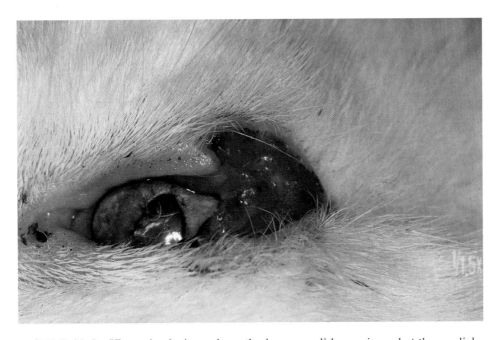

FIGURE 12-3. *Ulcerative lesions along the lower eyelid margin and at the medial canthus typical of adnexal squamous cell carcinoma in a 9-year-old white domestic Shorthair.*

therapy of choice for topical treatment of canine KCS, but its efficacy and safety in feline KCS have not been established. Parotid duct transposition in the cat has been described, but this procedure is reserved for those cases in which medical therapy is either impractical or unsuccessful.

DISEASES OF THE CONJUNCTIVA, NICTITATING MEMBRANE, AND CORNEA

Because of the frequent, concurrent involvement of the feline conjunctiva, nictitating membrane, and cornea, diseases of these tissues are discussed together here.

CONGENITAL AND DEVELOPMENTAL DISORDERS

Ocular dermoids occur only infrequently in the cat, but they have been described in the domestic Shorthair, Burmese, and Birman breeds. Bilateral limbal dermoids, with congenital swelling of the nictitans gland, occur in Burmese cats. **Complete excision by lamellar keratectomy is the treatment of choice (see Chapter 7).**

Nictitating membrane disorders also occur only rarely in the cat. Prolapse and eversion of the nictitans gland are uncommon, and they have been reported only in the Burmese breed. This condition can be corrected by a variety of surgical techniques, which include suturing the prolapsed gland to orbital fascia, extraocular muscle, or Tenon's capsule or sclera. Because the nictitans gland contributes secretions to the aqueous tear film, total surgical excision is not recommended. Eversion of the nictitans cartilage occurs in the Burmese cat, and treatment consists of excising the abnormal portion of the cartilage through a small, conjunctival incision on its posterior (i.e., bulbar) surface.

Protrusion of the nictitans commonly occurs secondary to changes in globe position, particularly enophthalmos; systemic diseases, the common causes of which are atrophy of the orbital fat in aged animals; and globe retraction associated with ocular pain. Protrusion of the nictitans also occurs secondary to orbital diseases (described later, as third-eyelid dysautonomia [see Chapter 16, p. 457]).

THE CONJUNCTIVITIDES

Most conjunctivitides in the cat are primary infections that are associated with specific causes.

Herpesvirus Conjunctivitis

Feline herpesvirus-1 is ubiquitous among the world's cat population, with similar (but serologically distinct) varieties having been isolated

from nondomestic felids. In domestic cats, primary infection is character-ized by diffuse replication of the virus in the epithelium of the upper respira-tory tract (i.e., turbinates, nasal mucosa, tonsils). Clinical manifestations result from a direct, viral cytopathic effect on the infected tissues and may be pro-longed by secondary bacterial infection. **Conjunctival infection consistently occurs during primary infection, and though not apparent clinically, lim-ited viral replication also occurs in the corneal epithelium. Stress asso-ciated with development of another disease, introduction of a new cat into the household, moving, and so on may trigger recurrences.**

The typical clinical syndrome of primary FHV-1 infection is an acute, conjunctival-respiratory infection in neonatal and adolescent cats. Neonatal ophthalmia has also been associated with FHV-1. Sneez-ing as well as ocular and nasal discharge typify the disease, and a course of 10 to 14 days is the rule. Both the incubation time and the duration of the illness, however, vary with the quantity of virus inoculum. **Conjunctivitis from FHV-1 is characterized by a bilateral, conjunctival hyperemia and a serous ocular discharge (Fig. 12-4). The ocular discharge becomes**

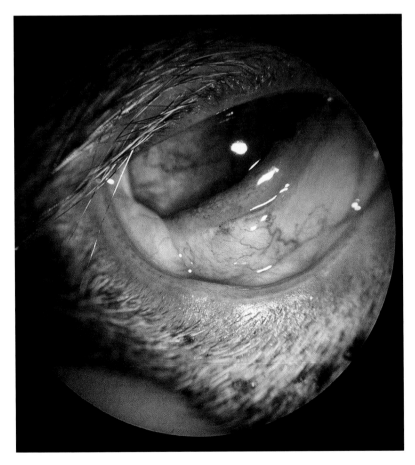

FIGURE 12-4. *Acute herpetic conjunctivitis characterized by bilateral conjunctival hyperemia and serous ocular discharge.*

mucoid to mucopurulent, and the conjunctiva swells as the disease progresses. Chemosis, however, is not a prominent feature of FHV-1 conjunctivitis. **Corneal microdendritic ulcers may be seen in acute primary infection, but their identification requires vital staining with rose Bengal.** Rose Bengal should not be used if virus isolation is anticipated, however, because it may significantly inhibit FHV-1 recovery. Fluorescein stain often is not retained, because the cytopathic effect may not reach the depth of the corneal epithelial basement membrane. Even so, topical fluorescein may affect the results of immunofluorescent antibody tests in the cat and produce in false-positive results.

In most cases, **primary infection resolves with no residual ocular lesions. In very young cats, symblepharon formation may be a sequela. After recovery from primary FHV-1 infection, an estimated 80% of cats become latently infected, and in 45% of these, the latent virus will spontaneously reactivate, manifesting either as asymptomatic virus shedding or recrudescent clinical disease.** A general characteristic of alpha herpesviruses is the tendency to establish latency in the sensory (i.e., trigeminal) ganglia.

In addition, FHV-1 may cause conjunctivitis in adult cats that presumably have been exposed to, and already recovered from, the virus earlier in life. Signs of respiratory infection are therefore often absent. Like the acute respiratory syndrome, FHV-1 conjunctivitis in adult cats tends to be bilateral and to affect young animals (mean age, 2.9 year). Concurrent infection with FeLV or feline immunodeficiency virus (FIV) is associated with increased rates of chronic conjunctivitides.

The clinical signs of FHV-1 conjunctivitis in adult cats are nondiagnostic. The conjunctiva is hyperemic, and there is intermittent blepharospasm. Ocular discharge is usually mild and serous in nature. In adult cats, FHV-1 conjunctivitis further contrasts with the acute respiratory syndrome in its tendency to be chronic and recurrent in nature. The persistence of ocular disease without respiratory signs is explained by the inability of FHV-1 to stimulate an effective local immunity. Infection with FHV-1 is uncommonly associated with inadequate tear production and, perhaps, decreased corneal sensation (see the previous section on lacrimal/tear disorders).

The clinical diagnosis of acute FHV-1 infection is established on the basis of the characteristic ocular and respiratory signs. The laboratory diagnosis is summarized in Table 12-2. Treatment of acute FHV-1 conjunctivitis is nonspecific and directed at controlling secondary bacterial invaders. Tetracycline ophthalmic ointment, such as Terramycin (Pfizer) and Achromycin (Lederle), is indicated because of its efficacy against _Chlamydia_ and _Mycoplasma_ sp., and it should be applied four times daily. Cats may find this medication topically irritating, however. Other potentially useful antibiotics are chloramphenicol and erythromycin. Specific antiviral therapies usually are reserved for herpetic keratitis but can also be used for chronic conjunctival infections.

Corticosteroids are contraindicated in most cases of feline conjunctivitis, and especially in those caused by FHV-1. Vaccination with modified live or killed vaccines effectively minimizes—or even prevents—the clinical signs of infection, and it may also limit establishment of the car-

TABLE 12-2

LABORATORY DIAGNOSIS OF FELINE HERPESVIRUS-1 INFECTION IN THE CAT

Test	Advantages/Limitations
Conjunctival cytology	Limited value, except in primary FHV-1 conjunctival infections. Intranuclear inclusion bodies of FHV-1 appear with primary FHV-1 infections but are not identifiable with the Wright-Giemsa cytology stain.
IFA testing	Commonly used to confirm FHV-1 infection. Uses the indirect method in which the cytologic specimen is reacted with a nonconjugated polyclonal antibody. Detects a variety of IFA reactions, but lacks sensitivity.
Virus isolation	Virus isolation has been the "gold standard" for diagnosis of FHV-1 infection. Used in the research laboratory, but results are markedly influenced by delayed handling, variable refrigeration, and repeated thawing. Less useful as well as insensitive for chronic FHV-1 infections.
Antigen-capture immunoassays	Herpesvirus enzyme-linked immunosorbent assay test employs a solid phase in which a capture antibody (either mono- or polyclonal) is bound. Not available to date for FHV-1.
Serology	Serum-neutralizing titer has not been useful clinically in diagnosis of FHV-1 infection. In chronic, low-grade infections, serum-neutralizing titers tend to become stable rather than increase. Often, FHV-1 titers are low after primary infections and vaccinations, and serum-neutralizing titers in reactivation of latent and recrudescent infections may rise.
Polymerase chain reaction	Permits small amounts of DNA to be amplified exponentially and detected. For FHV-1, a segment of DNA is amplified by the thymidine kinase gene. Sensitivity for FHV-1 detection appears to be vastly superior to those of other available techniques and is 80% more sensitive than viral isolation at detecting virus shedding in conjunctival swabs from asymptomatic cats. The high sensitivity for FHV-1 has caused some difficulties, however, with its interpretation in clinical patients.

IFA, immunofluorescent antibody; *FHV-1,* feline herpesvirus-1.

rier state. Vaccination does not necessarily prevent infection, however, and it probably has little value in a cat that is already infected with or a latent carrier of FHV-1.

Three other modes of therapy have been investigated for FHV-1 infection. Orally administered valacyclovir, 60 mg/kg, was used for experimentally induced, primary FHV-1 infections. In that study, treated cats became lethargic and dehydrated between 6 and 9 days. At 12 days, the therapy could not be continued because of the animals' poor conditions. **Hence, cats appear to be highly sensitive to the toxic effects of systemic vala-cyclovir, and these high doses do not appear to suppress FHV-1 replication in acutely infected cases.**

Oral L-lysine, 250 mg/day, has been recently suggested to either prevent or reduce the severity of recurrent FHV-1 infections in the cat. In vitro tests with L-lysine and arginine suggest that arginine is required for the replication of FHV-1, and that depletion of arginine in the culture media causes a profound reduction in viral growth. At 300 mg/mL, lysine reduces FHV-1 replication in the presence of low arginine concentrations, but these viral inhibitory effects are negated at higher arginine concentrations. On the basis of these results, in vivo tests with oral lysine, 250 to 500 mg/day, will be necessary to demonstrate any effectiveness.

Recombinant human interferon-α, 5 to 25 IU/day administered orally and topically, has also been recommended for FHV-1 infection on the basis of in vitro results that are suggestive of possible efficacy. Clinical observations, however, are still incomplete at this time.

The prognosis for recovery from acute ocular infection with FHV-1 is excellent. In adult cats with chronic or recurrent infections, however, the prognosis for permanent recovery is guarded.

CHLAMYDIA PSITTACI CONJUNCTIVITIS

Chlamydia psittaci **is a common pathogen in the cat that primarily affects the conjunctiva. Respiratory infection does occur, but only infrequently is this apparent clinically.** The zoonotic potential is considered to be low, though transmission of *C. psittaci* from the cat to humans has been suspected on several occasions.

The typical clinical syndrome in the cat is one of unilateral conjunctivitis, with eventual involvement of the fellow eye. Cats of all ages may be affected. In acute infection, the characteristic clinical appearance is that of conjunctival hyperemia, chemosis, and serous ocular discharge, which may become purulent with chronicity. Conjunctival follicle formation occurs during chronic infections. **Cytologically, the disease is characterized by the presence of intracytoplasmic inclusions within the conjunctival epithelial cells between days 7 and 14 of infection.** At conjunctival cytology, neutrophils predominate initially, but after 14 to 21 days of infection, all cell types (i.e., neutrophils, macrophages, lymphocytes) are equally present.

The diagnosis can be confirmed by conjunctival cytology during the first 2 weeks of the primary disease, either by detecting antigen on conjunctival scrapings using the fluorescent antibody technique or by isolating the organism in embryonated eggs. Tetracycline ophthalmic ointment, applied four times daily, generally is effective at arresting the clinical signs. If tetracycline is too irritating, topical chloramphenicol or erythromycin may be substituted. *Chlamydia* sp. are resistant to many routine antibiotics, however, including gentamicin, bacitracin, and neomycin, and chronic infections have been reported that required long-term systemic tetracycline therapy to control. Newer antibiotics (e.g., doxycycline, azithromycin) may be useful. Recurrent infections and a latent carrier state have been suggested as well. *Chlamydia psittaci* also infects the feline gastrointestinal tract, and in one recent study, ocular infection resulted in persistent urogenital and gastrointestinal infection. The relationship between ocular disease and gastrointestinal infection in natural disease, however, is not yet clear. The efficacy of chlamydial vaccines is difficult to establish because of conflicting results. In the most recent and thorough experimental study, use of a live vaccine decreased the severity of the ocular disease, but it had no effect on the shedding of organisms or on their ability to infect and to persist at other sites (i.e., gastrointestinal, urogenital).

Mycoplasmal Conjunctivitis

Mycoplasma felis and *M. gatae* have been incriminated as causes of feline conjunctivitis. Clinical signs include unilateral or bilateral conjunctivitis characterized initially by epiphora and papillary hypertrophy of the conjunctiva. Associated abnormalities include conjunctival follicles, chemosis, and formation of conjunctival pseudomembranes composed of thick, white exudate. Cytologically, polymorphonuclear leukocytes predominate, and small basophilic inclusion bodies may be seen at the level of the epithelial cell membrane. The diagnosis is confirmed by isolating the organism in specific media. The disease responds dramatically to topical application of appropriate antibiotics four times daily. *Mycoplasma* sp. are susceptible to most routinely used antibiotics. Because of its efficacy against *Chlamydia* sp., however, which may be a concurrent pathogen, tetracycline is most often used.

Other Causes

Potential miscellaneous causes of feline conjunctivitis include other bacteria, reovirus, salmonellosis, and calicivirus.

Neonatal Conjunctivitis

Neonatal conjunctivitis is a syndrome of acute conjunctival inflammation that occurs among neonatal kittens. Copious ocular discharge (usually mucopurulent) is the consistent finding. If infection develops before resolution of physiologic ankyloblepharon at 10 to 14 days of age, the eyelids take on a characteristic, distended appearance. The causes of neonatal conjunctivitis probably include most of the agents discussed earlier as well as common bacterial pathogens. **The problem usually resolves promptly after topical therapy with broad-spectrum antibiotics. If the eyelid margins are adhered, the palpebral fissure should be opened by inserting the blade of a small scissor into the medial canthus and then sliding the blade laterally.** If the kitten is younger than 10 to 14 days, tear production and the blink reflex may be inadequate when the ankyloblepharon is opened; in these patients, topical antibiotics, artificial tears, and even temporary, incomplete closure of the eyelids may be indicated.

Lipogranulomatous Conjunctivitis

Older cats (mean age, 11.9 year) can develop either unilateral or bilateral lipogranulomatous conjunctivitis. Some cats also have concurrent ocular or periocular neoplasia, marked goblet cell hyperplasia, or both. The conjunctival disease consists of large amounts of deposited lipid, with an associated granulomatous inflammation that is refractory to medical therapy.

Symblepharon

Symblepharon is the adhesion of any portion of the conjunctiva to itself or to the cornea. **Symblepharon appears to develop primarily in young cats. The cause remains speculative, but most cases occur after severe conjunctival inflammation, often with characteristics suggestive of FHV-1 infection.** Treatment depends on the extent of the adhesions. If adhesions obscure vision or impair eyelid function, they can be treated surgically using combinations of keratectomy and conjunctival repositioning procedures. Other therapies include mitomycin (as an antifibrotic agent), beta radiation, and cyclosporin A.

Miscellaneous Conjunctival Disorders

The cat occasionally develops conjunctivitis unrelated to micro-organisms. For example, feline conjunctivitis can be associated with the nematode *Thelazia californiensis*. The clinical signs are mild conjunctival hyperemia and ocular discharge, and the parasite is easily removed from the conjunctival fornix using forceps. Allergic conjunctivitis is rare in the cat, but hypersensitivity reactions to ophthalmic preparations of tetracycline, idoxuridine, trifluridine, and neomycin can occur.

KERATITIS

The prevalence of conjunctival bacterial flora is lower in the cat than in other domestic species. Organisms commonly isolated from normal cats include *Staphylococcus epidermidis* and *Mycoplasma* sp. Cytologic examination of the normal feline conjunctiva reveals predominantly epithelial cells, which sometimes contain melanin granules. Lymphocytes, monocytes, plasma cells, and neutrophils are seen uncommonly, however, and eosinophils and basophils are not seen at all. Goblet cells are found only in scrapings from the fornix. The prevalence of fungal flora in the cat also appears to be limited.

Bacterial Keratitis

In all animal species, bacterial keratitis is initiated by a traumatic disruption of the corneal epithelium that allows bacteria to gain a foothold. Because of the paucity of primary adnexal diseases with the potential to irritate the feline cornea, however, bacterial keratitis is relatively uncommon. The clinical signs, diagnostic approach, and treatment of feline bacterial keratitis are similar to those in the dog (see Chapter 7).

Feline Herpesvirus-1 Keratitis

Feline herpesvirus-1 is the only known viral cause of keratitis in the cat (Fig. 12-5), and it appears to cause corneal disease through two different mechanisms. First, corneal ulceration may result from its direct cytopathic effects in the corneal epithelium. When this occurs, characteristic branching (i.e., dendritic) lesions may be produced. Therefore, dendritic keratitis can be subtle in appearance, and because the epithelial lesions

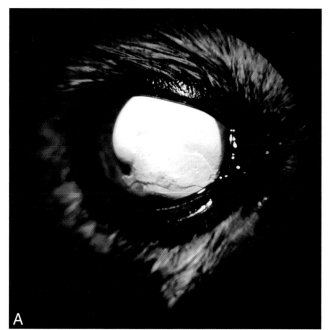

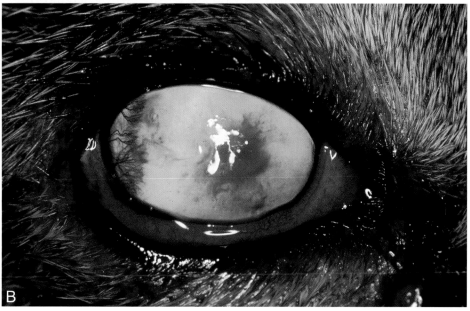

FIGURE 12-5. *The effects of feline herpesvirus-1 on the feline cornea.* **A.** *Outline of a geographic herpetic corneal erosion can be seen in the central cornea of this 7-month-old domestic Shorthair.* **B.** *Stromal keratitis in the cat. Note the generalized stromal opacification.*

often do not reach the depth of the corneal epithelial basement membrane, their identification can be difficult without the use of vital stains (e.g., rose Bengal). During primary ocular infection, FHV-1 corneal dendrites tend to be small and numerous; such lesions are termed *microdendritic* (for more details the reader should consult the third edition, pp. 1004–1008).

Feline herpesvirus-1 also may cause corneal stromal damage unrelated to direct viral replication. In FHV-1–related stromal keratitis, suppression of the local immune responses appears to allow the virus access to the corneal stroma, and the subsequent keratitis is mediated by an immune response to the viral antigen. Topical corticosteroids seem to enhance the development of experimental FHV-1 stromal keratitis. Deep corneal ulcers sometimes are associated with FHV-1 infection, especially in young cats. Corneal melting and loss of collagen, however, probably relate to concomitant bacterial infection.

In young animals, the source of corneal infection undoubtedly is the extension of a primary conjunctival infection, but in adults, the source is probably the reactivation of latent virus. As mentioned, sensory ganglia are the most likely sites of clinically relevant viral latency (the cornea may also be a potential site). Virus reactivation and recrudescence of clinical disease occur after numerous forms of endogenous stress and after exogenous administration of corticosteroids.

The clinical signs of FHV-1 keratitis vary depending on the chronicity and the depth of infection. Acute dendritic keratitis is accompanied by mild to moderate conjunctivitis, invariably by blepharospasm, and usually by serous to mucopurulent ocular discharge. In chronic cases, the corneal stroma may be mildly edematous in the area of the lesion, and areas of fibrosis and superficial vascularization may occur as well. Stromal keratitis may occur with or without overlying epithelial lesions, but ulceration is the rule, often in an irregular or a maplike (i.e., geographic) pattern. A diagnosis of stromal keratitis is justified when corneal edema is more severe than can be explained by the epithelial ulceration alone or when extensive, deep vascularization or cellular infiltration (or both) is evident. Eventually, FHV-1 stromal keratitis can culminate in significant stromal scarring and impaired vision. Both the epithelial and the stromal keratitis forms of the disease may be unilateral. As with chronic FHV-1 conjunctivitis, respiratory signs are usually absent.

A diagnosis of FHV-1 keratitis can usually be presumed on the basis of the characteristic clinical signs. Application of rose Bengal stain helps to identify dendrites that are insufficiently deep to stain with fluorescein. The presence of dendritic lesions is considered to be pathognomonic for FHV-1 infection. Confirmation of FHV-1 infection requires laboratory detection of viral antigen (see the previous section on infectious conjunctivitis). As with chronic FHV-1 conjunctivitis, demonstrating viral antigen in cases of chronic FHV-1 keratitis is often difficult.

The response of FHV-1 keratitis to treatment is unpredictable at best. Acute epithelial keratitis carries the best prognosis, however, and it often responds dramatically to ophthalmic antiviral medications (see Appendix E). Most cases have little need for prophylactic topical antibiotics. Topical treatment should be continued for at least 2 weeks or until the clinical signs have been absent for longer than 1 week. The response to antiviral therapy in cases with stromal involvement typically is poor. Corticosteroids may be indicated on the basis of the postulated immunologic basis of the keratitis, but these agents can aggravate FHV-1 infections as well as stimulate the transition of epithelial to stromal keratitis. Hence, corticosteroids may be indicated in severe cases, but they should not administered without concomitant antiviral therapy. Likewise, cyclosporin A adversely affects the course of active ocular herpesvirus infections (for more details, the reader should consult the third edition, pp. 1011–1013).

Mycotic Keratitis

Keratomycosis is rare in the cat and usually represents an opportunistic infection after disruption of the normal corneal physiologic and anatomic integrity. Corneal infection by *Cladosporium* sp. has been reported in one cat.

Other Corneal Infections

Corneal abscessation that was presumed to be bacterial in origin has been described in a cat. The probable cause was a penetrating injury. The cornea was white in appearance and densely vascularized, and treatment using subconjunctival and topical administration of gentamicin was curative. Corneal infection with protozoa *Encephalitozoon* (*Nosema*) sp. has been described in a single cat, and this infection was associated with blepharospasm and numerous stellate, superficial corneal opacities that resembled lipid deposits. The diagnosis was established on the basis of histopathologic results, and keratectomy was curative.

CORNEAL DYSTROPHIES AND DEGENERATION

Corneal dystrophy is defined as a primary, inherited corneal disease that typically manifests early in life, is bilateral, and shows a preference for the central cornea. **Feline corneal diseases that conform to this definition are rare. A syndrome of progressive stromal edema without endothelial disease has been described in the Manx cat, however, and it may affect other breeds as well. Edema of the anterior stroma (evident as early as 4 months of age) is associated with swelling and disintegration of the collagen fibers.** Eventually, fluid vesicles and bullae form. The course is progressive, and the entire cornea eventually is affected. The success rate of feline corneal transplantation appears to be comparable with that of humans, thus suggesting this condition should be treated with penetrating keratoplasty.

Corneal degenerations are the extracellular deposition of lipids and, less commonly, calcium in the corneal stroma secondary to some other disease. In the cat, corneal degenerations are uncommon, but several cases of lipid degeneration have been described. In a domestic Shorthair cat, lipid degeneration was also a sequel to corneal ulceration (for more details, the reader should consult the third edition, pp. 1013–1014).

CORNEAL SEQUESTRATION

Corneal sequestration is a disease that is unique to the cat. It is characterized by degeneration of collagen and accumulation of a brown

FIGURE 12-6. *A history of recurrent herpetic ulceration preceded development of a dark-brown sequestrum in the axial cornea of this 3-year-old domestic Shorthair. The adjacent cornea appears normal.*

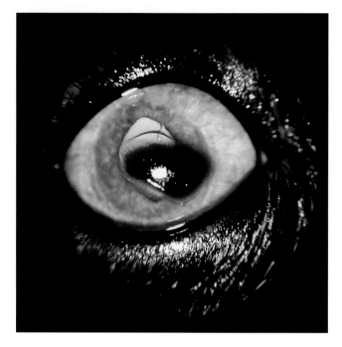

pigment. Other names for this condition include corneal black spot, corneal nigrum, corneal mummification, and focal corneal degeneration. Corneal sequestration occurs in all breeds, but the Persian, Himalayan, and Burmese appear to be predisposed.

The clinical appearance of this condition is characteristic. The lesion usually occurs in the central or the paracentral cornea, is circular or oval in shape, and invariably appears pigmented (Fig. 12-6). The intensity of the pigmentation, however, is extremely variable. Some cases have an extremely subtle, tan discoloration of the superficial stroma; others involve a lesion that is nearly black. Tan lesions may be covered by intact epithelium, whereas darker lesions are ulcerated. Loose, edematous epithelium is often visible at the periphery of the lesion as well. The cornea typically is affected only to the midstroma, but sequestra may extend as deep as the Descemet's membrane. Corneal vascularization, perilesional stromal edema, and inflammation are common with chronicity. Histopathologically, the sequestra are composed of degenerative collagen and fibroblasts, with a surrounding zone of inflammatory cells.

The cause of corneal sequestration is unknown, but heredity, ocular irritation (i.e., entropion, lagophthalmia, and corneal microtrauma), and infection with FHV-1 have been proposed. The pigment, which appears to be water soluble and not melanin, may be passively absorbed by the damaged stroma from the tears, but pigment in the stroma of an otherwise normal-appearing cornea is suggestive that a pathologic role is also possible.

The choice of treatment for corneal sequestration varies depending on the stage of disease and the lesion depth. An effort should first be made to identify and then correct any underlying causes. Because some superficial sequestra may slough spontaneously, the conservative approach of observation may be selected for these lesions. **An early keratectomy,**

however, may quickly relieve the discomfort and prevent superficial sequestra from becoming deeper. If the surgical wound is deeper than half the cornea, the defect may be covered with a sliding corneoconjunctival graft, which provides a more transparent result than that with a pedicle conjunctival graft. Sequestration can recur after surgery, especially if the excision was incomplete or the corneal surface was left ulcerated. Covering the keratectomy site with a corneoconjunctival or a conjunctival pedicle graft has been reported to prevent recurrence of the sequestrum (for more details, the reader should consult the third edition, pp. 1014–1016).

PROLIFERATIVE KERATOCONJUNCTIVITIS (EOSINOPHILIC KERATITIS)

Proliferative eosinophilic keratitis also appears to be unique to the cat and has also been termed *proliferative keratoconjunctivitis.* The typical lesion is a proliferative, white to pink, edematous, irregular, and vascularized mass (or masses) that most commonly originates from the nasal or the temporal limbus, the peripheral cornea, or the adjacent bulbar conjunctiva (Fig. 12-7). The nictitating membrane may be affected as well, and with chronicity, the entire cornea can become affected. Initially, the condition is usually unilateral, but bilateral involvement often eventually occurs. Signs of ocular discomfort are inconsistent. Dermatologic lesions that are typical of the eosinophilic complex are absent.

The cause of proliferative keratitis is unknown. Recent polymerase chain reaction results, however, have revealed that FHV-1 may also be important in the pathogenesis of this disease, because in that study, 76.3% of surgical specimens from cats with proliferative keratoconjunctivitis were positive for FHV-1. Histopathologically, proliferative

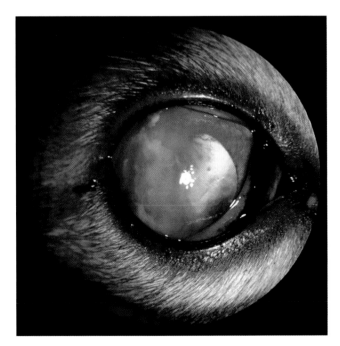

FIGURE 12-7. *Focal white plaques, cellular infiltrates, stromal edema, and superficial vascularization characterize the lesions of eosinophilic keratitis, as seen in the temporal cornea of this young domestic Shorthair.*

keratitis is a chronic, granulomatous inflammatory response that is characterized by an inflammatory cell infiltrate of plasma cells and lymphocytes, variable areas and amounts of eosinophils, and occasionally, histiocytes and mast cells. In cytologic preparations collected by corneal scraping, eosinophils are usually (but not always) the most conspicuous type of cell. Hematologic evaluation may reveal eosinophilia.

Feline proliferative keratoconjunctivitis usually responds dramatically to topical therapy with 0.1% dexamethasone ophthalmic ointment or 1% prednisolone acetate suspension. Treatment should be initiated at a frequency of at least four times daily and then, after several weeks, be reduced to maintenance therapy of one or two times daily. Megestrol acetate is also effective at an oral dose of 5 mg/day for 5 days, which is then reduced to 5 mg every other day for 7 days, and then to 5 mg/week for maintenance. Megestrol is not recommended as the initial choice of therapy, however, because of its serious potential systemic side effects (e.g., diabetes mellitus).

Florida Keratopathy ("Florida Spots")

"Florida spots" occur in the cat (and also the dog) in the southeastern United States. They appear clinically as focal, gray-white opacities within the anterior stroma. The lesions vary in diameter from 1 to 8 mm, and they typically are multiple and usually bilateral. The condition is usually asymptomatic and either slowly progressive or nonprogressive. The cause was suspected to be the fungal organism *Rhinosporidium* or mycobacterial. Topical antibiotics and corticosteroids usually do not produce any resolution.

ACUTE BULLOUS KERATOPATHY

Acute bullous keratopathy is a rare disease of young cats. There has been no reported history of systemic disease and trauma, but anterior uveitis may be present. **All corneas are variably edematous, with either focal edema or involvement of the entire cornea with iris prolapse. Treatment has consisted of conjunctival grafts or enucleation.** The cause of this condition has not been determined, but it appears to be a possible stromal defect rather than a focal to diffuse corneal endothelial dysfunction.

INFLAMMATORY MASSES AND NEOPLASIA OF THE NICTITANS, CONJUNCTIVA, AND CORNEA

Neoplasms of the nictitating membrane are rare, but single cases of fibrosarcoma and adenocarcinoma have been reported. Lymphosarcoma may also infiltrate the nictitans; however, it is not known if these tumors are primary to the nictitans or simply the extension of an orbital lesion. Except for squamous cell carcinomas that invade from the eyelids, feline conjunctival neoplasms are rare. When they do occur, however, they include malignant melanoma and lymphosarcoma.

A proliferative stromal lesion that was diagnosed as being fibrous histiocytoma has been described in a domestic Shorthair cat. Like its counterpart in the dog, this lesion began at the temporal limbus and was characterized histopathologically by lymphocytes, plasma cells, and histiocytes and by active fibroplasia. Keratectomy was curative.

Neoplasms affecting the feline cornea and sclera are rare but include squamous cell carcinomas and limbal melanomas. The limbal melanomas arise in the superficial sclera, are slow growing and minimally invasive, and can be treated conservatively, with surgical resection or cryosurgery.

DISEASES OF THE ANTERIOR UVEA

Diseases of the feline anterior uvea include congenital and developmental disorders as well as anterior and posterior uveitis. Inflammations of the feline uveal tract are commonly seen in clinical practice and often associated with systemic diseases.

CONGENITAL AND DEVELOPMENTAL DISORDERS

The Siamese and Blue Irides

The Siamese breed has blue irides, convergent strabismus or esotropia, and nystagmus. Siamese cats also demonstrate decreased stereopsis compared with normal cats. These clinical findings are associated with neuroanatomic abnormalities in which the major retinal pathways travel an abnormal route and nearly all projections cross to the pretectum and superior colliculus. Thus, binocular vision is denied to this breed, and stereopsis is impaired. Convergent strabismus therefore is presumed to result from a limited ability to process spatially coordinated binocular information (an ability on which normal ocular alignment depends). Esotropia also may result from a conscious attempt to position the functional temporal visual fields from the nasal retinas to a more frontal position, because the extensive crossing-over of the axons from the temporal retinas at the optic chiasm are suppressed. Normally, the optic nerve axons of the temporal retina remain ipsilateral, but crossing to the contralateral side of the brain occurs in the Siamese. Input from the abnormally routed axons is thus suppressed. Siamese cats also have a lower percentage of Y- to X-type ganglion cells (8%) than normal cats (32%). Misrouted projections of the central visual pathways are present in cats with the Chédiak-Higashi syndrome as well.

Blue Irides and Other Diseases

Blue irides, deafness, and white coat color occur as a dominantly inherited condition in the domestic cat. This condition is similar (but not analogous) to Waardenburg's syndrome in humans. Features that are absent or not recognizable in the feline condition are dystopia canthorum, a prominent nasal root, and hyperplastic medial eyebrows. The hearing deficit has been linked to bony alterations in the modiolus and membranous changes in the labyrinth.

Chédiak-Higashi syndrome is an autosomal recessive disease that is characterized in the cat by partial oculocutaneous albinism, bleeding tendency, and increased susceptibility to infection. Affected cats have lightly colored irides, reduced pigmentation of the nontapetal fundi, and congenital cataracts. The characteristic histopathologic feature is enlarged cytoplasmic granules that include lysosomes and melanosomes. Postnatal tapetal degeneration also is a feature. The diagnosis is established on the basis of identifying compatible clinical signs and demonstrating enlarged melanin granules in hair shafts examined using light microscopy.

Iris Cysts and Pupillary Membranes

Congenital iris and ciliary body cysts occasionally are seen in the cat. They are identified by their spherical shape, tendency to be attached at the pupillary margin, and translucency when illuminated with a focal light source. As in other species, iris cysts in the cat rarely threaten vision; however, their surgical removal and laser rupture have been described.

Iridal colobomas, usually in the 6-o'clock position, may occur as part of the colobomatous syndrome in cats with eyelid agenesis. These colobomas allow for direct inspection of the exposed ciliary body and peripheral lens. They also produce an obvious, irregularly shaped pupil with a less-than-complete response to mydriatics. In themselves, iridal colobomas do not impair vision, but when coupled with other ocular anomalies, they may be associated with blindness.

Persistent pupillary membranes occur only rarely in the cat. They do not appear to be inherited, and they may occur in eyes that are otherwise normal or that have multiple ocular anomalies. Persistent pupillary membranes consist of thin, translucent to heavily pigmented tissues extending from the iridal collarette to other areas of the iris, the posterior cornea, or the anterior lens capsule. Most persistent pupillary membranes require no treatment, but medical therapy using long-term mydriatics or surgical or laser transection may be used.

Partial anterior segment cleavage syndrome occurs in the cat as well. This syndrome appears as a broad adherence of the iris to the posterior cornea, with loss of the anterior chamber, focal corneal edema, and distortion of the pupil. The globe is often microphthalmic, but other anomalies are usually absent. The condition is nonprogressive, and treatment is not indicated. The cause is unknown, though in utero influences late during development of the globe appear to be likely.

ANTERIOR AND POSTERIOR UVEITIS

Anterior uveitis, with or without chorioretinitis, is the most frequent and significant intraocular disease in the domestic cat. Both the direct and secondary effects of anterior uveitis (especially the chronic types) may be destructive to the eye and to the maintenance of vision. In the cat, serious—and often fatal—systemic diseases may first be presented to the veterinarian with only the ophthalmic signs of anterior uveitis. Hence, in the clinical evaluation of all feline patients with uveitis, a thorough physical examination, clinical pathology, and selected serology are recommended. (For more details, see Chapter 17.)

Causes of Uveitis

The causes of uveitis in the cat are summarized in Box 12-1. **In recent reports, approximately 38 to 70% of affected cats have had concurrent systemic diseases.** Infection with FIV causes chronic immunosuppression and a mild to moderately severe, chronic uveitis. Coinfection with *Toxoplasma gondii* increases the possibility of ocular disease.

Feline infectious peritonitis (FIP), which is caused by a coronavirus, produces a chronic and progressive anorexia, depression, weight loss, fluctuating fever, variable peritoneal and thoracic involvement, and debility. The anterior uveitis may develop with or without concurrent systemic signs (Fig. 12-8). Survival after the onset of clinical signs is usually less than 1 year, but survival is slightly longer among cases with only ocular involvement and the noneffusive forms. Feline infectious peritonitis produces a pyogranulomatous uveitis that affects the intraocular

---

BOX 12-1

Causes of Uveitis in the Cat

Trauma

Blunt

Penetrating

Infectious

Feline immunodeficiency virus

Feline infectious peritonitis

Feline leukemia virus

Toxoplasma gondii

Cryptococcus neoformans

Histoplasma capsulatum

Coccidioides immitis

Candida albicans

Neoplastic

Diffuse iridal melanoma

Primary ocular sarcomas

Primary ciliary body adenomas and adenocarcinomas

Metastatic uveal neoplasms (mainly adenocarcinomas)

Lens

Cataract-induced

Lens luxations

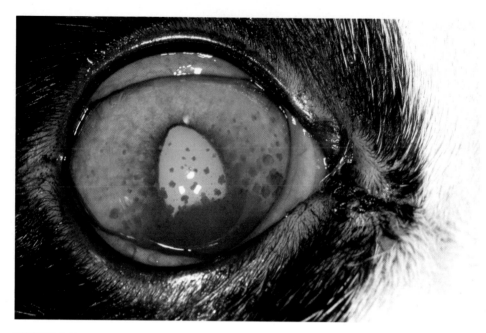

FIGURE 12-8. *Anterior uveitis in a 2-year-old domestic Shorthair with feline infectious peritonitis. Note the character of the inflammatory exudate within the anterior chamber adhering to the posterior cornea.*

blood vessels and the blood–aqueous barrier. It also affects the posterior segment but can be masked by the anterior uveal involvement. Changes in the posterior segment consist of a pyogranulomatous chorioretinitis and retinal vasculitis demonstrated clinically as chorioretinitis, perivascular cuffing, exudative retinal detachments, and optic neuritis.

The FeLV complex causes both direct and indirect lymphosarcoma (i.e., lymphosarcoma-related) uveitis in the cat. The ophthalmic involvement of FeLV can involves orbital masses, eyelid masses, subconjunctival and nictitating membrane masses, anterior chamber and anterior uveal tumors (i.e., lymphosarcomas), iridocyclitis with or without hypopyon, secondary glaucoma, chorioretinitis, chorioretinal masses, and retinal detachments.

Toxoplasma gondii **also produces posterior segment disease (i.e., granulomatous chorioretinitis and retinal vasculitis) as well as anterior segment disease (Fig. 12-9).** Granulomatous anterior uveitis is less frequent, however, and often is combined with concurrent chorioretinitis. In addition, granulomatous anterior uveitis has been associated with cryptococcosis, histoplasmosis, blastomycosis, and coccidioidomycosis. Ocular involvement with these organisms seems to be hematogenous except in cryptococcosis, in which extension from the central nervous system and the optic nerve seems to be likely. Other, less frequent causes of feline uveitis include lentivirus, *Candida* sp., intraocular parasites, and tuberculosis.

CLINICAL SIGNS

The clinical signs of anterior uveitis in the cat are the same as those in other species. They include ciliary flush, nictitating membrane protrusion, aqueous flare and fibrin, hypopyon, "mutton fat" keratic precipitates, iridal hyperemia, iridal nodules, decreased intraocular pressure (IOP), cellular infiltrates in the anterior vitreous, and variable involvement of the posterior segment. **These clinical signs are not pathognomonic for the known causes of feline anterior uveitis, but some do tend to occur more frequently with certain causes.** The "mutton fat" keratic precipitates, for example, occur most often with FIP and FeLV, and hemorrhage with inflammatory cells occurs with FIP. Iridal nodules occur most frequently in eyes with FIV or FeLV (Fig. 12-10). Obvious, white to pink masses both within the anterior chamber and adherent to the anterior iridal surface are usually associated with FeLV. Cellular infiltrates in the anterior vitreous (i.e., pars planitis) occur most often with FIV. With chronic FIV involvement, formation of posterior synechiae, cortical cataracts, and secondary glaucoma are likely. In eyes with FIP, the inflammatory condition gradually progresses to involve the entire inner eye (i.e., panuveitis/panophthalmitis), with diffuse and severe corneal edema, marked anterior uveitis, marked cellular infiltration of the vitreous (i.e., vitreitis), chorioretinitis, and inflammatory retinal detachments. The anterior uveitis of FeVL may progress to either diffuse inflammation of all the intraocular tissues or frank tumor formation.

Diagnostic Tests

In establishing the diagnosis of feline uveitis, infectious diseases, including FeLV, are first considered (Table 12-3).

Feline Sarcoma Virus

An oncogenic RNA virus, FeSV is thought to have evolved by mutation from FeLV. The virus is responsible for spontaneous tumor formation in

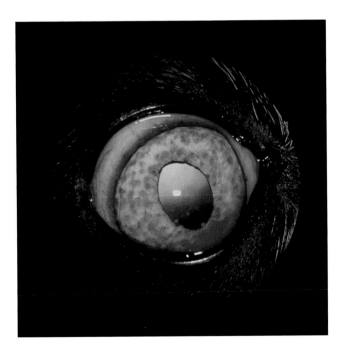

FIGURE 12-9. Toxoplasma *sp.–induced anterior uveitis, as in this 4.5-year-old domestic Shorthair, is characterized by iridal nodules, keratic precipitates, and a fibrin clot in the ventral anterior chamber. (Reprinted with permission from Ketring KL, Glaze MB. Atlas of feline ophthalmology. Trenton, NJ: Veterinary Learning Systems, 1994.)*

FIGURE 12-10. *Signs of idiopathic uveitis in a 4-year-old domestic Shorthair, including keratic precipitates and numerous iridal nodules.*

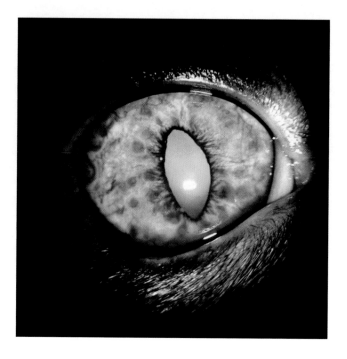

naturally infected cats. Experimental subcutaneous injection, however, induces a syndrome of anterior uveitis. In addition, bizarre transformed cells and large multinucleate cells (resembling sarcomatous changes) are also seen. A role for FeSV in naturally occurring feline uveitis has not been demonstrated.

Ophthalmomyiasis

Ophthalmomyiasis is also rare in the cat. The condition most commonly manifests as the migration of parasites both in and around the sensory retina, and most affected cats are asymptomatic. A *Cuterebra* sp. larva has recently been described as causing uveitis in a cat, in which the clinical signs were ocular pain, aqueous flare, and corneal edema.

Traumatic Anterior Uveitis

Anterior uveitis may follow both blunt and penetrating ocular trauma. Clinical signs include those of acute anterior uveitis plus hyphema, with the hyphema having variable amounts of fibrin. In cases of more intense anterior uveitis and additional fibrin, exit of the erythrocytes may be prolonged. In cases with limited blunt injury, the hyphema usually exits within a few days, but with considerable blunt trauma, the traumatic or resultant anterior uveitis may damage the iris, produce lens luxation, and result in cataract formation.

Penetrating ocular injuries may affect the cornea, lens, and posterior segment. When the lens and posterior segment cannot be visualized at slit-lamp biomicroscopy and ophthalmoscopy, ultrasonography is indicated. Treatment of traumatic uveitis is similar to that for the inflammatory types.

Corticosteroids are used to control the anterior uveitis and also to minimize formation of fibrin. The hyphema usually resolves within several days. If intravitreal hemorrhage occurs, however, the blood may require several months to exit the vitreous. If the lens capsule is penetrated, the lens itself should be removed sooner rather than later.

Lens-Induced Anterior Uveitis

Lens-induced anterior uveitis in the cat may be associated with cataract formation, hypermature cataracts, perforation of the lens capsule, and lens luxation. Perforation of the feline lens capsule usually follows lacerations by cat claws or foreign bodies. As in the dog, large or non-sealing anterior capsule lacerations (or both) expose the anterior uvea to progressively increasing amounts of lens material. Extracapsular lensectomy or phacoemulsification should be performed before the anterior uveitis becomes medically uncontrollable and threatens vision.

TABLE 12-3

LABORATORY TESTS FOR FELINE ANTERIOR UVEITIDES

Disease	Laboratory Tests
FIV	ELISA detects antibodies to FIV as early as 2 weeks. Aqueous cytology: plasmacytes and lymphocytes.
FIP	Coronavirus antibody titers tend to cross-react (FIP test only a guide). Pleural or peritoneal effusions: straw colored, high in fibrin and specific gravity. Hyperproteinemia (polyclonal gammopathy in 50% of cats with effusive FIP and 70% of cats with noneffusive FIP). Aqueous cytology: fibrin, red blood cells, monocytes, and neutrophils.
FeLV	FeVL titers, bone marrow aspiration, lymph node biopsy, and direct biopsy of intraocular masses. Aqueous humor cytology: lymphocytes and occasional plasmacytes and neutrophils. Abnormal or atypical lymphocytes are infrequent.
Toxoplasmosis	Organisms in the uveal tissues, and measurement of immunoglobulin G and M antibodies. ELISA test (Immunoglobulin M antibodies) greater than 1:256 is considered to be suggestive. PCR (B1 gene) tests for *Toxoplasma gondii*–specific Immunoglobulin M and G in both serum and aqueous humor samples.
Mycotic	Hematology, clinical chemistries, and aqueous and vitreous paracentesis. Lymph node and bone marrow aspirations (histoplasmosis). Cerebrospinal fluid aspirates for cryptococcosis.

ELISA, enzyme-linked immunosorbent assay; *FeLV,* feline leukemia virus; *FIP,* feline infectious peritonitis; *FIV,* feline immunodeficiency virus; *PCR,* polymerase chain reaction.

Lens luxations in young cats may follow trauma. In cats younger than 10 years, anterior and intravitreal lens luxations can occur, but the role of trauma versus aging is unknown. Glaucoma is usually present, however, and the relationship between the lens luxation and the glaucoma may be primary as well as secondary. Lens luxations in the cat can be removed early in the genesis of the glaucoma, and such removal may be curative of the elevated IOP.

Therapy and Ophthalmic Complications

Therapy for feline anterior uveitides is summarized in Table 12-4. **Several complications from anterior and posterior uveitis may develop in the cat. Usually, these complications relate directly to the duration and the cause of the uveal inflammation.** Glaucoma may result from peripheral anterior synechiae, iridocorneal angle and sclerociliary cleft closure, complete posterior synechiae with iris bombé, and development of preiridal membranes. **Secondary glaucoma may develop in 50% of eyes having uveitis with systemic diseases and in 28% of eyes having uveitis without systemic diseases. Cataracts (often with multiple posterior synechiae) occur in approximately 36% of cats with lymphoplasmacytic uveitis but in only 22% of cats with anterior uveitis and concurrent systemic diseases.** In cases with *T. gondii* infection, 70% of eyes develop secondary glaucoma. The end-stage sequela may be an enlarged, absolute glaucomatous globe or an atrophied globe (i.e., phthisis bulbus). In one re-

---

TABLE 12-4

THERAPY FOR FELINE UVEITIDES

Drugs	*Recommendations*
Mydriatics	Use 1% atropine ointment (less chance of salivation than solution). Administer to effect and maintain mydriasis.
Corticosteroids	Topical (and occasionally systemic) 1% prednisolone or 0.1% dexamethasone. Monitor aqueous flare and intraocular pressure to adjust frequency and duration.
NSAIDs	Can partially substitute for corticosteroids.
Antibiotics	For *Toxoplasma gondii* clindamycin (25 mg/kg daily in divided oral doses), with and without cortiscosteroids. Combination reported to improve the therapeutic response (86.7% with the corticosteroid–clindamycin combination versus 42.9% with corticosteroids alone).
Antifungals	For cryptococcosis and histoplasmosis, ketoconazole (10 mg/kg given orally twice per day).

NSAIDs, nonsteroidal anti-inflammatory drugs.

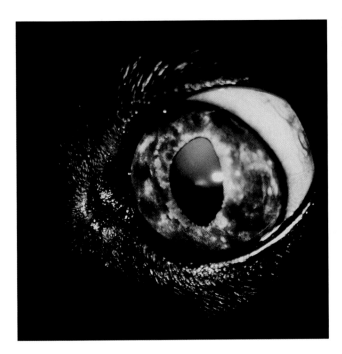

FIGURE 12-11. *Diffuse iris melanoma produced a change in both the color and contour of the iris over an 8-month period in this 4-year-old domestic Shorthair. (Reprinted with permission from Ketring KL, Glaze MB. Atlas of feline ophthalmology. Trenton, NJ: Veterinary Learning Systems, 1994.)*

port, blindness or visual impairment occurred in 72% of cats with uveitis and systemic diseases, but uveitis responded to therapy in only 33% of cats. Idiopathic uveitis as well as uveitis occurring secondary to infection with FIV were more responsive (<56%) to therapy than those uveitides associated with other systemic diseases (<33%).

ANTERIOR UVEAL NEOPLASMS

Both primary and secondary uveal neoplasms occur in the cat, and these neoplasms generally tend to be more aggressive in this species than in the dog. Of the feline intraocular neoplasms, anterior uveal tumors appear to be the most frequent and generally affect cats older than 10 years of age. No predisposition regarding breed or sex has been reported. The two different types that occur in the cat are the more common, diffuse iris melanoma and the infrequent melanoma (which histopathologically is similar to that in the dog).

Diffuse Iridal Melanoma

The diffuse iridal melanoma of the cat manifests as a progressive pigmentation of the iris that occurs over months to years (Fig. 12-11). The pigmentation may develop simultaneously in several areas on the anterior iridal surface. Generally, both the extent and amount of pigmentation increase with time. Changes in both the shape and the mobility of the pupil may result as the iridal thickness increases. Glaucoma secondary to tumor infiltration of the filtration angle is indicative that the condition is quite advanced in that patient. These tumors also have presented, albeit rarely, as amelanotic melanomas. Metastasis may occur as late as 1 to 3 years after enucleation, and it usually involves the liver and the lungs. The metastatic rate may be as high as 63%, but metastasis sometimes is not noted until death occurs.

Both clinical and histopathologic parameters have been developed to assist veterinarians with the clinical management of these patients. One report, which was based on histopathologic findings, suggested that prognostically poor indications include a high mitotic index, larger tumor size, tumor infiltration of the stroma, and invasion of the scleral venous plexus. Another report was indicative that cats with advanced melanoma and aggressive infiltration of the iris, posterior epithelium, and ciliary body had shortened survival times, and that death almost always was suggestive of a metastatic disease.

One dilemma for veterinarians is when removal of the eye will benefit the patient. Pigmentary changes may progress over several months to several years. **Enucleation may be justified on the basis of increased amounts and sizes of pigmented areas, any pigmented mass within the iridocorneal angle and sclerociliary cleft at gonioscopy, changes in the shape and mobility of the pupil, and elevated IOP.**

Trauma-Associated Sarcomas

Primary ocular sarcomas are second in frequency of occurrence among the cat (diffuse iridal melanomas being the first), and they are highly malignant neoplasms. Ocular trauma seems to be the inciting event. Affected cats range in age from 7 to 15 years, and time from trauma to detection of tumor averages 5 years. Risk factors include trauma to the lens, chronic uveitis, intraocular surgery (perhaps), and gentamycin injections to destroy the ciliary body during treatment of advanced absolute glaucoma. Presenting clinical signs include chronic uveitis, glaucoma, intraocular hemorrhage, and possible single or multiple, white to pink masses. Because cartilage and bone formation may occur within this tumor, ultrasonography and radiography may be helpful. **Early enucleation with exenteration of the orbit is recommended, because involvement of the optic nerve and regional lymph nodes as well as distant metastasis occurs.** After diagnosis and surgical removal of the affected globes, however, most cats will unfortunately die from neoplasm-related causes within several months.

Primary Ciliary Body and Metastatic Uveal Neoplasms

Primary ciliary body adenomas and adenocarcinomas are rare in the cat. They present as nonpigmented masses within the pupil that originate from the ciliary pars plicata, and they often produce secondary glaucoma. They usually grow slowly and seldom penetrate the sclera. Once the diagnosis is established, enucleation is recommended.

Most feline metastatic neoplasms involve the uveal tract, but such neoplasms are rare. Reported types include adenocarcinomas with a mammary or uterine origin, hemangiosarcoma, and squamous cell carcinomas from various sites. Anterior uveal involvement usually presents as masses of the ciliary body. The choroidal masses produce retinal hemorrhages and detachments.

Ocular Involvement with Feline Leukemia Virus

Lymphosarcoma is the most frequent intraocular tumor in cats presented to small animal clinics. Anterior uveal involvement occurs in nearly all globes as an anterior uveitis, an intraocular mass, or a combination of both (Fig. 12-12). Typically, there is a pink to white mass in the anterior chamber or within the anterior uvea. Signs of inflammation include miosis, reduced IOP, aqueous flare, keratic precipitates, and hypopyon. Secondary glaucoma as evidenced by an enlarged globe may result from neoplastic obstruction of the aqueous humor outflow pathways. Posterior uveal involvement seems to be less frequent. In some FeLV-positive cats without any other clinical signs (see chapters 16 and 17), a "D" or "reverse-D" pupil may signal the disease. The diagnosis of FeLV is summarized in Table 12-3.

Treatment of intraocular lymphosarcoma usually is not attempted, but topical or subconjunctival corticosteroids (or both) can temporarily reduce the size of the intraocular mass. Treatment of the secondary glaucoma is usually medical and consists of topical or systemic carbonic anhydrase inhibitors as well as topical β-antagonists (e.g., 0.5% timolol).

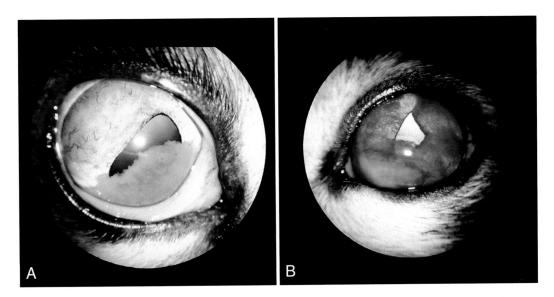

FIGURE 12-12.   **A.** *Early uveal infiltration in ocular lymphosarcoma has altered the color and contour of the temporal iris in this adult domestic Shorthair. A large fibrin clot occupies the nasal anterior chamber as well.* **B.** *In this 7-year-old domestic Shorthair with advanced ocular lymphosarcoma, swelling of the iris and posterior synechiae distort the shape of the pupil, and a fibrin clot obscures the iris surface. Serology results for feline leukemia virus were positive. (Reprinted with permission from Ketring KL, Glaze MB. Atlas of feline ophthalmology. Trenton, NJ: Veterinary Learning Systems, 1994.)*

IRIDAL DEGENERATIONS AND CYSTS

Degenerations and Acquired Cysts

Iridal degenerations occur in the cat less frequently than in the dog. In old cats, the iridal stroma may thin and thus permit partial transillumination with an intense light source. Iridal degenerations may be focal, and some color changes may be evident. The cause, however, is unknown. Iridal and ciliary cysts in the cat can also be acquired, and they usually are pigmented, transilluminate with an intense light source, and generally are attached to the posterior aspects of the pupillary margin. Iridal cysts may be confused with early melanomas. They readily transilluminate, however, and their surfaces are very smooth. Treatment usually is not necessary.

FELINE GLAUCOMA

The prevalence of glaucoma in the cat is less than in the dog, and most feline glaucomas appear to be secondary. **Several different types of glaucoma occur in the cat (Box 12-2), but those secondary to anterior uveitis are the most frequently presented.** The gonioscopic appearance of the normal feline iridocorneal angle and ciliary cleft reveals long, slender, and slightly branching pectinate ligaments that usually are the same color as the iris and a pigmented trabecular meshwork.

BOX 12-2

Types of the Glaucomas in the Cat

Primary glaucomas

  Open/normal angle, with and without collapsed cleft (Siamese breed)

  Narrow/closed angle (chronic)

Secondary glaucomas

  Uveitic (chronic anterior uveitis)

  Lens luxations (trauma/age)

  Phakolytic/phacoclastic uveitis (lens perforation)

  Hyphema (rare)

  Intraocular neoplasia (primary/secondary neoplasms)

Congenital glaucomas

  Secondary to outflow anomalies

Congenital glaucomas are rare, occur in kittens, can be either unilateral or bilateral, and may result from developmental abnormalities of the aqueous humor outflow pathways. Primary glaucomas also are rare, but the Siamese breed may be predisposed. Most glaucomas are secondary and associated with intraocular neoplasia, chronic anterior uveitides, and intraocular neoplasms. The feline uveitides that tend to become protracted (e.g., those with FIV or FeLV) are more apt to induce secondary glaucoma. The cause of the glaucoma appears to be secondary to the obstruction of aqueous humor outflow through the iridocorneal angle and the ciliary cleft by inflammatory cells, peripheral anterior synechiae, and collapse of the cleft. Concurrent involvement of the trabecular meshwork with chronic uveitis may also reduce outflow of the aqueous humor. At gonioscopy, the iridocorneal angle may be closed or appear to be unusually wide (because of angle recession and enlargement of the globe). The ciliary cleft is collapsed, however, and peripheral anterior synechiae may be scattered among some of the pectinate ligaments.

Another, less frequent cause of the secondary glaucomas is lens luxation. In one study, lens displacements were overly represented in the Siamese breed, age at presentation was 7 to 9 years, and male cats were disproportionately affected. Uveitis was the most frequent intraocular disease that was associated with lens displacement, which may have been indicative of concurrent zonulary disease in these eyes. Alternatively, the slight and early globe enlargement secondary to the onset of uveitic glaucoma also might contribute to zonulary disinsertion and lens instability. Lens luxations are common in cats with advanced glaucoma and buphthalmia, but determining the exact pathogenesis of the lens displacement is not possible.

Making the diagnosis of glaucoma in the cat is the same as in other animal species, but the clinical signs may be more subtle, especially with the chronic and the uveitic types. Buphthalmia, exposure keratitis with vascularization, and lens luxation (usually subluxation and anterior luxation) are common sequelae to chronic intraocular hypertension. Buphthalmia, however, is often overlooked, because the orbit and the eyelids effectively camouflage the enlarged globe.

Retinal degeneration is recognized ophthalmoscopically by vascular attenuation and tapetal hyperreflectivity. Because the small optic papilla of the cat normally lacks myelin, optic nerve cupping is often difficult to visualize. Even so, the atrophic optic nerve head is darker than normal in color.

The diagnosis of glaucoma is confirmed by elevated IOP as measured using applanation or Schiotz tonometry. Therapy for feline glaucoma generally follows the same guidelines as those in other species. The foremost consideration is to correct, if possible, the underlying cause. Glaucoma secondary to idiopathic uveitis sometimes is effectively treated using aggressive anti-inflammatory therapy with topical and subconjunctival corticosteroids (described earlier). These corticosteroids offer both benefits and limitations, however, because long-term topical dexamethasone can elevate the IOP in normal cats. If lens luxation or rupture is the cause, lens extraction is beneficial. Medical therapy with antihypertensive agents generally is indicated only when the underlying cause is correctable or manageable and there is a possibility of preserving vision. In contrast to the dog, the cat seems to tolerate antiglaucoma medical treatments

poorly, especially when they are administered systemically. When the IOP is greater than 50 mm Hg and accompanied by mydriasis, a hyperosmotic agent generally is indicated to lower the IOP and to preserve the optic nerve and retinal functions. **Useful topical medications include the lower concentrations of pilocarpine and epinephrine ophthalmic solutions (with some irritation), β-antagonists or β-blockers, and topical carbonic anhydrase inhibitors.** Clinical studies are lacking, but experimental data are indicative that β-blockers lower the production of aqueous humor in normal cats. Effectiveness of the new topical prostaglandins (e.g., prostaglandin $F_{2\alpha}$) for the feline glaucomas has not been reported. Surgical treatment has received little interest among veterinary ophthalmologists, probably because most feline glaucomas are associated with inflammations. (For more details, see Appendices A, G, J, and K.)

DISEASES OF THE LENS
AND CATARACT FORMATION

CONGENITAL CATARACTS
AND LENS ANOMALIES

Multiple ocular defects rarely occur in the cat, but all reported cases have included some form of lenticular abnormality. Microphakia has been described in a Siamese and a domestic Shorthair, and bilateral aphakia associated with retinal detachment has been described in a domestic Shorthair kitten. Congenital cataracts are uncommon, and affected breeds include the Persian, Birman, and the domestic Shorthair.

Primary and Secondary
Cataract Formation

Most feline cataracts are secondary, and in contrast to the dog, primary and inherited cataracts are rare in the cat. To date, all reported feline cataracts that have been presumed to be hereditary were present congenitally. Secondary cataracts may be divided into those associated with trauma, lens luxations, anterior uveitis, or glaucoma. Traumatic cataracts are relatively common in the cat and often are sequela to perforating ocular injury, particularly from cat claws. Traumatic cataracts tend to be unilateral, focal, and primarily in the region of the insult. They often are associated with focal posterior synechia as well. Traumatic cataracts generally are slowly progressive. When the rupture of the lens capsule is sufficiently large, lens proteins may escape, thereby causing severe uveitis. Cataracts also frequently occur as sequelae to lens luxation in the cat and appear as diffuse, subcapsular cortical opacities. The most common cause of secondary feline cataracts is anterior segment inflammation (especially the chronic types), and they are also associated with posterior synechiae, rubeosis iridis, periridal and pupillary inflammatory membranes, and slow progression (Fig. 12-13).

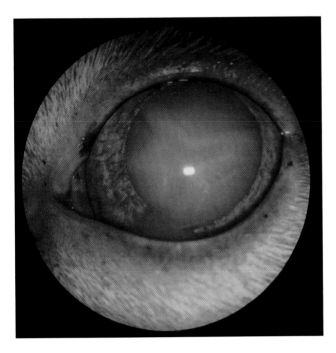

FIGURE 12-13. *Subtle iridal vascular congestion and a small fibrin clot are testaments to the chronic, low-grade anterior uveitis that preceded cataract development in this adult domestic Shorthair.*

Four types of metabolic/toxic cataracts have been reported in the cat:

1. Those that consist of diffuse anterior and posterior lens opacification as well as vacuolation of the posterior "Y"-sutures in kittens fed commercially available kitten milk replacer;
2. Diabetic cataracts, which are uncommon and appear as equatorial lens vacuoles;
3. Those related to nutritional secondary hyperparathyroidism and hypocalcemia, which appear as axial posterior subcapsular opacities; and
4. Those resulting from long-term topical treatment with 0.1% dexamethasone, which appear as subcapsular, presumably posterior opacities.

Lens Luxations

Feline lens luxations have been associated with trauma, chronic uveal inflammatory disease, and glaucoma (Fig. 12-14). The mechanism appears to be zonular damage. An apparently primary zonular degeneration may occur in aged felines, but no breed predilection exists to suggest any hereditary basis. As in other species, complications of lens luxation in the cat are direct corneal endothelial cell damage, secondary glaucoma, and persistent uveal inflammation. **Treatment involves intracapsular lens extraction using either a cryoprobe or lens loop, and the prognosis depends on both the duration and the underlying cause.** The prognosis in other types is less favorable, however, but lens luxation secondary to idiopathic uveitis can be successfully treated with surgery if appropriate therapy for the underlying uveitis is concurrently provided.

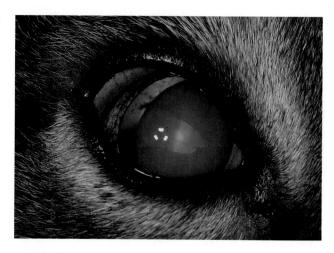

Cataract Surgery and Lensectomy

Feline cataract surgery is performed in a manner identical to that of canine cataract surgery, but reports of clinical operative series are not available in the literature. Extracapsular extraction and phacoemulsification are effective procedures (see Chapter 10). The success rate for cataract surgery in the cat appears to be better than that in the dog. The power of a prototype posterior chamber intraocular lens has been determined to be 53 to 55 diopters, which is substantially higher than that in the dog.

DISEASES OF THE POSTERIOR SEGMENT

The posterior segment includes the vitreous, the ocular fundus, and the optic nerve. As in other species, the ocular fundus in the cat is divided into the tapetal fundus, the nontapetal fundus, the optic nerve head or optic disc, and the retinal vasculature. **The feline vascular pattern is holangiotic, with three major pairs of cilioretinal arterioles and larger veins that emerge near the periphery of the optic nerve head. The tapetal fundus appears to be more consistent in the cat than in the dog, appearing as a highly reflective, usually yellow-green triangular area in the dorsal fundus.** Partial to complete lack of the tapetal fundus occasionally occurs in blue-eyed cats. The "area centralis," which has high cone concentrations, is located approximately 3-mm lateral to the optic nerve head. Conus or peripapillary hyperreflective areas as well as pigmented areas immediately adjacent to the optic disc are not uncommon. Usually, the nontapetal fundus is heavily pigmented, appearing as a brown-black area surrounding the tapetal fundus. In color-dilute cats, the nontapetal fundus is less pigmented focally or diffusely (i.e., tigroid nontapetal fundus), thereby allowing visualization of the deeper choroidal vasculature at ophthalmoscopy. The optic nerve head or optic disc usually is situated in the tapetal fundus; it is small, circular, nonmyelinated to permit visualization of the scleral lamina cribrosa, and somewhat gray. Occasionally, myelination of the nerve fiber layer may occur, either focally or diffusely, around the optic disc.

CONGENITAL AND DEVELOPMENTAL DISORDERS

Focal retinal and optic disc colobomas are rare in the cat, and they generally occur in association with the colobomatous syndrome in cats who are presented with eyelid agenesis. In some eyes, focal retinal dysplasia is also present, and vision may (or may not) be impaired. Both heredity and in utero infections have been suggested as causes.

Retinal dysplasia is loosely defined as anomalous retinal development with resultant aberrant organization of retinal elements to form rosettes, folds, and gliosis. **The causes of retinal dysplasia are numerous, but in the cat, the condition is typified by having only been described as resulting from intrauterine or early neonatal intraocular viral infection.** When injected intraocularly or systemically (i.e., intraperitoneally) into fetal or neonatal kittens, FeLV produces a syndrome of retinal dysplasia that is characterized by disorganization and necrosis of the retinal tissue, with reorganization into cell clumps and dysplastic rosette structures. Impaired development of retinal, cerebral, and cerebellar tissues has been associated with perinatal feline panleukopenia infection, and bilateral optic nerve aplasia has been described in a Longhair kitten.

NUTRITIONAL RETINAL DEGENERATION (TAURINE DEFICIENCY)

Taurine is a sulfur-containing amino acid that is essential to the cat, because this species has a limited ability to synthesize it from cysteine, which is a precursor amino acid in most animal species. A dietary taurine level of 500 to 750 ppm has been suggested as being necessary to prevent retinal disease. Nutritional retinal degeneration and feline central retinal degeneration appear to be identical and associated with inadequate levels of dietary taurine. As a result of these studies, commercial feline diets now contain sufficient levels of dietary taurine, and the disease is rarely encountered. **The ophthalmoscopic appearance of taurine deficiency retinopathy is considered to be pathognomonic, especially during its early stages. The earliest lesion consists of an increased granularity in the area centralis (Fig. 12-15) that progresses to an ellipsoidal, hyperreflective lesion. A second hyperreflective lesion then becomes visible nasal to the optic papilla, and the two lesions eventually coalesce to form a large, band-shaped area of hyperreflectivity dorsal to the optic papilla. The end stage is a generalized retinal degeneration with attenuation or loss of retinal vessels.** Because taurine deficiency has been linked with feline cardiomyopathy, cardiac function should be evaluated in all cats with these ophthalmoscopic abnormalities. (For more details, the reader should consult the third edition, pp. 1035–1036.)

FIGURE 12-15. *Stage 2 of taurine deficiency retinopathy is character-ized by an elliptical, hyperreflective lesion temporal to the optic disc. (Reprinted with permission from Ketring KL, Glaze MB. Atlas of feline ophthalmology. Trenton, NJ: Veterinary Learning Systems, 1994.)*

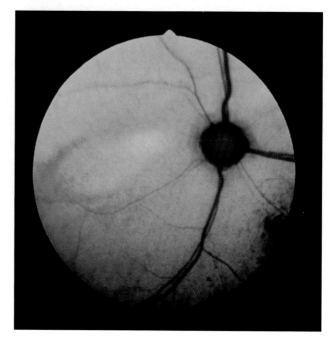

INHERITED CONE-ROD DYSPLASIA AND DEGENERATIONS

Except for those disorders with a nutritional basis, retinal degenerations are relatively rare in the cat, as evidenced by the infrequent reports in the literature. Photoreceptor degeneration, which is characterized ophthalmo-scopically by tapetal hyperreflectivity and vascular attenuation, was de-scribed in several related Persian cats. The mode of inheritance in this re-port was suspected to be autosomal recessive.

Rod-Cone Dysplasia in the Abyssinian

An autosomal dominant rod-cone dysplasia has been described in the Abyssinian breed. Affected kittens as young as 4 weeks may show my-driasis and nystagmus, which is variable, intermittent, and often rapid. At ophthalmoscopy, the first lesions consist of dullness and loss of de-tail in the tapetal fundus, and they occur in kittens by 8 to 12 weeks of age. Progression of the disease is fairly rapid and manifests by tapetal fundus hyperreflectivity, loss of pigmentation in the nontapetal fundus, and retinal vascular attenuation. The disease is very advanced by 1 year of age. Secondary cataracts have not been observed.

Rod-Cone Degeneration in the Abyssinian

The second form of feline progressive retinal degeneration also affects the Abyssinian breed. This disease does not begin until 1.5 to 2.0 years of age, but then progresses to complete degeneration during the next

2 to 4 years. There is no predilection for either sex, and the mode of inheritance is autosomal recessive. Ophthalmoscopic changes include (in order):

1. A subtle, gray discoloration of the peripapillary area on one or both sides of the optic disc;
2. A more diffuse, gray tapetal discoloration that usually is associated with mild vascular attenuation;
3. The development of hyperreflective areas in a diffusely discolored tapetal fundus with prominent vascular attenuation; and
4. A generalized hyperreflectivity with severely attenuated or absent retinal vessels.

OTHER RETINAL DEGENERATIONS

An isolated case of retinal degeneration has been described that has similarities to the rare human condition of gyrate atrophy. Concurrent administration of methylnitrosourea and ketamine hydrochloride also causes severe retinal degeneration in the cat.

INFLAMMATIONS

Chorioretinitis refers to inflammatory conditions that arise in the choroid and extend into the retina. Retinochoroiditis refers to inflammations that originate in the retina and, eventually, involve the choroid. **Active retinal inflammations are characterized ophthalmoscopically by edema, hemorrhages, inflammatory or neoplastic infiltrates, mycotic and parasitic granulomas, and exudates that both decrease the neurosensory retinal transparency and obstruct the intraretinal blood vessels and underlying retinal pigment epithelium in the nontapetal fundus as well as the tapetal reflection in the tapetal fundus. At ophthalmoscopy, chronic or previous retinitis appears as areas of hyperreflectivity, with or without pigment deposition in the tapetal fundus and areas of increased or decreased pigment in the nontapetal fundus.** Chorioretinitis in the cat has been associated with viruses (e.g., FIP, FIV, FeLV); bacteremias associated with dental diseases, tuberculosis, and other systemic diseases; fungal diseases such as cryptococcosis, histoplasmosis, blastomycosis, coccidioidomycosis, and candidiasis; and parasitic infections such as toxoplasmosis and dipteran larvae. (For more details, see the discussion of anterior uveal inflammations in this chapter and Chapter 17.)

HYPERTENSIVE RETINOPATHY

Hypertensive retinopathy has become a common disease among older cats with acute loss of vision. Because most cats are presented for the loss of vision, ophthalmologists are often the first clinicians to encounter this disease. The condition occurs most commonly in cats older than 10 years of age and with a typical presenting complaint of acute vision loss. Ophthalmic examination reveals hyphema, glaucoma secondary to hyphema, intravitreal hemorrhage, retinal

vascular tortuosity, sub- and intraretinal hemorrhages, and varying degrees of retinal detachment (Fig. 12-16). The probable mechanism of the retinal disease is precapillary vasoconstriction of the retinal arterioles, which leads to vascular smooth muscle necrosis, vascular dilatation and leakage, and perhaps, similar events affecting the choroidal vessels. Serous retinal detachments occur secondarily.

Systolic arterial blood pressure in cats with hypertensive retinal disease typically is greater than 160 mm Hg. Other frequent abnormalities include elevated blood urea nitrogen and creatine levels. Affected animals may also have cardiomegaly and left ventricular hypertrophy. The cause-and-effect relationship of these abnormalities, however, remains uncertain. Both cardiac and renal abnormalities may occur secondary to prolonged hypertension; conversely, primary renal disease may cause hypertension through disturbance of the renin-angiotensin regulatory system. Other concurrent abnormalities may include hyperthyroidism and hyperglycemia after the administration of megestrol acetate. High-salt diets have also been reported among affected cats.

Prompt resolution of the retinal detachments associated with feline hypertensive retinopathy by lowering the systemic blood pressure are critical to preserve as much retinal function as possible and to increase the probability for return of vision. Treatment of feline systemic hypertension has markedly improved with the introduction of more effective drugs and the calcium channel blocker amlodipine (0.625 mg/once daily,

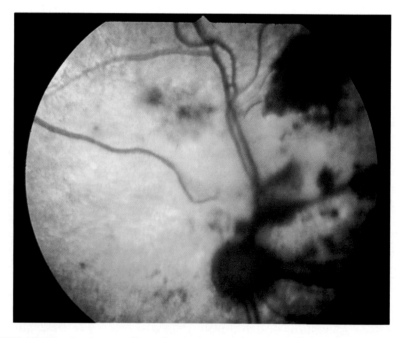

FIGURE 12-16. *Ocular manifestations of systemic hypertension in an aged domestic Shorthair. Note the intraretinal and preretinal hemorrhages as well as the focal retinal detachment immediately above the optic disk.*

sometimes administered in a vitamin solution (see question list). This therapy effectively lowers the blood pressure, and the rate of retinal reattachment sufficient for the return of at least some clinical vision is 50% or greater.

LIPEMIA RETINALIS

The term *lipemia retinalis* describes the presence of lipids or lipoproteins (or both) in the retinal blood vessels at ophthalmoscopy. Like the dog, the cat may also be affected. The condition is of diagnostic significance only, because an elevated blood lipid level has not been demonstrated to affect retinal tissue adversely. The condition has been experimentally induced in neonatal kittens using parenteral administration of large doses of methylprednisolone. Lipemia retinalis also occurs in the cat secondary to primary, familial hypercholesterolemia.

ANEMIC RETINOPATHY

The cat also demonstrates an anemic retinopathy that manifests by coexistent anemia and retinal hemorrhages. Hemorrhages occur at all depths in the retina and with equal frequency in both the tapetal and the nontapetal fundus. The mechanism of retinal hemorrhage formation is thought to be anemia-induced hypoxia of the retinal vessels, which is followed by compensatory venule dilation to maintain retinal perfusion and then a subsequent increase in capillary fragility, which ultimately leads to hemorrhage. Anemic retinopathy occurs in a high percentage of cats with hemoglobin levels of less than 5 g/dL, and the condition is aggravated by concurrent thrombocytopenia, which most commonly is attributable to infection with FeLV.

DIABETIC RETINOPATHY

Retinal manifestations of diabetes mellitus are considered to be rare in animals, but a case of presumed diabetic retinopathy has been described in a 10-year-old cat. Both retinal and vitreal hemorrhages as well as retinal detachments were the prominent changes at ophthalmoscopy, and microaneurysms were present as well.

HYPERVISCOSITY RETINOPATHY

The retina of the domestic cat is sensitive to the effects of increased serum hyperviscosity, but the prevalence of such diseases appears to be low. Ocular changes have been described in a cat with serum hyperviscosity syndrome caused by an IgG-secreting myeloma. In that report, the ophthalmoscopic changes were retinal hemorrhages, optic disc swelling, and partial retinal detachment. Serum hyperproteinemia (i.e., 14 g/dL) was attributable to a significant increase in the gamma globulin fraction. The ophthalmologic manifestations of serum hyperviscosity are ascribed to a decrease in the retinal blood flow, thus causing secondary hypoxic damage to the retinal capillaries.

OPHTHALMOMYIASIS INTERNA POSTERIOR

Ophthalmomyiasis interna involves the intraocular migration of parasites, and the term *posterior* indicates that the posterior segment is involved. Affected cats are usually asymptomatic. Ophthalmoscopic examination reveals multiple, criss-crossing, curvilinear tracks in the sensory retina. The tracks are of uniform width, have distinct margins, and occur in both the tapetal and the nontapetal fundus. Tapetal hyperreflectivity with foci of pigment deposition typify the tapetal lesions, whereas those in the nontapetal fundus demonstrate pigment loss and clumping. Retinal hemorrhage and edema have been interpreted as indicative of recent migration. The actual parasite may (or may not) be seen at ophthalmoscopy. No larvae from feline cases of ophthalmomyiasis interna posterior have been recovered for speciation, but their clinical appearance is suggestive of the order Diptera, which includes the parasites thought to cause most human cases. If active signs of inflammation are absent, no treatment is indicated; otherwise, systemic corticosteroids may be beneficial. Surgical intervention (either parasite extraction or laser coagulation) also may be attempted, but the parasite should not be killed within in the posterior segment.

RETINAL FOLDS AND DETACHMENTS

Retinal folds occur as congenital lesions but are also recognized in the cat as being secondary to other ocular diseases. **Retinal detachments or separation of the sensory and epithelial retina of the cat has been described in association with many ophthalmic and systemic abnormalities, including hypertension, hyperviscosity syndromes, periarteritis nodosa, toxoplasmosis, trauma, cryptococcosis, blastomycosis, histoplasmosis, coccidiomycosis, FIP, ethylene glycol toxicosis, polycythemia, and primary as well as secondary intraocular neoplasms.** The specific pathologic mechanisms of detachment appear to be similar to those in other animal species.

POSTERIOR SEGMENT NEOPLASIA

An astrocytoma of retinal origin has been described in one cat. The presenting signs were leukocoria and a vascularized mass visible within the pupil. Histopathologically, the tumor infiltrated the optic nerve head, choroid, and vitreous humor.

LYSOSOMAL STORAGE DISEASES

Storage disorders are a group of progressive, inherited diseases caused by the deficiency of a specific lysosomal enzyme. Such disease ultimately results from abnormal accumulation of the deficient enzyme's substrate within the lysosomes of affected cells. Lysosomal storage diseases that have been reported to have ophthalmic manifestations are mucopolysaccharidosis I and IV, GM_1- and GM_2-gangliosidosis, and mannosidosis. (For more details the reader should consult Table 29.5 in the third edition, p. 1044.)

Equine Ophthalmology

WHAT DOES THE HORSE "SEE"?

The horse has a total visual field nearly 350° when its head is pointed forward, with only a small blind spot near its tail. A small, frontal binocular field of 65° to 70° develops postnatally. Large uniocular fields of 146° result in a total visual field of approximately 215° per eye. The nasal extension of the retina, the lateral position of the orbits, and the horizontal shape of the pupil allow this increased peripheral vision to exist. The peripheral vision of the horse is more an adaptation to detect motion, but horses can also use monocular depth cues in judging distance. A horse viewing an object at a distance of 20 feet has, approximately, the visual acuity of a person viewing the object at 33 feet, or 20/33 vision (21.2 cpd). The horse has 0.6 times the acuity of humans, 1.5 times that of the dog, and 3.0 times that of the cat. The fibrous tapetum of the dorsal fundus is an adaptation for night vision. Despite the retinal photoreceptors in the horse being primarily rods, and despite yellow pigment in the lens that severely limits the transmittance of short-wavelength light, the horse is believed to be dichromatic, with the ability to detect the colors red and blue but not the colors yellow and green. The horse has a weak dynamic accommodative ability of the lens, but only small changes in refraction (≈2.0 diopters [D]) are necessary to maintain a focused image on the retina. Changes in head orientation, dynamic accommodation, and the equine retinal "area centralis" also aid in near vision.

EXAMINATION OF THE EQUINE EYE

Adequate restraint of the animal is important when evaluating the equine eye. **Topically applied anesthetics, supraorbital sensory and**   337

auriculopalpebral motor nerve blocks, a nose or ear twitch, and intravenous sedation all facilitate examination of the injured equine eye, and the fluorescein dye test should be an integral part of every ocular examination in the horse as well. A focal light source (e.g., a transilluminator) and a direct ophthalmoscope are essential pieces of equipment for such examinations.

OCULAR PROBLEMS IN THE EQUINE NEONATE

Ocular disorders of the equine neonate may be congenital, inherited, or acquired. **Normal embryogenesis of the foal eye results in a fully developed globe and adnexa at birth; low tear secretion, a round pupil, reduced corneal sensitivity, lack of menace reflex during the first 2 weeks postpartum, and lagophthalmos may be found in neonates. Hyaloid artery remnants in foals may contain blood for several hours after birth, but these generally disappear by 3 to 4 months of age.** Lens "Y" sutures are often prominent in foals and should not be mistaken for a cataract.

MICROPHTHALMOS

Microphthalmos (i.e., a congenitally small globe) is common in foals and may be unilateral or bilateral. It may be spontaneous and idiopathic, or it may be secondary to uterine infection or drug toxicity. **Thoroughbreds appear to have an increased risk.** Microphthalmos can be an isolated finding or associated with other ocular abnormalities (e.g., cataracts, retinal dysplasia). **The microphthalmic eyes of most foals are blind, and a small palpebral fissure and prominence of the nictitans may be noted in affected foals (Fig. 13-1).** Entropion may be caused by a lack of support from the small globe and be associated with mild to severe ulcerative keratitis. Corneal ulceration resulting from entropion and microphthalmia may necessitate entropion repair or even enucleation of nonvisual globes. As the foal ages, the bony orbit and skull containing the microphthalmic globe may become malformed as well.

ORBIT

Development of the bony equine orbit is influenced by development of the globe. **Facial asymmetry because of an underdeveloped bony orbit can be associated with congenital microphthalmia or with phthisis bulbi resulting from severe globe trauma in a young foal.** Fractures of the orbit caused by trauma from kicks or accidents may require surgical correction in foals.

STRABISMUS

Strabismus refers to a deviation of the globe from its normal position. In the neonatal foal, the horizontal axis of the pupil and the globe deviates slightly

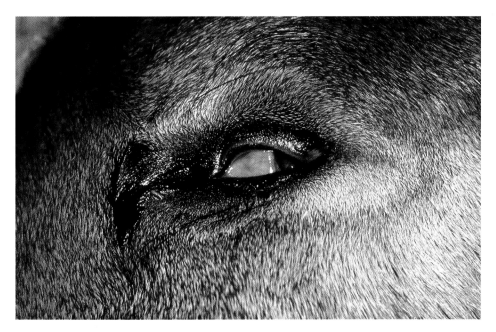

FIGURE 13-1. *Protrusion of the nictitans in a microphthalmic Thoroughbred foal.*

medially and ventrally, with the eye reaching a normal adult position by 1 month of age. **Congenital strabismus (i.e., hyperopia) and dorsomedial strabismus have been reported in Appaloosa foals and may be associated with equine congenital stationary night blindness.** Esotropia has been reported in the mule, with an incidence of 0.5%. Surgical correction of strabismus by rectus muscle transposition has been reported in horses.

BLEPHARITIS

Alopecia, excoriation, and depigmentation are associated with fly-bite blepharitis in foals. Fly repellants containing pyrethrins may be applied frequently, or slow-release insecticide strips can be attached to the mane or halter. Fenthion, 1 mL of 20% solution per 50 kg of body weight to a maximum of 10 mL per horse, is a safe and effective fly repellant when applied to the hair. Dermatophytosis, dermatophilus, and staphylococcal folliculitis can affect the eyelids of foals as well, and juvenile Arabian leukoderma (or "pinky" syndrome) is a cutaneous condition involving depigmentation that affects Arabian horses from 6 to 24 months of age. Lesions may undergo cyclic depigmentation and repigmentation, and the condition may be inherited.

ENTROPION

Inversion of the lower or the upper eyelid may occur in foals as a primary anatomic condition or secondary to microphthalmia, dehydration, malnutrition, prematurity/dysmaturity, eyelid trauma, or cicatricial formation after eyelid trauma. Ocular pain may exacerbate the degree of anatomic entropion. **The entropion may cause increased lacrimation, blepharospasm, conjunctivitis, or corneal ulceration. Temporary**

treatment in young foals includes eversion of the eyelid with temporary, nonabsorbable sutures in a vertical mattress pattern (4-0 silk); eversion with surgical staples; or injection of a subcutaneous bleb of procaine penicillin adjacent to the entropic region. Permanent reconstructive entropion surgeries should be reserved for larger, older foals.

EYELID TRAUMA

Traumatic eyelid lacerations and forehead trauma can also occur in foals. Upper eyelid lesions are more serious than lower eyelid injuries, however, because upper eyelid movement distributes tear film and, thus, prevents exposure keratitis. Excision of the lacerated pedicles of eyelid marginal tissue should be avoided. Wounds should be gently cleansed with 1:50 povidone-iodine solution, and systemic antibiotics should be administered. Two-layer closure of skin–orbicularis muscle and the tarsoconjunctival layers is recommended. Surgical repair of the upper eyelid is imperative.

DERMOIDS

Dermoids (i.e., choristomas) of the eyelids, nictitans, cornea, and conjunctiva have been reported in foals. Corneal and conjunctival dermoids may appear to be aberrant pigmentation when associated with a lack of hair follicle development. Treatment depends on location. Superficial to deep keratectomy is indicated for corneal dermoids, and blepharoplasty for eyelid dermoids, to remove the dermoids before the hairs can grow, thereby causing ocular irritation.

NASOLACRIMAL SYSTEM ATRESIA

Agenesis of the distal nasolacrimal duct occurs occasionally in foals. The clinical signs are a unilateral or bilateral, chronic mucoid and, eventually, mucopurulent ocular discharge in a young horse. The discharge is often copious, because a dacryocystitis generally develops. Contrast dacryocystorhinography using 4 to 6 mL of radiopaque solution may be necessary to confirm the diagnosis. Atresia of the nasal puncta may be presumed, however, by noting the lack of a distal opening to the nasolacrimal duct within the nares at the mucocutaneous junction, failure of the irrigating solution to exit the nasal puncta during flushing of the proximal nasolacrimal system through the palpebral lacrimal puncta, and distention of the nasal vestibular floor in response to irrigation. Once the atretic site has been identified, a cutdown through the eyelid conjunctiva or nasal mucosa will establish patency. A stent of polyethylene tubing or silicone will also need to be placed in the nasolacrimal system for several weeks to allow for epithelialization of the new duct and puncta and for resolution of the dacryocystitis.

HETEROCHROMIA IRIDIS

Heterochromia iridis is a variation in the normal, dark-brown iridal color. It may be a combination of white and blue iridal color with brown corpora nigra (i.e., "wall eye") or a white iridal color with brown corpora nigra (i.e., "china eye"). Heterochromia iridis is common to the Appaloosa as well as to palomino, chestnut, gray, spotted, and white horses.

IRIDAL ABNORMALITIES

Aniridia (i.e., complete absence of the iris) has been reported with congenital cataracts in Thoroughbreds and alone in Quarter horses and Belgians. Aniridia in foals is usually bilateral and associated with a pupil so dilated that the lens equator and the ciliary processes become visible. Photophobia and blepharospasm may be present as well. Iridal hypoplasia and iridal as well as ciliary body cysts may mimic one another. **Hypoplasia of the corpora nigra and iris associated with macrocornea, ciliary cysts, and cataract as well as lens luxation occur in the Rocky Mountain horse. Large corpora nigra and iridal cysts may be successfully deflated with transcorneal neodymium:yttrium-aluminum-garnet (Nd:YAG) laser treatment.**

Remnants of the anterior tunica vasculosa lentis, or persistent pupillary membranes, are rare in foals. These membranes generally regress during the first 6 to 12 months of life, and they require no treatment.

THE LENS

Lens sutures are apparent in many foals and may gradually disappear during the first year of life. The anterior suture has a "Y" configuration, with the posterior suture varying in shape from "Y," sawhorse, to stellate patterns. **Cataracts are a frequent congenital ocular defect in foals, and most are bilateral. Heritable, traumatic, nutritional, and postinflammatory causes have been proposed, and a dominant mode of inheritance has been reported in Belgian as well as in Thoroughbred horses. Morgan horses have nonprogressive, nuclear, and bilaterally symmetrical cataracts that do not seriously interfere with vision. Cataracts and lens luxation are associated with anterior segment dysgenesis in the Rocky Mountain horse.** Healthy foals with cataracts, visual impairment, the personality to tolerate administration of topical therapy, and without uveitis are candidates for cataract surgery. The preoperative evaluation for these foals is identical to that in small animals, and it includes ocular ultrasonography and electroretinography. **The most common technique for removing congenital cataracts in foals is phacoemulsification, which has a reported success rate of nearly 80%. Aphakic foals should be quite farsighted postoperatively, but the amount of vision after successful cataract surgery both in adult horses and in foals is functionally normal.**

CONJUNCTIVITIS AND SUBCONJUNCTIVAL HEMORRHAGE

Conjunctivitis resulting from environmental irritants (e.g., hay, sand, dirt, ammonia) is common among neonates, with recumbent foals being especially at risk. Conjunctival inflammation secondary to pneumonia

usually occurs among older foals (age, 1–6 months). Causative agents include adenovirus, equine herpesvirus (EHV)-1, equine viral arteritis, influenza virus, *Streptococcus equi* subspecies *equi* (strangles), *Rhodococcus* sp., and *Actinobacillus* sp. Therapy begins by flushing the conjunctival sacs to remove any underlying irritant. Patency of the nasolacrimal duct should then be established, because duct obstructions can exacerbate conjunctivitis. **Broad-spectrum antibiotic ophthalmic ointments or eye lubricants are used as indicated, and if no corneal ulcer is present, corticosteroid ophthalmic preparations are useful.**

Subconjunctival or episcleral hemorrhages can result from birth trauma; however, these generally resolve in 7 to 10 days and require no treatment. Traumatic hemorrhages usually are quite large and must be differentiated from the petechial or ecchymotic hemorrhages that are suggestive of a coagulation disorder. Scleral hemorrhages also are associated with neonatal maladjustment syndrome in foals.

SUPERFICIAL CORNEAL OPACITIES

Superficial, irregular epithelial opacities may be found in one or both eyes among Thoroughbred foals. They do not appear to be painful, and they resolve with age.

CORNEAL ULCERS IN FOALS

Corneal ulceration in foals requires early clinical diagnosis, laboratory confirmation, and appropriate medical as well as surgical therapy. Both bacterial and fungal keratitis may present with a mild, early clinical course. They require prompt therapy, however, to avoid serious ocular complications (for more details, the reader should consult the third edition, pp. 1058–1060).

IRIDOCYCLITIS IN NEONATES

Systemic disease can cause blinding iridocyclitis in foals; therefore, the cause must be diagnosed early and treated aggressively. The iridocyclitis may be immune mediated, with sterile hypopyon, or result from direct invasion of an organism that creates an infectious endophthalmitis. Organisms associated with equine anterior uveitis include *Salmonella* sp., *Rhodococcus equi*, *Escherichia coli*, *Streptococcus equi* subspecies *equi*, *Actinobacillus equuli*, adenovirus, and equine viral arteritis.

Lacrimation, blepharospasm, and photophobia can occur in eyes with iridocyclitis or anterior uveitis. Corneal edema, conjunctival hyperemia, ciliary injection, aqueous flare, hyphema, fibrin, and hypopyon are also observed in eyes with iridocyclitis. Miosis usually is a prominent sign in cases of anterior uveitis, and it can result in a misshapen pupil as well as in anterior and posterior synechiae. Fibrin and pigment deposition on the anterior lens capsule as well as cataract formation are sequelae to anterior uveitis in foals.

The major goals when treating foals with anterior uveitis are to preserve vision and to decrease pain. A fluorescein dye test should be employed immediately to differentiate a painful eye with anterior uveitis resulting from ulcerative keratitis from an eye with anterior uveitis and no corneal ulcer or abscess. Corticosteroids are the treatment of choice for anterior uveitis, but they can lead to rapid demise of an eye that also has a corneal ulcer. **Treatment includes systemic antibiotics and nonsteroidal anti-inflammatory drugs (NSAIDs) as well as topically administered mydriatic/cycloplegics, antibiotics, and corticosteroids (see Appendixes D, F, H, I, and L). Anti-inflammatory medications, specifically corticosteroids and NSAIDs, are used to control the intense intraocular inflammation, which can lead to blindness. The medications are administered every 1 to 6 hours, depending on the severity of the disease, and then tapered as the problem resolves.** Mydriatics/cycloplegics effectively stabilize the blood–aqueous barrier. Relaxation of the ciliary muscles also eliminates ciliary spasm, which is a major factor causing ocular discomfort. Pupillary dilatation protects the visual axis from occlusion and minimizes the development of synechiae. Atropine can last several days in the normal eye but only a few hours in the inflamed foal eye. Gut motility should be monitored when using ocular atropine as well; if the motility decreases during treatment, atropine should be discontinued before a hypomotile colic develops. Shorter-acting mydriatics such as tropicamide can be used if necessary. Use of broad-spectrum antibiotics (e.g., chloramphenicol) with good corneal penetration is advised for the prophylaxis and treatment of infections in the anterior chamber. Depending on the cause, the overall prognosis of the animal with anterior uveitis is usually guarded. The owner should be educated immediately about the potentially severe nature of this disease and the possibility for loss of vision.

EQUINE NEONATAL GLAUCOMA

Congenital glaucoma has been reported in foals and been associated with developmental anomalies of the iridocorneal angle (i.e., goniodysgenesis). **No particular predisposition regarding breed has been reported for glaucoma among equine neonates. The clinical signs of early glaucoma include generalized corneal edema, deep linear corneal band opacities, lens luxations, optic nerve cupping, as well as a fixed and dilated pupil. The linear corneal band opacities are a consistent feature of equine glaucoma, and histopathologically, they represent thin areas of Descemet's membrane. Buphthalmia will occur if the intraocular pressure (IOP) remains elevated. Therapy for equine neonatal glaucoma aims to preserve vision and to minimize discomfort. Glaucoma can be treated medically, but surgical therapy may be best for goniodysgenic foals. Medical treatment is directed at decreasing the IOP by reducing the production of aqueous humor or, more importantly, by increasing its outflow.** Surgical therapy for equine glaucoma is directed at reducing the production of aqueous humor by damaging the ciliary body using nitrous oxide (i.e., cyclocryotherapy) or laser energy (i.e., cyclophotocoagulation). Chronically painful and blind, buphthalmic globes should be enucleated or implanted with an intrascleral prosthesis.

DISEASES OF THE RETINA/OPTIC NERVE IN EQUINE NEONATES

Congenital abnormalities of the equine neonatal fundus that affect vision are uncommon. Variations of the normal equine neonatal fundus

are numerous, however, and relate primarily to coat color. Color-dilute neonates may have light-yellow zones of tapetal color with red "Stars of Winslow." White horses may have an entire tapetal region that appears yellow.

Neonatal maladjustment syndrome is commonly associated with ocular abnormalities. These lesions include small and round retinal hemorrhages, hemorrhages on the optic disc, pupil asymmetry, corneal edema, and ulcerative keratitis. Hemorrhages associated with neonatal maladjustment syndrome disappear in several days—if the foal survives.

Retinal dysplasia in foals is generally bilateral, is not heritable, and is often associated with other congenital ocular problems. Retinal dysplasia can appear clinically as either single or multiple, linear or geographic regions. Retinal detachments may be either unilateral or bilateral and can be observed through the dilated pupil as a floating veil of opaque tissue in the vitreous. If the detachment is bilateral, the foal will be blind since birth and also may have nystagmus. Congenital, inflammatory, and traumatic causes have been reported.

Congenital stationary night blindness of Appaloosas and Quarter horses has been reported in the United States. In these horses, the fundus appears to be normal, with characteristic, a-wave–dominant electroretinographic patterns serving to confirm the diagnosis. A defect in neural transmission between the photoreceptor layers and the bipolar cells is suspected. Vision is severely diminished at reduced light levels, with day blindness also being reported (though infrequently). Microphthalmia, strabismus, and nystagmus may be present as well. The mode of transmission is thought to be recessive or sex-linked recessive, with the defect occurring on the X chromosome.

The diagnoses of optic nerve hypoplasia and optic nerve atrophy are established on the basis of direct ophthalmoscopic results in foals and may occur secondary to developmental or inflammatory processes. Foals with optic nerve hypoplasia display smaller-than-normal discs, have slow pupillary light reflexes, and may retain some vision (depending on the degree of hypoplasia). (For more details, the reader should consult the third edition, pp. 1063–1064.)

EQUINE ORBIT

The adult equine orbit is 62.1 mm in width, 59.4 mm in height, and 98.3 mm in depth. The globe diameter is larger in the horizontal (48.4 mm) than in the vertical (47.6 mm), and the mean anterior-to-posterior diameter is 43.7 mm. The volume ranges from 45.0 to 50.9 mL. Orbital disease processes can occur within the extraocular muscle cone (i.e., intraconal), between the muscle cone and the periorbital sheath, or external to the periorbital sheath (i.e., subperiosteal). **Infectious, traumatic, inflammatory, or neoplastic disease processes involving the eyelids, paranasal sinuses, tooth roots, guttural pouch, or nasal cavity may extend into the orbit, thereby causing exophthalmus or strabismus (or both). Fractured walls of the para-**

nasal sinuses can result in orbital emphysema, and tooth-root abscesses may produce sinus and orbital disease. As in small animals, equine orbital disease processes can result in exophthalmos because of space-occupying orbital lesions or enophthalmos if the volume of the orbital contents decreases through malnutrition or pathology. Orbital diseases may be diagnosed using several procedures (Table 13-1).

SURGICAL TECHNIQUES

Enucleation (i.e., surgical removal of the globe, conjunctiva, and nictitating membrane) is the most frequently performed orbital surgical procedure in the horse. It is indicated for severe corneal infection and endophthalmitis, corneal or adnexal neoplasia, orbital neoplasia, or severe ocular trauma causing a painful, blind eye. The transpalpebral technique is most useful in cases of severe corneal infection or of conjunctival, nictitating membrane, or corneal neoplasia, but it does leave a larger orbital soft-tissue defect than occurs with the subconjunctival technique (see Chapter 2).

Orbital exenteration is a surgical technique to remove malignant tumors of the orbit that are unresponsive to chemotherapy or radiation therapy (or both). In this procedure, the entire orbital contents, including the periorbita, are surgically removed. The intrascleral prosthesis (or intraocular silicone prosthesis) has been used in the horse as a cosmetic alternative to enucleation. The prosthesis replaces the intraocular

TABLE 13-1	
DIAGNOSTIC PROCEDURES FOR DISEASES OF THE EQUINE ORBIT	
Technique	*Indications/Limitations*
Radiography	Increased soft-tissue densities and lytic bone changes are associated with neoplasia and chronic inflammatory diseases, and soft-tissue calcification can occur in orbital cellulitis. Special contrast-enhancement procedures may be worthwhile.
CT and MR imaging	Limited access. Size of the animal is important (foals, ponies, and small horses). Aspiration of fluid. Usually requires anesthesia; provides guidance culture, cytology, and histopathology or biopsy.
Ultrasonography	Noninvasive, painless procedure that can both qualitatively and quantitatively evaluate various ocular and orbital abnormalities. Helps in the differentiation of solid, soft-tissue masses versus cystic orbital masses; determination of the size of various globe or orbital components; and localization of many types of foreign bodies.

CT, computed tomography; *MR,* magnetic resonance.

contents, which are removed by evisceration. Implants with a diameter of 38 to 44 mm are recommended for adult horses, but they should not be placed in eyes with severe corneal disease, intraocular neoplasia, or infectious panophthalmitis.

Orbitotomy is indicated when the orbital conditions are unresponsive to medical therapy or the cause of the disease cannot be ascertained (or both). Orbital exploration is indicated for the biopsy or excision of orbital masses, drainage of infectious processes, and retrieval of foreign bodies. Orbital surgery also may be necessary in the horse to repair periorbital fractures.

ORBITAL DISEASES

Inflammatory, infectious, and neoplastic diseases of the sinuses and the guttural pouch, teeth problems, foreign bodies, and trauma can result in orbital cellulitis or abscess formation (or both). **Orbital cellulitis manifests as blepharoedema, swelling of the supraorbital fossa, exophthalmos, orbital pain, epiphora, and nictitans protrusion, and it can quickly damage the globe and the optic nerve. Topical and systemically administered broad-spectrum antibiotics are indicated.**

ORBITAL TRAUMA

Even though the complete bony orbital rim of the horse protects against traumatic globe proptosis, this problem still occasionally occurs after orbital injuries. The proptosed globe should be evaluated for integrity, hyphema, pupil size, corneal dessication, and ocular venostasis resulting from eyelid entrapment of the globe. Miosis with severe hypotony and hyphema is indicative of severe trauma as well as of poor prognosis for a viable globe. Corneal ulcers and keratomalacia can be minor or severe. The equine eye tolerates little disruption of its intraocular blood supply, and severe intraocular hemorrhage usually results in phthisis bulbi. The proptosed globe should be replaced into the orbit with the horse under general anesthesia. A temporary tarsorrhaphy will protect the cornea, and topically applied antibiotics and atropine as well as systemically administered NSAIDs and antibiotics will decrease the swelling and also minimize the risk of infection.

Fractures of the orbital bones can manifest through asymmetry of the globes or face, epistaxis, exophthalmos, proptosis, eyelid and conjunctival swelling, depression or concavity of the periorbital region, crepitus, and sometimes, pain on periorbital palpation. Damage to the intraosseous nasolacrimal duct, globe, optic nerve, paranasal sinuses, or some combination of these can also occur. All cases of suspected orbital fractures should be examined and evaluated using radiography. Ophthalmic complications include corneal ulcers, iridocyclitis, entrapment of the globe by bone fragments, and blindness. Periorbital fractures should be repaired quickly, because fibrous union of the fractured pieces begins within 1 week of the injury, thus making elevation and realignment difficult. Minor orbital rim fractures may not require surgical correction unless fracture fragments are impinging on the globe or perfect cosmesis is required.

Horses may injure the orbital region on the race track, in trailers or pastures, by rearing and hitting stall ceilings or starting gates, from gunshots or kicks from other horses, or when being disciplined. Orbital fractures, panophthalmitis, and orbital cellulitis as well as abscesses can result from orbital trauma. Pain, fever, blepharoedema, swelling of the supraorbital fossa, nictitating membrane protrusion, corneal edema, and chemosis can occur as well. In addition, severe intraocular trauma can result from penetrating wounds or blunt trauma. As mentioned, the equine globe does not tolerate much intraocular hemorrhage and, in many cases, will develop phthisis bulbi if this occurs. The treatment for panophthalmitis or a severely damaged globe is enucleation. In several traumatized globes, the enucleation should be performed without undue delay, because bacteria can spread along the optic nerve to the brain (for more details, the reader should consult the third edition, pp. 1067–1069).

ORBITAL MASSES

Orbital fat may herniate through weakened episcleral fascia or because of trauma, thereby causing lobular, subconjunctival masses that mimic tumors. Aspiration, biopsy, and cytology of these masses reveal the presence of adipose cells, and the affected tissue can usually be excised and the wound sutured to prevent recurrent herniation. Tumors of the equine orbit include most histopathologic types and produce progressive exophthalmos, orbital swelling, blindness, strabismus, anisocoria, and behavioral abnormalities. In Europe, hydatid cysts have also been reported in the equine orbit.

DISEASES AND SURGERY
OF THE EYELIDS

Entropion is an inward rolling of the eyelid margin. It can be a primary anatomic problem in foals, or it can be secondary to dehydration and weight loss in "downer foals." Entropion may be cicatricial from previous eyelid trauma, or it may be acquired or spastic secondary to chronic, irreversible ocular irritation that causes spasms of the orbicularis oculi muscle. **Clinical signs include epiphora, blepharospasm, conjunctivitis, and ulcerative keratitis, but these signs may vary with the extent of the entropion.**

Surgical correction of entropion in neonatal foals generally is not recommended. Foals should be managed medically using ocular lubricants or temporary sutures as they mature and grow. Nonabsorbable vertical mattress sutures to evert the eyelid margin in foals can be placed for 10 to 14 days and provide positive therapeutic results. The amount of surgical correction for entropion in mature horses must be estimated, however, before general anesthesia is provided. **The modified Hotz-Celsus procedure is simple and can be adapted for use with most types of entropion in the horse (see Chapter 3).**

Eyelid lacerations are common in the horse (Fig. 13-2). Damage to the upper eyelid is more significant, however, because most lid movement occurs here. Medial canthal lacerations may cause damage to the nasolacrimal canaliculi. Lid lacerations may be accompanied by orbital cellulitis, periorbital fractures, and minor to severe corneal ulceration. Careful examination of the globe for corneal integrity, anterior chamber clarity and depth, and scleral continuity is essential to rule out the presence of any additional damage.

Eyelid lacerations must be repaired quickly to avoid lid infection, to reduce eyelid edema, and to minimize scarring of the lid as well as corneal dessication and ulceration. Because of the abundant vasculature in the eyelids, minimal (or no) debridement of a laceration generally is necessary. Accurate two-layer closure of the tarsoconjunctiva and skin–orbicularis muscle aids the healing process by minimizing for formation of scar tissue and lid deformity and by encouraging the quick return of normal eyelid function.

SQUAMOUS CELL CARCINOMA

Squamous cell carcinoma (SCC) is the most common tumor of the equine eye and adnexa. The cause may relate to the ultraviolet component of solar radiation, periocular pigmentation, or an increased susceptibility to carcinogenesis. There is an increased prevalence of ocular/adnexal SCC, presumably resulting from increased exposure to ultraviolet radiation, with increasing altitude, longitude, and mean annual solar radiation. **Prevalence rates in the horse increase with age; one report lists the mean age at diagnosis as 11.1 ± 0.39 years. Belgians, Clydesdales, and other draft horses have a high prevalence of ocular SCC, followed by Appaloosas and Paints. The lowest prevalence of ocular SCC is found in Arabians, Thoroughbreds, and Quarter horses.** White, gray-white, and palomino hair colors predispose to ocular SCC, with a lower prevalence occurring among horses with bay, brown, and black hair coats.

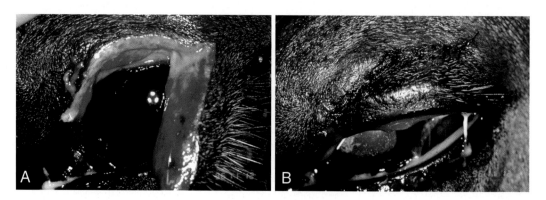

FIGURE 13-2. *An eyelid laceration of the upper margin (A) is sutured without debridement (B).*

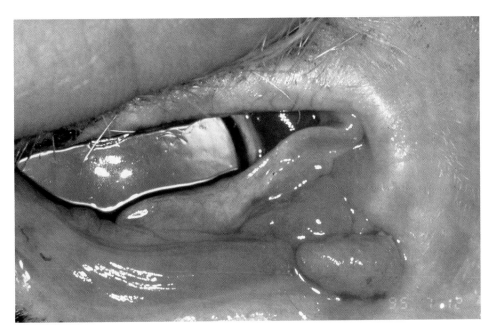

FIGURE 13-3. *Medial canthal squamous cell carcinoma may involve the nasolacrimal system*

The eyelids, nictitans, conjunctiva, and limbus are commonly affected (Fig. 13-3). Ocular SCC must be differentiated from other tumors (e.g., papilloma), inflammatory masses from parasites (e.g., habronema, onchocerca, thelazia), focal infections, granulation tissue, and foreign-body reactions. **Treatment depends on the tumor location, tumor size, extent of invasion, visual status, the animal's purpose, available equipment, and the owner's financial constraints.** Untreated ocular SCC can invade the local soft tissues, bony orbit, sinuses, and brain, and it can metastasize to the regional lymph nodes, salivary glands, and thorax. The tumor recurrence rate is highest in the eyelid or the nictitans. **Surgical excision of equine ocular SCC should be followed by radiation therapy, cryotherapy, radiofrequency hyperthermia, or intralesional chemotherapy (for more details, the reader should consult the third edition, pp. 1070–1073).** Chemotherapy with intralesional, slow-release cisplatin has recently been reported to yield effective results, with or without surgical debulking, in large eyelid and orbital SCC. Reported 1-year relapse-free rates for SCC treated with cisplatin approach 90%. Four sessions at 2-week intervals with 1 mg/cm^3 for tumors 10 to 20 cm^3 in size are necessary, and cisplatin, 3.3 mg/mL (10 mg of cisplatin in 1 mL of water and 2 mL of purified, medical-grade sesame oil), is also used. Topical 5-fluorouracil, 1% solution applied three times a day, or topical mitomycin C, 0.02% solution applied four times a day, may be effective therapy for corneal intraepithelial carcinoma in situ and be beneficial among animals with extensive, periocular SCC. Lid tattooing may decrease the incidence and the recurrence of SCC.

SARCOIDS

Sarcoids are solitary or multiple tumors of the eyelids and the periocular region in the horse. Clinical types include hyperkeratotic fibropapilloma (i.e., verrucous), fibrosarcoma or fibroblastic fibropapilloma, and mixed forms. The fibroblastic form is more aggressive, and intervention can convert the verrucous to the fibroblastic form. Retroviruses and papilloma viruses may be involved as causative factors. Flies may also initiate sarcoid formation by translocating sarcoid cells into the open wounds of horses. Sarcoids are generally found in horses younger than 7 years of age.

Treatment is surgical resection of necrotic tissue and adjunctive immunotherapy with the immunostimulant, bacille Calmette-Guérin (BCG)–attenuated *Mycobacterium bovis* cell wall in oil. Surgical debulking alone carries a high recurrence rate, but success rates approach 100% if debulking is combined with BCG. Using a 25-gauge needle, 1 mL of BCG for each square centimeter of tumor surface area is injected into the lesion; the sarcoid should be saturated, especially around the border. Therapy is repeated every 2 to 4 weeks for as many as six injections and may cause a mild to severe inflammatory tissue reaction. Anaphylaxis may occur, but this can be minimized with systemic administration of flunixin meglumine, 1.1 mg/kg intravenously, and corticosteroids before the treatment itself begins.

Cryotherapy, hyperthermia, carbon dioxide laser excision, and radiation therapy can also be effective treatments. Interstitial brachytherapy with iridium-192 has an 87 to 94% success rate. Intralesional cisplatin or 5-fluorouracil have been effective in approximately 80% of sarcoids treated, and anecdotal evidence is suggestive that autogenous vaccines can be effective as well (Fig. 13-4).

MELANOMA

Eyelid melanomas are found in gray horses, with Arabians and Percherons also having an increased risk. Melanomas may be single or multiple, and treatment is usually surgical excision and cryotherapy. Systemically administered cimetidine has been effective for cutaneous melanomas in the horse, but its efficacy for periocular melanomas has not yet been evaluated.

BLEPHARITIS

Primary bacterial blepharitis is uncommon in the horse. Eyelid abscesses associated with foreign bodies, subpalpebral lavage systems, and bony sequestra are observed, however, and dermatophytosis resulting from *Trichophyton* or *Microsporum* sp. is associated with blepharitis. Miconazole (2%) or thiabendazole ointments are administered topically. *Histoplasma farciminosus* and *Cryptococcus mirandi* cause equine blepharitis and require systemic antifungal therapy.

Equine papillomas resulting from a papovavirus are common among immature horses. They may regress spontaneously, or they may require surgery, cryotherapy, or autogenous vaccination. Lymphosarcoma is associated with lid swelling and conjunctivitis.

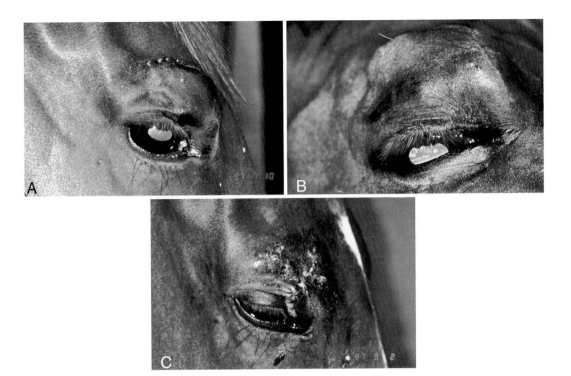

FIGURE 13-4. *Surgical debulking and intralesional cisplatin effectively resolved this neurofibrosarcoma of the upper eyelid and superior orbital rim during a 2-month period. Initial lesion (**A**) increased in size (**B**) until resolution by lid and facial scarring (**C**).*

Habronemiasis is a common cause of equine granulomas in the eyelids, conjunctiva, lacrimal caruncle, medial canthus, and nictitans. Nonhealing, elevated, and ulcerated periocular granulomas with fistulous tracts and a yellow, caseous exudate having gritty foci of necrotic mineralized tissue are found on horses during the warm-weather months, because house and stable flies both serve as vectors. Dying microfilaria are believed to incite immune hypersensitivity. Scrapings reveal numerous eosinophils, mast cells, polymorphonuclear cells, and plasma cells; because the larvae are rarely located, however, it can be difficult to differentiate habronemiasis from mastocytoma, nodular necrobiosis, or fungal granulomas. Topical therapy for solitary, focal lesions involves a mixture containing 135 g of nitrofurazone ointment, 30 mL of 90% dimethyl sulfoxide (DMSO), 30 mL of 0.2% dexamethasone, and 30 mL of 12.3% oral trichlorfon solution. Multifocal lesions should be treated with ivermectin, 200 g/kg orally. In addition, intralesional corticosteroid injection (i.e., triamcinolone) can reduce the size of granulomas.

The spiruroid nematode *Thelazia lacrimalis* is a commensal parasite that inhabits the equine conjunctival fornices and nasolacrimal ducts. Most horses are asymptomatic, but signs can include mild lid swelling, conjunctivitis, superficial keratitis, and dacryocystitis. Demodex may cause meibomianitis, lid alopecia, and papulopustular dermatitis.

DISEASES OF THE CONJUNCTIVA

Conjunctivitis is a nonspecific indicator of ocular inflammation (Table 13-2). The conjunctiva becomes inflamed during both infectious and noninfectious diseases of the lids, cornea, sclera, anterior uvea, nasolacrimal system, and orbit as well as with several systemic diseases.

In adult horses, onchocerciasis is associated with temporolimbal conjunctival thickening and depigmentation as well as with corneal edema, vascularization, and stromal cellular infiltration. Keratitis, conjunctivitis, and keratouveitis may also be present. The causative organism is *Onchocerca cervicalis,* and the vector is the female *Culicoides* sp. midge. Conjunctival biopsy specimens placed in saline may demonstrate free microfilaria, and large numbers of eosinophils and lymphocytes, with or without microfilaria, are found in conjunctival histopathologic specimens. At present, this disease does not appear to be common in the United States. Treatment involves systemically administered ivermectin and topical anti-inflammatory agents.

Lymphoma, papilloma, SCC (most common), hemangioma, and hemangiosarcomas are all tumors that involve the equine conjunctiva. Jaundice and anemia may change the conjunctival color to yellow and pale pink, respectively.

DISEASES OF THE NICTITATING MEMBRANE

The most common neoplasm of the equine nictitans is SCC. The diagnosis is confirmed on the basis of biopsy results, and treatment is surgical resection of the nictitans, combined with cryotherapy or chemotherapy. Protrusion of the nictitans is associated with several conditions (Box 13-1).

TABLE 13-2
CONJUNCTIVITIS AND SYSTEMIC DISEASES IN THE HORSE

Neonate	Neonatal maladjustment syndrome, neonatal septicemia, and immune-mediated hemolytic anemia.
Adult	Keratoconjunctivitis sicca, lymphosarcoma, multiple myeloma, infection with *Moraxella equi* or *Streptococcus equi,* leptospirosis, equine herpesvirus-4, adenovirus, equine infectious anemia, equine viral arteritis, influenza type A_2, polyneuritis equi, equine protozoal myeloencephalitis, vestibular disease syndrome, African Horse sickness, and epizootic lymphangitis.

BOX 13-1

Conditions Producing Nictitans Protrusion

Pain (usually from conjunctivitis, corneal ulcers, or anterior uveitis)

Tetanus

Inflammation because of bacteria, trauma, parasites, and tumors

Enophthalmos because of pain, microphthalmos, and phthisis bulbi

Protrusion of orbital fat

Horner's syndrome (see Chapter 16)

Hyperkalemic, periodic paralysis, and foreign bodies

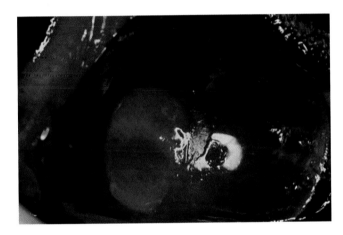

FIGURE 13-5. *A large, pseudomonal ulcer with evidence of gelatinous "melting."*

DISEASES OF THE CORNEA

CORNEAL ULCERATION

Equine corneal ulceration is a potentially sight-threatening disease that requires early clinical diagnosis, laboratory confirmation, and appropriate medical as well as surgical therapy. Bacterial and fungal keratitis may present with a mild, early clinical course, but they both require prompt therapy to avoid serious ocular complications. Ulcers can range from simple, superficial ulcers or abrasions to full-thickness perforations with iris prolapse. Corneal infection and iridocyclitis are always major concerns in cases of even the slightest corneal ulcerations (Fig. 13-5). The type of medical or surgical treatment (or both) is determined by the type and extent of the corneal disease and by any ocular complications that have occurred. All corneal injuries should be fluorescein stained to detect corneal ulcers.

Pathogenesis

The environment of the horse is such that the conjunctiva and cornea are constantly exposed to bacteria and fungi. **The conjunctival microbial flora of the horse varies, however, depending on the season and the geographic area.** Many bacterial and fungal organisms that are normally found in the equine conjunctival flora are also potential ocular pathogens. In one study of horses from Missouri, Gram-negative bacteria, especially *Pseudomonas* and *Enterobacter* sp., were found responsible for most cases of ulcerative keratitis. *Fusarium* and *Aspergillus* sp. are both common causes of ulcerative fungal keratitis among horses in the United States, and Gram-negative bacteria known to be associated with equine corneal ulcers include *Pseudomonas* sp. and assorted coliform bacteria. *Staphylococcus* and *Streptococcus* sp. are Gram-positive bacteria that are found in cases of infectious equine keratitis. Mixed bacterial and fungal infections can be present as well.

Total corneal ulceration ultimately requires the degradation of collagen, which forms the framework of the corneal stroma. Most evidence indicates that true corneal collagenolysis results from the proteases produced by the polymorphonuclear cells. Bacterially derived proteases probably cannot degrade intact collagen fibrils, but they can contribute to stromal collagenolysis once the initial collagen breakdown has been initiated by a true collagenase.

Clinical History and Appearance

Many early cases of equine ulcerative keratitis initially present as minor corneal epithelial ulcers or infiltrates, with slight pain, blepharospasm, epiphora, and photophobia. At first, anterior uveitis and corneal vascularization may not be pronounced clinically; however, a slowly progressive, indolent course often belies the seriousness of the condition. The healing of a small epithelial defect can also result in the isolation of organisms in the stroma, thus causing a severe, deep, interstitial keratitis. Both superficial and deep corneal vascularization as well as painful uveitis may occur. Extensive intrastromal lesions, vascularization, conjunctival injection, and corneal edema then may become evident. Corneal collagen breakdown or "melting" appears as a gelatinous, gray opacity to the margins or the central regions (or both) of an ulcer. Deep penetration of the stroma to Descemet's membrane with corneal perforation is a possible sequela to all cases of equine corneal ulcers.

Diagnostic Techniques

Each case of equine ulcerative corneal disease must be approached in a systematic manner. **Any ulcers that are not responding to the usually effective therapy or that are rapidly progressing require cytology as well as culture and sensitivities for bacteria and fungi.** Vigorous corneal scrapings at both the edge and base of the lesion to detect bacteria and deep hyphal elements can be obtained with use of the blunt, handle end of a sterile scalpel blade and topical anesthesia. Superficial swabbing cannot be expected to yield the organism (or organisms), however, in a high percentage of cases, because these organisms are deep within the ulcer.

Therapeutic Methods

Horses with corneal ulcers often are in pain, and topical treatment usually is difficult. **In a horse that is fractious or has a painful eye needing frequent therapy, subpalpebral (i.e., a length of silicone tubing with a single hole and footplate positioned in the superior palpebral fornix) or nasolacrimal lavage treatment systems are employed (Fig. 13-6).** Minimal equipment is required, and the tubing can be removed without sedation. A standard needle holder, a 12-gauge needle with the hub removed, 1 to 2 m of silicone tubing (0.065-inch, in the right eye), and standard dermal suture material are also required. Sedation, eyelid akinesia, sensory eyelid blocks, and topical anesthesia generally are sufficient to place this tubing system.

Medical and Surgical Therapy

Medical therapy almost always comprises the major thrust of treatment to control an ulcer, albeit tempered by judicious use of adjunctive surgical procedures (Fig. 13-7). This pharmacologic attack should be intensive enough to satisfy the therapeutic objectives and be modified according to its efficacy (Table 13-3; see Appendixes D, F, H, I, and L). Treatment frequently needs to be sustained for weeks or, occasionally, even months. (For more details, the reader should consult the third edition, pp. 1076–1088.)

CORNEAL LACERATIONS/PERFORATIONS

Corneal lacerations in the horse are always accompanied by varying degrees of iridocyclitis. Medical therapy should be sufficient for superficial, nonperforating lacerations, and use of topically applied broad-spectrum antibiotics, mydriatics/cycloplegics, and serum are recommended. Topically applied serum reduces enzymatic collagen breakdown of the cornea, and use of systemic NSAIDs is strongly indicated as well.

   Full-thickness corneal perforations are usually associated with iris prolapse, a shallow anterior chamber, and hyphema. If the corneal lesion extends to the limbus, the sclera should also be checked carefully for perforation, because the sclera can be obscured by conjunctival chemosis and hemorrhage. Failure to detect such a scleral tear can result in chronic hypotony and atrophy of the globe (i.e., phthisis bulbi) being allowed to develop. **Deep or irregular corneal lacerations require surgical support of the cornea and more aggressive therapy for iridocyclitis. Direct corneal suturing and conjunctival flaps are also indicated to more rapidly restore the corneal integrity. Topically applied antibiotics and mydriatics/cycloplegics as well as systemically administered anti-inflammatory agents are used until healing is complete (for more details, the reader should consult the third edition, pp. 1082–1083).**

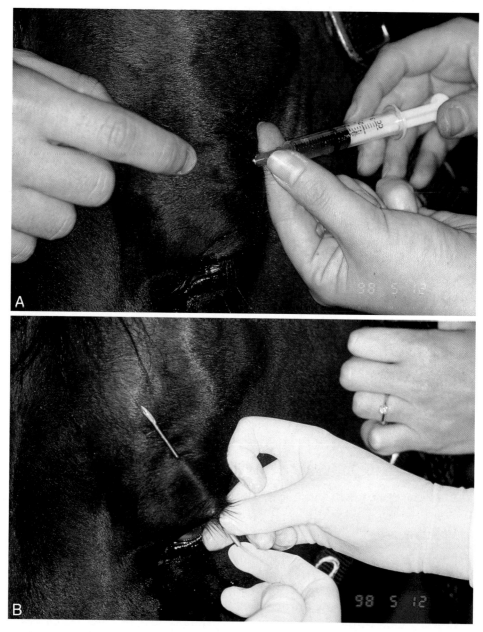

FIGURE 13-6. *Placement of the subpalpebral system to medicate an equine eye.*
A. The supraorbital nerve block is performed, thereby providing local anesthesia
and akinesia to the central upper eyelid. **B.** *A 12-gauge hypodermic needle (without*
its hub) is carefully inserted under the upper eyelid as well as through the upper
conjunctival fornix and the entire lid.   *continued*

EQUINE ULCERATIVE KERATOMYCOSIS

Fungi are normal inhabitants of the equine conjunctival microflora,
but they can become pathogenic after a corneal injury. Keratomycosis
is common in the horse but very rare in animals such as the dog, cat,

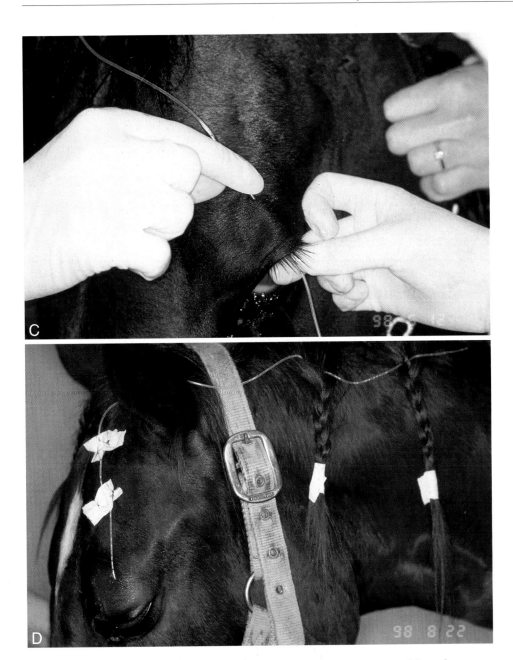

FIGURE 13-6—(continued) *C. The subpalpebral system is threaded into the needle, and the needle is then exited through the lid, leaving the subpalpebral system in place (with the footplate in the conjunctival fornix). **D.** Sutures or medical white tape (or both) are used to secure the subpalpebral system to the upper forehead and mane. Ophthalmic solutions are periodically injected (using a 1- to 3-mL syringe) through the tubing.*

and cow. In the horse, keratomycosis manifests clinically as an ulcerative keratitis (see the previous discussion of corneal ulcerations), an interstitial keratitis known as stromal abscessation, and iris prolapse. A stromal abscess results from stromal inoculation with bacteria or

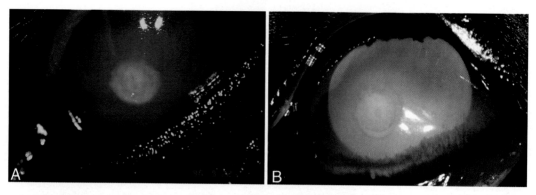

FIGURE 13-7. *A. A cellular infiltrate creates a white appearance to this corneal ulcer, which has edema, vascularization, and hypopyon. B. Three days after initiation of medical therapy with antibiotics, atropine, and autogenous serum, the pupil is dilated, the uveitis and corneal edema are lessened, and the ulcer is nearly healed. The white opacity that still remains is caused by disruption of the collagen lamellae.*

fungi through a corneal defect. The organisms become encapsulated in the corneal stroma after re-epithelialization of the corneal ulcer over the infection site. Therapy for ulcerative keratitis, iris prolapse, and stromal abscess varies, but all cases of iris prolapse require surgical repair and most cases of deep stromal abscess require penetrating keratoplasty.

Ulcerative keratomycosis is a serious, sight-threatening disease in the horse. Vision after keratomycosis in the horse may be retained in as few as 50% of eyes, with nearly half the eyes having ulcerative keratomycosis being reported to become blind or to require enucleation (or both). Aggressive surgical therapy early in the course of ulcerative keratomycosis is most effective (Fig. 13-8). Treatment must be directed against the fungi as well as the corneal and the intraocular inflammatory responses that occur after fungal replication and hyphal death (see Appendix F). The levels of ophthalmic antifungal drugs in the cornea needed to achieve fungicidal effects are so difficult to obtain, however, that many such agents, including miconazole, generally are considered to exhibit fungistatic activity only—even though the loss of corneal epithelium results in increased corneal and aqueous concentrations. Long duration exposure to antifungal drugs is required for complete fungal destruction and resolution of the clinical signs. Frequency of treatment is another important aspect in using antifungal agents. Topically administered antifungal therapy for equine keratomycosis with topical miconazole or natamycin, applied three to four times per day over the first few days. This frequency of treatment was determined empirically, because the intensity of iridocyclitis is often noted to be magnified dramatically on the day after topical administration of miconazole at frequencies higher than this. Sudden death of stromal fungi because of the initiation of antifungal drug therapy can result in acute and intense iridocyclitis; topical administrations of antifungal medications are then increased to six times per day on subsequent days.

Combined medical and surgical therapy is indicated if the ulcers are extremely deep, are not responding to medical treatment, or are

worsening despite medical treatment. In one report, approximately half the horses were treated with combined medical and surgical therapy. Surgeries for keratomycosis include conjunctival pedicle grafts, bridge grafts, hood grafts, island grafts, and full-thickness penetrating keratoplasty (for more details, the reader should consult the third edition, pp. 1083–1088).

TABLE 13-3

TREATMENT OF CORNEAL ULCERS IN THE HORSE

Class of Drugs	*Recommendations*
Antibacterials	Appropriate antibiotics such as chloramphenicol, gentamicin, ciprofloxacin, or tobramycin ophthalmic solutions may be used topically to treat bacterial ulcers. Amikacin, 10 mg/mL, may also be used topically. Apply topically or with subpalpebral system.
Antifungals	**Topical:** Miconazole, 1%; natamycin. **Systemic (infrequent and expensive):** Ketoconazole, 30 mg/kg orally once or twice a day (in 0.2-N HCl); fluconazole, 4 mg/kg orally once a day; thiabendazole, 44 mg/kg orally once a day; itraconazole, 3 mg/kg orally twice a day.
Control of uveitis	Systemic phenylbutazone or flunixin can be used orally or parenterally at anti-inflammatory dosages. Topical anticholinergics (e.g., 1–2% atropine) help stabilize the blood-aqueous barrier, relax the ciliary muscles (ciliary spasm), and provide pupillary dilatation (maintains visual axis and minimizes development of synechiae). Horses on topical atropine should be watched closely for symptoms of colic and mydriasis of the fellow eye.
Prevention of collagenolysis	Topical autogenous serum. Replaced by new serum every 3 to 5 days. Ten percent acetylcysteine or 0.05% potassium EDTA can also be administered until stromal liquefaction diminishes.
Adjunctive surgery	To augment medical therapy. **Keratectomy** to remove necrotic tissue speeds healing, minimizes scarring, and decreases the stimulus for iridocyclitis. **Conjunctival grafts** for deep, melting, and large corneal ulcers; descemetoceles; and perforated corneal ulcers both with and without iris prolapse. Conjunctival flaps are best mobilized from the bulbar conjunctiva. **Nictitating membrane flaps** provide more support to a diseased cornea than a temporary, complete tarsorrhaphy.
Inappropriate therapy	Corticosteroid therapy by all routes is contraindicated.

EDTA, ethylenediaminetetraacetic acid.

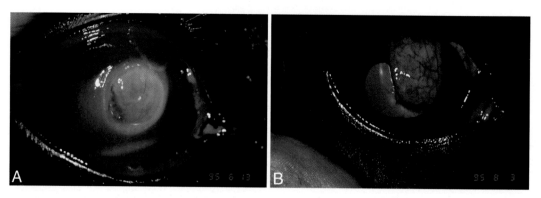

FIGURE 13-8. *A. A midstromal fungal ulcer with keratomalacia, deep corneal vascularization, and hypopyon. B. A pedicle conjunctival graft was curative but produced a large scar. The base of the pedicle flap was transected 6 weeks postoperatively.*

CORNEAL STROMAL ABSCESS

Corneal stromal abscess can be vision-threatening sequelae to apparently minor corneal ulcerations in the horse. A corneal abscess may develop after epithelial cells that are adjacent to a small epithelial puncture defect divide and migrate over the wound and, thereby, seal infectious agents or foreign bodies in the stroma. This re-epithelialization forms a barrier that protects the bacteria or fungi from both topically and systemically administered antimicrobial medications. As mentioned, corneal stromal abscesses can be infected by bacteria or fungi, but they also can be sterile.

The diagnosis of stromal abscessation is established on the basis of a focal, yellow-white, stromal infiltrate with associated corneal edema. Single or multiple abscesses may be present, and a mild to fulminating iridocyclitis occurs secondary to what initially appears to be a relatively benign corneal disease, thus causing severe pain and, possibly, blindness. Corneal vascularization is variable at presentation. Most cases have initial clinical signs that are suggestive of minor corneal trauma. Fluorescein dye retention is either negative or positive over an area much smaller than the diameter of the corneal lesion.

Stromal abscesses often require combined medical and surgical therapy. Many superficial stromal abscesses will initially respond to medical therapy but then gradually worsen clinically, thus requiring surgical intervention. Repeated scrapings to remove the corneal epithelium may allow for better drug penetration in superficial stromal abscesses. If the signs associated with a stromal abscess do not improve significantly within the first 48 to 72 hours of intense and appropriate medical therapy, surgery can improve these results and also reduce the duration of medical therapy. Medical therapy includes antibiotics (see Appendix D), antifungals (see Appendix F), mydriatics (see Appendix L), and NSAIDs (see Appendix I). Surgery includes deep lamellar and penetrating keratoplasties. Intraocular injection of miconazole and fluconazole (0.1 mg in a 0.1-mL solution), which can be performed during surgery, has been an effective adjunctive treatment in deep fungal stromal abscesses. Placing a conjunctival pedicle graft over a deep lamellar keratectomy site rapidly restores the physical integrity of the cornea by supplying fibrovascular tissue that fills in the stromal defect. It also delivers a focal, direct blood supply such that the need for vascularization is met and angiogenic factors no longer are required to stimulate ingrowth of the limbal blood vessels. In addition, conjunctival grafts allow plasma, leukocytes, antibodies, and systemically administered antibiotics to reach the diseased cornea (for more details, the reader should consult the third edition, pp. 1083–1088).

OTHER KERATOPATHIES

Nonulcerative Keratouveitis

Nonulcerative keratouveitis is an unusual corneal disease that is characterized in the horse by a nonulcerated, fleshy, stromal infiltrate involving the limbus. Signs of iridocyclitis are prominent. This may be an immune-mediated disease, because no organism has been cultured from the affected sites or noted in the biopsy specimens reported to date. Treatment consists of topically administered corticosteroids, cyclosporin A, or beta radiation therapy, or some combination thereof, plus systemic NSAIDs. Enucleation often becomes necessary because of the inability to control pain.

Eosinophilic Keratitis

Eosinophilic keratitis is associated with blepharospasm, chemosis, conjunctival hyperemia, mucoid discharge, and corneal ulcers covered by raised, white, subepithelial, and necrotic plaques. Both keratoconjunctivitis sicca and lacrimal gland adenitis can occur. The diagnosis is established on the basis of clinical signs and cytologic findings of numerous eosinophils and a few mast cells, lymphocytes, and plasma cells. Histopathologically, the plaques consist of coalescing foci of eosinophilic, degenerating collagen fibers that have been infiltrated by eosinophils, polymorphonuclear cells, lymphocytes, and plasma cells, which in turn are surrounded by a layer of eosinophilic, acellular granular material. Eosinophilic keratitis in the horse possibly is an allergic, immune-mediated, or inflammatory manifestation of chronic ivermectin administration for parasitic microfilaria control, but the specific cause of this disorder is not known.

Treatment is often prolonged. Topical corticosteroids are beneficial during the early stages of disease, despite corneal ulceration, but medical therapy in conjunction with superficial lamellar keratectomy to remove the plaques significantly speeds healing. Topical antibiotics, atropine, and phospholine iodide in combination with systemic NSAIDs and corticosteroids can also be effective.

Herpes Keratitis

Multiple, superficial, white, punctate or linear opacities of the cornea, with or without fluorescein dye retention, are found with viral keratopathy in the horse. Varying amounts of ocular pain, conjunctivitis, and iridocyclitis are present, and the punctate opacities may retain rose Bengal stain. **Equine herpesvirus-2 has been cultured from such**

lesions. Idoxuridine and trifluorothymidine have been used successfully as treatment, but recurrence is common.

Burdock Pappus Bristle Keratopathy

Persistent corneal ulcerations caused by burdock pappus bristle foreign bodies embedded in the conjunctiva are common among horses in the northeastern United States. For treatment, conjunctivalectomy of the bristle foreign body and the surrounding tissue is recommended.

Calcific Band Keratopathy

Calcific band keratopathy occurs as a complication of uveitis in the horse. The corneal lesions are dense, white, dystrophic bands in the interpalpebral region of the central cornea. Scattered areas of fluorescein dye retention can be present, and calcium deposited at the level of the corneal epithelial basement membrane may accumulate and disrupt the epithelium, thereby producing painful ulcers. Superficial keratectomy is generally necessary to remove the calcium deposits and thus eliminate the pain caused by the ulcers, but topically administered calcium-chelating drugs (e.g., 0.05% Na- or K-ethylenediaminetetraacetic acid [EDTA]) can also be beneficial.

LENS OPACITIES

Cataracts are the most frequent congenital ocular defect in foals (discussed earlier).

ACQUIRED CATARACTS

In the horse, cataracts secondary to equine recurrent uveitis (ERU) or trauma are frequently seen, whereas juvenile-onset cataracts are uncommon. True senile cataracts that interfere with vision occur in horses older than 20 years of age. Increased cloudiness of the lens, or nuclear lenticular sclerosis, is also common among older horses. Because nuclear sclerosis is not a true cataract, however, vision in these horses is clinically normal.

LENS LUXATION

Contusional or perforating injuries of the globe can produce changes in the lens position (i.e., luxation, subluxation). **Injuries to the globe that are sufficient to cause lens luxation also may result in cataracts and other ocular as well as cranial lesions. Both ERU and glaucoma are causes of equine lens luxation as well (Fig. 13-9).**

CATARACT SURGERY

Most veterinary ophthalmologists recommend surgical removal of cataracts in foals younger than 6 months of age if the foal is healthy,

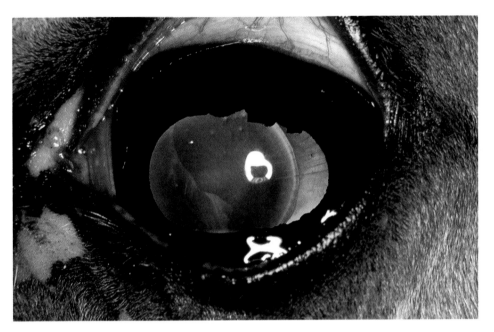

FIGURE 13-9. *A lens luxation associated with glaucoma in a horse.*

will tolerate aggressive topical therapy, and has no uveitis or other ocular problems. Adult horses with visual impairment because of cataracts are also candidates for surgery. Surgery in foals is easier, however, because the globe is small enough that standard cataract surgical equipment is satisfactory in size, general anesthesia carries less risk, and foals heal very quickly after cataract surgery. Early return of vision is paramount in foals to ensure development of the higher visual centers. The preoperative ophthalmic evaluation in foals is identical to that for small animals. **Phacoemulsification is an extracapsular technique most useful for equine cataract surgery, because it involves a small corneal incision (3.0–3.2 mm).**

Most reliable reports of vision after successful cataract surgery in the horse are indicative that postsurgical vision is functionally normal. From an optical standpoint, the postoperative aphakic eye should be quite farsighted or hyperopic and, in one study, was 19.94 D. Images close to the eye should be blurry and appear to be magnified. Such loss of accommodation, however, could be severely debilitating to some horses. (For more details, the reader should consult the third edition, pp. 1094–1097.)

EQUINE GLAUCOMA

The glaucomas are a group of diseases resulting from alterations in the aqueous humor dynamics that increase the IOP to greater than that compatible with normal function of the retinal ganglion cells and the optic nerve. **Primary bilateral glaucoma has been rarely reported in the** horse; secondary glaucoma resulting from anterior uveitis and intraocular neoplasia is most commonly recognized. **Congenital glaucoma is reported in foals, and it is associated with developmental anomalies of the iridocorneal angle (e.g., goniodysgenesis).**

Glaucoma in the horse is being recognized with increased frequency, but the actual prevalence of equine glaucoma is surprisingly low (e.g., 0.07% in the United States) given the horse's propensity for ocular injury and marked intraocular inflammatory responses. **Horses with previous or concurrent ERU, those older than 15 years of age, and Appaloosas have an increased risk for glaucoma. Glaucoma is an uncommon complication of ERU, but the presence of active or even inactive uveitis appears to be a major factor in its development among horses.**

The presence of corneal striae (or corneal endothelial "band opacities") in nonbuphthalmic equine eyes warrants a high degree of suspicion for elevated IOP, but corneal striae also may be found in eyes that are normotensive at examination. Corneal striae are linear and often interconnecting, white opacities deep in the cornea. They are caused by stretching or rupture of the Descemet's membrane, and they may be associated with increased IOP (Fig. 13-10). Accurate measurement of IOP in the horse requires the use of applanation tonometry. The mean equine IOP ranges from 17 to 28 mm Hg, with the IOP of the individual eyes in a given horse being within 5 mm Hg of each other. The pupils are often only slightly dilated, and overt discomfort is uncommon. Afferent pupillary light reflexes, corneal striae, decreased vision, lens luxations, mild iridocyclitis, and optic nerve atrophy/cupping also may occur.

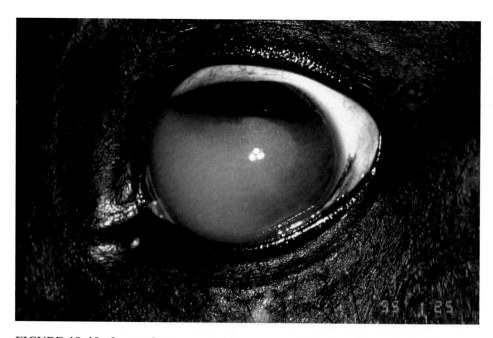

FIGURE 13-10. *Incomplete corneal edema and a dilated pupil in a foal with glaucoma and an intraocular pressure of 50 mm Hg. Laser cyclophotoablation was unsuccessful at reducing the level of pressure.*

THERAPY

Therapy for equine glaucomas is complicated by the lack of information regarding the drugs traditionally used during therapy for these diseases. The systemically administered carbonic anhydrase inhibitors acetazolamide and dichlorphenamide (see Appendix G); the topical miotics phospholine iodide, 0.12 to 0.25% given twice a day, and pilocarpine, 2% given four times a day (see Appendix K); and the β-blocker timolol maleate, 0.5% given twice a day (see Appendix A), have been used with varying degrees of success to lower equine IOP. The most successful drugs have been those that reduce formation of the aqueous humor formation (i.e., β-adrenergic antagonists and carbonic anhydrase inhibitors). Topical carbonic anhydrase inhibitors (e.g., dorzolamide) can be beneficial in horses with glaucoma.

Paradoxically, glaucoma in some horses may respond to topical corticosteroid and atropine therapy even if active uveitis is not clinically evident. Anti-inflammatory therapy, consisting of both topically and systemically administered corticosteroids with or without topically and systemically administered NSAIDs (e.g., phenylbutazone, 1 mg/kg orally twice a day, or flunixin meglumine, 250 mg orally twice a day), also appear to control the IOP. A nonselective β-adrenergic antagonist, timolol maleate, 0.5% given twice a day, is effective at lowering IOP in the horse and may be used either alone or in combination with other drugs. Oral carbonic anhydrase inhibitor therapy using dichlorphenamide, 1 mg/kg orally twice per day, or acetazolamide, 1 to 3 mg/kg orally four times per day, also may be beneficial in lowering the IOP when combined with β-adrenergic antagonists and miotics.

When medical therapy is inadequate, Nd:YAG or diode laser cyclophotoablation may be a viable alternative for long-term control of the IOP. Cyclophotoablation with the Nd:YAG laser is very effective at controlling the IOP and maintaining vision in the horse. For contact Nd:YAG laser cyclophotoablation in the horse, 55 laser sites per eye placed 5- to 6-mm posterior to the limbus at a power setting of 10 W for a duration of 0.4 seconds per site are recommended. Diode lasers may be used at 55 to 60 sites for 1500 mW at 1500 msec per site. Chronically painful and blind buphthalmic globes should be enucleated or have an intrascleral prosthesis implanted. (For more details, the reader should consult the third edition, pp. 1097–1101.)

EQUINE RECURRENT UVEITIS

Equine recurrent uveitis is a common cause of blindness in the adult horse. A multitude of terms have been assigned to ERU, including *periodic ophthalmia, moon blindness,* and *iridocyclitis,* but *ERU* remains the most descriptive (albeit an umbrella) term for this set of diseases characterized by episodes of active uveitis alternating with varying intervals of clinical quiescence.

CLINICAL SIGNS

Horses with ERU display increased lacrimation, blepharospasm, and photophobia to varying degrees. Subtle amounts of corneal edema, conjunctival hyperemia, and ciliary injection are present initially and, as the condition progresses, can become prominent. Aqueous flare, hyphema, intraocular fibrin, and hypopyon may be observed with a bright, focused light or slit beam (Fig. 13-11). Miosis is usually a prominent sign in horses with ERU and can produce a misshapen pupil and posterior synechiae. Delayed or failed pharmacologic mydriasis is common when uveitis is active. The IOP in affected hoses is generally low, but ERU may also be associated with intermittent and acute elevations. Fibrin and iris pigment may be deposited on the anterior lens capsule. Cataract formation may occur if the inflammation does not subside quickly. The fundus should be evaluated for active or inactive chorioretinitis (Fig. 13-12). Choroiditis may be associated with leakage of plasma or blood from the choroidal and retinal blood vessels, thereby resulting in focal or diffuse, nontapetal, exudative retinal detachments. Retinal vascular congestion can occur as well. The vitreous may develop "haziness" from the leakage of proteins and cells from the retinal and choroidal vessels, and the optic nerve head can appear to be congested.

Corneal vascularization, permanent corneal edema, synechiation, cataract formation, and iris depigmentation or hyperpigmentation can result in chronic cases. Secondary glaucoma leading to chronic hypotony and phthisis bulbi can also occur. In addition, vitreous liquefaction as well as retinal degeneration, as indicated by focal to generalized peripapillary regions of depigmentation in the nontapetal fundus, can result. Irreversible blindness is a common sequela to ERU and results from cataract formation or severe chorioretinitis.

PATHOGENESIS

The pathogenesis of ERU is enigmatic, but it is undoubtedly immune mediated, with hypersensitivity to infectious agents such as *Leptospira*

FIGURE 13-11. *Hyphema and a miotic pupil in a horse with equine recurrent uveitis.*

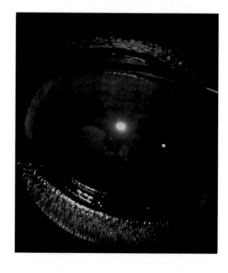

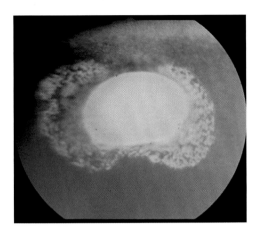

FIGURE 13-12. *Peripapillary depigmentation caused by previous chorioretinitis.*

interrogans **serovar** *pomona* **commonly being implicated as a possible cause.** All major serogroups of *L. interrogans* have been isolated from the horse, and all these may be involved with initiating ERU. The serovars *pomona, grippotyphosa, icterohaemorrhagiae, canicola, hardjo,* and *sejroe* have been reported to cause ERU in the horse. Affected horses develop circulating antibody titers against *L. interrogans,* with the titer rising during the active phases of the disease and decreasing during the quiescent phases. The anti–*Leptospira* sp. antibodies are found in the serum, the tears, and the aqueous humor of infected horses. The equine cornea and lens share antigenic properties with the *Leptospira* organism, and the antigenicity the equine corneal antigens share with leptospiral surface molecules allows for the binding of anti–*Leptospira* sp. antibodies to the cornea, activation of complement, and initiation of the mechanisms of tissue damage. The presence of living leptospiral organisms, however, is not necessary to produce the disease itself. Major histocompatibility complex (MHC) class II antigen–expressing cells and nodules of predominantly B and, less so, T lymphocytes are found in the iris, ciliary body, and pineal body of horses with ERU. The nonpigmented ciliary epithelium and retina both express MHC-II antigen in horses with ERU as well. Extensive pineal gland infiltration may accompany active uveitis, and it may regress with resolution of the uveitis. Exposure to exogenous proteins results in the expression of MHC-II antigen and may perpetuate the immune/inflammatory response, thus contributing to the recurrent nature of ERU. Horses that are seropositive to *L. interrogans* serovar *pomona* (titers, <100) are 13.2 times more likely than seronegative horses to show signs of uveitis. Seropositive horses with uveitis are 4.4 times more likely to lose vision than seronegative horses with uveitis. Seropositive Appaloosas are 8.3 times more likely than other breeds to develop uveitis and 3.8 times more likely to lose vision after uveitis has developed.

Toxoplasmosis, brucellosis, salmonellosis, streptococcus hypersensitivity, *Escherichia coli, Rhodococcus equi,* borreliosis, intestinal strongyles, onchocerciasis, parasites (e.g., *Halicephalobus deletrix*), and viral infections have also been implicated as causes of ERU, but no consistency has been found in the isolation of these organisms from affected horses. Viral organisms suspected of playing a role in ERU include equine influenza virus, EHV-1, EHV-4, equine arteritis virus, and possibly, the equine infectious anemia virus. *Onchocerca cervicalis* has been implicated as a cause of ERU as well. Conjunctivitis, nonulcerated keratitis, keratouveitis, and signs of both anterior and posterior uveitis may be seen, and dead or dying microfilaria may release antigens to incite ERU after vascular migration of living microfilaria to the eye.

LABORATORY TESTING

Laboratory testing may be beneficial in assessing the horse with ERU. Serum biochemical profiles and complete blood counts may detect major organ abnormalities or active systemic infection (or both). Serologic testing for leptospirosis, brucellosis, and toxoplasmosis should be considered as well. Serologic results can be difficult to interpret, however, because many horses have "positive" titers without clinical evidence of ocular or systemic disease. Leptospiral titers for the serovars *pomona, bratislava,* and *autumnalis* should be requested for horses in the United States; a positive titer for serovars at dilutions of 1:400 or greater are of clinical importance. A higher titer in the aqueous humor than in the serum is indicative of antibody production and supportive of a leptospiral cause for the uveitis.

TREATMENT

The major goals in the treatment of ERU are to preserve vision, to decrease pain, and to prevent or minimize the recurrence of uveitis. Specific prevention and therapy are often difficult, however, because in many cases, the cause is not identified. Treatment should be aggressive and prompt to maintain transparency of the ocular structures. Therapy can last for weeks or months, and it should not be stopped abruptly. Otherwise, there may be recurrence. Medications should be slowly reduced in frequency once the clinical signs abate (Table 13-4; see Appendices H, I, and L).

PROGNOSIS

Recurrence of anterior uveitis caused by immunologic mechanisms is the hallmark of ERU. Overall, the prognosis is usually poor. Treatment can be both time-consuming and expensive, but saving the horse's vision is worth attempting for as long as possible. The owner should be educated immediately about the potentially blinding nature of this disease and the possibility of enucleation to remove a painful eye if vision is lost. The role of pars plana vitrectomy in the long-term clinical management of ERU is currently under study, and the preliminary results appear to be promising. (For more information, the reader should consult the third edition, pp. 1101–1105.)

POSTERIOR SEGMENT DISEASES

Correctly interpreting the normal appearance of the equine fundus requires considerable practice, because there is much normal variation. **Examination**

TABLE 13-4

TREATMENT OF EQUINE RECURRENT UVEITIS

Drug Group	*Recommendations*
Active/acute Corticosteroids	**Administer topically** (every 4–6 hours): prednisolone acetate, 1%, or dexamethasone, 0.1%. **Subconjunctival injections:** methylprednisolone acetate, 40 mg every 1–3 weeks, or triamcinolone acetonide, 40 mg every 1–3 weeks. **Sytemically:** orally, intramuscularly, or intravenously. Systemic steroids may be beneficial in severe, refractory cases, but they do pose some risk of inducing laminitis and should be used with caution.
NSAIDs	**Administer topically:** flurbiprofen, indomethacin, diclofenamic acid, or suprofen 4–6 times daily. **Systemically:** flunixin meglumine 0.25–1.0 mg/kg orally twice a day; phenylbutazone, 1 g intravenously or orally twice per day; or aspirin, 25 mg/kg orally twice per day.
Mydriatics	Decrease potential formation of synechiae by inducing mydriasis, and alleviate some of the pain by relieving ciliary body muscle spasms. Atropine, 1–3%, or tropicamide, 1%, is instilled to effect and maintain mydriasis. Gut motility should be strictly monitored by abdominal auscultation and observing signs of abdominal pain when using topically administered atropine in both adult horses and foals. Should gut motility decrease during treatment with topical atropine, discontinue the drug or change to the shorter-acting tropicamide. A combination of topically administered phenylephrine, 2.5%, and atropine, 1%, can also be used to obtain maximum dilation in the inflamed eye. Topically administered phenylephrine does not achieve mydriasis when used alone in the horse, however, and it does not cause cycloplegia. Injectable atropine can be administered subconjunctivally for a repository effect (5–10 mg per injection) in difficult-to-manage horses, but gut motility must be monitored closely.
Antibiotics	Systemically or topically administered: should be broad-spectrum and appropriate for the geographic location of the patient. The efficacy of antibiotic treatment for horses with positive titers for leptospirosis remains speculative (streptomycin may be a good choice). Penicillin and tetracycline at high dosages may be beneficial during acute leptospiral infections.
Chronic/inactive	Long-term topical/systemic corticosteroids/NSAIDs. Pars plana vitrectomy has been used successfully to remove vitreal debris to improve vision, delay progression of the clinical signs, and reduce the frequency of "attacks."

NSAIDs, nonsteroidal anti-inflammatory drugs.

in a dark area with mydriasis using 1% tropicamide is recommended. The direct ophthalmoscope provides the most magnified view of the equine fundus, with a lateral magnification of ×7.9 and an axial magnification of ×8.4. Indirect ophthalmoscopy with a 14-D lens provides a magnified view with a lateral magnification of ×1.18 and an axial magnification of ×1.86, whereas a 20-D lens minifies the fundic view with a lateral and an axial magnification of ×0.79 and ×0.84, respectively. A 20-D lens provides a nice panoramic, screening view of the equine fundus, but it is not satisfactory for detailed, highly magnified observations.

The retinal vasculature is classified as being paurangiotic, with 50 to 80 small-diameter retinal arterioles and venules arising from the edge of the disc and extending only a short distance from the optic nerve head (Fig. 13-13). The equine retina primarily depends on the choroid for its blood supply. Vascularized remnants of the hyaloid artery may be seen in the central area of the optic disc. The retina itself is divided into dorsal tapetal and ventral nontapetal regions. The nontapetal region is usually brown to dark brown in color because of melanin in the retinal pigment epithelium (RPE), but this pigment may be absent depending on the horse's coat and iris coloration. The tapetal fundus is usually yellow to blue-green, but

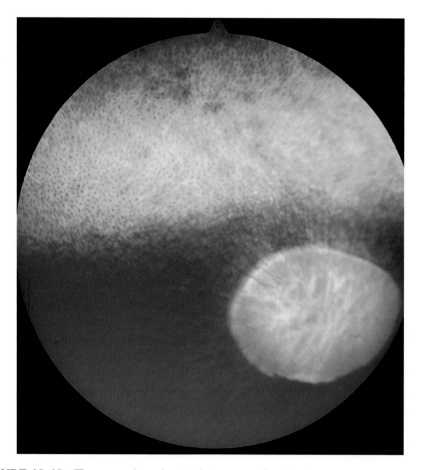

FIGURE 13-13. *The normal equine optic nerve and retina.*

variation can occur because of, again, the horse's coat or iris color. Color diluents, subalbinotic or albinotic coat-colored horses, or horses with heterochromia iridis or blue irides may have no tapetum, areas of tapetal thinning, or lack of pigment in the nontapetal retina such that choroidal vessel patterns can be observed. **Small dots (i.e., "Stars of Winslow") distributed in a uniform pattern throughout the tapetal fundus represent end-on views of the choroidal capillaries that penetrate the tapetum.**

The optic nerve head (or optic disc) is oval to round in the horse, and it is located slightly temporal, in the inferior quadrant of the nontapetal fundus. It is somewhat pink to orange in color. The equine optic disc is easily differentiated into the optic cup and the neuroretinal rim regions, with the visible fenestrations in the central region of the optic disc being the lamina cribrosa. The cup:disc ratio in the horse is quite large (average, 0.61).

Congenital alterations of the equine ocular fundus are uncommon. Atypical retinal colobomas have been noted, both singly and in groups, in both the tapetal and the nontapetal fundic regions and have been reported to be unilateral. Visual hemifield deficits were reported in one horse with a large coloboma near the optic nerve head. Congenital retinal detachments are associated with blindness and may be unilateral or bilateral. They also may be hereditary or associated with multiple ocular abnormalities. Retinal dysplasia or folds within the retinal layers, peripheral retinal cysts, and optic nerve hypoplasia have been reported in foals, and chorioretinitis has been noted in foals born to mares with respiratory disease during the late gestational period.

CHORIORETINITIS

Chorioretinitis manifests in the equine eye as "bullet-hole lesions," diffuse chorioretinal lesions, nontapetal "horizontal band" lesions, and peripapillary chorioretinitis. **"Bullet-hole" chorioretinitis may be seen as white, focal or multifocal, circular lesions ventral to the optic disc that typically have a hyperpigmented center surrounded by a white, depigmented zone.** Viral-mediated infarctions of the choroid result in RPE depigmentation at the periphery of the infarct and RPE hypertrophy at the central region. Regarding the pathogenesis of these lesions, EHV-1 has been implicated. Acute lesions demonstrate foci of gray-white retinal edema. A few "bullet-hole" lesions probably have little significance, but 20 or more focal lesions in one eye may produce subtle to obvious visual loss.

Diffuse chorioretinal lesions are less common and manifest as circular, band-shaped, or vermiform lesions in the tapetum or nontapetum. Tapetal lesions are associated with tapetal hyperreflectivity, and nontapetal lesions are associated with RPE depigmentation and hyperpigmentation. Widespread retinal or choroidal inflammation (or both), choroidal infarction, massive blood loss, or severe head trauma may induce these lesions. Varying degrees of optic nerve degeneration and atrophy may occur as well.

"Horizontal band" lesions in the nontapetum occur one to two optic disc diameters ventral to the optic nerve head, and they radiate across the posterior pole from the nasal ora ciliaris retinae to the temporal ora. They are associated with visual deficits or complete blindness and may result from vascular infarction. There is no treatment.

Active peripapillary chorioretinitis is associated with ERU and may result in focal "bullet-hole" lesions or larger, "butterfly"-shaped lesions adjacent to the optic nerve head. Active lesions also may be associated with optic neuritis and can develop into secondary retinal detachments because of vitreoretinal adhesions. Identifying inactive peripapillary scars in visual eyes during purchase examinations can be confusing, at least in terms of their significance. If no anterior segment lesions are associated with the scars, ERU can probably be removed from consideration as a cause of the retinal lesions. Many horses have small to large peripapillary scars, with no visual deficits or evidence of ERU.

PROGRESSIVE RETINAL ATROPHY

Progressive retinal atrophy is uncommon in the horse, but it can be observed in Thoroughbreds. Clinical signs include progressive visual impairment, multifocal depigmented areas with hyperpigmented centers (primarily in the nontapetal fundus), nyctalopia early in the disease, and optic atrophy late in disease.

CONGENITAL STATIONARY NIGHT BLINDNESS

Congenital stationary night blindness is found in the Appaloosa breed, in which it is possibly inherited as a sex-linked recessive trait. It is also noted, however, in Thoroughbreds, Paso Finos, and Standardbreds. Clinical signs include visual impairment in dim light (with generally normal vision in daylight), behavioral uneasiness and unpredictability at night, and a normal ophthalmoscopic examination. Foals may appear to be disoriented, stare off into space, and have a bilateral dorsomedial strabismus. This disease rarely progresses, but in a few case, it can produce poor photopic vision. The diagnosis is established on the basis of electroretinography, with decreased scotopic b-wave amplitude and a large, negative, monotonic a-wave potential. The true incidence of this disease in Appaloosas is not known. There is no treatment, and affected horses should not be used for breeding.

EQUINE MOTOR NEURON DISEASE RETINOPATHY

Accumulation in the RPE cells of a substance with the characteristics of ceroid lipofuscin is associated with the neurodegenerative condition known as equine motor neuron disease (EMND). A mosaic pattern of dark to yellow-brown pigmentation in the tapetum of affected horses is noted in association with a horizontal band of pigmentation at the tapetal–nontapetal junction. Consistent evidence of vitamin E deficiency (<1.799 μg/mL) in horses with EMND is suggestive that the RPE, retinal, and spinal lesions result from oxidative injury associated with a deficiency of nutritionally derived antioxidants. Supplementation with vitamin E, 6000 IU/day, in horses with EMND may stabilize the neurologic signs, but whether this will affect the RPE and the retinal changes is not known.

RETINAL DETACHMENTS

Retinal detachment (or separation from the RPE) is associated with slowly progressive or acute blindness in the horse. Exudative and traction detachments are also found. Clinically, total retinal detachments are seen as free-floating, undulating, opaque veils overlying the optic disc. The tapetum is hyperreflective as well. **Retinal detachments are a complication of the posterior segment inflammation from ERU, head trauma, or perforating globe wounds, and they also may occur secondary to tumors. The surgical treatment of retinal detachments in the horse has not been reported.**

OPTIC NERVE HYPOPLASIA

Optic nerve hypoplasia in the horse is characterized by varying degrees of visual impairment (or total blindness), mydriasis with slow to absent pupillary light reflexes, small and pale optic discs with absent optic disc vessels, and posterior depression of the optic disc by several diopters. The cause is a congenital lack of retinal ganglion cell development or excessive destruction of the embryonic ganglion cells.

OPTIC NERVE ATROPHY

Optic nerve atrophy in the horse occurs secondary to the inflammation of optic neuritis and ERU or from noninflammatory causes such as trauma, glaucoma, toxicity, and blood loss.

PROLIFERATIVE OPTIC NEUROPATHY

Proliferative optic neuropathy is a condition found primarily in older horses. **It is characterized by a slowly enlarging, yellow-white mass protruding from the optic disc and into the vitreous that has only a minimal effect on vision.** This lesion is unilateral, and histopathologically, it resembles a schwannoma. There is no therapy.

EXUDATIVE OPTIC NEURITIS

Exudative optic neuritis occurs rarely and is found in older horses. It manifests as a sudden onset of total blindness, and it is a bilateral condition. The optic discs are swollen, and retinal as well as optic disc hemorrhages may occur. The cause is not known.

ISCHEMIC OPTIC NEUROPATHY

Used for the treatment of epistaxis caused by guttural pouch mycosis, ischemic optic neuropathy resulting from arterial occlusion of the internal carotid, external carotid, and greater palatine arteries can result in sudden, irreversible blindness to the eye on the surgically operated side. Possibly, only the maxillary artery should be occluded on each side of the lesion; regardless, however, the risk of ischemia to the optic nerve remains. Optic nerve head congestion and nerve fiber layer involvement are prominent lesions. Severe blood loss may cause bilateral blindness in horses, though the exact mechanism for this is not yet understood.

DISORDERS OF THE VITREOUS

Vitreitis is common among horses with ERU. Exudates of cells and fibrin from the choroid accumulate in the vitreous, thereby causing vitreal opacities. The vitreous may appear to have a yellow-green color as a result of the fibrin and porphyrin metabolites. Severe vitreal inflammation promotes vitreous syneresis, and it may contribute to cataract formation. Vitreal fibrin also may form traction bands, thus causing retinal detachments. Most horses older than 6 years of age have vitreal degeneration that manifests by vitreal floaters and strands. Asteroid hyalosis is an incidental finding among older horses.

PHOTIC HEADSHAKING

Photic headshaking (i.e., head tossing) behavior in the horse has been described. The role of light in this behavior has been assessed by blindfolding the horses, placing them in darkened environments, or placing eye masks over their eyes. Headshaking behavior improved significantly when the amount of light striking the horses' eyes was diminished. Most horses were asymptomatic during the winter months; the headshaking behavior was commonly initiated with the onset of exercise. A condition in these horses similar to the photic sneeze of humans has been suggested as the causative mechanism. Otitis media/interna, guttural pouch disease, upper respiratory tract disease, and oral as well as ocular diseases, however, must be ruled out as a cause. The mechanism for photic headshaking in the horse may be a form of optic-trigeminal nerve summation, in which optic nerve stimulation produces referred sensation to the nasal cavity. Sunlight may stimulate parasympathetic activity in the infraorbital nerve, or the facial sensory branch of the trigeminal nerve, and thereby produce irritating nasal sensations that explain the rubbing, sneezing, and flipping of the nose and the head as seen in photic headshaking behavior. **A favorable response to oral cyproheptadine, which is an antihistamine serotonin antagonist given at a dose of 0.3 mg/kg twice daily, occurs in most horses, and melatonin therapy may be beneficial as well.** Bilateral infraorbital neurectomy can be used for medically refractory cases if infraorbital nerve blocks ameliorate the behavior.

THE PREPURCHASE OPHTHALMIC EXAMINATION

A complete ocular examination of both eyes using a focal light source (e.g., a transilluminator and a direct ophthalmoscope) should be part of every overall examination of the performance horse. The eye examination before purchase is performed by a veterinarian who represents the buyer, and it is designed to detect any congenital or hereditary ocular abnormalities as well as any active disease that might lead to decreased vision (e.g., cataracts, uveitis). Minor signs of eye disease that are overlooked at this examination may lead to vision loss, rider injury, and lawsuits. The purpose for which the horse is to be used determines the emphasis to be placed on any ocular problems that may be noticed; for example, a horse with a large corneal scar may be unsuitable for young children but satisfactory for more mature riders. Some horses also may need to be re-examined before their suitability can be determined (Box 13-2). The cornea should be clear, smooth, and shiny; corneas that appear to be dull and roughen may be ulcerated, edematous, or scarred. Corneal scars from previous injuries or ulcerations may pose no problem for the horse's vision if they are small or located near the limbus. Large scars in the central cornea, however, may be associated with less-than-satisfactory vision and should be evaluated carefully. The presence of corneal striae or corneal endothelial "band opacities" in nonbuphthalmic equine eyes warrants a high degree of suspicion for equine glaucoma.

Cataracts or lens opacities are always important, because they may be progressive and be associated with visual impairment. Lens opacities are best seen when the pupil is dilated and the examination is performed in complete darkness. Normal aging of the equine lens will produce cloudiness of the lens nucleus (i.e., nuclear sclerosis) beginning at 7 to 8 years of age, but this should not be confused with a true cataract.

Equine recurrent uveitis is the most common cause of blindness in the horse. Buyers should be made aware of any evidence concerning previous episodes of active ERU, because the clinical signs may recur. Corneal scarring, iris synechiae and depigmentation, cataracts, aqueous flare, vitreal floaters, and chorioretinal degeneration manifesting as "butterfly lesions" are common indications of uveitis. The nontapetal region ventral to the optic disc should be carefully examined with a direct ophthalmoscope, because this is where the focal retinal scars are seen. Large areas of retinal depigmentation and degeneration are suggestive that the animal has a blind spot of at least the size of the scar and, therefore, may have reduced vision as well.

Retinal detachments may be congenital, traumatic, or secondary to ERU, and they are serious faults because of their association with loss of vision. Vitreal floaters can develop with age or be sequelae to ERU, may cause some headshaking (in a few horses), but generally are benign in nature. Optic nerve atrophy can relate to ERU, glaucoma, or trauma, and it can also be associated with blindness. Proliferative lesions of the optic nerve may be noted among older horses but usually are not sight- or life-threatening.

Vision should be assessed during the examination using ophthalmoscopy as well as the dazzle and menace reflexes. Appaloosas should be examined in both the light and the dark to detect any evidence of night blindness. Maze testing with blinkers alternatively covering each eye also may provide information regarding any subtle or unilateral visual deficits.

To avoid litigation, inform the potential buyer of what was—and was not—done during the examination because of the limitations of the

---

BOX 13-2

Classification of Equine Lesions

   I. *Suitable:* No visible lesion or a nonprogressive lesion. No loss of vision or vision-threatening disease detected.

  II. *Unsuitable:* Eye disease leading to insufficient vision for safety. Inherited disorder in a breeding animal.

 III. *Provisionally suitable:* Suspicious disease or lesion. Suggest examination by an ophthalmologist.

 IV. *Reexamine:* After therapy or after no therapy.

  V. *Unsuitable lesions:*

    Blindness for any reason (one or both eyes).

    Mature cataract.

    Acute or chronic lesions of uveitis (anterior or posterior synechiae and small or large peripapillary chorioretinal scars).

    Large corneal scar in the visual axis.

    Ocular neoplasia.

    Corneal striae or "band opacities."

    Posterior subcapsular cataract (often progressive).

    Partial or total retinal detachment in one eye.

    Large numbers of vitreal floaters.

    Optic nerve atrophy.

---

equipment available. In most cases, the veterinarian is examining an eye without any overt clinical signs. The findings of the ocular examination should be related to the intended use of the animal, and the possibility that any lesion noted could progress to interfere with vision should be assessed. The intended functions of the horse must be considered when determining whether any ocular lesions that may be present are unimportant or "safe" for the horse and its rider, and whether the horse can satisfactorily perform its intended functions. Some eye problems might not preclude use of that horse in a manmade arena, in which unexpected visual stimuli are unlikely to be present and the rider is both experienced and aware of any specific shortcomings in that horse's vision. Many examples of horses with varying degrees of blindness can perform at a high level in various types of equestrian competitions; horses with "suspicious" or subtle signs of ocular disease should not necessarily be excluded. The importance of ocular lesions with an uncertain significance may be determined if the horse is reexamined over a period of several months. If the horse is a brood mare, the genetic nature of any ocular lesion should be considered as well.

14

Food Animal Ophthalmology

Ophthalmic diseases of cattle, sheep, goats, and pigs are as variable as those in other species. **Ophthalmic diseases with a significant financial impact can be very important in food animals.** For example, in 1988, ocular squamous cell carcinoma (OSCC) was the leading cause (17%) of carcass condemnation at slaughterhouses inspected by the U.S. Department of Agriculture. In 1984, infectious bovine keratoconjunctivitis (IBK) resulted in an economic loss in the United States that was conservatively estimated at $200 million.

INCIDENCE OF OPHTHALMIC DISEASES IN FOOD ANIMALS

The incidence of ophthalmic disease among food animals is estimated on the basis of information derived from slaughterhouse material, veterinary medicine teaching hospitals, and disease outbreaks. **In one study of Brown Swiss cattle, 18.8% showed ocular abnormalities, and the incidence increased with age. In cattle 6 years of age or younger, the incidence was 3%. In those between 7 and 14 years of age, it increased to 43%, and in still older animals, as many as 75% were affected. In another report that used abattoir-derived data, the incidence of acquired ophthalmic lesions (not including the eyelids) was 14.6%, and of these affected animals, 6.3% had neoplastic lesions and 9.2% inflammatory conditions.** Herefords also had significantly more ocular lesions, both neoplastic and inflammatory, than other breeds of cattle. **Congenital ocular lesions (as a percentage of congenital defects) varied from 3.5% in sheep to 5.5% in swine (including cyclopia, anophthalmia, and microphthalmia) to 18.7% in cattle.** In cattle albinism (either complete or

377

incomplete), blindness, anophthalmia, heterochromia iridis, microphthalmia, and retinal dysplasia are the most frequent anomalies. Entropion is the most common congenital eye disease in sheep, and among severely affected flocks, approximately 80% of lambs may be affected. In swine, microphthalmia and anophthalmia are the most common defects.

DISEASES OF THE ORBIT AND GLOBE

Microphthalmia is one of the more frequent eye defects among food animals. It is sometimes reported as anophthalmos, thereby suggesting a deficiency of the forebrain neural ectoderm before the optic sulci has formed. Closer inspection of these eyes, however, usually reveals microphthalmia, which is the presence of rudimentary ocular tissue resulting either from a deficiency in the optic vesicle or, later, from the failure of normal growth and expansion by the optic cup. **Microphthalmia usually is combined with other ocular defects, and these may include corneal opacities, cataracts, aniridia, corectopia, persistent pupillary membranes, and various retinal abnormalities, such as folds, retinal nonattachment, and retinal detachment (Fig. 14-1).** Congenital anophthalmia/ microphthalmia syndrome with malformations of the posterior vertebral column occurs in dairy and beef cattle, and though the exact cause is known, but some cases have been speculated to have an hereditary basis. Congenital microphthalmia (i.e., anophthalmia) with caudal vertebral anomalies such as wedge vertebra, hemivertebra, and sagittal cleft verte-

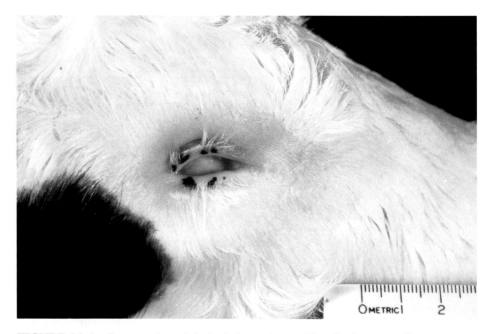

FIGURE 14-1. *Severe microphthalmia in an Angus-Hereford cross-calf.*

bra has been reported in Japanese Brown cattle. Microphthalmia has also been reported in sheep and swine, but no cause has been determined in those cases.

TERATOGENIC AGENTS

Several agents may impair ophthalmic development in food animals. Some of these agents also have critical "windows" of time during ophthalmic development for the teratogenic effect to occur.

Veratrum californicum

The common names of *Veratrum californicum* include skunk cabbage, western hellebore, false hellebore, and wild corn, and teratogenic ocular defects may occur with ingestion of *V. californicum* in sheep. **Various globe abnormalities, such as anophthalmia, cyclopia, and synophthalmia, may be induced in lambs by the maternal ingestion of *V. californicum.*** The incidence of malformations may be as great as 25% and occur by feeding sheep both fresh and dried *V. californicum*. The specific agents responsible are a group of alkaloids (e.g., jervine, pseudojervine, isorubijervine, veratrosine) that occur throughout the plant but are concentrated in the roots.

Sheep embryos are highly susceptible to the teratogenic agents in *V. californicum* when the plant is eaten by the ewe on gestational day 14. In cases of cyclopia, this timing corresponds to the period of gastrulation and formation of the neural plate before separation of the optic fields. Ewes fed these plants on gestational days 11, 12, 13, 15, and 16 had normally developed fetuses or normally developed embryos that died between the eighteenth and the twenty-third day of embryonic development. Teratogenic effects of *V. californicum* have also been reported in cattle and goats.

Apholate

Congenital orbital anomalies in sheep have been associated with a polyfunctional alkylating agent, apholate, that is used as an insect chemosterilant. The congenital anomalies have consisted of anophthalmia, absence of the orbital cavities, and defective formation of the cranial and the facial bones. In these reports, the liver was ectopic, and the spleen was malpositioned.

Selenium

Historically, selenium has been credited with causing "blind staggers" in livestock and with being a teratogenic agent. Reported findings at necropsy that have been attributed to ewes grazing on seleniferous pastures include microphthalmia with multiple cysts; corneal, lens, and iris deficits; and colobomas of various structures. The results of subsequent studies, however, are suggestive that many of these field cases involving "blind staggers" were, in fact, sulfur-related polioencephalomalacia (PEM). Plants that bioaccumulate selenium are often associated with waters that are high in sulfate content, and high sulfate levels have been linked with PEM.

Other Teratogens

Maternal vitamin A deficiency in piglets has been linked with anophthalmia, microphthalmia, macrophthalmia, retinal dysplasia, and other ocular abnormalities. The degree of eye changes varies between litters, animals from the same litter, and even the eyes in the same animal. Several infectious agents have been associated with congenital ophthalmic anomalies in food animals, and these include the blue tongue virus (in sheep) and bovine viral diarrhea.

ABNORMALITIES OF GLOBE POSITION AND MOVEMENT

Of the food animal species, cattle seem to be affected most frequently by abnormalities in the position of the globe. Most of these animals are presented with bilateral and convergent globes (i.e., esotropia), but occasionally, they are presented with unilateral and divergent globes (i.e. exotropia). Most defects in globe position are inherited, and other eye diseases are not concurrent. Divergent bilateral strabismus, however, has been associated with hydrocephalus. **Bilateral convergent strabismus with exophthalmia is an autosomal recessive defect in Jersey and, perhaps, Shorthorn cattle. In the German Brown Swiss breed, the presence of additively acting genes best explain the relationship of affected animals in these pedigrees, and a dominant autosomal gene may be responsible. Esotropia also occurs in the Holstein, Ayrshire, and German Brown Swiss breeds.** Clinical signs include a progressive exophthalmia and esotropia until maturity. Nystagmus may be present as well, and vision is compromised.

The onset of strabismus in growing and adult cattle may signal the presence of a serious disease. **Bilateral dorsomedial strabismus is suggestive of PEM, and affected calves are frequently blind and exhibit opisthotonus. Listeriosis causing inflammation of the brainstem may impinge on the abducens nucleus, which can result in medial strabismus through loss of function in the lateral rectus muscle.** Unilateral strabismus or exophthalmia (or both) in cattle also may result from space-occupying orbital lesions that consist of inflammations and neoplasia.

ORBITAL NEOPLASIA

In cattle, lymphosarcoma affecting the retrobulbar tissues is the most frequent cause of bilateral exophthalmos, with and without strabismus. Other unilateral retrobulbar orbital neoplasms include metastatic squamous cell carcinoma and adenocarcinoma.

ORBITAL INFLAMMATIONS

Inflammatory orbital disease is common among cattle and involves the orbital tissue or tissues adjacent to the orbit. **Causes include traumatic wounds, chronic frontal sinusitis, puncture wounds of the eyelids or conjunctiva, foreign-body migration from the mouth to the retrobul-**

bar space, actinobacillosis, and panophthalmitis. Treatment involves identification of the underlying cause, topical and systemic antibiotics (possibly), hot packing, drainage and lavage for any nidi of infection, and if panophthalmitis is present, enucleation.

NYSTAGMUS

Nystagmus is an involuntary, rhythmic oscillation of the eyeball, either with equal movements (i.e., pendular) or with quick and slow phases (i.e., jerk), that can occur in any plane. The quick phase occurs in the direction of the rotation, can be elicited in normal animals, and is termed *physiologic* or *normal nystagmus*. In cattle, nystagmus may be either congenital or acquired. **A congenital rapid pendular nystagmus, which usually is horizontal, is observed among Holstein-Friesians especially and in other breeds as well. Clinical vision is not significantly affected, but the animals are affected for life. Other causes for acute-onset nystagmus include brain tumors and abscesses; intoxication by chemicals, plants, and heavy metals; cerebral anemia and vascular disease; and congenital or early postnatal blindness.**

EYELID DISEASES

Eyelids diseases are uncommon in cattle, goats, and pigs, but they occur frequently in sheep. Anatomic defects that cause corneal disease usually are treated with surgery. Entropion is an inversion of part (or all) of the eyelid margins, and it may result from congenital, spastic, and cicatricial causes. **Congenital entropion is relatively frequent among small domestic ruminants, and it usually affects the lower lid. The incidence of congenital entropion in sheep varies markedly between flocks, ranging from 1.0 to 80.0% (Fig. 14-2). In sheep, entropion may be inherited as a polygenic trait as well. With uncontrolled progression of the disease, an initial, serous epiphora may become mucopurulent. Secondary corneal ulceration and vascularization, keratouveitis, and endophthalmitis may develop as well. Treatment involves eversion of the affected eyelid, and a variety of techniques can be used.** Mechanical eversion using two or three metal wound clips adjacent to the eyelid margin or vertical mattress sutures may be used. When many lambs are involved, the staples or sutures are allowed to slough off several weeks later. If only a few lambs are affected by severe entropion and corneal disease, however, or if highly valuable individual animals are affected, a modified Hotz-Celsus technique is effective. Affected lambs should not be retained for breeding.

The pot-bellied pig also develops entropion, particularly when this animal becomes overweight. Surgical intervention is usually required, and successful use of a modified Hotz-Celsus procedure has been reported. A modified brow sling using either mersilene mesh or polyester suture coated with polybutilate can be effective in some cases. The large suture or mesh

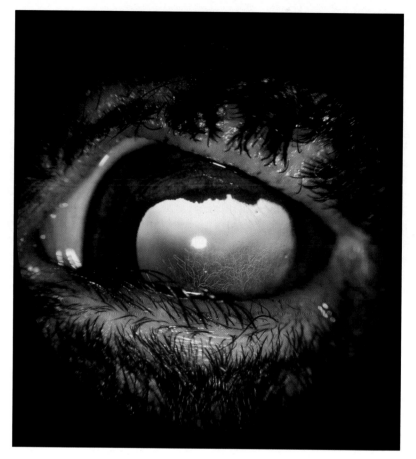

FIGURE 14-2. *Lower entropion and secondary keratitis in a lamb.*

acts as a scaffold for the attachment of fibroblasts, thereby facilitating development of a more permanent adhesion. Postoperative control of the animal's weight is important for long-term success of the surgery.

Entropion in cattle is rare, but it has been reported in the Simmental breed. Spastic and cicatricial entropion is more common than congenital entropion in this species, and surgical correction with the modified Hotz-Celsus procedure can be used for treatment.

ECTROPION

Ectropion (i.e., eversion of the eyelid) is less dangerous than entropion to the eye, but it can produce chronic keratitis, conjunctivitis, keratoconjunctivitis, epiphora, and tear staining as well as scalding of the eyelids. Ectropion may result from developmental, cicatricial, trauma, neurologic, and postoperative causes. **Congenital ectropion is rare, but it has been recorded in Piebald sheep.** Affected animals exhibit a gross deformity or notching of the upper eyelid. Ectropion occurs at the notch, with entropion occurring on either side. Surgical intervention is recommended when secondary ophthalmic disease results (see Chapter 3).

EYELID TRAUMA

Eyelid lacerations occur infrequently among food animals. The basic principles of eyelid closure, however, apply when such lacerations occur (see Chapter 3).

BLEPHARITIS

Inflammation of the eyelids may result from bacterial, fungal, parasitic, allergic, traumatic, and neoplastic causes. Most generalized skin diseases also may affect the periocular region and the eyelids. Causes and conditions of blepharitis among food animals include *Actinobacillus lignieresii*; clostridial diseases, especially *Clostridium* novyi; dermatophilosis (i.e., streptothricosis) from *Dermatophilus congolensis*; *Trichophyton* sp. in all food-producing animals; *Microsporum* sp. in pigs, sheep, and goats; and *Candida albicans* as a cause of optical eczema in Jersey cattle. Viral diseases that have been implicated in eyelid disease include pox viruses (in sheep and goats), ulcerative dermatosis virus, and papilloma virus. Primary blepharodermatitis may result from ectoparasites (e.g., mites, lice, ticks, keds). Sarcoptic mange results from *Sarcoptes scabiei*, with a subspecies being specific for each host species. The disease is uncommon in the United States, however, and is reportable. Treatment of all affected as well as exposed animals is indicated. Topical application of or dipping with lime sulfur, trichlorphon (0.2%), fenchlorphos, phosmet (20%), amitraz (0.1%), and coumaphos (0.1%) has been recommended. Ivermectin, 0.2 mg/kg, may be given orally to pigs or subcutaneously to cattle. *Demodex* sp. are host specific and may affect all food animals. The adult mites invade the hair follicles and sebaceous glands of the face, limbs, and back, which then become distended with the mites and inflammatory material. The disease tends to be generalized in goats and cattle, but the face is a site of predilection in pigs and sheep. In small ruminants, keds, lice, and ticks may cause pruritus and self-trauma.

Other miscellaneous causes, including photosensitization, also may produce blepharitis. Direct solar irritation (i.e., sunburn) may occur in food animals with little periocular pigmentation, but acute periocular dermatitis is more likely the result of photosensitization. If photosensitizing substances are present at sufficient concentration in the skin, dermatitis occurs when that skin is exposed to light. The causative photodynamic agents may be ingested in a preformed state (i.e., primary photosensitization), be the products of abnormal metabolism, or be the normal metabolic products that accumulate in tissues because of faulty hepatic excretion. Some of the primary photodynamic agents include hypericin in *Hypericum perforatum* (i.e., St. John's wort), fagopyrin in *Polygonum fagopyrum* (i.e., buckwheat), and perloline in *Lolium perenne* (i.e., perennial ryegrass). Miscellaneous agents include phenothiazine sulfoxide from phenothiazine as well as rose Bengal and acridine dyes. Treatment involves removing the affected animal from sunlight, preventing ingestion of further toxic material, and administering laxatives. Treatment of any underlying hepatic and biliary disease is also recommended. (For more details, the reader should consult the third edition, pp. 1124–1125.)

DISEASES OF THE NASOLACRIMAL SYSTEM

The nasolacrimal system is divided into the tear-producing glands and the tubular drainage apparatus. **In food animals, the tear-producing glands rarely have any primary abnormality, but epiphora and nasolacrimal drainage disorders do occur.** Epiphora is the most common abnormality among food animals, and it usually occurs secondary to irritative ocular disease. **Congenital abnormalities, including supernumerary openings of the nasolacrimal drainage apparatus, occur in cattle, with the Brown Swiss and the Holstein-Friesian breeds being affected. The openings on the face vary in distance from the medial canthus, but all the openings are connected in the proximal third of the nasolacrimal duct.** Dacryocystorhinography has been extremely useful in diagnosing anatomic defects in the nasolacrimal ducts.

DISEASES OF THE CONJUNCTIVA AND CORNEA

The conjunctiva and cornea are common sites for ophthalmic disease in food-producing animals, and such diseases can have profound economic effects. In cattle, IBK and squamous cell carcinomas dominate. In sheep and goats, infectious mycoplasma and chlamydia keratoconjunctivitis occur.

CONGENITAL ANOMALIES

Dermoids, which are a noncystic, developmental malformation characteristically containing components of the skin, occur principally (≤2% affected) in cattle, but they can occur in other species of food animals as well. The defect in Herefords is inherited, with the characteristics of autosomal recessive and polygenic inheritance. In cattle, the site predilection of ocular dermoids is, in decreasing order, the limbus, third eyelid, canthus, eyelid, and conjunctiva. Dermoids rarely appear bilaterally, except in certain lines of Hereford cattle. In some cases, other congenital defects may exist concurrently as well. **Surgical removal of dermoids is recommended if vision is impaired or the condition is causing pain.**

Inherited Corneal Dystrophy

Primary endothelial disease is extremely rare in food animals, but an autosomal recessive corneal disease has been reported among Holsteins and other cattle. Affected animals show bilateral corneal edema either at or soon after birth. The condition is not amenable to treatment, and affected animals should not be used for breeding. These conditions are as-sumed to result from a primary endothelial cell defect; however, low num-bers of endothelial cells have not been reported. If significant visual com-promise occurs, the affected animal should be culled. In addition, the recessive nature of the disease implies that parents of affected animals should not be used for breeding.

INFECTIOUS KERATOCONJUNCTIVITIS IN SHEEP AND GOATS

Infectious keratoconjunctivitis in sheep and goats has been associated with decreased twinning rates in ewes, increased rates of pregnancy toxemia, starvation, weight loss, blind ewes trampling offspring, and decreased economic return. Numerous infectious agents have been implicated; there-fore, the terms *pink-eye* and *heather blindness* or *blight* are used somewhat broadly, especially among small ruminants. (For more details, the reader should consult the third edition, pp. 1127–1131.)

Keratoconjunctivitis Associated with *Chlamydia* sp.

Chlamydia sp. of ophthalmic importance include *C. psittaci,* which is a di-verse group containing strains from a wide variety of animal sources. *Chlamydia* sp. may be the cause of primary ocular disease in several animal species, including sheep, goats, and swine, but they have also been isolated in cattle. **Chlamydia sp. in sheep are associated with an infectious ker-atoconjunctivitis that occurs worldwide. These strains of chlamydia organisms causing conjunctivitis and polyarthritis in sheep belong to the C. psittaci group. They are closely related to each other, but not to the abortion or the fecal strains.** Outbreaks usually occur during the lambing season, when ewes and lambs are confined and have maximal opportunity for contact and stress. Carrier animals may be reservoirs for the disease.

The pathogenesis of the organism is probably multifactorial, with the animal's immune status, secondary infection, and other factors all playing a role. Clinically, immunity appears to be of short duration, because ani-mals may be infected repeatedly.

Clinical signs begin within 4 days of infection, and initially, they in-clude epiphora, chemosis, and conjunctival hyperemia. By 11 days, the serous conjunctival exudates become more purulent, and blepharo-spasm occurs. Lymphoid follicles begin to develop by 23 days, but they can also develop as early as 6 days after inoculation with *Chlamydia* sp. and *Branhamella ovis*. The follicular reaction is not unique to this dis-ease. Approximately 10% of patients develop interstitial keratitis approxi-mately 1 week after the initial signs develop, along with deep vasculariza-tion and edema of the cornea. Permanent scarring and pigmentation of the cornea are infrequent complications.

The diagnosis of chlamydia is established on the basis of scrapings from the infected conjunctival epithelial cells early during the course of disease. New methylene blue, Wright's, or Giemsa stains reveal typical cytoplasmic inclusions in the infected cells. In one report, 80% of lambs had chlamydiae cultured at 14 days after experimental inoculation, but by 18 days, chlamydiae usually could not be isolated. Immunofluorescent antibody tests, however, could detect chlamydial antigens 5 weeks after infection; thus, fluorescent antibody tests may be more sensitive than culture for detecting chlamydiae.

Culture during the latter stages of chlamydia-induced ocular disease may show a variety of commensals, such as *B. ovis*. Failure to culture chlamydiae during the latter part of the disease process, however, does not necessarily preclude *Chlamydia* sp. as the initial causative agent. **Treatment efficacy is also difficult to evaluate with a self-limiting disease, but systemic tetracyclines do shorten the course.**

Keratoconjunctivitis Associated with *Mycoplasma* sp.

Mycoplasma **sp. cause keratoconjunctivitis in goats and sheep, both clinically and experimentally. Subclinical carrier states of *Mycoplasma* sp. exist as well. In some animals, *Mycoplasma conjunctivae* is not associated with clinical disease.** This may result from differences in the pathogenicity of individual strains, or the samples studied may have been obtained just before the development of clinical signs. **The respective conjunctival isolates for goats and sheep were *M. mycoides* var *capri* and *M. conjunctivae* var *ovis*.** Concurrent presence of *B. ovis, Escherichia coli,* and *Staphylococcus aureus* may enhance the severity of the disease.

Clinical signs may vary slightly between goats and sheep. **There is an initial hyperemia of the palpebral and conjunctival vessels, serous lacrimation, and blepharospasm. Keratitis with superficial and deep vascularization usually develops as well. In more advanced cases among sheep, a mucopurulent conjunctivitis, occasional follicular conjunctivitis, iritis with hypopyon, and corneal ulceration occur (Fig. 14-3). Phthisis bulbi rarely results, however, and the disease usually lasts between 1 and 4 weeks.** Generally, older sheep are more severely affected. Goats usually do not develop corneal ulcers or hypopyon, but permanent corneal opacity and blindness may result.

The diagnosis of infection with *Mycoplasma* sp. is established on the basis of the clinical signs and the results of conjunctival cytology, culture, and serology. Cytologic preparations can use Giemsa stain, carbol basic fuchsin stain of Gimenez, or Gram's stain. In acute mycoplasmal keratoconjunctivitis, there are large numbers of neutrophils but no plasma cells. Intracytoplasmic coccobacillary and ring-shaped bodies may be observed in the epithelial cells with *Mycoplasma* sp. infection, and bright-field as well as dark-ground examination of Giemsa-stained smears demonstrate *Mycoplasma* sp. in scrapings from the conjunctivae of affected (and even healthy) sheep.

The organism can also be cultured—provided that special nutrient requirements and incubation methods are used. Previous use of antibiotics, however, can interfere with growth of the organism on culture. Serology, including complement fixation, indirect hemagglutination, and enzyme-linked immunosorbent assays (ELISA), may be helpful in establishing the

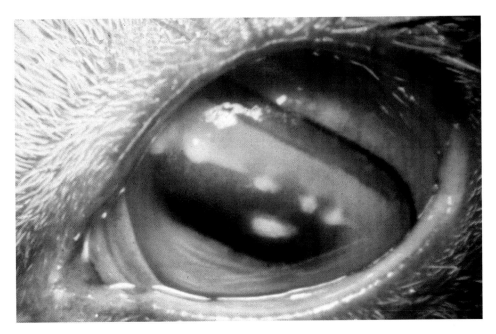

FIGURE 14-3. *Keratoconjunctivitis associated with mycoplasmal infection approximately 7 to 10 days after the onset of clinical signs. Note the focal corneal abscesses and the neovascularization.*

diagnosis. ELISA tests in goats may be used to detect subclinical mycoplasmal infection and individual carriers, which may assist in determining control measures.

Mild infections are often self-limiting, but therapy with antibiotics (e.g., tetracycline) can shorten the course of disease and is indicated among cases with considerable corneal involvement. **Treatment may not eliminate *M. conjunctivae*, however, and may even promote a carrier state. Oxytetracycline, either topically or intramuscularly 20 mg/kg, is the drug of choice.** Minimal inhibitory concentrations as well as minimal mycoplasmacidal concentrations of various antibiotics are suggestive that tylosin, streptomycin, and chlortetracycline as well as oxytetracycline should be recommended for use.

Development of immunity to subsequent infection may be possible. Lambs experimentally infected with *M. conjunctivae* have shown evidence of both local and systemic antibody production, and seroconversion has been shown in adult ewes inoculated with *Mycoplasma* sp. Diseases that may be concurrent with mycoplasmal conjunctivitis include mastitis, pleuropneumonia, and arthritis in sheep and goats. *Mycoplasma agalactiae* has been associated with mastitis, arthritis, and conjunctivitis, with pregnant animals being more severely affected than nonpregnant animals. *Acholeplasma oculi* has been implicated as the cause of keratoconjunctivitis in sheep, with approximately 25% of affected animals also exhibiting blepharospasm, conjunctivitis, keratitis, and pannus in one report. Subsequently, approximately half the flock was affected, and treatment with subconjunctival oxytetracycline was successful.

Bacterial Keratoconjunctivitis in Sheep and Goats

Cases of keratoconjunctivitis in sheep and goats have been attributed to *B. ovis* (formerly known as *Neisseria ovis*), either alone or in combination with other micro-organisms. The role of *Branhamella* sp. as a primary pathogen has been questioned by some authors, however, because this organism may be a common component in the conjunctival flora of normal eyes. *Branhamella ovis* is found in conjunctival scrapings from affected as well as healthy sheep, and both smooth and rough types of *B. ovis* have been identified. Experimentally, these colonial variants have been used, either alone or together with *M. conjunctivae* and *C. psittaci*, to induce conjunctivitis.

CHLAMYDIAL KERATOCONJUNCTIVITIS IN SWINE AND CATTLE

Pigs with chlamydial keratoconjunctivitis show a combination of conjunctivitis and keratoconjunctivitis, with or without mucopurulent rhinitis. *Mycoplasma bovoculi* has also been reported in the microflora of normal cattle and, in addition, to be associated with ocular disease. Herd outbreaks with conjunctivitis and epiphora resulting from infection with *M. bovoculi* and *Ureaplasma* sp. have occurred; however, cattle younger than 2 years are more frequently infected with *Mycoplasma* sp. (62.5%) than older cattle (19.4%).

INFECTIOUS BOVINE KERATOCONJUNCTIVITIS

Infectious bovine keratoconjunctivitis, which is also known as pinkeye, contagious ophthalmia, and New Forest disease, has received considerable attention because of its worldwide distribution and economic impact. Financial losses result from decreased weight gain, cost of feeding during the nongaining or the weight loss period, and treatment costs for affected animals. **In 1984, the economic loss was conservatively estimated at $200 million in the United States alone. Similarly, an estimated $23.5 million was lost each year during the early 1980s in Australia because of lost production and treatment costs.**

Incidence

Infectious bovine keratoconjunctivitis occurs worldwide. **The prevalence may be as great as 4.5% of adults and 10% of calves, and with 45% of farms being affected by the disease. In a 5-year study, the average infection rate was 75% for calves and 63% for cows; however, only 58% of the infected calves and 16% of the infected cows developed clinical signs of disease.** This significantly lower rate of clinical disease despite the high rate of infection is suggestive that a limited immunity can be developed.

Infectious bovine keratoconjunctivitis occurs primarily during the summer months, though winter outbreaks can occur. This seasonal fluctuation may result from the increased presence of hemolytic *M. bovis*, the fly population, and increased solar radiation during the summer months. The decline through the fall season may result from the lack of susceptible calves, fewer vectors, and decreased intensity of the enhancing factors.

Etiology

Moraxella bovis, **which is a Gram-negative bacillus, is considered to be the cause of IBK.** Other pathogens that may contribute to the severity of IBK, however, include infectious bovine rhinotracheitis (IBR) and *Mycoplasma* sp. Concurrent infection with the IBR virus may occur and cause more severe clinical signs than those of IBK alone. An increased prevalence of IBK also may occur in animals that have been vaccinated for IBR. *Mycoplasma* sp. have been speculated to play an ancillary role in IBK as well. The morphology of in vitro *Moraxella bovis* colonies is either rough or smooth. Clinical cases of IBK are associated with the rough type, which have cell-surface pili, autoagglutinate in distilled water, and hemagglutinate. *Moraxella bovis* colonies are easy to identify, and they do not require complex growth media . Characteristic growth patterns may be used to aid in bacterial differentiation, and β-hemolytic variants are usually associated with clinical disease. Spontaneous transformation from the rough to the smooth colony type also occurs in the laboratory.

Electron microscopy has revealed that cells from the rough colonies of *M. bovis* are piliated, whereas those from the smooth colonies are nonpiliated. The capsular pili, which promote cellular adhesion, enhance the ability to overcome host defenses, and they have been used in the production of IBK vaccines. **Electron microscopic studies have shown that the piliated form can result in disease, but that the non-piliated form is nonpathogenic.** Colonies that stain with crystal violet (i.e., the rough type) contain pili. As a general rule, the piliated, hemolytic form is found in acute cases of IBK, and proportionately more smooth, nonpiliated, and nonhemolytic isolates are recovered from convalescent and clinically normal carrier cattle. Pilus biotyping is possible using immunofluorescence and immunogold electron microscopy. The pili are classified into seven different groups, and isolates show little antigenic variation.

Transmission

The source of infection within a herd is usually a new animal or a previously affected one. The nonhemolytic *M. bovis* may reside in the herd during the winter months and produce no clinical signs. With the onset of spring and increased ultraviolet (UV) radiation, however, a reversion to the pathogenic, hemolytic form can occur, along with subsequent infection of susceptible calves. *Moraxella bovis* is transmitted by animal handlers or by direct contact with infected animals, contact with fomites, and mechanical vectors such as flies (e.g., face fly [*Musca autumnalis*], house fly [*Musca domestica*], and stable fly [*Stomoxys calcitrans*]).

Predisposing Factors

All breeds of cattle may be affected, but breed-related differences in susceptibility occur as well. *Bos indicus* breeds are more resistant than *Bos taurus* breeds, and Herefords as well as Hereford crossbreeds appear to have a much higher susceptibility, as do Murray Grays. The increased risk of clinical disease among younger cattle as well as the increased severity of disease among calves, however, are

consistent findings. Older cattle are more resistant and less severely affected than younger cattle. Developmental immunity is also suggested by observations of infected calves that develop disease while their dams, which are also infected, fail to develop any clinical signs. Even so, older animals are still infected at high rates. Cattle younger than 2 years of age have the highest morbidity rate, however, and also the most severe clinical signs.

Increased levels of UV radiation have been linked to the development of IBK, because a high correlation exists between the annual peak incidence of IBK and the annual peak levels of UV radiation. In addition, calf corneas subjected to UV radiation and *M. bovis* infection are more damaged than corneas subjected to UV radiation alone. Ultraviolet radiation also causes degeneration of the corneal epithelium and enhances *M. bovis*–induced keratitis in mice. The effect of UV light on the immune response in bovine eyes, however, is unknown.

The number of face flies present also correlates well with the infection rate and with the number of new isolates. Once the number of flies exceed 10 per animal, IBK spreads from one herd to another. Other environmental factors, such as mechanical irritants to the conjunctiva and cornea and the ingestion of aflatoxin, have also been suggested as enhancing factors.

Development of IBK additionally relates to the intrinsic virulence factors associated with *M. bovis,* such as the presence or absence of pili and hemolysin. Pili enhance the attachment of bacteria in vitro and enable maintenance of an established infection. Different strains of *M. bovis,* however, as well as different isolates of the same strain, may vary in virulence. This pleomorphism may explain the variation in disease expression and the unpredictable response to vaccinations that have been observed.

Pathogenesis

During clinical outbreaks of IBK, *M. bovis* can be isolated from most affected cattle. **The initial corneal lesions probably result from bacterial cytotoxicity, whereas the advanced lesions may be associated with bacterial/host inflammatory interaction.** *Moraxella bovis* does not produce collagenase, but gelatinase and DNAase have been detected in whole cultures. Numerous neutrophils surround the corneal lesions as well, and these may contain phagocytosed organisms. *Moraxella bovis* has a marked cytotoxicity for bovine neutrophils and corneal epithelial cells. The pathophysiology of IBK likely is associated with collagenase release from the damaged epithelial cells, fibroblasts, and neutrophils, not from *M. bovis.*

Clinical Signs

In 75% of cases, the ocular involvement is unilateral, but subsequent bilateral involvement also is frequent. **Affected animals are reluctant to compete for food or position, milk production is reduced, and weight gain is suppressed, usually in direct relation to the severity of the lesion.** Considerable variation among disease expression may be evident between animals, however. In young cattle, the disease is usually more severe, with a longer recovery period (2–6 weeks), than in older cattle. **The earliest signs are varying degrees of epiphora, blepharospasm, and photo-**

phobia, but conjunctival hyperemia and chemosis also occur. Within 24 to 48 hours after the onset of clinical signs, the axial cornea may develop small epithelial defects, which often are visible only at slit-lamp biomicroscopy (Fig. 14-4). **A small, pale, yellow to white raised abscess may appear near the center of the cornea, and during the following 24 to 48 hours, the corneal opacity may increase in size or slough, thus leaving a shallow, round to oval, superficial ulcer with perilesional edema. Ulceration may be preceded by small corneal vesicles. During the next few days, the corneal ulcer may expand and deepen (Fig. 14-5).**

Marked, circumcorneal hyperemia of the conjunctival vessels and initiation of superficial corneal vascularization occur as well. The eye is painful, thereby making both the ophthalmic examination and treatment difficult. Mild to moderate anterior chamber aqueous humor flare and iridocyclitis are present, and the conjunctival exudate becomes mucopurulent, with matting of the eyelashes. Superficial corneal vascularization proceeds rapidly toward the primary central lesion, and by 7 to 9 days after infection, the well-delineated corneal ulcer is surrounded by an area of inflammation and large networks of superficial corneal blood vessels extending centrally from the limbus. When the superficial vascularization reaches the center of the cornea, the corneal opacity tends to clear, from the periphery toward the center. **The ulcer then epithelializes, and the facet gradually reduces through stromal regeneration, thus leaving a slightly raised, dense scar. In 2 to 3 weeks, corneal healing is well advanced, and in 1 to 2 months, only a faint, localized, central corneal opacity may remain.** The keratoconjunctivitis may, however, result in secondary iridocyclitis, hypopyon, synechiae, and even panophthalmitis.

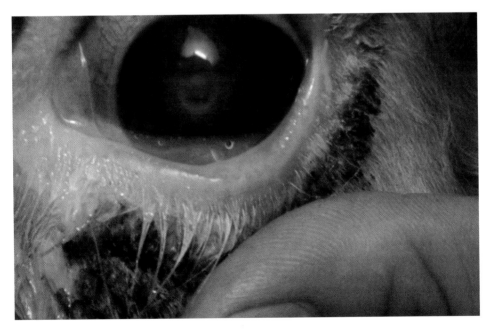

FIGURE 14-4. *Early, faint fluorescein retention in a central cornea affected with infectious bovine keratoconjunctivitis.*

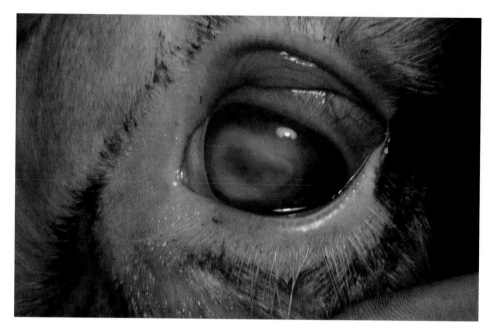

FIGURE 14-5. *Large, central corneal ulcer surrounded by a cellular infiltrate associated with infectious bovine keratoconjunctivitis.*

Infrequently, perforation of the corneal ulcer results in iris prolapse, in which case blindness may result. In addition, the eye may become buphthalmic (from secondary glaucoma) or phthisical.

Medical Treatment

A plethora of information exists regarding appropriate therapy for IBK. Unfortunately, however, most studies are hindered by a lack of suitable controls and by the self-limiting nature of the disease itself. **Therapy for IBK is recommended to relieve pain, to enable animals to remain as productive as possible, and to prevent further spread of the disease. Fortunately, *M. bovis* is sensitive to most antibiotics, but differences among regions and strains in susceptibility patterns necessitate culture and sensitivity testing to select a specific antibiotic, especially during a severe outbreak.** Penicillin, ampicillin, oxytetracycline, ormetoprim-sulfadimethoxine, furazolidone, gentamicin, neomycin, and erythromycin have all been recommended. *Moraxella bovis* usually is resistant to tylosin, lincomycin, and erythromycin, however, and it has variable susceptibility to cloxacillin. **The major difficulty generally is the administration of antibiotics for a sufficient period of time to ensure completely elimination of the *M. bovis*. Dairy operations therefore may chose procaine penicillin because of the short milk-withdrawal times, whereas nonlabor-intensive beef operations may opt for long-lasting parenteral medications such as tetracycline.**

Other medical treatments to be considered in therapy for severe cases of IBK include atropine and nonsteroidal anti-inflammatory drugs. These medications will relieve intraocular pain and decrease the incidence of inflammatory-induced ocular lesions (e.g., synechiae, secondary glaucoma, cataracts). Some reports have detailed use of corticosteroids in IBK-affected eyes without any detrimental effect, but the potential for developing collagenases and prolonging corneal healing times must be considered. Therefore, until conclusive data show otherwise, corticosteroids are best avoided in cases of IBK.

The duration of the carrier stage (i.e., a normal eye with hemolytic *M. bovis*) can be reduced by two injections of long-acting tetracyclines at 20 mg/kg each. Additional steps in treatment may include segregating the affected animals, performing herd management practices during the cool time of the day, using insecticides to control face flies, and practicing personal disinfection between treatments of affected and noninfected animals.

Surgical Treatment

Nictitating membrane flaps and complete temporary tarsorrhaphies have been used in the treatment of deep and perforated corneal ulcers in IBK. These methods have been modified from the surgical procedures used in small animals (see chapters 3 and 6). Often 0-0 or 1-0 chromic gut sutures are used in beef animals so that suture removal can be avoided.

Vaccination

Several vaccines for *M. bovis*, including those based on live or formalin-killed cells, ribosomes, and pili, have been tested. Early vaccines provided only limited protection, but the more recent vaccines appear to be more (but not totally) preventative. Passive immunity from vaccinated animals also may occur. Calves of vaccinated cows or calves fed colostrum from vaccinated animals show a reduced incidence of IBK, reduced severity of clinical signs, and delayed onset of clinical signs. Vaccination with homologous strains reduces both the incidence and the severity of disease, whereas heterologous strain vaccines against IBK have had only limited success. Endemics of IBK have been associated with *M. bovis* isolates possessing novel pili types; therefore, multivalent vaccines with the inclusion of pili from one representative strain of each serogroup should be effective. **Further refinements include use of a relatively low dose of pili produced by recombinant DNA technology to develop an effective vaccine, the preliminary results of which are extremely encouraging.**

Vaccination guidelines often include recommendations to vaccinate 6 weeks before onset of the expected disease season. Calves should be vaccinated at 21 to 30 days of age, with a second vaccination being given 21 days later. (For more details, the reader should consult the third edition, pp. 1131–1138.)

PARASITIC KERATOCONJUNCTIVITIDES

Infestation with *Estrus ovis* in sheep may cause conjunctivitis if the larvae invade the ocular mucous membranes. The adult flies deposit eggs around the mucous membranes of the face, and when the eggs hatch, the larvae migrate to the nasal cavity, turbinates, and the maxillary and frontal sinuses. The larvae may, however, also progress to the nasolacrimal duct and eye. These larvae are large (2.5 cm), spiny, and cause irritation; secondary infection, epiphora, and conjunctivitis may result as well. The larvae mature within several weeks to months and then return to the nostril, where they are sneezed onto the ground to pupate. Treatment usually involves physical removal of the larvae and systemic organophosphates. Ivermectin, 50 mg/kg, may be effective, and treatment is best performed during the fall months (when the larvae are small).

Thelazia sp. nematodes are small, slender, white worms. Males range from 7 to 13 mm in length and females from 12 to 18 mm. More female than male worms (ratio, 2:1) have been recovered from cattle. The worms are found in the conjunctival sac and the nasolacrimal ducts, and they move rapidly in the preocular tear film. *Thelazia californiensis* occurs in sheep, deer, and other species; *T. rhodesi, T. gulosa, T. skrjabini,* and *T. lacrymalis* affect cattle. Mixed infections of two or more genera of parasites have also been reported.

In North America, unilateral, chronic, and follicular or mucoid conjunctivitis is most common, with irregularities occurring in the lining of the ducts of the nictitans gland. Other clinical signs include profuse epiphora, photophobia, and ulcerative keratitis. The clinical examination should include a careful gross examination of the entire lacrimal apparatus and conjunctival surfaces for embryonated eggs, larvae, or immature worms using specialized techniques. Treatment modalities range from simple lavage; mechanical removal after topical anesthesia; oral administration of levamisole, 5 mg/kg or 1% solution topically, or fenbendazole; and topical administration of ivermectin or echothiophate iodide.

PHENOTHIAZINE-ASSOCIATED CORNEAL DISEASE

Phenothiazine is used as a prophylactic for controlling manure-breeding insects and as an anthelmintic in livestock. **Corneal edema and keratitis have been associated with phenothiazine toxicity, but this condition is seen mainly in calves and, to a lesser extent, in pigs and goats. Most ophthalmic cases result from a high dose of phenothiazine, but low daily doses may produce ophthalmic disease as well.** In both calves and sheep, phenothiazine is absorbed from the rumen as the sulfoxide, and it is conjugated in the liver to form leucophenothiazine ethereal sulphate, which is then excreted into the urine and the bile. Cattle are unable to detoxify all the phenothiazine sulfoxide, however, so a proportion enters the systemic circulation and the aqueous humor of the eye, thereby causing photosensitization.

Beginning with lacrimation, the clinical signs of phenothiazine toxicity may occur unilaterally or bilaterally within 12 to 36 hours after treatment. They consist of edema in variable parts of the cornea, depending on where the cornea is exposed to light, as well as subsequent photophobia, blepharospasm, and keratitis. Eyelid edema has also been reported.

Treatment for this condition is symptomatic, but affected animals may show no clinical signs—and even recover spontaneously—if access to sunlight is restricted, especially for 12 to 36 hours after treat-

ment. Affected animals may recover within 5 to 7 days, but recovery can be prolonged as well (60–90 days).

CONGENITAL PORPHYRIA AND PROTOPORPHYRIA

Congenital defects of porphyrin metabolism in cattle and swine are characterized by excessive deposition of porphyrin isomers in the tissues, and these defects are inherited as an autosomal recessive trait. The metabolic defect probably results from an abnormal synthesis of heme resulting from enzymatic insufficiency at the stage of converting pyrrol groups to series 3 porphyrins. Excess series 1 porphyrins are produced as a result and deposited into the tissues. These high levels of porphyrins then sensitize the skin and the eyes to light. The incidence is higher in females than in males, but the disease is rare overall. Even so, it has been recorded in Shorthorn, Holstein, Black and White Danish, Jamaica Red and Black cattle, and in Ayrshires. In pigs, the inheritance is uncertain, but it may result from one or more dominant genes.

Protoporphyria is a less common, milder disease than porphyria, and it is thought to be inherited in cattle as well. This disease involves deficient activity of the enzyme ferrochalase, thereby resulting in excessive synthesis of protoporphyrin.

Ocular clinical signs relating to abnormal porphyrin metabolism result from photosensitization. These includes photophobia, edema, inflammation, and necrosis of the eyelids and the periocular skin. Therapy for photosensitization consists of maintaining the affected animal indoors.

CORNEAL DISEASE SECONDARY TO SYSTEMIC DISEASES

Corneal edema is a common clinical sign associated with corneal ulcerations, keratitis, anterior uveitis, and many systemic diseases (see Chapter 17).

TUMORS OF THE CONJUNCTIVA AND CORNEA

Of the food animal species, cattle are most frequently affected by neoplasia of the ocular and the periocular regions. **Primary tumors of any site, including the eye, are rare in sheep, goats, and swine (incidence, 0.64%). In cattle, however, the most common neoplasia is ocular squamous cell carcinoma (OSCC).** In fact, OSCC is second only to lymphosarcoma in terms of economic loss resulting from condemnation or reduction in salvage value and a shortened productive life span. Of all the bovine tumors reported at slaughter, 80% have been OSCC.

Incidence

In the general cattle population of the United States, the incidence of OSCC varies from 0.8 to 5.0%. In the Netherlands, however, the incidence is 0.04%. In some breeds (e.g., the Hereford), the incidence may be much higher. Results of logistic regression analyses are indicative that age and corneoconjunctival pigmentation are significant risk factors.

Geographic Distribution

Bovine OSCC occurs worldwide, but the occurrence of OSCC is associated with the geographic location. For example, the incidence increases significantly with increases in altitude and mean annual hours of sunlight and with decreases in latitude. Results of subsequent studies have confirmed these observations of an increased risk for OSCC with an increased level of solar radiation.

Signalment

The onset of OSCC is related to age, with older cattle having a significantly greater risk. The tumors are uncommon in cattle younger than 5 years of age, and they are rare in cattle younger than 3 years. The average age of cattle with OSCC is 8.1 years. The incidence of OSCC is significantly higher in *Bos taurus* than in *Bos indicus* breeds, and though other cattle breeds have been documented with OSCC, the Hereford is overrepresented. This association also relates, at least partially, to the periocular skin depigmentation that is typical of the breed. Ayrshires are the most susceptible dairy breed and have a corresponding predilection for squamous cell carcinoma of the vulva. The sites of OSCC may be single or multiple, unilateral or bilateral. In one report, both eyes were affected in 35%. There is probably no sex difference in the incidence of OSCC.

Genetic Predisposition

Considerable evidence is suggestive of a genetic basis for OSCC, as indicated by the variable morbidity rates among breeds of cattle, lines of sires, and increased rates in the progeny of affected compared with those of unaffected parents, especially in the Hereford breed. Lesion development is not heritable per se, but to a large extent, the genetic effect on periocular pigmentation indirectly determines the degree to which the eye is susceptible to some carcinogenic agent. A negative association exists between eyelid pigmentation and the occurrence of OSCC. Eyelid pigmentation is highly heritable, and pigmentation of the eyelid margins clearly has an inhibitory effect on eyelid lesions. Such pigmentation, however, seems to have little effect regarding development of the more frequent, conjunctival OSCC.

Causes

A specific carcinogenic agent causing OSCC has not been identified, and several coexisting factors likely contribute to its development. Factors that have been implicated include age, gender, breed, circumocular and corneoscleral pigmentation, exposure to UV radiation, viral infection, and nutrition.

Clinical Signs

Approximately 75% of OSCC and precursor lesions affect the bulbar conjunctiva and cornea, and of these, 90% involve the limbus and 10%

the cornea. The remaining 25% of OSCC lesions are distributed in the palpebral conjunctiva, nictitating membrane, and eyelid skin. Limbal lesions occur more frequently in the horizontal than in the vertical meridian, which could be the result of greater exposure at these areas to irritation by foreign matter and sunlight. Bovine OSCC often has a characteristic progression through a series of benign stages and then, possibly, to a malignant stage. On the globe and the third eyelid, the initial lesion is a plaque. **Plaques may progress to a papilloma, then to a noninvasive carcinoma (i.e., carcinoma in situ), and finally, to an invasive carcinoma.** In the eyelids, however, extensive keratosis (i.e., keratoma) may occur, particularly near the mucocutaneous junction, either at or near the hairline. This keratosis may appear as a cutaneous horn and be the precursor to carcinoma. The keratotic lesions are moistened by tears, collect debris, and become brown. They can be easily removed as well, thereby leaving a bleeding surface.

The plaque is a small area of hyperplastic epithelium, and most conjunctival OSCC lesions can be linked to this. Plaques may be single or multiple, raised, of various shapes, and found in the conjunctiva following the curvature of the limbus (Fig. 14-6). The surfaces are smooth or irregular, and the consistency may be firm (because of keratinization). Plaques also appear opaque and grayish-white. **Papillomas are distributed in a manner similar to plaques, and they may be thrown up into fronds.** They have a core of connective tissue with multiple, hard, spinelike

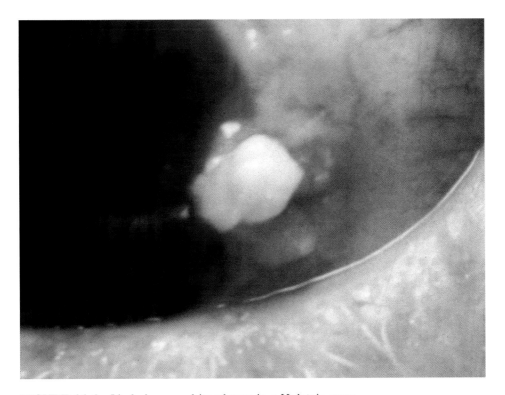

FIGURE 14-6. *Limbal gray-white plaque in a Holstein cow.*

projections of variable size, and they may be sessile or pedunculated. Papillomas often merge with the underlying plaques as well.

Noninvasive carcinomas follow the plaque-to-papilloma sequence, and they arise directly from plaques (Fig. 14-7). Noninvasive carcinomas are characterized microscopically as the stage before the neoplastic cells have penetrated the lamina propria of the epithelium, thereby becoming a squamous cell carcinoma. Grossly, they resemble papilloma and exhibit no invasive tendencies. Invasive carcinomas generally are large and protrude through the palpebral fissure. They can invade the anterior chamber and even, eventually, infiltrate the entire globe. **Carcinomas arising from the nictitating membrane commonly replace this structure. These carcinomas seldom invade the cartilage, but they may infiltrate the medial or the ventromedial orbit. Secondary changes such as necrosis, ulceration, hemorrhage, and inflammatory cell infiltration occur in more than 40% of cases involving the invasive carcinomas.**

Metastatic Potential

Systemic metastases occur late in the course of OSCC; however, the local invasion may be particularly aggressive. As the carcinomas penetrate the lamina propria, they extend "fingers" of neoplastic cells into the surrounding tissues. **Corneal OSCC shows less inward invasion, however, which results from resistance by the stroma and Descemet's membrane.** Even so, the anterior chamber of the eye may still be involved, and in one series, intraocular extension was reported in 14% of the carcinoma cases. The posterior segment rarely is affected. **A greater percent-**

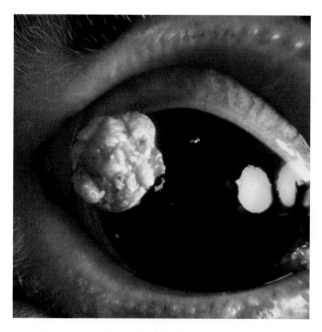

FIGURE 14-7. *Noninvasive limbal squamous cell carcinoma in a mature Hereford cow.*

age of systemic metastases occur from tumors of the lid, lacrimal lake, and nictitating membrane than from limbal and corneal lesions. Cows with OSCC demonstrate metastases involving the regional lymph nodes, orbital bones, maxilla, and the orbital parts of the frontal bones. Intracranial metastasis (probably by extension through the foramen orbitorotundum) has been reported, and intracranial invasion via the cranial nerves (i.e., optic nerve and ophthalmic branch of trigeminal nerve, with progression to the trigeminal ganglion nerve) has been documented. **Systemic metastasis usually occurs via the parotid lymph node and then spreads to the regional lymph nodes, including the atlantal, retropharyngeal, submaxillary, mandibular, and cervical nodes. Once the metastatic cells gain access to the thoracic duct, they spread hematogenously via the venous circulation. Metastases can affect the lungs, heart, pleura, liver, kidney, and bronchial as well as mediastinal lymph nodes.**

Diagnosis

Cytology should not be used as an alternative to histopathology. Instead, cytology should be used to establish a preliminary clinical diagnosis and to permit the clinician to develop a therapeutic approach. Cytologic and histopathologic diagnoses have a strong correlation. High rates of agreement (86.5%) between the two diagnostic modalities have been reported, and anecdotal reports of 90% have also appeared. Well-differentiated OSCCs show a marked predominance of large, markedly angular, nucleated squamous cells that have nuclear features of malignancy (e.g., hyperchromatic chromatin and large, multiple nucleoli of various shapes).

Histopathology of the plaque reveals an area of hyperplastic conjunctival epithelium. As this epithelial cell hyperplasia develops, the underlying connective tissue proliferates into the overlying epithelium. At this stage, the plaque becomes a papilloma. When fully developed, the papilloma consists of multiple papillary projections (i.e., fronds) that are covered by proliferative epithelium and supported by vascular connective tissue stalks. The covering epithelium also exhibits different extents of hyperkeratosis.

The noninvasive form of the OSCC exhibits malignant transformation of the epithelial cells in the basilar layer or, less commonly, in the stratum spinosum. These cells display hyperchromatic nuclei, increased numbers of mitotic figures, pleomorphism, and loss of polarity. The neoplasm also may show signs of early invasiveness, and infiltration by mononuclear cells is common at these sites. Invasive carcinomas have been graded on the basis of the World Health Organization classification of tumors, and they generally include whorls, with intensely eosinophilic, keratinized centers (i.e., pearls). The cells are frequently arranged in cords or nests. Few whorls are present, but some of these contain little eosinophilic cornified material. Cells with intercellular bridges are infrequently seen.

Treatment

Before therapeutic intervention, the extent of invasion should be evaluated. Extensive systemic invasion may preclude further treatment because of financial or prognostic reasons. In one report, examination of slaughterhouse material revealed that 5% of animals had metastatic lesions. In addition, animals with invasive carcinoma of the eye or eyelids had an even higher level of metastasis (11%). A thorough physical examination, with emphasis on early lesions and concentrating on chest and regional lymph node abnormalities, is essential. Routine blood and serum biochemistry profiles are also suggested, and orbital palpation is necessary, especially in those animals with eyelid masses. If indicated and the owner's finances allow, orbital radiography may be useful in determining any bony involvement; dorsal oblique radiography provides the most useful information. If present, bony involvement carries a very guarded prognosis.

When deciding on treatment strategies, it is important to realize that not all precancerous lesions progress. Approximately 50% of the precursor lesions (e.g., plaque, papilloma, keratosis) show only minor changes in size, but approximately 30 to 50% regress spontaneously.

If treatment is undertaken, the options include curative or cytoreductive surgery before adjunctive therapy, cryotherapy, hyperthermia, immunotherapy, radiation therapy, and possibly, chemotherapy. **The most common treatment is surgery, and when combined with other treatment modalities (often cryothermy), the success rates are quite good.**

Several surgical procedures are available, and these range from local excision to enucleation and exenteration. The transpalpebral enucleation technique is the most frequently used, especially in cattle with extensive neoplasia of the globe, eyelids, nictitating membrane, and conjunctiva. Block resection, which involves removal of a block consisting of retropharyngeal lymph node, mandibular salivary gland, and parotid salivary gland/subparotid lymph node as well as performance of a transpalpebral enucleation, offers cure rates as high as 90%. Transpalpebral enucleation alone, however, may show a recurrence rate of 37%.

Eyelid and orbital surgery are performed most frequently in standing cattle, and regional anesthesia for most ocular surgeries in food animals can be achieved using a Peterson nerve block or a "four-point" block of the orbit. Clients should be informed that apnea, though rare, may occur 8 to 9 minutes after injection—and that death may occur after a Peterson nerve block. This may result from injection of the anesthetic agent directly into a blood vessel, which can obviously be avoided by aspirating first, or it may result from injection into the dural sheath.

The Peterson nerve block is a retrobulbar injection that blocks the optic, oculomotor, trochlear, abducens, and ophthalmic as well as maxillary branches of the trigeminal nerve. Lack of pupillary constriction is indicative of successful application of this block, in which a slightly curved, 10-cm, 18-gauge needle is inserted at the caudal angle between the supraorbital process and the zygomatic arch. The concavity of the curvature is directed posteriorly, thereby allowing passage of the needle anterior to the anterior border of the coronoid process of the mandible. To achieve this, the needle may need to be "walked off" the coronoid process anteriorly. The needle is advanced slightly ventral to the pterygopalatine fossa and the foramen orbitorotundum, and complications may be avoided if the needle is not advanced to the bony floor of the pterygopalatine fossa. At this point, aspiration is performed, and approximately 15 to 20 mL of lidocaine (2%) are injected.

A "four-point" block may achieve sufficient anesthesia as well. In this block, a 6-cm needle is inserted transconjunctivally adjacent to the globe at the 12-, 3-, 6-, and 9-o'clock positions, and 5 to 10 mL of lidocaine are injected at each site. A variation of this technique is to direct the needles in similar positions through the eyelids rather than through the conjunctiva.

Akinesia of the eyelids is obtained by the auriculopalpebral nerve block, in which local anesthetic is injected subcutaneously 5- to 7-cm caudal to the supraorbital process, where the nerve crosses the zygomatic arch. Eyelid anesthesia is achieved using local anesthetic infiltrated at the anticipated incision sites. Injecting lidocaine (2%) in a line before the advancing needle minimizes both patient discomfort and the number of injection sites that are required.

Postoperative Management

After enucleation, most animals do not require systemic postoperative treatment with antibiotics; however, an injection of flunixin meglumine, 1 mg/kg, will decrease postoperative pain and swelling. Antibiotics may by placed in the orbit at the conclusion of the enucleation procedure. In cases with marked sepsis, administration of appropriate systemic antibiotics for several days is indicated. Packing the orbit with sterile gauze after enucleation is not recommended, however, unless uncontrollable hemorrhage occurs. If used, the gauze should be gradually removed from between the sutures during a 3- to 4-day period; the opening for the gauze removal is then sutured to prevent fistula formation.

Surgery for eyelid neoplasms may involve simple "V" or four-sided, full-thickness excision of the neoplasm as well as apposition of the eyelid margins. With larger, lower-eyelid OSCC, the "H"-plasty or sliding skin graft provides excellent results in cattle. Tumors larger than 50 mm in diameter or with ill-defined margins are suitable candidates. In one study, 12 of 14 animals treated had no recurrence at a 6-month follow-up examination. All wounds were cosmetically acceptable, and all wounds had healed by primary intent. In addition, all but two animals had normal eyelid function after surgery. These high success rates resulted from the large excisions that can be performed using this technique. Surgery for neoplasms of the nictitating membrane ranges from focal excision (for small lesions) to total excision of the structure (with large masses). In this area, however, OSCC may frequently recur after surgical removal as well, and it may invade the orbit by the hematogenous route or by direct infiltration. Surgery for neoplasms of the conjunctiva varies in scope. During the early stages, these tumors may be amenable to local excision, and conjunctival lesions may be excised by scalpel, electrocautery, or carbon dioxide laser. Surgery for limbal and corneal neoplasms usually involves superficial keratectomies to remove masses limited to the outer layers of these tissues; postoperative corneal scarring is not a significant problem in cattle. Limbal lesions affecting the cornea and adjacent bulbar conjunctiva are similarly removed. With a No. 64 Beaver blade, a delineating incision is made into the cornea and the sclera around the periphery of the lesion. Then, with the blade held flat against the globe, the entire lesion is undermined along a lamellar plane, thus leaving an underlying bed of normal corneal tissue. To cover the surgical defect, a conjunctival grafting procedure may be performed using 7-0 absorbable suture.

Cryotherapy involves the controlled application of a cryogen to destroy selected tissues, and it is a popular treatment of OSCC in cattle. High success rates have been achieved as well. In one study using a double freeze–thaw technique (to −25°C) , 97% of OSCCs regressed, including 73% of those larger than 20 mm in diameter. Large OSCCs should be "debulked" surgically to reduce the extent of cryotherapy that is required. Nitrous oxide and liquid nitrogen are the cryogens most commonly used, and several different cryosurgical units are available. Microthermocouple needles attached to a recorder are placed 0.5 cm from the tumor margin and at the base of the mass are recommended to monitor the freezing of larger masses.

Ionizing radiation has also been used to treat OSCC in food animals. The expense and legal requirements necessary to possess such radioactive materials, however, result in low usage of radiation as a treatment modality (except at veterinary institutions).

Hyperthermia has been successfully used in the treatment of bovine OSCC as well. Often, hyperthermia is combined with some other treatment modality, such as surgical debulking or immunotherapy. In one study of 45 tumors, 80% regressed completely and 16% partially after a single treatment. In another study with 3- to 12-month follow-up periods, 96% of tumors either disappeared (53%) or were only represented by suspicious scar tissue (43%), which could be retreated. Neoplastic cells are selectively destroyed with hyperthermia. In this technique, radiofrequency (i.e., 2 MHZ) electric current is passed between two electrodes using a small, handheld radiofrequency device (Western Instrument Company). The electrodes of the treatment device are placed directly on the tumor, and the resistance of the tissue to the flow of electric current generates heat in that tissue. The temperature of the tumor tissue is raised to approximately 50°C, and temperature control is maintained through monitoring with a temperature-sensitive device (i.e., a thermistor) that is built into one electrode. Thirty seconds are allowed to elapse after the tissue temperature reaches the 50°C (122°F) target temperature.

Hyperthermia is not recommended for tumors that extend deeper than 3 mm or have a diameter larger than 4 cm. Surgical debulking may reduce the size of the tumor sufficiently to allow for adequate treatment results using hyperthermia. Follow-up care at 30 days is generally recommended, with further treatment being possible if needed.

Immunotherapy

Immunotherapy in the treatment of bovine OSCC is not common, but antibodies to tumor cells have been demonstrated in sera. Successful use of immunotherapy has also been reported in the treatment of bovine OSCC, with arrest and resolution of the tumor in 78 to 94% of cases within 8 weeks after a single, intramuscular injection of a concentrated saline-phenol extract of fresh tumor tissue, which consisted primarily of tumor nucleoproteins. The response to treatment is dose dependent. Recently, use of peritumoral interleukin-2 has shown promise as well. In one report, complete regression of OSCC tumors was observed in 67% of cases at 20 months using 10 injections of 200,000 U of interleukin-2; lower doses were associated with higher rates of relapse.

Prevention and Control

Results of some studies are indicative that selective breeding can be used toward the control of OSCC. **To achieve this goal, animals with increased amounts of lid and corneoconjunctival pigment should be selected, but the latter pigmentation is not fully expressed until 5 years of age.** Selection on the basis of eyelid margin pigmentation leads to a slight reduction in the incidence of OSCC, however, because the eyelids are the sites for only approximately 10% of these tumors. In purebred herds, the offspring of affected animals should be culled, and bulls with a history of this tumor should not be used as a sire.

THE GLAUCOMAS

Glaucoma is an optic neuropathy that is usually associated with elevated intraocular pressure. **The incidence of glaucoma in cattle is less than 1%, and the types of the glaucomas that occur include congenital, hereditary, and secondary glaucomas (from inflammatory or neoplastic processes).** Endogenous inflammatory episodes (e.g., those seen with neoplastic or granulomatous processes) may cause both peripheral anterior and posterior synechiae, which in turn may impede aqueous outflow to a degree sufficient to elevate the intraocular pressure. Perforated corneal ulcers, especially from IBK, may result in globe rupture, iris prolapse, and synechiae, which also may result in glaucoma. **Clinical signs in cattle with glaucoma are like those in other species. Successful treatment of glaucoma in cattle, however, has not been reported.**

DISEASES OF THE UVEA

The uveal tract includes the iris and the ciliary body (i.e., anterior uvea) as well as the choroid (i.e., posterior uvea), and it is affected by both local and systemic diseases. Systemic diseases have a tendency to manifest in the uvea because of its large vascular supply. Of the uveal diseases reported, most result from secondary association of the uvea rather than from primary involvement.

CONGENITAL DISORDERS OF THE ANTERIOR UVEA

Congenital disorders of the anterior uvea in food animals are not, for the most part, clinically significant. **Such anomalies include persistent pupillary membranes, heterochromia, aniridia and iris hypoplasia, polycoria,** cysts, pigment nevi, and colobomas. Among cattle reported in one study, heterochromia iridis represented almost 10% of the ocular defects found. Persistent pupillary membranes appear to be rare in food animals.

Heterochromia irides is a difference in the coloration of the iris. It may be unilateral or bilateral, and it may be complete or partial. Iridal pigmentation may vary between white, light pink, blue, gray, and brown. In some cases, heterochromia irides may be associated with other ocular anomalies (e.g., tapetal fibrosum hypoplasia) and with colobomas of the fundus (Fig. 14-8). Both dominant and recessive forms of inheritance have been reported. Heterochromia irides have been reported in various breeds, including Herefords, Ayrshires, Holsteins, Angus, Brown Swiss, and Guernseys. In most cases, vision is unaffected; however, photophobia and nystagmus have been reported. In Guernseys, the condition has been suggested to be inherited recessively. Heterochromia irides with incomplete albinism is inherited as an autosomal dominant trait with variable expressivity in Herefords. These cattle usually are totally white, though some have occasional patches of pigmentation on the shoulder and the hip. Most irides have a white periphery and a medium-blue center, but a few exhibit distinct zones of blue, white, and tan. Ocular anomalies of the fundus, including typical optic disc colobomas, are present as well.

Heterochromia irides also occur in miniature swine, with a higher incidence in white miniature pigs (38.3%) compared with that in miniature pigs having a variety of coat colors (15.8%). The abnormality is inherited as an autosomal recessive trait with variable expressivity. Both the frequency and bilateral involvement of heterochromia irides depend on heterochromia in the parents.

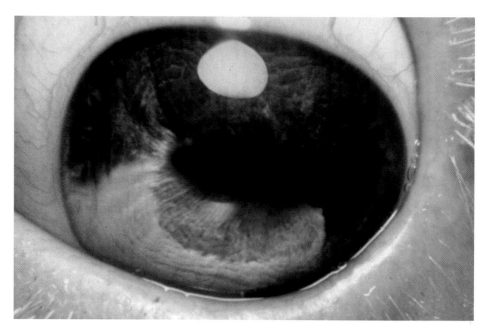

FIGURE 14-8. *Tricolored heterochromic iris (brown, blue, and white) of a Hereford bull with dominant albinism.*

An autosomal recessive, hereditary iridal defect occurs in Jersey calves as part of multiple eye defects. Affected animals may show bilateral aniridia or iridal hypoplasia in association with microphakia, cataracts, and ectopia lentis. The calves can also exhibit visual impairment and even blindness.

Defects in the anatomy of the iris, which are termed *essential iris atrophy,* **have been described among purebred Shropshire sheep in Pennsylvania.** The affected animals are apparently not born with iridal defects, but by 1.0 to 1.5 years of age, they may be affected with full-thickness holes in the iris stroma. **The corpora nigra is rudimentary or absent, and the animals are affected bilaterally though not symmetrically.** Reported lesions have not been associated with any previous inflammatory episodes. (For more details, the reader should consult the third edition, pp. 1153–1154.)

UVEITIS

The term *uveitis* refers to inflammation of the uveal tract. Anterior uveitis includes the iris and ciliary body, and posterior uveitis includes the choroid. The association of uveitides with systemic diseases are numerous (see Chapter 17). **Specific reported causes of uveitis in cattle have included neonatal infections; bacterial septicemia associated with severe mastitis, metritis, or traumatic reticuloperitonitis; malignant catarrhal fever; tuberculosis; IBK; thromboembolic meningoencephalitis; leptospirosis; toxoplasmosis; listeriosis; and lymphoma.**

In sheep and goats, neonatal pyosepticemia from various bacterial agents, listeriosis, mycoplasmosis, toxoplasmosis, thiamine deficiency, trypanosomiasis, blunt trauma, retroviral, and toxic causes for uveitis have been reported. In pigs, bacterial, viral, and parasitic causes of uveitis, some of which are exotic to North America, have also been reported.

UVEAL TUMORS

Primary tumors of the anterior and the posterior uvea are rare in food animals. Sarcomas and ciliary body epitheliomas do occur in cattle, however, and a malignant melanoma has been reported in a sheep and a congenital intraocular melanoma in a Charolais cross-calf. Secondary intraocular tumors of the uveal tract can occur by extension from the orbit, conjunctiva, and cornea. The sclera is resistant to external invasion, but it may be breached by squamous cell carcinomas in cattle. Intraocular lymphosarcoma is rare.

DISEASES OF THE LENS

Cataracts are rarely reported in food animals; however, the actual incidence may be much higher than that indicated by the literature. Lens luxations appear mainly to occur in enlarged globes with glaucoma. Careful inspection of the lens is not routinely performed, however, unless the food animal has a history of visual impairment. Small, focal lens opacities usually do not result in visual impairment, but they usually are missed unless mydriasis is induced before the ophthalmic examination. Among food animals, congenital cataracts (with or without associated ocular anomalies), secondary cataracts (from metabolic, postinflammatory, or traumatic causes), and cataracts of unknown origin have been described.

Congenital cataracts have been reported in cattle, sheep, and pigs but have rarely been reported in goats. Congenital bilateral cataracts are inherited by an autosomal recessive mechanism in several breeds of cattle, including the Jersey, Hereford, and Holstein-Friesian. Congenital nuclear cataracts have been observed in sheep and goats. **Other ocular abnormalities occurring in association with cataracts have been described in the Hereford, Holstein-Friesian, Jersey, and Shorthorn breeds. Microphthalmia and cataracts with retinal lesions may be seen in calves exposed in utero to bovine viral diarrhea at 76 to 150 days of gestation.**

Secondary cataracts have some precedent cause, which in food animals usually relates to an inflammatory episode. In such cases, changes observed in the eye should be compatible with an inflammatory episode, such as posterior synechiae, iridal changes, pigment deposition on the lens, and possibly, secondary glaucoma and cataracts.

Cataracts, goiter, and infertility have been reported as a result of an exclusive diet of *Leucaena leucocephala* in cattle. The filarid worm *Elaeophora schneideri* has induced cataracts among domestic sheep in the western United States, and diabetes mellitus has been implicated as the cause of cataracts in ram lambs. Bilateral cortical opacities have been described in mature sows, and in that report, hygromycin B, which was used as a food additive, was the suspected cause.

Cataract surgery has been successfully performed in food animals using the same techniques as used in small animals. (For more details, the reader should consult the third edition, pp. 1156–1158.)

DISEASES OF THE OCULAR FUNDUS

In food animals, the ocular fundus includes the retina, the choroid (including the tapetum fibrosum, except in swine), and the optic nerve head (Figs. 14-9 through 14-11). The ocular fundus may show signs arising from both primary and secondary diseases. Fundic examination in food animals is facilitated by mydriasis induced using tropicamide (1%). With adequate restraint of the animal's head as well as mydriasis, both direct and indirect ophthalmoscopy can be easily performed in food animals, because eye movements are limited. (For more details, the reader should consult the third edition, pp. 1158–1160.)

CONGENITAL DISORDERS

Congenital fundus abnormalities are unusual, but when they do occur, they may mimic acquired lesions. **Complete albinism is rare but has been documented in both cattle and sheep. More commonly, however, a partial albinism (i.e., subalbinism) is described. In complete albino cattle, the**

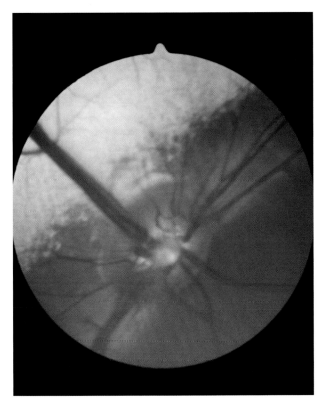

FIGURE 14-9. *Normal bovine ocular fundus. The optic disc is predominantly in the nontapetal fundus, and the large, primary blood vessels emerge from the surface of the optic disc.*

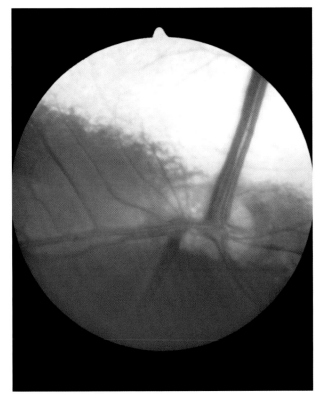

FIGURE 14-10. *Normal ovine ocular fundus. The kidney-shaped optic disc is at the junction of the tapetal and nontapetal fundi.*

FIGURE 14-11. *Normal caprine ocular fundus. The round optic disc is at the junction of the tapetal and nontapetal fundi.*

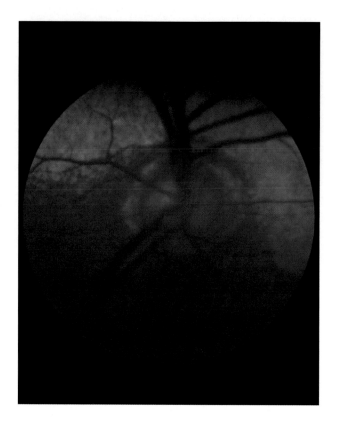

fundus contains a yellow tapetal fundus but a nonpigmented nontapetal fundus. With incomplete albinism in cattle, the tapetal fundus is often blue-green and the nontapetal fundus partially pigmented. In Icelandic sheep, albino animals have occurred among both white and nonwhite strains.

Colobomatous Malformations

Colobomatous defects in the ventral 5- or 6-o'clock quadrants (i.e., typical colobomas) may result from failed closure of the optic fissure. Colobomas of the choroid are common among cattle (Fig. 14-12), with various estimates indicating a prevalence rate of from 1 to 2%. Typical colobomas of the optic disc occur in the dominant form of incomplete albinism among Hereford cattle and in Charolais cattle as well. The defects are bilateral and often small, though not symmetrical, and they generally are restricted to the posterior segment. Larger colobomas involve the entire optic disc and, occasionally, extend into the choroid and sclera in other areas of the ocular fundus. With some extreme cases, calves have been born blind, with grossly affected eyes. The pattern of inheritance for typical colobomas in Charolais cattle is suggestive of a dominant mode, but the results of test breedings are suggestive of a polygenic inheritance.

Retinal Dysplasia

Infectious agents such as bovine virus diarrhea–mucosal disease in cattle or bluetongue in sheep have been implicated as causing retinal

dysplasia, as have inherited multiple ocular anomalies, including retinal dysplasia and internal hydrocephalus, in Shorthorn cattle. Clinically, the dysplastic retinas are often detached.

Osteopetrosis-Induced Ocular Fundus Disease

Osteopetrosis in cattle is a generalized skeletal disease that is characterized
by the absence of bone cavities because of defective bone remodeling. The
disease is expressed as an autosomal recessive trait in North American
Black Angus cattle. The clinical signs resulting from this condition include
fragile bones, brachygnathia, hypoplastic foraminae, and various neurologic defects (e.g., blindness). Most animals are premature at birth and
stillborn. The ocular complications of osteopetrosis include defects in the
retina and the optic nerve.

INFLAMMATIONS OF THE OCULAR FUNDUS

Various infectious agents have been implicated as causing posterior segment inflammatory changes in food animals. **Cattle have been affected by
neonatal septicemic infections (*Escherichia* and *Pasteurella* sp.), thromboembolic meningoencephalitis (*Hemophilus somnus*), rabies and other
viral causes, toxoplasmosis, tuberculosis, and listeriosis. Small domestic ruminants have been reported to experience posterior segment**

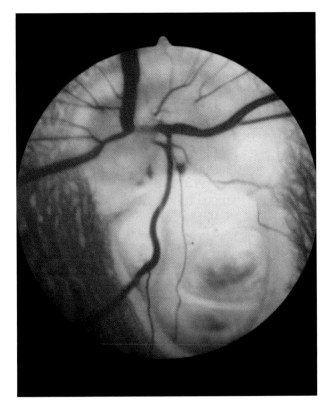

FIGURE 14-12. *Typical coloboma
of the optic disc and the nontapetal
fundus. The multiple-depth defect is
traversed by a large venule and a
smaller arteriole.*

changes related to bacterial and parasitic causes (i.e., mycoplasmosis, listeriosis, elaeophorosis, trypanosomiasis, toxoplasmosis) as well as viral causes (i.e., bluetongue, scrapie). Swine may have chorioretinal lesions resulting from pseudorabies (i.e., Aujeszky's disease), hog cholera, listeriosis, toxoplasmosis, Glasser's disease, ocular cysticercosis, Teschen encephalitis, and swine erysipelas.

DEGENERATIONS OF THE OCULAR FUNDUS

Most documented retinal degenerations in food animals are acquired, and they may arise from the ingestion of forage material. Ocular defects, however, are usually only one of several systemic signs in such cases. Chronic inflammatory diseases also may result in degenerative retinal disease. Retinal degenerations, which possibly are genetically based (as seen among some of the domestic species), have also been reported in goats and cattle. Possible hereditary retinal degeneration occurs in cattle as well. Initially, the clinical signs include pupils that are poorly responsive to light stimulation and nyctalopia with subsequent blindness. Examination of the fundus reveals signs that are typical of retinal degeneration. Tapetal hyperreflectivity, small vessel attenuation (but preservation of larger vessels until late in the disease), and minimal optic nerve abnormalities characterize the disease initially, whereas the end stage shows diffuse pigmentation of the tapetal fundus.

Retinal degeneration has been reported in Toggenburg goats. The posterior segment abnormalities consist of generalized tapetal hyperreflectivity and retinal vessel attenuation.

Vitamin A deficiency may cause blindness, abnormal bone growth, abnormal epithelial function, and embryologic maldevelopment in cattle. Ingestion by cattle of *Dryopteris felix mas* (i.e, male fern) is associated with possible permanent loss of vision because of retrobulbar optic nerve disease. Bilateral blindness is the main presenting sign, but weakness, malaise, and constipation can also occur. In severely affected animals, optic nerve atrophy occurs as well, with subsequent retinal degeneration. Fundoscopy reveals hemorrhage either on or about the optic disc as well as various amounts of papilledema. Chronically affected animals exhibit blindness, optic nerve atrophy, reduced retinal vasculature, and tapetal degeneration.

In sheep and goats, a similar syndrome of retrobulbar optic nerve neuropathy and retinal degeneration occurs after ingestion of *Stypandra glauca* (i.e., blind grass). Field evidence is suggestive that *S. glauca* is toxic during the flowering stage. Affected animals die after an acute illness with signs of neurologic disturbances, or they survive and become permanently blind. Funduscopy has revealed multifocal tapetal and peripapillary hyperpigmented foci interspersed with other areas of tapetal hyperreflectivity in these animals. Optic nerve atrophy may be present as well.

Polioencephalomalacia (or cerebrocortical necrosis), may result from thiamine deficiency, which in turn may result from primary or secondary causes. Primary deficiency is uncommon among ruminants because of the rumen synthesis of thiamine, but it may occur in swine. Secondary deficiencies resulting from the ingestion of thiaminase-containing plants such as bracken fern (*Pteris aquilina*), however, are more likely. In addition, PEM has been caused by water deprivation and ad libitum access to sulfur. Treatment of sulfur-induced cases with vitamin B_1, dexamethasone, and antibiotics has been associated with a prolonged recovery time. The basic lesion of PEM is necrosis of the cerebrocortical neurons, with associated perineuronal and pericapillary edema; this results in a variety of ocular and neurologic signs. Neurologic signs are associated with increased cerebrospinal fluid pressure, and impaired vision may be an early sign. **The blindness is cortical, but the ocular signs of papilledema and decreased pupillary light reflexes may occur. Treatment consists of thiamine hydrochloride, 6 to 10 mg/kg injected either intramuscularly or intravenously.** Corticosteroids also may benefit cases early during the course of disease. Recovery from neurologic signs may be slow, however, and decreased vision or blindness may persist as well.

Bracken fern (*Pteris aquilina*) has been associated with a progressive degeneration of the outer retinal layers in sheep. Affected animals have variously been called "bright blind," "moonlight blind," "clear blind," or simply "glass eyed." This terminology has arisen on the basis of the abnormal shine (i.e., tapetal reflection through a dilated pupil) of the affected eyes in semidarkness. The disease is limited to certain geographic areas, including northern England, Scotland, and possibly, Wales. Clinically, the sheep are permanently blind. Affected animals have dilated pupils and sluggish pupillary responses, and the earliest ophthalmoscopic sign is an increased tapetal fundus reflection. The optic disc is normal, though with chronicity, this should change. Attenuation of the retinal blood vessels also occurs, however, as do hyperreflective, pale tapetal fundi.

Poisoning with locoweed (*Astragalus mollissimus*) causes retinal degeneration in cattle, sheep, and other species. Poisoned animals show disturbances of vision as well as dry, lusterless eyes. Water hemlock (*Cicuta* sp.) causes an acute syndrome that is associated with sudden death. In addition, a new, fatal mycotoxicosis of cattle has been recognized in Australia, and feeding trials have demonstrated a previously unknown mycotoxic species of *Corallocytostroma* that grows on Mitchell grass (*Astrebla* sp.). *Kochia scoparia* (i.e., Mexican fireweed, summer cypress, burning bush) can produce blindness and nystagmus. *Sarcostemma* sp. cause neurologic disease among sheep in Africa and also may be associated with visual impairment. Darling pea (*Swainsonia galegifolia*) causes signs similar to those of locoweed in cattle and sheep, and *Amaranthus retroflexus* and *Chenopodium albuim* cause neurologic signs and decreased vision in pigs.

Arsanilic acid toxicity may result in blindness among pigs. Arsanilic acid is used therapeutically for swine dysentery and as a growth stimulant. Clinical signs appear if arsanilic acid is given in excess, for a prolonged period of time, or during times of restricted water intake. Affected swine show blindness, weakness, torticollis, and incoordination. The pupillary light reflexes are absent, and the ophthalmoscopic examination reveals bilateral optic disc atrophy that is characterized by pallor, well-defined margins, and narrowed retinal arterioles. (For more details, the reader should consult the third edition, pp. 1163–1167.)

INHERITED LYSOSOMAL STORAGE DISEASES

A variety of inherited lysosomal storage diseases with ophthalmic implications have been reported among food animals. These include

FIGURE 14-13. *Papilledema and retinal degeneration secondary to avitaminosis A in a yearling Angus steer.*

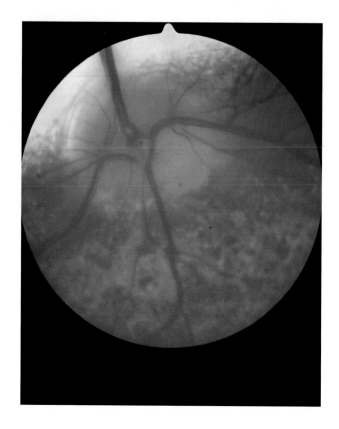

GM$_1$-gangliosidosis (i.e., leukodystrophy), GM$_2$-gangliosidosis (i.e., lipodystrophy), mannosidosis, and ceroid lipofuscinosis. The inherited lysosomal storage diseases are summarized in Chapter 17.

OPTIC NERVE DISEASES

The term *papilledema* refers to a descriptive clinical finding, not to a specific disease entity. It is a noninflammatory swelling of the optic disc that can be caused by various conditions, and it may signal increased intracranial pressure. **Papilledema is commonly encountered among cattle and sheep. Causes can include avitaminosis A, acquired and congenital hydrocephalus, space-occupying brain lesions, meningitis, coenurosis, encephalitis, and hexachlorophene toxicity. The margins of the optic disc appear to be hazy, and the physiologic depression is lost. The disc also becomes thickened and swollen and appears to be grayish-white, with striations. The retinal veins and arteries show a distinct kink as they pass down over the edge of the disc and onto the retina. The retinal venules may be dilated and engorged peripherally but hidden centrally within the swollen disc (Fig. 14-13).** Many more fine veins are visible. The arterioles are a brighter red and more threadlike than the congested venules. Eventually, if the cerebrospinal fluid pressure remains elevated, the optic nerve and disc will atrophy.

15

Exotic Animal Ophthalmology

Exotic animal ophthalmology includes those species that are the unusual or nontraditional pets. This chapter summarizes the chapters on laboratory animal ophthalmology, animal models for ophthalmic diseases in humans, and exotic animal ophthalmology in the third edition (pp. 1209–1236, 1237–1272, and 1273–1305, respectively). Zoo animals usually are presented only infrequently to practicing veterinarians and more commonly to specially trained zoo veterinarians. **This chapter discusses the most common eye diseases of nontraditional pets that may be presented for veterinary care.**

EYE DISEASES OF AMPHIBIANS

OPHTHALMIC ANATOMY

The anatomy of amphibian eyes varies with the order (i.e., Anura versus Urodel) as well as with the developmental stage (i.e., larval versus adult). The eyes of larval anurans (i.e., frogs and toads) have poorly developed eyelids, with the false nictitating membrane being formed by an elastic, translucent fold of conjunctiva in the lower fornix. When the globe is retracted, it passively covers the eye. Superior eyelid glands and a harderian gland are also present. The nasolacrimal duct, however, is absent. The retractor bulbi is the most important extraocular muscle; it retracts the globe and aids in swallowing. The globe is spherical, with hyaline cartilage in the inner sclera from the posterior pole as far as the equator. The cornea has the mammalian pattern, and a ciliary body is present, with hypertrophied folds dorsally that extend to the pupillary border and form pupillary nodules. A protractor lentis muscle arises from the peripheral cornea to insert on the ciliary folds; contraction of this muscle moves the lens forward to effect accommodation for distance vision. The iris is thin and often highly colored by various stromal pigments. Myoepithelial sphincter and dilator muscles are present as well, as

413

are pupillary excursions. Resting pupil size and shape are remarkably variable, but the pupil is spherical when dilated. The avascular retina derives its blood supply from the vascular choroid alone in urodeles and from both the choroid and membrana vasculosa retinae in the vitreous on the retinal surface in anurans. The optic disc is either circular or elongated. The retina contains at least four types of photoreceptors as determined on the basis of visual pigments in the rods and cones. Oil droplets are present at the distal end of the ellipsoid of some cones. Anuran photoreceptors have been the subject of extensive research involving photochemistry, renewal, and electrophysiology.

OPHTHALMIC DISEASES

Severe panophthalmitis and otitis interna have been reported in a large group of recently imported, fire-bellied toads (*Bombina orientalis*). Corneal stromal infiltrates, scleritis, hyphema, hypopyon, iridocyclitis, cataract, and chorioretinitis were prominent, and opisthotonus, circling, head tilt, and loss of righting reflexes were associated with otitis interna. Several bacterial strains were cultured from both the affected eyes and from normal viscera. These strains included *Aeromonas hydrophila, Citrobacter freundii, Providencia alcalifaciens, Klebsiella oxytoca,* and an unidentified, oxidase-positive, Gram-negative bacilli that was resistant to tetracycline. Both *A. hydrophila* and *C. freundii* have been implicated as causes of red-leg septicemia in anurans. Treatment of affected fire-bellied toads with oxytetracycline, 26 mg per 1 L of water, was not effective; however, it may have prevented infection among other, normal toads. Topical treatment of presumptive or proved bacterial ocular infections in amphibians must be undertaken with recognition of the potential for systemic toxicity. Gentamicin, diluted to 2 mg/mL, has been recommended. Parenteral antibiotic or corticosteroid administration may be preferable, however, because an exact dosage can then be delivered.

Corneal opacities in amphibians have several potential causes. The most extensively reported and investigated disorder is lipid keratopathy. Originally discovered in Cuban tree frogs (*Osteopilus septentrionalis*), it has since been identified among species of hylid, leptodactylid, and ranid frogs, either as a corneal and hepatic lesion or as part of a generalized xanthomatosis affecting the brain, some viscera, the peripheral nerves, periarticular soft tissues, and digital pads. Hypercholesterolemia has been noted in animals with disseminated xanthomatosis. **Clinically, dense and white stromal opacities are seen, and these opacities are often raised, with corneal thickening and surface epithelial irregularity. Stromal neovascularization and superficial pigmentation may be present as well. In advanced cases, the densest opacities occur in the central cornea.**

EYE DISEASES OF REPTILES

Four of the five orders within the class Reptilia (i.e., lizards, chelonians, crocodilians, and the tuatara) have anatomically similar eyes. The fifth order, snakes, lost the prototype reptilian anatomic pattern during a fossorial period in their evolution, only to re-evolve eyes with certain differences from those of other reptiles.

OPHTHALMIC ANATOMY

The features of the external eye and adnexa have great clinical significance. Except in snakes and certain ablepharine skinks, the upper and lower eyelids in reptiles are well-developed, with the lower eyelid being the more mobile. The eyelids of chameleons are constricted around the cornea and move with the very mobile globe. In some lizards of the families Lacertidae, Scincidae, and Teidae, the lower lid is variably transparent. **Snakes, ablepharine geckos, and skinks possess a spectacle covering the cornea that developed from fused eyelids and is separated from the cornea by an epithelial-lined, subspectacular space. This tertiary spectacle contains an extensive vascular network that is optically transparent but demonstrable using microsilicone injection. The anterior layers of the spectacle are shed during normal ecdysis with the rest of the skin. Before ecdysis, the spectacle becomes cloudy because of thickening and breakdown of the skin layers, with fluid accumulating between the new and the old surface layers of the spectacle. The spectacle is transparent, however, immediately before its surface is shed. During the period in which the spectacle is cloudy, the animal is blind, and many species become more irritable and aggressive during this period. The spectacle is impervious to topically applied medications; thus, topical ocular therapy is ineffective.** The ocular surface in reptiles is bathed by fluids secreted from the lacrimal (except in snakes) and harderian glands. The latter are large in chelonians, especially among marine species, and the lacrimal gland functions as an extrarenal site of salt excretion. The nasolacrimal duct, which is absent in chelonians, drains from the medial canthus to the roof of the mouth to emerge at the base of or behind the vomeronasal organ.

Anatomic features of the globe that distinguish reptiles include poorly developed rectus muscles (except in lizards), a well-developed retractor bulbi muscle (except in snakes), and limited rotational movements (except in chameleons). Hyaline cartilage is present in the sclera of lizards and chelonians from the equator to the posterior pole, with scleral ossicles extending anteriorly from the equator to the limbus (Fig. 15-1). These ossicles form a sclerocorneal sulcus, thereby giving shape to the anterior segment and apposing the ciliary body to the lens equator, which in turn provides leverage for action of the ciliary muscle. Snakes lack both scleral ossicles and cartilage, and crocodilians lack scleral ossicles. The soft, pliable lens in both crocodilians and lizards has an equatorial pad, which is absent in snakes and poorly developed in chelonians. Accommodation in most reptiles occurs through pressure exerted by the ciliary body, which is mediated by the ciliary muscle, against the lens equator to increase the anteroposterior diameter of the lens. Unlike the eyes of other vertebrates, the lenses of chameleons (*Chamaeleo dilepis*) have a negative refractive power and are capable of very rapid accommodation (60 diopters [D] per second) with very broad accommodative range (45 D). Accommodation in snakes

FIGURE 15-1. *The lacertilian eye.*

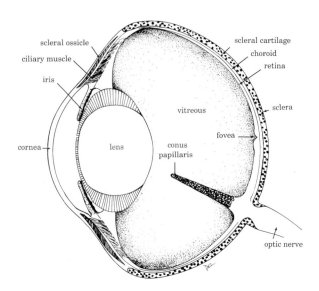

appears to occur through forward movement of the lens, which is accomplished indirectly though increased pressure on the vitreous applied by the ciliary muscle.

Iris color, pupil shape, and uveal vascular pattern in reptiles are variable, and ciliary processes are present in all reptiles except for lizards. Mydriasis, however, can be achieved using general anesthesia or intracameral injection of curariform drugs; topical application of these same drugs rarely achieves mydriasis (for more details, the reader should consult the third edition, pp. 1279–1280). The avascular retina is supplied by the choroid in all reptiles, and all reptiles have a choriocapillaris and, during ocular development, a transient intravitreal hyaloid vascular system.

OPHTHALMIC DISEASES

Reported ocular disorders among reptiles include malformations, infections, nutritional disorders, degenerations, neoplasia, and trauma. Some diseases are more common, however, and this discussion centers on those diseases.

Herpesvirus infection in mariculture-raised green sea turtles (*Chelonia mydas*) between 56 days and 12 months of age causes extensive, proliferative, and ulcerative skin lesions that frequently involve the eyelids. Intranuclear inclusions have been noted at histopathologic examination. Secondary bacterial infections have required antibacterial therapy.

Bacterial infections have been associated with several ocular disorders. For example, bacterial blepharitis with abscess formation commonly occurs; these abscesses are usually focal and contain inspissated pus. Both Gram-negative (i.e., *Escherichia coli, Pseudomonas* sp.) and acid-fast organisms have been incriminated. Surgical excision or draining and curettage are indicated.

Subspectacular abscesses are either unilateral or bilateral and develop secondary to ascending infection from the oral cavity through the nasolacrimal duct, penetrating injuries to the spectacle, or systemic in-

fections. Chronic stomatitis may be a predisposing factor in the former. Clinical signs include distention of the spectacle to cause apparent buphthalmos or exophthalmos and cloudiness. White or yellow exudate is often visible below the spectacle. Therapy aims to establish drainage through careful excision a 30° wedge of inferior spectacle, culture and cytology of expressed exudate for antibiotic-sensitivity testing, and flushing of the space with antibiotic solutions. Bacterial isolates have included *Pseudomonas* and *Proteus* sp. as well as *Providencia rettgeri*. Hemoprotozoa are sometimes identified in the material, but their presence is considered to be incidental and probably facilitated by inflammation of the spectacular blood vessels. A complete physical examination is warranted to identify any oral abnormalities or systemic infections. Some cases resolve spontaneously and without treatment, whereas others progress to corneal perforation and panophthalmitis despite appropriate therapy.

Blockage of the nasolacrimal duct occurs in snakes associated with congenital malformation, inflammation associated with necrotic stomatitis and subspectacular infections, and pressure from nearby tumors and granulomas. It sometimes is termed *pseudobuphthalmos* because of the protruding but clear spectacle. Some cases may resolve without treatment. Discriminating a blocked nasolacrimal duct from subspectacular abscess is potentially difficult at visual inspection, except that simple obstruction causes spectacle distention at first, with either clear or slightly turbid fluid. Abscess formation may occur after "simple" obstruction. If spontaneous resolution does not occur within a reasonable period of time, drainage by partial excision of the spectacle is indicated, as for a subspectacular abscess. Recurrence is possible, but the risk has not been reported.

Fibromas, fibropapillomas, and fibrosarcomas that develop on the integument of green sea turtles are not uncommon. These tumors may, however, be part of a proliferative, connective tissue response to the eggs of the trematode *Laraedius laraedii* (which lodge in the small vessels of the skin and conjunctiva after hematogenous release from the parasite), herpesvirus, or unknown factors. The tumors may involve the eyelids and conjunctiva as well, and they also may impair vision.

Retained Spectacles

Retained spectacles in snakes present a challenge for treatment. Causes of retained spectacles include generalized integumentary disease, dry environment, local injury to the spectacle, mite or tick infestation, and systemic illness (Fig. 15-2). During several ecdysis cycles, a thick layer of old spectacles accumulates. Spectacle opacification may render the snake blind in one or both eyes as well as possibly unable or unwilling to feed. Conservative treatment is often effective. Such treatment is also the safest and consists of increasing the environmental humidity through misting or soaking the snake and then allowing natural shedding to occur during the next cycle. If this is unsuccessful or the spectacle has been previously damaged and is unlikely to be shed, application of acetylcysteine (Mucomyst; Mead Johnson Pharmaceutical Division) to the spectacle may loosen it sufficiently to allow for atraumatic removal with forceps. Extreme care must be taken, however, to avoid injury to the cornea.

FIGURE 15-2. *A python snake with distension of the subspectacular space because of nasolacrimal duct obstruction from necrotic stomatitis.*

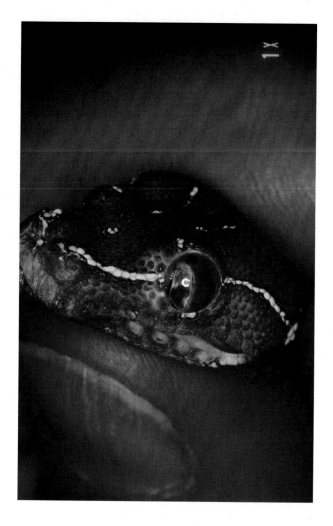

Vitamin A Deficiency

Hypovitaminosis A is commonly recognized in chelonians. This deficiency occurs most frequently among aquatic species, and especially among rapidly growing, young turtles fed diets of meat and insects, and it causes squamous metaplasia of the orbital glands and their ducts (Fig. 15-3). The glands increase in size as desquamated cells block their ducts. The eyelids then become edematous, and blepharoconjunctivitis ensues. In addition, the palpebral fissure closes, and secondary bacterial conjunctivitis as well as keratitis are common. Concomitantly, squamous metaplasia of renal, pancreatic, gastrointestinal, and respiratory epithelia progress to a fatal consequence. **During the early stages of the disease, when the affected animal is still eating, a change of diet to commercial trout pellets supplemented with cod liver oil can reverse the problem, at least initially. Later, parenteral vitamin A (Aquasol-A; USV Pharmaceutical), 1000 to 5000 IU, is recommended for weekly administration until resolution. Topical antibiotic ointment is recommended to control bacterial infection.**

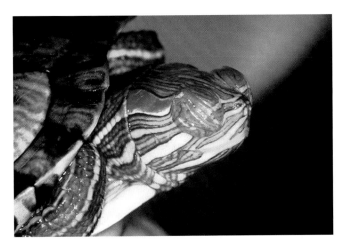

FIGURE 15-3. *A young red-eared slider with blepharoconjunctivitis because of hypovitaminosis A.*

EYE DISEASES OF BIRDS

OPHTHALMIC ANATOMY

Both upper and lower eyelids as well as membrana nictitans are present in birds. The lower lid is more mobile than the upper, however, and usually contains a fibroelastic tarsal plate. The nictitans is well developed, actively mobile, nearly transparent, thin, and covered by a papillary layer of epithelium. Drawn from the nasal canthus, the nictitans moves through contracture of the pyramidalis muscle that originates from the posterior pole of the sclera, where it loops through a sling formed by the quadratus muscle. Both muscles are innervated by cranial nerve VI and may derive from the crocodilian retractor bulbi muscles, which are otherwise absent in birds. The oblique and rectus muscles are thin and relatively poorly developed. Meibomian glands are absent as well. The lacrimal gland is located inferotemporal to the globe, and a harderian gland is located adjacent to the posterior sclera, near the base of the nictitans (but not as part of it). Two lacrimal puncta drain lacrimal secretions into a nasolacrimal duct and, thence, to the nasal cavity. The orbit is incomplete, large, open, and can be evaluated radiographically.

The globe is very large relative to the size of the body (Fig. 15-4), and the posterior segment is much larger than the anterior segment. Three basic shapes are typical:

1. Flat, with a short anteroposterior axis and a flat or partly concave ciliary region;
2. Globose, in which the ciliary region protrudes further from the posterior segment though remains somewhat concave in many diurnal birds, including raptors, needing high-resolution distance vision; and
3. Tubular (i.e., the owl), in which the intermediate segment is elongated anteroposteriorly, forming a tube.

The shape of the globe is formed and maintained by hyaline cartilage in the sclera of the posterior segment and by 10 to 18 scleral ossicles (sometimes

FIGURE 15-4. *The raptor eye.*

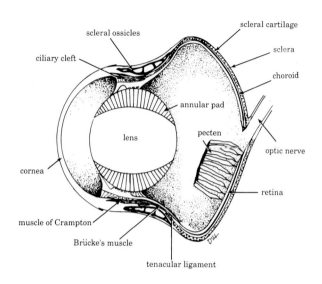

pneumatic) in the sclera of the intermediate segment. The iris contains striated sphincter and dilator muscles as well as myoepithelium and smooth muscle, and its stroma harbors several pigments that are responsible for variable iris coloration. The circular pupil is subject to influence by retinal stimulation as well as to voluntary control. Iris vascularization is similar to that in lizards. The iridocorneal angle is well developed and is drained by two annular channels. The lens is soft, pliable, and of variable shape, being spherical in nocturnal species and flattened anteriorly in some diurnal species. An equatorial annular pad formed by modified lens fibers is present as well and may be very prominent. Accommodation in birds involves changes in the corneal curvature, anterior movement of the lens, and lens deformation. Lens power is increased by contraction of the striated meridional ciliary muscles (i.e., Brücke's muscle posteriorly and Crampton's muscle anteriorly) that insert on the peripheral cornea, move the ciliary body axially, and thus compress the lens by exerting pressure on the annular pad. Contraction of Crampton's muscle may flatten the peripheral cornea. The retina is avascular and atapetal, but it does have a well-developed choroid and pecten. The pecten itself is a highly vascular, pigmented structure of greatly variable size that extends into the vitreous from—and obscures during visual examination—the optic nerve head.

OPHTHALMIC EXAMINATION

Clinical examination of avian eyes uses the same instrumentation and diagnostic techniques as that in mammals. **Avian responses to eye-related reflexes differ from those of mammals in some respects. Palpebral response is present, with the lower lid covering the globe more extensively than the upper lid, and membrana nictitans excursions are prominent. Menace responses seem to be inconsistent, however, even in birds with evidently normal vision. Thus, an absent menace response has little diagnostic significance.** Avoidance behavior is a more reliable indicator of vision. Because the retractor bulbi muscles are absent in birds, being replaced by the quadratus and pyramidalis muscles that subserve motility of the membrana nictitans, globe retraction is not a feature of eye-related reflex responses. The corneal reflex is present, however, manifesting as blinking, nictitans excursion, and avoidance behavior. **Direct pupillary light reflex is present as well, though its assessment is often problematic because of the presumptive voluntary control of the striated components of the iris musculature and the emotional state of the bird. Slight, intermittent, dynamic anisocoria may be normal. Because of the complete decussation of the optic nerve fibers, consensual pupillary light responses are not expected in birds.** Artefactual consensual responses may be induced by inadvertent stimulation of the retina in the fellow eye when eliciting the direct pupillary response through the posterior pole of the stimulated eye and the thin interosseus septum that separates the two orbits.

Posterior segment examinations in birds are confounded by the difficulty of achieving mydriasis. Parasympatholytic agents are ineffective because of the complex muscular arrangement of the iris. **Predominantly striated in nature, the iris muscles may be partially paralyzed by neuromuscular paralyzing agents, and intracameral injection of D tubocurarine, which is a nondepolarizing, neuromuscular-blocking agent, causes consistent, moderate to maximal mydriasis in pigeons and several raptor species.** (For more details, the reader should consult Appendix L as well as the third edition, pp. 1286–1287.)

OPHTHALMIC DISEASES

Avian ocular disorders generally may be categorized, albeit imperfectly, as malformations, inflammations, infections, degenerations, neoplasia, nutritional disorders, and traumatic injuries. **Developmental malformations have been reported only infrequently. In one series of ocular anomalies among 16 raptors, the most common lesion was microphthalmia.**

Ocular inflammation in birds originates from infections, including both primary ocular and systemic diseases; nonseptic inflammation, including presumptively immune-mediated processes; and traumatic injuries. (For more details, the reader should consult the third edition, pp. 1288–1291.)

Traumatic ocular injury occurs frequently in raptors and wild passerine birds. Such injuries, however, often are not confined to the eyes. They also may be complex and involve the external eye as well as the anterior segment or posterior segment (or both). Even the bony scleral ossicles are subject to injury and fracture. Perhaps because of the relatively large size of the raptor eye, evaluation of the fundus is relatively easy in these birds, and a high prevalence of posterior segment injuries has been found, including retinal edema, tears, and detachment; intravitreal hemorrhage, especially surrounding the pecten; and perforation of the posterior segment (Fig. 15-5). Secondary glaucoma occasionally results as well. If present, globe enlargement is usually subtle as the rigid sclera probably limits the extent of buphthalmos. Enucleation in birds may be performed by a lateral or a transaural approach. In some birds, incision and collapse of the globe facilitates its removal. In owls, their very large tubular eyes may be more easily enucleated if the

FIGURE 15-5. *Ocular fundus of great horned owl after head trauma. Note the intravitreal hemorrhage from the pecten that overlies a large area of retinal edema and detachment.*

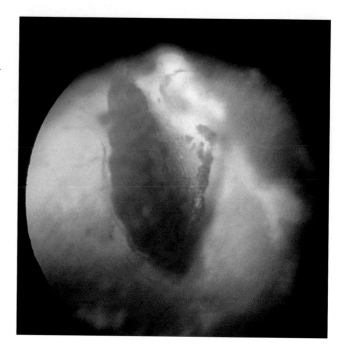

auricular skinfold bordering the external ear is transected. During enucleation, traction on the optic nerve must be avoided, however, because the fellow optic nerve can be easily avulsed because of its close proximity.

EYE DISEASES OF THE MOUSE AND RAT

The small size of rodent eyes renders ophthalmoscopic examination more difficult in this species than in the rabbit, dog, cat, and nonhuman primates. **Slit-lamp biomicroscopy of the adnexa, cornea, and anterior segment is relatively straightforward, whereas fundoscopy can be difficult, especially in pigmented strains, among which mydriasis is exceptionally difficult to achieve. Indirect ophthalmoscopy is readily performed in lagomorphs and primates, and with practice, it can be mastered in rodents as well. Some prefer to use a 90-D lens in conjunction with a table-mounted slit lamp; others prefer to use a 28-D lens and an indirect headpiece.** Still others find a 2.2 panretinal lens to be useful in the latter context. Photography is by the Kowa laboratory animal retinal camera or the Topcon fundus camera with an attached 2.2 panretinal lens. Mydriasis using tropicamide greatly facilitates fundoscopy, with a 1% solution being used in the rabbit and nonhuman primates and the 0.5% solution in rodents and lagomorphs. In pigmented rodents, drug-induced mydriasis is difficult to achieve, but 10% phenylephrine can be combined with 1% atropine.

Collecting blood samples may be important in animals with certain diseases. One of the optimum sites for collecting small venous blood samples in several rodent species has been the orbital venous sinus. A 23-gauge needle or capillary tube can be inserted under the upper eyelid at the lateral canthus and then directed medially while compressing the jugular vein. Repeated collections, however, have been associated postbleeding exophthalmos, hemorrhages and subsequent inflammatory foci along the puncture track, and dark focal areas in the nasal fundus subsequent to orbital bleeding in the rat that may be sequelae of orbital hemorrhage. In animals without tail veins (e.g., the hamster) or with pigmented tail skin (e.g., the gerbil), the venous sinus behind the eye is a good site for sampling under anesthesia (in experienced hands).

When interpreting ocular findings, one must consider the prevalence of inherited disease as a background against which other ocular disease is noted. This is particularly important among inbred strains, in which recessive genes may occur in a given strain not being used to study that specific trait.

CHROMODACRYORRHEA

Both the rat and the mouse have an intraorbital tear gland, an extraorbital tear gland, and a harderian gland, and the latter is associated with the nictitating membrane. **Many rodents, but particularly rats, exhibit red crusting around their eyes in cases of ocular irritation, upper respiratory tract infection, and general stress (Fig. 15-6). Porphyrin-pigmented and lipid-laden tears are produced in normal amounts by the harderian glands in several rodent species. In the rat, however, excess tear production with characteristic red deposits on the periorbital fur, nose, and paws after wiping of the eyes are regularly seen.** Several causes for parasympathetic stimulation of the harderian glands that results in this secretion are known, and the condition can be blocked using parasympatholytics such as atropine. **Diseases such as mycoplasmosis and sialodacryoadenitis, nutritional deficiencies, and other physiologic stresses**

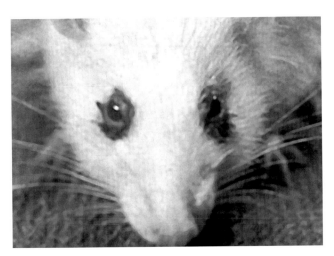

FIGURE 15-6. *Chromodacryorrhea in a rat. (Courtesy of L. Black.)*

are factors that may cause chromodacryorrhea. The incidence of this condition during restraint and transport are indicative that its development should be noted rapidly and appropriate remedial action taken.

SIALODACRYOADENITIS

Coronavirus infection in the rat causes ocular irritation with conjunctivitis and periorbital swelling, which are followed by sneezing, edematous cervical swelling, and enlarged lymph nodes as well as salivary glands. This can be a highly contagious, though self-limiting, disease in rat colonies. The classic epizootic disease has a high morbidity but a low mortality rate. The acute form is rarely seen; the subacute or chronic form is much more common. Ocular signs may be primary or occur secondary to reduced tear production. Primary signs include blepharospasm, photophobia, and eye rubbing. Lacrimal gland involvement (e.g., reactive hyperplasia) leads to reduced tear production and, hence, keratitis, conjunctivitis, periorbital swelling aggravated by self-mutilation, and chromodacryorrhea (discussed earlier). Occasionally, more severe signs of anterior uveitis and glaucoma can also occur, but the prevalence of these intraocular complications is low. The disease itself is usually self-limiting within 1 week, whereas resolution of the secondary signs may take as long as 1 month. The diagnosis can be established on the basis of observing the classic pathognomonic signs, but detection of coronavirus antigen and serologic testing of animals are also possible.

CONJUNCTIVITIDES

Inflammation of the conjunctiva can occur as one sign of a more severe disease affecting the whole eye, may relate to upper respiratory tract infections, or be the sole clinical abnormality. Both in the rat and in mice, the most common cause of conjunctivitis unrelated to intraocular signs is mycoplasmal respiratory disease, though other agents can be involved as well. Numerous infectious agents may be isolated from the conjunctival sac of affected animals. Interpreting these bacteriologic findings is difficult, however, because little evidence will be suggestive that any of these organisms is causing the conjunctival inflammation. One report strongly suggested that *Corynebacterium* sp. were an important causative factor in keratoconjunctivitis of varying severity among a large group of aging C57BL mice, but not among young animals, in the same colony.

During some outbreaks of conjunctivitis, as many as 50% of stock may be affected soon after weaning in conditions of poor ventilation or other stressors. Discharge and reddening of the conjunctiva can be readily noted in many animals, though some may have subtle lesions. Some cases of more overt, purulent conjunctivitis have been reported to be associated with opportunist *Pasteurella* sp. infections in rats already exhibiting signs of chronic respiratory disease. Other infectious agents are likely to be causal factors in other cases. Such conditions respond to topical antibiotics.

CORNEAL DYSTROPHIES

Corneal dystrophies occur in several experimental rodent strains. One report documented spontaneously occurring corneal lesions among nine strains of mice, including BDF1, B6C3F1, and C57BL/6. Corneal dystrophies in the C3H/He and DBA/2 mice were characterized by deposition of basophilic material in the subepithelial stroma, with subsequent vascularization and leukocyte infiltration. ICR-n/n mice showed neutrophil and lymphocyte infiltration as well as vascularization in the stroma without basophilic deposition, whereas ICR and ICR-n/1 mice showed no such lesions. CD-1 and CF-1 mouse strains exhibited a dystrophy that was seen as a characteristic elliptical corneal opacity. Sprague-Dawley and F344 rats have been reported as having subepithelial mineralization in 5 to 15% of males and in 6 to 10% of females between 7 and 26 weeks of age. In some rats, this mineralization was reported to manifest as fine, basophilic granules at the epitheliostromal interface, whereas in others, a coarser deposit was noted in either the subepithelial stroma or the epithelium itself. In Wistar rats, similar lesions have been noted.

KERATITIS

Several causes of corneal inflammation exist; therefore, recognition of the lesion is important. Opacities in the nasal part of the cornea are common among rats, and though they may relate to anterior segment inflammation, they may also relate to orbital gland inflammation.

UVEAL NEOPLASIA

Intraocular melanomas have been reported in the F344 rat arising both from the iris and from the ciliary body. Ciliary body spindle cell melanomas and schwannomas can also occur in the Sprague-Dawley strain.

THE LENS AND CATARACT FORMATION

Several inherited cataracts occur in mice and the rat, and they are often strain specific. Though infrequent in pet stock, some types may surface through inbreeding. The inherited types are summarized in Table 15-1.

CONGENITAL POSTERIOR SEGMENT ABNORMALITIES

Most congenital lesions of the rat and mouse fundus are either abnormalities of the retinal and the hyaloid vasculature or colobomatous defects of the retina or the optic disc. A small number of other anomalies also occur. In rats from 5 to 6 weeks of age, persistence of the hyaloid vasculature is common. This may consist of a single vessel or, more commonly, three to four branches of the hyaloid artery traversing the vitreous posteriorly from the posterior lens capsule. These vessels regress over the next few months, but during this period, considerable vitreal hemorrhage may occur. Unless very marked, these hemorrhages resolve and leave little in the way of a remnant. Yellow to brown pigment, however, may be visible as

TABLE 15-1

INHERITED CATARACTS IN THE RAT, MOUSE, GUINEA PIG, AND DEGU

Strain	Age of Onset	Characteristics	Inheritance or Cause
Fraser mouse	Congenital	Anterior cortical opacity	Autosomal semidominant
Emory mouse	6–8 months	Posterior cortical opacity	Autosomal dominant
Lop mouse	Congenital	Anterior subcapsular opacity	Autosomal semidominant
Lop 2 mouse	Congenital	Nuclear/perinuclear opacity	Autosomal recessive
Lop 3 mouse	Congenital	Nuclear/perinuclear opacity	Autosomal semidominant
Nakano mouse	3 weeks	Nuclear opacity	Autosomal recessive
Balb/c-nct/nct mouse	30 days	Cortical opacity	The Nakano gene bred into the Balb/c line
Nop mouse	Congenital	Nuclear opacity	Autosomal dominant
Philly mouse	5–6 weeks	Nuclear/subcapsular opacity	Autosomal recessive
Swiss-Webster mouse	Congenital	Equatorial opacity	Autosomal dominant
SAM-R/3	Females: 10 weeks Males: 32 weeks	Posterior cortical opacity	Unknown
Cts mouse	Congenital	Anterior polar opacity with microphthalmia	Autosomal fully penetrant semidominant
RCS rat	7–8 weeks	Posterior subcapsular opacity	Associated with retinal degeneration and probably linked to toxic aldehydes after rod outer segment peroxidation
Sherman rat	4 months	Anterior cortical opacity	Unknown
Sprague-Dawley rat	Congenital	Anterior capsular and subcapsular opacity	Autosomal recessive with associated skull malformation

continued

TABLE 15-1

INHERITED CATARACTS IN THE RAT, MOUSE, GUINEA PIG, AND DEGU—*continued*

Strain	Age of Onset	Characteristics	Inheritance or Cause
Wistar rat	Congenital	Anterior capsular opacity, then cortical with posterior capsular rupture in some cases	Autosomal recessive x-ray–induced, with the predominant biochemical change being sulphydryl-to-disulphide oxidation
	Senile	Posterior subcapsular opacity	Unknown
Dahl salt-sensitive rat	Congenital	Capsular opacity	Autosomal, but unclear whether dominant or recessive
WBN/Kob rat	15–20 months	Cortical opacity	Associated with diabetes
KUdR rat	Congenital	Nuclear opacity	Associated with maternal BUdR exposure
ICR rat	3–4 months	Posterior subcapsular opacity	Associated with abnormal lens oxidation
SHR rat	Congenital	Nuclear cloud of white dots or spherical nuclear opacity	—
	21 weeks	Posterior subcapsular opacity followed by anterior subcapsular opacities and posterior cortical involvement	Associated with hypertension
Brown-Norway rat	—	—	A model strain for cataractogenesis by streptozotocin-induced diabetes, naphthalene, or ultraviolet B radiation
Guinea pig 13/N strain	Congenital	Early nuclear changes followed by cortical involvement	Autosomal dominant, associated with the zeta crystallin
Degu	Diabetic cataract	Total diabetic cataract	Associated with high lens aldose reductase level
	Congenital	Posterior cortical cataract	Inherited by mode unknown
Deer mouse	Before 90 days	Early equatorial changes	Autosomal recessive trait in both types of cataract associated with hindlimb syndactyly
	1 year	Posterior subcapsular opacity	

the hemorrhage or hemosiderin (or both) are removed by the vitreal macrophages. Other posterior segment vascular anomalies include preretinal loops; in one study, 12% of rats had such an anomaly. Retinal and chorioretinal colobomas have been reported as well.

INHERITED RETINAL DYSTROPHIES AND DEGENERATIONS

Inherited retinal dystrophies and degenerations might be thought to occur only among experimental animals bred specifically to study their particular retinal disease; however, they may also occur among inbred stains. The *rd* gene, for instance, is seen in the C57BL/6J, CBA, C3H, and various outbred albino mouse strains. The rat has comparatively fewer examples of hereditary retinal dystrophy or degeneration. The Royal College of Surgeons (RCS) rat with its retinal epithelial dystrophy is one such example, as is the Osburne-Mendel rat with its retinal degeneration.

ACQUIRED RETINAL ABNORMALITIES

Some retinal lesions in young laboratory rodents might be considered to be congenital, but careful examination has shown that their incidence increases from 0.3% in weanling rats to 3% at 14 weeks of age. Thus, they may more accurately be considered to be early acquired lesions. Laboratory rodents are also sensitive to the toxic effects of light on the retina. The lesions caused by light-induced retinal degeneration can be severe and obscure other lesions, and they may cause blindness as well. This condition can occur in albino rats exposed to as little as 2 to 3 weeks of constant illumination with fluorescent or incandescent lights, but environmental and body temperatures also are important. Even in standard lighting, more than 11% of 2-year-old rats had lesions in one study, though the relationship between light-induced and age-related retinal degeneration was not entirely clear. Retinal changes such as alterations in vessel caliber, fundal reflectivity, and optic disc pallor could be observed ophthalmoscopically after 7 days of continuous light in one report, but electroretinography demonstrated changes after only 1 day.

OPTIC NERVE ABNORMALITIES

Colobomas of the optic nerve head are regularly reported among laboratory rodents, either as a sporadic finding or as an inherited trait. Typical colobomas, with or without involvement of the peripapillary choroid, have been reported in Sprague-Dawley rats as well. A small number of these optic disc colobomas are associated with iridal colobomas. They also may occur with colobomatous microphthalmos, which has been reported to be an inherited trait in mice.

EYE DISEASES IN THE RABBIT

The rabbit, which is a common laboratory animal, has more recently also become a popular household pet in many countries. The bacteria

Pasteurella multocida **is frequently associated with infectious ophthalmic disorders in this species.** A more commonly occurring condition is orbital cellulitis and retrobulbar abscessation associated with *P. multocida* infection in the rabbit.

ENTROPION

Entropion, which is most commonly seen in the rabbit, is rarely of sufficient interest to warrant reporting in the literature. The few reports that have appeared, however, confirm that this lesion can be severe and only corrected by surgery.

BLEPHARITIS

Blepharitis in the rabbit may be associated with *Treponema cuniculi*, which is the agent of rabbit syphilis (i.e., a condition transmitted to neonates by the genitally infected dam). The diagnosis is established on the basis of identifying the spirochaete on conjunctival-scrape cytologic specimens. The treatment is three injections of penicillin G at 40,000 IU/kg and given at 7-day intervals. Considering that prolonged β-lactam antibiosis can cause fatal dysenteribiosis in the rabbit and in rodents, this treatment should be given with care, and it should be stopped if any diarrhea is noted.

DACRYOCYSTITIS

Understanding the anatomic relationship between the nasolacrimal duct, the orbit, and the roots of the upper incisor and molar arcades is important regarding oculodental disease, particularly in lagomorphs and hystricomorph rodents such as the rabbit and the chinchilla. The rabbit also has only one nasolacrimal punctum, with a nasolacrimal duct that follows a tortuous route through the lacrimal and the maxillary bones. Sudden duct narrowing results in specific sites at which material can collect and cause obstruction. Obstruction can results from oil droplets without infection, in which case epiphora alone is noted, or with infected purulent material, in which case epiphora with dacryocystitis is noted. **Chronic epiphora can cause severe nasofacial dermatitis.** The nasolacrimal duct passes close to the roots of both the premolar and the incisor teeth, and this apposition is important in the development of duct obstruction when associated with dental disease or maxillary osseous change secondary to nutritional hyperparathyroidism. What appears at first examination to be purulent conjunctivitis in the rabbit more often than not is dacryocystitis (Fig. 15-7). This can sometimes be shown by expressing purulent material from the nasolacrimal punctum using pressure just ventral to the punctum, cannulation of the nasolacrimal canaliculus, and flushing with sterile saline. **Epiphora and dacryocystitis result from close apposition of the nasolacrimal duct to the incisor and the molar roots.** Malocclusion of the molar arcades in particular results in retropulsion of the tooth into the weakened maxillary bone, with subsequent nasolacrimal occlusion; incisor malocclusion can, and perhaps more commonly does, produce this same result.

   Treatment of dacryocystitis in the rabbit involves cannulation of the single nasolacrimal punctum and flushing of the duct. If cannulation

FIGURE 15-7. *Purulent discharge in a rabbit with dacryocystitis.*

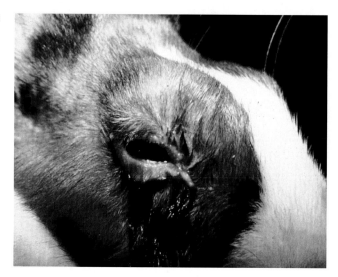

from the ocular punctum is difficult, cannulation of the duct opening at the nasal meatus is possible; however, the small diameter of the duct at its nasal end renders this procedure difficult. The proximal end of the nasolacrimal duct can also be difficult to visualize in rabbits when dacryocystitis has extended to produce a florid conjunctivitis. Pressing on the lower eyelid will often manifest the duct as a pair of lighter pink lips that are "pouting" through the darker red, inflamed conjunctiva. In most cases, cannulation and flushing of the duct with a drug such as ofloxacin or gentamicin will resolve the problem. When this does not have the desired effect, however, the duct can be cannulated in a more permanent manner using fine monofilament nylon.

CONJUNCTIVITIS

In the rabbit, conjunctivitis must be distinguished from dacryocystitis. Purulent ocular discharge with conjunctival hyperemia often relates not just to conjunctivitis but also to nasolacrimal duct and lacrimal sac infections. The diagnosis of infective conjunctivitis and dacryocystitis must be considered with an understanding of the normal bacterial flora in the conjunctival sac. ***Pasteurella* sp. are considered by many to be the most common bacterial pathogen in the rabbit, but *Staphylococcus aureus* should not be forgotten. In one survey of staphylococcal disease in the rabbit, more than 60% had nasal exudate with conjunctivitis.** In a recent survey of conjunctival flora in rabbits with conjunctivitis and dacryocystitis, *Pasteurella* was not the species most commonly isolated. Bacteria were isolated from 78% of swabs, with *Staphylococcus* sp. being found in 42% of isolates whereas *Pasteurella* sp. were only detected in 12%. **Blepharoconjunctivitis, which is characterized by mucopurulent ocular discharge with thickening and crusting of the eyelids, has reportedly been associated with localized *S. aureus* infection. Topical and parenteral gentamicin was curative in that re-**

port. In other rabbits with staphylococcal conjunctivitis, an autogenous vaccine was useful in ameliorating ocular signs. *Haemophilus* sp. have also been reported to be conjunctival pathogens in the rabbit.

Conjunctival disease in the rabbit can result from viral as well as from bacterial agents. The myxoma virus causes inflammatory and edematous lesions of the lids and conjunctiva as well as of the mouth, anus, and genitals.

ABERRANT CONJUNCTIVAL OVERGROWTH

An unusual—and apparently unique—abnormality in the rabbit is an aberrant overgrowth of conjunctiva that produces a type of ankyloblepharon. Though widely seen among individual rabbits, this condition has been poorly documented in the literature. Other terms for this disease have included *precorneal membranous occlusion, pseudopterygium,* and *conjunctival centripetalization.* The fold of conjunctival tissue arises from the limbus, is nonadherent to the palpebral corneal, and may appear to be a thin annulus or to cover a considerable portion of the cornea. Surgical removal results only in reformation of the aberrant tissue, whereas suturing the fold to the sclera or using topical cyclosporin A postsurgically is a more effective method of preventing recurrence and possible visual impairment.

CORNEAL DISEASES

Corneal epithelial dystrophy in the rabbit has been reported as a peripheral lesion that was characterized histopathologically by areas of epithelial thinning adjacent to areas of epithelial cell hyperplasia. Another report described a plaquelike, paracentral, granular stippling in American Dutch belted rabbits that was characterized histopathologically by an irregularly thickened epithelial basement membrane similar to that seen with epithelial basement membrane dystrophy or Reis-Buckler's dystrophy among humans.

Lipid keratopathy has been documented in rabbits fed cholesterol-rich diets specifically designed to produce atheromatous lesions for research. It also has been documented in rabbits fed a 10% fish meal maintenance diet and in one pet rabbit fed a predominantly milk-based diet.

ANTERIOR UVEITIS

The two most common causes of anterior uveitis in the rabbit are *Pasteurella* sp. and the protozoan *Encephalitoxoa cuniculi*. Cases associated with *Pasteurella* sp. often are not associated with rapid cataract formation but, instead, with a more classic uveitis that is characterized by episcleral congestion, miosis, and hypopyon.

Lens-induced uveitis and cataract formation may be linked to capsular rupture caused by intralenticular infection with the protozoan *E. cuniculi*. Given the lens-induced nature of this inflammation, the treatment is lens removal, predominantly by phacoemulsification, with concurrent topical anti-inflammatory medication.

CONGENITAL GLAUCOMA

Hereditary glaucoma in the New Zealand white rabbit has been known since the 1960s. Neonatal bu/bu homozygotes have normal intraocular pressure (15–23 mm Hg), but after 1 to 3 months of age, the pressure rises to between 26 and 48 mm Hg. Gonioscopic and histopathologic features are indicative of goniodysgenesis involving the pectinate ligaments and trabecular meshwork among the affected eyes. These eyes become buphthalmic with cloudy corneas. Vision is lost at this stage, but the eyes do not appear to be painful, probably because of the increased globe size accompanying the raised pressure (Fig. 15-8). Over a period of several months, pressure returns to either normal or near normal, which is associated with ciliary body degeneration. Medical treatment for this condition has been investigated with an experimental model and is also useful in affected pet rabbits.

The *bu* gene is a recessive trait that is also semilethal, with heterozygotes giving birth to small litters of unthrifty pups. The New Zealand white rabbit is considered to be the predominant lagomorph strain with the bu/bu trait, but other white and pigmented strains of pet rabbits also show the classical signs of this same condition.

DISEASES OF THE LENS
AND CATARACT FORMATION

Congenital cataracts have been documented in a litter of rabbits, and in this case, the lenticular opacities were nuclear in most cases, with persistent pupillary membranes in some of the affected animals as well. The cataracts were shown not to be inherited.

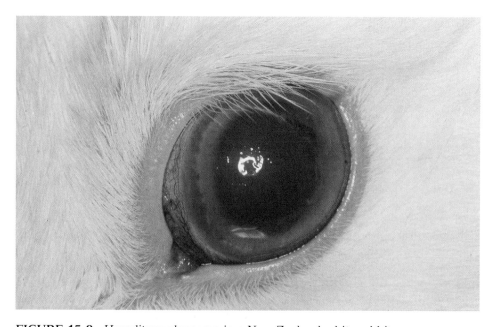

FIGURE 15-8. *Hereditary glaucoma in a New Zealand white rabbit.*

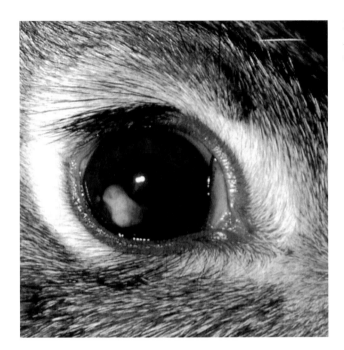

FIGURE 15-9. *White peripupillary lesion of lens-induced uveitis in a dwarf rabbit.*

The rabbit lens is also affected by the microsporidial parasite *Encephalitozoan cuniculi,* which is transmitted vertically and, thus, presumably enters the lens during its formation (Fig. 15-9). Given that the parasite invades tissue by a fine, sporoplasmic discharge tube, intralenticular introduction is unlikely in the adult, which has a lens capsule of 50 to 70 μm. Therefore, lens involvement is presumed to occur in utero. *Encephalitozoan cuniculi* would appear to be overtly cataractogenic only infrequently, but it has the subclinical effect of rupturing the lens capsule.

THE NORMAL OCULAR FUNDUS IN THE RABBIT

The rabbit ocular fundus varies in pigmentation depending on whether the animal is albino or pigmented. **The rabbit has a merangiotic retina, with the retinal blood vessels and myelinated nerve fibers emerging from the optic disc at the 9-o'clock and the 3-o'clock positions, respectively. The deep physiologic cup of the normal rabbit optic disc is often confused with colobomata (Fig. 15-10).**

EYE DISEASES IN THE GUINEA PIG

Conjunctivitis in the guinea pigs has been regularly associated with *Chlamydia psittaci* since the early 1960s. Some animals have only slight reddening of the eyelid margins, whereas others have a thick, purulent exudate. Infection in young animals is characterized by inclusion bodies in the

FIGURE 15-10. *Merangiotic fundus of a normal albino rabbit.*

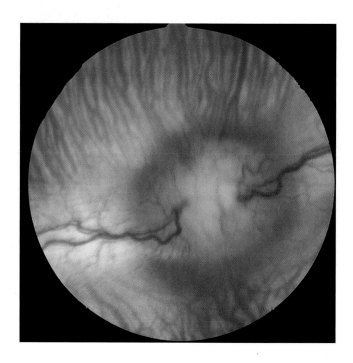

conjunctival epithelial cells with leukocytic infiltrates, but in many cases, it resolves spontaneously in 1 month. Dermoids have been reported several times in the both standard and the hairless guinea pig.

The guinea pig also develops a particularly severe keratoconjunctivitis when infected with *Listeria monocytogenes,* which produces only mild disease in other rodents, the rabbit, and in nonhuman primates. Another infectious cause of conjunctivitis in the guinea pig is salmonellosis. In addition, infectious agents are not the only causes of conjunctival lesions in this species. For example, because it cannot form its own vitamin C, the guinea pig is at considerable risk of scurvy, one of the early signs of which is conjunctival disease.

Bony spicules surrounded by a fibrous envelope have been reported in the ciliary body of the guinea pig. Heterotopic bony metaplasia and calcification occur in healthy tissue and are regularly seen among guinea pigs at various nonocular sites. In one recent report, a link was suggested between secondary glaucoma with buphthalmos and osseous choristoma.

Congenital cataracts have been reported in a litter of guinea pigs that was also affected with urogenital abnormalities after the treatment of pregnant sows with the antibiotic tylan. An inherited cataract also occurs in the guinea pig. In this instance, the affected strain is 13/N, and the congenital cataract appears as early nuclear opacities followed by cortical involvement and is inherited as an autosomal dominant trait.

EYE DISEASES IN THE FERRET

The depth of the orbit in the ferret renders detection of an orbital space–occupying lesion difficult until it has reached a considerable size. Exophthalmos has been reported in two ferrets with orbital involvement of multifocal lymphoma. Even with use of radical orbital exenteration and meticulous antibiotic coverage, however, these cases can often recur, with euthanasia then being the only option. A large, poorly encapsulated zygomatic salivary gland is located posteroinferior in the orbit of the ferret, and head trauma may result in salivary mucocoele with associated exophthalmos.

Ferrets are affected by conjunctivitis associated with human influenza, canine distemper, and systemic salmonellosis. Canine distemper in this species may cause serous oculonasal discharge, which becomes mucopurulent, with associated chemosis and corneal ulceration. Brown crusts form around the mouth and the eyes and often causes ankyloblepharon. These animals may appear to be photophobic. The diagnostic signs are a skin rash, occurring days later, and hyperkeratosis of the foot pads. Death is almost inevitable in this condition, but with influenza, the early signs, which are almost identical, often resolve. Conjunctival scrapings may be useful in establishing a diagnosis. Intracytoplasmic eosinophilic inclusions that often contain refractile particles may be detected during routine cytology in animals with distemper, or indirect immunofluorescence may be used to arrive at a definitive diagnosis.

CATARACT FORMATION

Cataracts have been reported several times in the ferret. In one report, two groups were documented in a single ferret colony. One group manifested a continuum of lens changes, from fine, multifocal punctate lens opacities through cortical change to complete, mature cataracts. The second group manifested cataracts associated with microphthalmos and, in some cases, unusual periodic acid-Schiff–positive material in the lens capsule.

EYE DISEASES IN ZOOLOGIC MAMMALS

Ocular examination in exotic mammals often requires manual restraint or chemical immobilization. Many—if not most—ocular disorders afflicting domestic carnivores and herbivores at least occasionally involve exotic species. In addition, both husbandry and management practices play direct roles in the development of ocular disease in some species (e.g., marine mammals). Delivery of effective therapy is often difficult and inconsistent, and it sometimes requires inventive compromises.

Malformations, infections, inflammatory disorders, nutritional disorders, neoplasia, and trauma are important causative factors in ocular disorders. They are also all of variable importance in different orders of mammals. In general, information about ophthalmic diseases can be transferred from domestic mammals to their zoologic relatives, and some examples are noted here (for more details, the reader should consult the third edition, pp. 1293–1299).

OPHTHALMIC MALFORMATIONS

In one report, the brain of a white tiger with strabismus showed abnormal lamination of the lateral geniculate nucleus, which was similar to abnormalities that have been noted in other animals with reduced pigmentation. Eye agenesis, other ocular colobomas (e.g., iris, optic nerve), and retinal dysplasia with a probable genetic origin have been reported in captive snow leopards on two continents.

OPHTHALMIC INFLAMMATIONS AND INFECTIONS

Most reported ocular inflammatory disorders have been infectious in nature; however, a few have not. **Keratoconjunctivitis has been reported among both wild and captive koalas in Australia because of infection with *Chlamydia psittaci*. Acute unilateral or bilateral infection may affect as many as 30% of wild populations and most commonly occur during the summer months.** Serous ocular discharge, conjunctival injection, and blepharospasm are followed by chemosis with eyelid eversion. By 3 weeks after infection, corneal neovascularization is evident, and this may progress and impair vision. The diagnosis is established on the basis of culturing the organism or a positive specific immunofluorescence of epithelial cells collected by conjunctival or urogenital swab.

The infectious keratoconjunctivitides of wild ungulates share many of the same causes as those in domestic cattle, sheep, and goats. Chlamydial keratoconjunctivitis can affect bighorn sheep and has a significant mortality rate. Keratoconjunctivitis in wild mule deer has been associated with infection by *Chlamydia* sp., *Moraxella* sp., and *Thelazia californiensis*.

Keratitis among reindeer in Scandinavia appears to be identical to that in animals with infectious bovine keratoconjunctivitis in North America. Summer epizootics occur in forest herds. Results of microbiologic evaluation have documented the presence of *Neisseria ovis*, *Colesiota* sp.–like organisms, and other bacteria, but the definitive causative agent has not been conclusively determined. Corneal injury from first instar larvae of *Cephenomyia trompe* (i.e., the nostril fly) in the conjunctival sac may be a predisposing factor.

Exotic felids are susceptible to infection with feline herpesvirus and calicivirus. As in domestic cats, these respiratory pathogens also cause conjunctivitis in these animals, and ulcerative keratitis may be caused by the rhinotracheitis virus. In a cheetah cub with a history of conjunctivitis and corneal ulceration, facial and eyelid cutaneous ulcers were proved on the basis of culture and histopathologic results to be caused by infection with feline herpesvirus-1.

The filarid *Elaeophora schneideri* may cause unilateral or bilateral chorioretinitis in elk. A vascular parasite, this nematode infects and occludes the large arteries of the head and neck, thereby resulting in ischemic necrosis of the brain, eyes, and other tissues of the head. Calves and yearlings are most commonly affected. Blindness occurs with or without neurologic deficits and may be secondary to ocular lesions or central nervous system lesions (or both). Retinal and optic nerve atrophy may be visible at ophthalmoscopy through tonically dilated pupils. Retinal edema and necrosis, optic neuritis, and optic atrophy are present at histopathologic examination. Microfilariae may be seen in the ocular blood vessels as well.

In Texas, fire ant bites frequently cause blepharitis and ulcerative keratitis in white-tailed deer fawns. The severity of the corneal lesions varies from pinpoint erosions or subepithelial opacities to melting corneal ulceration and perforation. Topical antibiotic therapy is effective, but on occasion, conjunctival graft placement has been necessary.

CATARACT FORMATION

The causes of cataract include congenital defects (discussed earlier), advanced age, trauma, nutritional deficiencies and imbalances, inherited lens defects, metabolic disorders, and environmental effects. **In one report, cataracts with a suspected nutritional origin in timber wolf pups were ascribed to a deficiency or imbalance of arginine. Posterior subcapsular sutural opacification developed first in pups fed the commercial milk replacement diet from 9 to 10 days of age.** Anterior cortical cataract formation followed, and after 2.5 weeks of the diet, generalized cataracts had developed. When the milk replacement was discontinued in favor of commercial dog food, the lens opacities partially regressed, leaving perinuclear opacities. Arginine deficiency was suspected after dietary experiments with succeeding litters of wolves, and an age-related susceptibility to cataractogenesis was demonstrated. Pups receiving the deficient diet from 5 days of age were more severely affected than those receiving that same diet after 12 days of age.

Cataracts are common among both wild and captive pinnipeds. Many are unilateral, appear to be posttraumatic, and are often associated with corneal opacities. Lactose intolerance has been incriminated in cataracts among Steller's sea lions; however, the cause of bilateral cataracts in pinnipeds has been documented only rarely. Unilateral extracapsular cataract surgery has been performed on a fur seal, and problems in this case included poor preoperative mydriasis, postoperative corneal edema, and miosis.

Galactosemic cataracts have been reported in kangaroos, wallabies, wombats, Australian possums, and cus cus. Affected animals have been orphaned or handreared for other reasons and received cow's milk. These neonatal marsupials may be variably deficient in either galactokinase or galactose-1-phosphate uridyl transferase, which limits conversion of the galactose in cow's milk to lactose. Dulcitol accumulation in the lens causes an osmotic cataract, and these nutritional cataracts may be prevented by feeding proprietary milk substitutes designed for human infants with inherited galactosemia, who lack both galactose and lactose. Surgical lensectomy has generally been unsuccessful, because most affected animals have vitreous that has been opacified by an unidentified material. **The combination of endocapsular phacoemulsification, axial posterior lensectomy, and anterior vitrectomy, however, can be successful.**

DISEASES OF THE OCULAR FUNDUS

Central retinal degeneration, which is typical of taurine deficiency in the domestic cat, has been reported in a white Bengal tiger in the United States and in three unrelated cheetahs in Israel. Retinal degeneration of uncertain cause has been noted in captive Asian elephants and in culled wild African elephants with cataracts.

Trauma

Traumatic injury is no doubt a frequent cause of ocular disease in nondomestic animals. Conjunctivitis, keratitis, and corneal ulceration commonly afflict both wild and captive pinnipeds and cetaceans. Among 126 captive pinnipeds, 22% had ocular lesions, with corneal opacities being the most frequent. In captivity, these lesions may be associated with trauma incurred while moving the animals or from poor water quality. Transient, dense, focal to diffuse corneal edema and both superficial and deep corneal opacities are regularly encountered and described among pinnipeds and cetaceans. Trauma, anatomic factors, exposure to ultraviolet light, and water quality are suspected of being promotional factors.

Comparative
Neuro-Ophthalmology

Veterinary neuro-ophthalmology is a transitional clinical discipline be-tween veterinary neurology and veterinary ophthalmology. Like neurology, knowledge of specific neuro-ophthalmic anatomy, physiology, and phar-macology is essential for the diagnosis and treatment of these diseases. In the third edition, the chapter on this subject is both large (pp. 1307–1400) and comprehensive. Here, this chapter emphasizes the neuro-ophthalmic examination as well as specific diseases and syndromes that affect both the eye and the nervous system.

NEURO-OPHTHALMOLOGIC
EXAMINATION

The neuro-ophthalmic examination is divided into the patient history (Box 16-1) and the analysis of specific components of the eye, brain, and cranial nerves. These various tests are summarized in Box 16-2.

THE PUPILLARY LIGHT REFLEX

The pupillary light reflex (PLR) is a very common and useful reflex used in veterinary ophthalmology (Fig. 16-1). Determining pupil symmetry is the most important pupillary assessment when beginning to evalu-ate the PLR in the ambient light of an examination room. Pupil size is best measured in ambient light using a hole-sizing ruler or calipers. The di-rect and consensual (or indirect) PLRs are a basic part of each eye exami-nation. A further modification, the swinging flashlight test, assesses the in-tegrity of the entire PLR pathway and is best conducted in a darkened room. A strong, focal light source (e.g., a Finoff transilluminator, a halogen

---

BOX 16-1

Anamnesis Associated with Visual Loss

Refusal to move; sleeps all day; seems old

Runs into unfamiliar objects

Unwilling to jump or climb

Unable to locate moving or stationary objects (or both)

Refusal to move in darkness

Develops aggressive behavior

Seeks security

Altered gait

Head carried low

BOX 16-2

Components of the Neuro-Ophthalmic Examination

History: General medical, neurologic disturbances, vision (day/night/near/far/stationary objects/moving objects); medications; evidence of pain.

Evaluate pupil: Symmetry; pupillary light reflex and swinging flashlight/cover-uncover; dark adaptation test.

Evaluate eye movements: Range of eye movements; vestibulo-ocular reflex; saccadic movements; eye alignment.

Evaluate eyelid movement: Corneal blink reflex; dazzle reflex; menace response.

Eyeball retraction response and third-eyelid protrusion sign.

Estimate vision: Photopic and scotopic obstacle course; electroretinography; visual evoked response; visual cliff; visual placing reaction; visual fields.

---

power source, or ideally, a fiberoptic cable with its transformer set to the highest intensity) is alternately swung from one eye to the other, with the direct light being maintained in each eye for 2 to 3 seconds. This procedure is repeated back and forth (thus the "swinging flashlight") as often as necessary to ensure that both pupils constrict both directly and indirectly. If the pupil dilates during direct light stimulation instead of performing the expected constriction, the swinging flashlight test is considered to be positive for the eye with the dilating pupil. The test is also considered to be positive if, as the light shifts from the normal to the abnormal eye, the direct stimulus is no longer sufficient to maintain the previously evoked degree of pupillary constriction. Therefore, both pupils dilate while maintaining the relative anisocoria that usually is present in domestic animals with optic nerve disease. Sometimes, a normal pupil will also dilate slightly during direct light stimulation, but only after the initial contraction to that stimulation has occurred. This response is normal, and it is referred to as "pupillary escape." **A positive swinging flashlight test is pathognomonic for unilateral retinal disease or unilateral prechiasmal optic nerve disease**

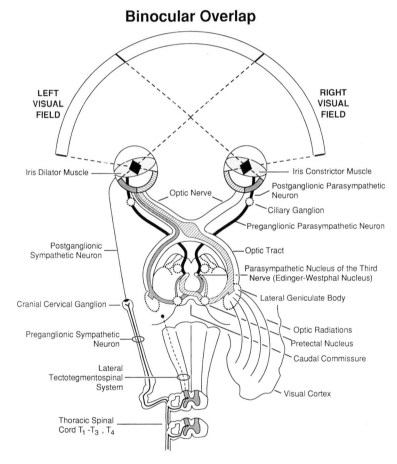

FIGURE 16-1. *Neural pathways for vision and control of pupillary behavior. The unequal distribution of optic fibers at the optic chiasm and caudal commissure differentiates the pupillary light reflexes of domestic animals from those of primates and humans. Regarding the "new" neuroanatomy of the EW (Edinger-Westphal) nucleus, the anteromedian nucleus extending rostrally from the EW nucleus and the ventral tegmental area bordering the descending root of the oculomotor nerve are newly identified sources of parsympathetic fibers going to the ciliary ganglion. The EW nucleus is the origin of the neurons to the spinal cord as well as to the cerebellar cortex and nuclei.*

(or both). Therefore, this test is used to differentiate lesions at these locations from other neurologic causes of anisocoria.

The final common neurologic pathway for eyelid closure of any type is mediated by the facial nerve (i.e., cranial nerve VII), which innervates the orbicularis oculi muscle. **The menace response, corneal blink reflex, and dazzle reflex represent the three types of eyelid blinks that are used in neuro-ophthalmologic evaluation, and each occurs in response to a different stimulus.** The blink response of all three types depends on an intact facial nerve and an afferent nerve supply. **The cranial nerves involved with the afferent pathways that mediate reflex blinking are primarily the optic nerve (i.e., cranial nerve II) and the ophthalmic branch of the trigeminal nerve (i.e., cranial nerve V).** Reflex closure also occurs after certain auditory stimuli mediated by the cochlear division of the vestibulo-cochlear nerve (i.e., cranial nerve VIII).

The corneal blink reflex is a subcortical reflex closure of the eyelids in response to a tactile or a painful stimulus to an unanesthetized cornea. The afferent pathway for the corneal blink reflex is the ophthalmic branch of the trigeminal nerve; the efferent (or final common) pathway for eyelid closure is the facial nerve. Lesion differentiation on the basis of the blink reflex is discussed in Table 16-1.

The dazzle reflex is a subcortical reflex that manifests as a bilateral, partial eyelid blink in response to a bright light directed toward one eye at a time. This reflex is characteristically a slight, bilateral, and often undetectable opening of the eyelids, which is followed by an obvious bilateral, secondary partial closure (i.e., a blink or squint). It occurs when the optic nerve is intact to the level of the midbrain, and particularly to the level of the reflex centers in the rostral colliculi (and, likely, the supraoptic nuclei of the hypothalamus) and with association fibers to the facial nucleus. The motor (i.e., behavioral) response (i.e., blink) requires an intact facial nerve.

The menace response is a cortically mediated eyelid closure (i.e., cortical blink) that may be accompanied by a degree of head withdrawal and eyeball retraction.

TABLE 16-1

LESION DIFFERENTIATION BY BLINK REFLEX

Lesion	Optic Reflex	Tactile Dazzle Reflex	Corneal Response	Menace Reflex
Cranial nerve II	−	+	−	−
Cranial nerve V	+	−	+	+
Cranial nerve VII	−	−	−	+
Visual cortex	+	+	−	−
Large cerebellum	+	+	−	+

The estimation of vision often involves a combination of tests, because each may have certain benefits and limitations. In small animals, an obstacle course evaluation (using four or more 4-inch × 24-inch gray, polyurethane foam cylinders or pylons) should be conducted in both ambient white light (i.e., a photopic course) and in darkness (i.e., a scotopic course). To obtain the most reliable information, the course should be evaluated both binocularly and monocularly. **If the retina appears to be normal in cases of blindness or the patient fails the scotopic or photopic obstacle course (or both), electroretinography (ERG) is needed to properly evaluate and document the function of the outer retina (i.e., photoreceptors).** The ERG will evaluate both scotopic (i.e., rod photoreceptor) and photopic (i.e., cone photoreceptor) functions and is a test of retinal, but not of visual, function. The pattern ERG is obtained using a stimulus whose overall luminance does not change and whose pattern is either a grating or a checkerboard pattern, and it appears to test for the inner retinal layers (especially the retinal ganglion cells). This pattern is phase-shifted by 180° (i.e., black-and-white components of the pattern are continuously exchanged) and at a moderate rate.

Spontaneous electrical activity emanating from the occipital cortex can be recorded, as can electrical activity in this region after brief flashes of light or stimulus patterns. This recorded occipital potential has been termed the *visual-evoked response, visual-evoked potential* (VEP) or *evoked potential,* and the *visually evoked cortical potential.* These small potentials, which are on the order of 5 μV, are embedded in the large-amplitude, randomly fluctuating electroencephalogram, which has a general amplitude of approximately 55 to 60 μV. Before the advent of computers and digital averaging, recording VEPs was not possible, because these small potentials were lost in the background of the higher-amplitude, random noise of the electroencephalogram itself.

In the visual cliff test, the sensitivity of monocular and binocular depth perception may be estimated. Visual placing reactions are used in the dog and the cat to test their ability to voluntarily move their legs in response to a visual stimulus.

Finally, the determination of visual fields is also used. This test is based on the general plan for the visual pathway that occurs in all mammalian species, in which optic nerve fibers from the nasal half of the retina decussate in the optic chiasm so that each optic tract contains the optic nerve fibers from the nasal half of one (i.e., crossed fibers) retina and from the temporal half (i.e., uncrossed fibers) of the other. The left temporal hemiretina, which views the contralateral (i.e., right) visual field in the area of binocular overlap, projects to the left hemisphere (and that of the right temporal hemiretina eye to the right hemisphere). In turn, the nasal hemiretinas project to contralateral hemispheres. In other words, the left nasal hemiretinal fibers go to the right cerebral hemisphere, and those of the right go to the left cerebral cortex. A target stimulus observed in the left half of the visual field (i.e., the left hemifield) is thus conveyed to the right dorsal lateral geniculate nucleus (dLGN) via the right optic tract from the ipsilateral nasal half of the retina (i.e., the left nasal hemiretina) and the contralateral temporal half of the retina (i.e., the right temporal hemiretina). The target stimulus information projects from the right dLGN to the right striate (i.e., area 17) and extrastriate visual cortex (i.e., area 18, 19, and others). (For more details, the reader should consult the third edition, pp. 1308–1323.)

NEUROLOGY OF INTRAOCULAR MUSCLES: THE PUPIL

The pupil is controlled by two muscles: the sphincter, and the dilator. In mammals, the intraocular smooth muscles were once thought simply to have parasympathetic innervation to the iris sphincter muscle and sympathetic innervation to the iris dilator muscle. Evidence from the dog, however, has convincingly demonstrated that the iris sphincter and dilator muscles receive functional, double reciprocal innervation by both the cholinergic and the adrenergic systems. In other words, stimulation of an iris muscle causes a reciprocal inhibition in its antagonist, which functionally means that cholinergic excitatory nerves to the sphincter cause it to contract but, at the same time, cholinergic inhibitory nerves to the dilator cause it to relax, thus enhancing miosis. The cholinergic inhibitory system to the dilator muscle has been demonstrated in the dog, cat, rat, ox, and in humans. On the adrenergic side, inhibition of the iris sphincter muscle has also been demonstrated. The final common pathway to the iris sphincter muscle (i.e., the efferent arm of the PLR) is a two-neuron pathway composed of neurons from the parasympathetic division of the autonomic nervous system. **Recent evidence is suggestive that the anteromedian nucleus, which is smaller than the Edinger-Westphal nucleus and extends rostrally from it, and the ventral tegmental area bordering the descending root of the oculomotor nerve are the source of most parasympathetics going to the ciliary ganglion.** The ciliary ganglion is a collection of postganglionic, parasympathetic cell bodies lateral to the optic nerve that give rise to the axons that innervate the iris sphincter muscle (and, because of dual reciprocal innervation, the iris dilator muscle) and become part of the short ciliary nerves. In the cat, only two short ciliary nerves arise from the ciliary ganglion; these are referred to as the malar (i.e., lateral) and nasal (i.e., medial) nerves. In birds, amphibians, and reptiles, the pupilloconstrictor muscle (i.e., the iris sphincter muscle) consists of striated muscle rather than the slower-acting, smooth muscle in the iris sphincter of mammals.

The afferent arm is a three-neuron pathway, with one neuron being linked in chainlike fashion to the next. The first neurons to be stimulated in this chain are the retinal chain neurons, which consist of the rod and cone photoreceptors, and the true first-order neurons, which consist of the retinal bipolar cells. The second, and longest, neurons in the chain are the optic nerve fibers, which originate from the retinal ganglion cells of the eighth retinal layer to form the ninth retinal layer (i.e., the nerve fiber layer). The nerve fiber layer then thickens centrally as the axons converge. The fibers become visible at ophthalmoscopy after their myelination at the optic disc before exiting the globe at the lamina cribrosa. The optic axons of both eyes then project posteriorly through the periorbita and the short optic canals to their point of meeting and decussation at the optic chiasm. **The extent of optic fiber decussation at the optic chiasm varies among domestic species. In large domestic animals such as the horse, ox, sheep, and pig,** decussation at the optic chiasm is estimated to be from 80 to 90%. This degree of decussation approaches that of nonmammalian species, such as most fish and birds, in which all optic fibers decussate. The cat most closely approaches the 50% decussation of primates, including humans. (For more details, the reader should consult the third edition, pp. 1323–1327).

SPECIFIC NEURO-OPHTHALMIC DISEASES AND SYNDROMES

Specific neuro-ophthalmic diseases or syndromes include several single and multiple neural and ophthalmic disorders. Because animals may present with specific medical histories and clinical signs, these diseases are presented here as a clinical guide. (For more details, the reader should consult the third edition, pp. 1328–1394.)

INTERNAL OPHTHALMOPLEGIA

Internal ophthalmoplegia may occur from impairment of the iris sphincter muscle with a resultant dilated pupil, atropinelike drugs in the eye, or defective parasympathetic innervation. Interruption of these parasympathetic fibers can occur without disturbing the motor efferents of the oculomotor nerve (i.e., cranial nerve III). In the dog, one neuroanatomic explanation for this selective vulnerability to injury is that these preganglionic, parasympathetic fibers are arranged superficially along the medial side of the nerve, which makes them preferentially vulnerable to injury during oculomotor nerve displacement or compression. The affected pupil is nonreactive to both direct and indirect light stimulation and is supersensitive to parasympathomimetic agents (ipsilateral). In the cat only, maximal and equal dilation of both eyes on dark adaptation occurs as well.

EXTERNAL OPHTHALMOPLEGIA

Because of the close proximity of the motor efferent nuclei in the oculomotor complex to the parasympathetic nuclei of the third nerve, and because the axons of these nuclei travel together in the trunk of the oculomotor nerve (i.e., cranial nerve III) as it exits the mesencephalon, oculomotor nerve damage not uncommonly results in external as well as internal ophthalmoplegia. **The clinical features of external ophthalmoplegia include ptosis (ipsilateral); lateral strabismus, with an inability to rotate the globe dorsally, ventrally, or medially; and the presence or absence of the signs of internal ophthalmoplegia.** External ophthalmoplegia more commonly occurs with central lesions and, thus, may provide localizing information.

HORNER'S SYNDROME

In the dog and the cat, Horner's syndrome, which results from interruption of the efferent sympathetic pupillomotor system anywhere along

its three-neuron pathway, produces several clinical signs (Table 16-2 and Fig. 16-2). A tentative diagnosis of Horner's syndrome requires pharmacologic confirmation. The classically described cocaine and epinephrine tests are sometimes used, but these tests rarely produce a clear localization of the lesion site. They can be used, however, to confirm a diagnosis of Horner's syndrome (Table 16-3).

TABLE 16-2

CLINICAL SIGNS OF HORNER'S SYNDROME IN ANIMALS

Clinical Signs	Further Explanations
Cats and dogs	
Miosis (ipsilateral)	For preganglionic lesions, the chance for recovery of pupillary function is better than that with postganglionic lesions. Recovery should not be expected beyond 6 months. Lesions that destroy the cranial cervical ganglion are permanent.
Anisocoria	Degree of anisocoria varies depending on the background illumination. Anisocoria becomes more pronounced in darkness and less apparent with increasing illumination.
Sympathetic ptosis	Sympathetic ptosis results from a loss of sympathetic supply to Müller's muscle, which is a smooth muscle of the eyelids. A topical sympathomimetic will transiently resolve a sympathetic ptosis but have no effect on ptosis from other causes.
Narrowed palpebral fissure	Sympathetic ptosis of the upper eyelid, either alone or in conjunction with reverse ptosis (i.e., elevation of the lower eyelid from decreased sympathetic supply to Müller's muscle in the lower eyelid), creates a narrowed palpebral fissure, which in turn often creates a false impression of enophthalmos.
Enophthalmos	Results from oculosympathetic denervation and subsequent relaxation of the orbital smooth muscles that encircle and are part of the periorbita.
Third-eyelid protrusion	Protrusion of the nictitans or the third eyelid results from denervation of the two smooth muscles of the third eyelid (i.e., medial and ventral smooth muscles of the third eyelid), at least in the cat.
Horses	In addition to the clinical signs seen in the dog and cat, regional sweating and hyperthermia (head and neck) are observed.
Cattle	In addition to those clinical signs seen in the dog and cat, vascular engorgement of the pinna, hyperthermia of the face and head, and absence of sweating on the planum nasale are observed.

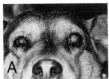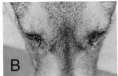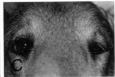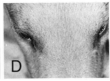

FIGURE 16-2. *Horner's syndrome. A and B. Horner's syndrome in the right eye without enophthalmos. Ptosis creates "apparent enophthalmos." C and D. Horner's syndrome in the left eye, with enophthalmos and marked ptosis.*

TABLE 16-3

PHARMACOLOGIC LOCALIZATION OF EFFERENT SYMPATHETIC LESIONS

Agent	Central Lesion	Preganglionic Lesion	Postganglionic Lesion
6% Cocaine	Impaired mydriasis	No dilation	No dilation
10% Phenylephrine	No dilation	No dilation	Mydriasis
1% Hydroxyamphetamine	Normal mydriasis	Normal mydriasis	Incomplete to no mydriasis

Horner's syndrome in large domestic animals also results from interruption of the oculosympathetic pathways. **Horner's syndrome is also associated with unilateral cutaneous facial and cervical hyperthermia, especially of the pinna in the horse, ox, sheep, and goat. Causes unique to the horse, however, include mycotic guttural pouch infections, traumatic lesions of the basisphenoid area, polyneuritis equi syndrome (i.e., cauda equina neuritis), equine protozoa myeloencephalitis of the cervical spinal cord, and esophageal rupture. Also unique, the horse has been reported to develop Horner's syndrome after intravenous injection of certain drugs, including xylazine, vitamin C/selenium, and phenylbutazone.** Horner's syndrome in the horse presents, in addition to those clinical signs listed in Table 16-2, with regional hyperthermia (e.g, head, cranial neck) and excessive ipsilateral facial sweating (Fig. 16-3). Sweating is also known to be increased by β_2-agonists, including clenbuterol (200 μg intravenously), isoprenaline (2 mg intravenously), or 10% phenylephrine applied locally.

The ophthalmic clinical signs of Horner's syndrome in cattle are similar to those in the horse. **In cattle, however, there is also a consistent, prominent vascular engorgement of the pinna.** Facial and cervical hyperthermia also occurs but, again in contrast to the horse, without profuse sweating. Sweating is absent on the planum nasale ipsilateral to the

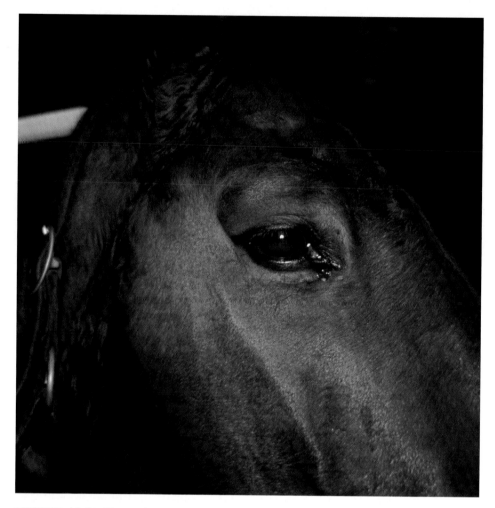

FIGURE 16-3. *Horner's syndrome in a horse. Note the regional sweating above the orbit.*

oculosympathetic lesion, which is detected if the entire nose is cleaned of nasal discharges and the entire surface wiped dry. Beads of moisture will be immediately observed to form on the normal, intact, sympathetic side, but they will not be observed on the denervated side.

OTITIS MEDIA AND SYMPATHETIC HYPERIRRITABILITY

The nature, location, and extent of lesions within the efferent sympathetic pupillomotor pathway largely determines which of the previously mentioned signs are present. **In ophthalmic practice, lesions of the postganglionic sympathetic fibers are most commonly encountered. The most frequent site of involvement for these fibers occurs in the middle ear secondary to chronic otitis media.** In early otitis media, when only irritation of the postganglionic sympathetics is present and before the interruption of nerve conduction, the pupil on the affected side is likely to dilate. The specific therapy depends on the cause.

FELINE DYSAUTONOMIA

Most clinical features observed with feline dysautonomia, which is a syndrome of unknown cause, result from dysfunctions of the parasympathetic or the sympathetic (or both) autonomic nervous systems. **Ocular signs, which include decreased lacrimation, dilated and unresponsive pupils, anisocoria, prolapsed third eyelids, photophobia, and blepharospasm, are seen in 70 to 90% of affected cats.** Establishing a definitive diagnosis requires histopathologic confirmation of lesions in the autonomic ganglia that are pathognomonic for feline dysautonomia.

FELINE SPASTIC PUPIL SYNDROME

Spastic pupil syndrome is a type of anisocoria in the cat that must be differentiated from afferent arm lesions and Horner's syndrome. **Affected cats retain vision and have no iris abnormalities, but their pupils either fail to dilate or do so incompletely in darkness. All affected cats test positive for the feline leukemia virus.** Since the widespread introduction and use of the feline leukemia vaccine, the occurrence of this condition, like that of the disease itself, has been reduced.

HEMIDILATED PUPIL IN THE CAT

In the cat, two short ciliary nerves arise from the ciliary ganglion and are referred to as the malar (i.e. lateral) and nasal (i.e., medial) nerves. They consist solely of postganglionic, parasympathetic fibers before penetration of the posterior globe, where they are joined by the long posterior nerves. **The malar nerve innervates the lateral half and the nasal nerve the medial half of the iris sphincter muscles. When either nerve is affected, the shape of the pupil is distorted, resulting in either a "D" or a "reverse-D" shape (Fig. 16-4).** Cats with hemidilated pupils are often positive for the feline leukemia virus. The hemidilated pupil should be

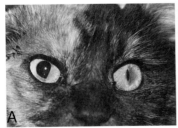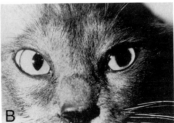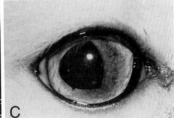

FIGURE 16-4. *Feline hemidilated pupil. **A.** Experimental transection of the right malar short ciliary nerve, resulting in a "reverse-D" pupil. **B.** Clinical lesion of the left malar nerve, resulting in a "D" pupil. **C.** A "reverse-D" pupil in a clinical case. (Part B courtesy of L. Campbell.)*

differentiated from a pupil distorted by posterior synechiae, feline spastic pupil syndrome, and feline dysautonomia.

NEUROGENIC KERATOCONJUNCTIVITIS SICCA

Injury to the parasympathetic nucleus of the facial nerve, pterygopalatine ganglion, preganglionic or postganglionic parasympathetic fibers, or some combination of these anywhere along their efferent pathway can lead to neurogenic keratoconjunctivitis sicca (KCS). Otitis media or petrositis (i.e., inflammation of the petrous temporal bone) from any cause can damage the preganglionic, parasympathetic fibers for lacrimal secretion as well as the facial nerve motoneurons, oculosympathetics, and glossopharyngeal nerve. Signs of facial palsy along with those of KCS are commonly observed. Horner's syndrome may be present as well, because the postganglionic, sympathetic nerves destined for the iris dilator muscle also travel through the middle ear of the petrous temporal bone. Lesions involving the preganglionic fibers or the pterygopalatine ganglion may cause KCS and xeromycteria, in association with anesthesia, in the lateral half of the upper and lower eyelids as well as the adjacent skin. **Lesions involving only postganglionic, parasympathetic fibers are more likely to manifest with KCS and anesthesia of the lateral half of the periocular area without xeromycteria or nasal cavity anesthesia.** The types of diseases that likely cause injury to the ganglion or the immediately adjacent pre- and postganglionic fibers include extraperiorbital sheath myositis (e.g., temporal muscle myositis, pterygoid muscle myositis), extraperiorbital sheath cellulitis, abscesses from penetrating foreign bodies through the soft-tissue floor of the orbit (i.e., soft palate of the mouth), caudal maxillary dental arcade apical abscesses, iatrogenic injury from dental manipulations, and orbital drainage procedures.

In cases of KCS with a known or a suspected neurogenic origin, a lacrimogenic modulator (e.g., cyclosporin A) is unlikely to have any effect. According to Rosenblueth and Cannon's law of denervation hypersensitivity, both pre- and postganglionic, parasympathetic denervation of a lacrimal or a salivary gland increases the excitability of cell membranes within the gland. **This physiologic response creates a clinical opportunity to re-establish lacrimation from a denervated lacrimal gland. Pilocarpine, which is a direct-acting parasympathomimetic agent, mimics the action of acetylcholine after injury to either pre- or postganglionic, parasympathetic nerves** (for more details, see Chapter 4).

ABNORMALITIES OF THE EXTRAOCULAR MUSCLES AND ASSOCIATED NERVES

Paralysis of the oculomotor (i.e., cranial nerve III), trochlear (i.e., cranial nerve IV), and abducens (i.e., cranial nerve VI) nerves may be produced by disorders affecting these nerves at any location, from their nuclear origin to their extraocular muscle termination. **Total paralysis of the oculomotor nerve or nucleus produces ptosis; inability to rotate the eye upward, downward, or inward; and a dilated, nonreactive pupil.** When the affected eye fixates straight ahead (i.e., the primary position of gaze), the eye is held in a position of divergence (i.e., divergent strabismus), but it can be returned to midline by directing the gaze to the side opposite the paralysis. **Lesions of the abducens (i.e., cranial nerve VI) nucleus cause ipsilateral palsy of the horizontal gaze. In this condition, the eyes do not cross the midline, because the abducens nucleus contains two groups of neurons: abducens motoneurons, which innervate the ipsilateral lateral rectus muscle; and abducens interneurons, which innervate the contralateral medial rectus motoneurons via the medial longitudinal fasciculus.** Abducens nuclear lesions will not result in eyeball retraction dysfunction, however, because the nucleus responsible for the eyeball retraction response lies in the accessory abducens nucleus and accessory abducens motoneurons are exclusively involved in eyeball retraction. **If a nuclear lesion occurs in the accessory abducens nucleus, innervation to the retractor bulbi muscles is lost.** Trochlear nerve paresis or paralysis will cause acquired vertical diplopia, with resultant diminished visual quality. During inward turning of the eye, the dorsal oblique muscle normally is a depressor of the eyeball; during outward turning, the dorsal oblique is an intorter. **Paralysis of the trochlear nerve (i.e., cranial nerve IV) results in extorsion of the eye, which becomes more marked as the gaze is directed outward because the dorsal oblique muscle serves as an intorter during outward gaze.** The unopposed ventral oblique muscle then extorts the eye.

CAVERNOUS SINUS AND ORBITAL FISSURE SYNDROMES

Because the cavernous sinus contains structures that continue through the orbital fissure, determining if the lesion is in the sinus or in the orbital fissure is often clinically impossible. **The most common clinical signs are ophthalmoparesis or ophthalmoplegia; mydriasis with a unilateral, fixed, and dilated pupil; decreased or absent corneal blink reflex, with or without neuroparalytic keratitis; and an absent eyeball retraction response.** Computed tomography or magnetic resonance imaging of the intracranial structures, however, can depict the location of the lesion. Involvement of the cranial nerve III axons as they course through the cavernous sinus or within the orbital fissure is frequently associated with the signs caused by lesions in cranial nerves IV, VI, and the first two branches (i.e., ophthalmic and mandibular) of V. **Space-occupying masses are the reported cause in the dog, whereas both neoplastic and inflammatory causes can result in either syndrome in the cat.** In general, cavernous sinus or orbital fissure syndrome should be considered as a diagnosis in any older dog or cat with ophthalmoparesis or ophthalmoplegia and a unilateral, fixed, and dilated pupil.

FELINE STRABISMUS

Strabismus can result from some accident or early abnormal visual experience. In the cat, strabismus is not uncommon, is usually congenital, and manifests primarily as esotropia. It has been well-documented in the Siamese breed (Fig. 16-5); however, many Siamese cats also

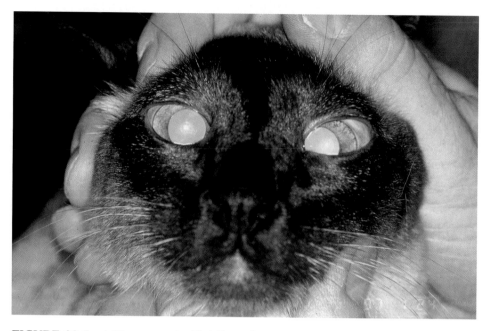

FIGURE 16-5. *A Siamese cat with bilateral unequal esotropia. Note that the corneal reflex (light spot) on each corneal surface is not in the same position, indicating unequal turning.*

have abnormalities in the central visual pathway and in the pigmentation of their eyes and coat color. Most non-Siamese cats with congenital strabismus are also esotropic, but they show no pigment abnormality in the eye or coat color. Strabismus can also be seen in the domestic Longhair, though it appears to be more common in the domestic Shorthair. In non-Siamese strabismus, the convergent nature may be noted within days of eyelid opening and persists throughout life, though it may become less marked with time. Non-Siamese cats with congenital esotropia have a clinical appearance and abnormal ocular dominance distribution of the (area 17) striate cortex similar to that of cats with artificial strabismus created by resection of the lateral rectus muscle.

SHAR PEI STRABISMUS (FIBROSING ESOTROPIA)

Shar Peis can develop a progressive juvenile esotropia that may lead to blindness in severe cases (Fig. 16-6). This condition can be unilateral but generally is bilateral, and neither gender seems to be preferred. The progressive nature of this condition usually ceases by 2 years of age. **Forced duction testing is generally indicative of the problem in this breed.** Passive forced duction tests are indicative of mechanical restriction, because the eyeball cannot be forced into the direction of gaze limitation, thereby indicating muscle entrapment or fibrosis of the muscle. Active forced duction tests reveal a lateral rectus muscle that can pull the eyeball caudally but cannot rotate it laterally. No active contraction can be felt on the medial side of the eyeball, thus indicating either entrapment or degeneration of the muscle. The condition appears to be a selective fibrosis of the medial rectus muscle and, possibly, other extraocular muscles as well. In humans, this condition has been reported to involve all the extraocular muscles.

EQUINE NEONATAL AND ADULT STRABISMUS

Neonatal foals have a ventromedial strabismus that slowly disappears by the time they are weaned. The position of the eyeball within the neonatal orbit presents with excess "scleral showing" of the lateral portion of the sclera. In addition, the horizontal pupil is slanted, with the lateral half being raised and the nasal half being depressed.

Strabismus in the adult horse and mule can be either congenital or acquired. Acquired lesions may cause esotropia or exotropia, and they usually result from traumatic injury to the orbit or from space-occupying masses within the periorbita or extraperiorbita (Fig. 16-7).

STRABISMUS IN CATTLE

A heritable strabismus associated with exophthalmos is seen in Jersey, Holstein, Brown Swiss, and Shorthorn cattle. This condition results in bilateral esotropia and exophthalmos in animals older than 6 months. Vision is diminished, as shown by the affected individuals have difficulty negotiating an unfamiliar environment. The nature of the inheritance is not known.

EYELID-OPENING ABNORMALITIES (PTOSIS)

An insufficient opening of the eyelids is termed *ptosis* or *blepharoptosis*. The drooping upper eyelid that manifests in ptosis may result from damage, at any level, to the motor pathways that are responsible for the control of eyelid position and elevation, from the cerebral cortex to the effector muscle. In those species exhibiting an "upward drooping or elevation" with

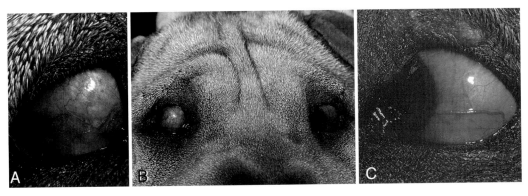

FIGURE 16-6. *Shar Pei strabismus (fibrosing esotropia).* **A.** *The anterior segment is not visible in the right eye of this 1-year-old Shar Pei. The right eye is also turned slightly downward.* **B.** *Progressive bilateral esotropia in this dog was so severe that it resulted in complete blindness.* **C.** *Only the lateral portion of the anterior segment of the left eye is visible.*

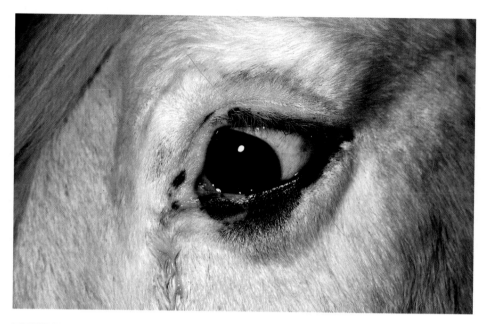

FIGURE 16-7. *Bilateral esotropia in a white horse. Excessive sclera is visible laterally.*

disease in the lower eyelid motor system, the ptosis is termed a *reverse ptosis.* The diagnosis depends on the character of the deficiency and the evidence of neuropathic, neuromuscular, or myopathic disease.

Oculomotor ptosis results from denervation of the levator palpebrae superioris muscle. Central lesions of the oculomotor nucleus are frequently associated with neighborhood neurologic signs, and such lesions usually lead to paralysis of the extraocular muscles with a ventrolateral strabismus, a fixed and dilated pupil, and a ptosis, which can be bilateral. Clinically, any progressive bilateral ptosis of neuropathic origin should be considered as likely to involve a nuclear lesion of the caudal midline structures.

HEMIFACIAL SPASMS

Hemifacial spasms in the dog result from unilateral spasms of the facial muscles, including the orbicularis, and lead to a narrowed palpebral fissure caused by partial closure of the eyelids. These muscle contractions also result in a wrinkled face on the involved side (Fig. 16-8). Horner's syndrome may accompany the facial spasms, and in the cases reported to date, the lesions have been secondary to otitis media. This condition, which begins as an irritation to the facial nerve, can lead to facial paralysis if the cause is not eliminated. Hemifacial spasm might be confused with facial paralysis in the normal, contralateral side, however, if the clinical examination is haphazard.

FACIAL NERVE PARALYSIS

When the eyelids fail to blink because of facial nerve disease, there is frequently an associated deficit in some, or even all, of the functions

served by this nerve. Thus, patients with weakness or loss of eyelid closure should be carefully examined for other signs of facial nerve disease. Important nonophthalmic signs of facial nerve dysfunction include ear movement, drooping of the upper and lower lip as well as the commissure of the mouth, drooling, food collecting in the buccal area, and lack of movement in the affected nostril during respiration. **Denervation of the orbicularis oculi, especially in the dog, leads to a widened palpebral fissure, increased visible sclera, and the illusion of proptosis (Fig. 16-9).** In all domestic animals, a Schirmer tear test should be performed to determine if the preganglionic, parasympathetic fibers for lacrimal secretion, which run with the facial nerve proximal to the genu of the facial canal, have been injured. Lesions of the parasympathetic nucleus of the facial nerve or of the facial nerve proximal to the genu of the facial nerve and facial canal may result in a dry eye along with motor neuron signs of facial nerve paralysis. Secretion of the lacrimal gland can be affected without signs of facial paralysis if the facial nerve is damaged distal to the genu of the facial canal of the petrous temporal bone, because these parasympathetic fibers leave the facial nerve at the genu of the facial

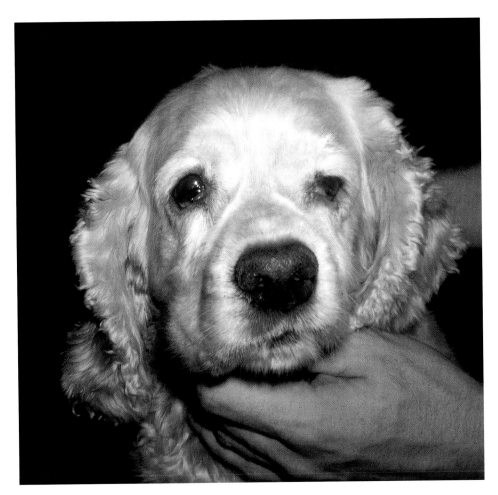

FIGURE 16-8. *Hemifacial spasms and contracture in an American Cocker Spaniel. Note the distorted face on the involved (left) side.*

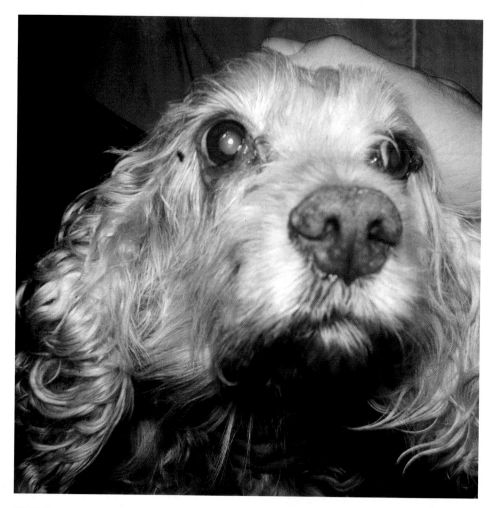

FIGURE 16-9. *Facial nerve paralysis in an American Cocker Spaniel. Note the widened right palpebral fissure and the illusion of proptosis.*

nerve and facial canal to form the major petrosal nerve, which in turn courses rostroventrally through the middle ear and is destined for the lacrimal gland. Facial palsy with normal tear production can infrequently lead to chronic exposure and subsequent ulcerative keratitis. **Short-term treatment aims to prevent corneal trauma and drying. Initially, topical antibiotics, artificial tear solutions and ointments, and oral pilocarpine are administered to stimulate tear production. If regeneration of the facial nerve has not occurred in 2 to 4 weeks, a temporary partial tarsorrhaphy for as long as 6 to 12 months is used to provide additional corneal protection. If regeneration of the facial nerve still does not occur, a partial permanent tarsorrhaphy, or even enucleation, may be necessary.**

NEUROTROPHIC KERATITIS

Corneal denervation because of injury to the trigeminal nerve results in a condition known as neuroparalytic (i.e., neurotrophic) keratitis.

In turn, the resulting corneal degenerative changes produce loss of corneal sensation and ulcerative keratitis. The blink reflex via the facial nerve, however, remains intact. If this condition is associated with Horner's syndrome and results from a single lesion, the lesion site must be distal to the trigeminal ganglion and along the ophthalmic branch of the trigeminal nerve. Neurotropic keratitis may occur after orbital trauma. Treatment consists of topical antibiotics, artificial tear solutions and ointments, and lacrimomimetics (either topical cyclosporin A or oral pilocarpine in the food) to moisten the cornea and to prevent ulcerations.

THIRD-EYELID DYSAUTONOMIA (HAW'S)

By definition in the *Webster's New Collegiate Dictionary,* "Haw's" is an "inflammation of the third eyelids of domesticated animals." In the dog and the cat, among which Haw's is observed, the third eyelids are not inflamed. Bilateral protrusion of the third eyelids is observed as an idiopathic condition. It is usually bilateral, and the protrusion is usually partial. Even so, the protrusion may be extensive enough to impair vision. It occurs more frequently in the cat but can be seen in the dog, and especially in the Golden Retriever. Most patients have no presenting history. Gastrointestinal dysfunction may antedate protrusion of the third eyelids or be concomitant. An imbalance in the oculosympathetic innervated smooth muscle system (i.e., active retraction mechanism) and the antagonistic passive protrusion system, which is mediated primarily by the extraocular muscles of the orbit, will lead to third-eyelid protrusion. The protrusion resolves over time, however, just as mysteriously as it arrived. If it is extensive enough to impair vision, the protrusion can be reduced with a topical sympathomimetic agent administered twice daily.

DISORDERS OF THE CENTRAL VISUAL PATHWAYS

Most diseases that affect the afferent visual pathway from the eyeball to the striate and parastriate visual cortex, or those oculomotor nerve lesions on the efferent side that affect the alignment of the optic axes, disrupt binocular overlap and stereoscopic dysfunction. In domestic animals, visual performance can be compromised by the loss of binocularity and stereopsis to such an extent that horses may not be able to safely clear a jump or canine retrievers to "mark." The visual pathways of predatory birds (e.g., owls) are anatomically different from those in mammals, yet the physiologic organization of their neural substrate for binocular vision has resulted in raptor stereopsis that is comparable to stereopsis in most mammals. The avian retinothalamotelencephalic pathway for vision is homologous to the mammalian retinogeniculocortical pathway. In the owl, as in all birds, total decussation of the optic nerve fibers occurs at the chiasm, but information from corresponding parts of each retina can still converge in the brains of owls and some other predatory birds to achieve stereopsis. The retinorecipient thalamic relay nuclei receive input solely from the contralateral eye because of the total decussation at the chiasm. Like the dLGN in mammals, the avian thalamic relay nucleus is the source of optic fiber projections to the highest visual centers.

The behavioral responses and physical signs associated with afferent visual pathway lesions depend not only on the nature of the optic stimuli used but also on the location, extent, and type of progression of the injury. Whether unilateral or bilateral, neoplasms generally are slow to progress, so the signs of neurologic deficits are also progressive. Seizures and elevated cerebrospinal fluid pressure may accompany blindness originating from such lesions. Traumatic lesions, however, are acute and often lead to severe central nervous system necrosis. Contralateral postural reaction deficits along with contralateral homonymous hemianopia may persist after this type of lesion, especially if an entire cerebral hemisphere is involved. In traumatic injury to the central nervous system, early posttraumatic signs generally are indicative of widespread cerebral injury; however, as the edema and hemorrhage subside, residual posttraumatic signs are confined to the areas of tissue necrosis.

Visual field defects are said to be homonymous when the visual loss is confined to one hemivisual field (i.e., the left or the right visual hemifield). Vision loss in portions of both fields is said to be heteronymous. Any unilateral lesion caudal to the chiasm (i.e., visual cortex, optic radiations, lateral geniculate body and optic tract) creates a homonymous loss of vision. With complete unilateral destruction of any one of these structures, the entire contralateral hemifield is lost, and this is referred to as a homonymous hemianopia. Lesions in the chiasm may cause different types of heteronymous visual field defects. Bilateral lesions at any level lead to bilateral visual field loss, and complete lesions lead to blindness.

Several specific diseases in domestic animals cause bilateral visual cortex lesions that lead to total blindness with normal subcortical neuro-ophthalmic reflexes. Unfortunately, one common, iatrogenically induced cause of total blindness is an overdosage of anesthetic agent. Prolonged apnea, either with or without cardiac arrest, may lead to a diffuse ischemic necrosis of the cerebral cortex, in which the only residual sign is total blindness. The subcortical neuro-ophthalmic reflexes (e.g., PLRs, dazzle reflex, corneal blink reflex) remain intact. In cattle and sheep, polioencepholmalacia, which is also known as polio and cerebrocortical necrosis, also leads to cerebral cortical tissue necrosis of the striate cortex, with resultant blindness. The metabolic changes initiating polioencephalomalacia relate to disturbances of thiamine (i.e., vitamin B_1) metabolism, and the resultant blindness reflects a decreased population of neurons capable of responding to photic stimulation. In affected animals, VEP studies have shown normal latency and decreased amplitude of the late peaks. In addition to blindness, affected animals may develop a variable nystagmus, strabismus (often dorsomedial), and head tilt. Lead intoxication in ruminants causes a similar acute necrosis of the cerebral cortex, with resultant total blindness. The subcortical neuro-ophthalmic reflexes, however, again remain intact. The storage diseases cause cerebral cortical blindness and are most common in the dog and the cat, and they result from a deficiency of specific degradative lysosomal enzymes, which leads to the accumulation of substrates (e.g., lipid, protein, carbohydrate) stored in the cytoplasm of neurons and, occasionally, in the glial cells, macrophages, and cells of organs.

Ocular Manifestations of Systemic Diseases

Ocular examination of animals with systemic disease is underused by veterinary clinicians. Ocular examination may provide an inexpensive method that helps to categorize as well as limit the number of diagnostic possibilities regarding a systemic disease process. In addition, the visual prognosis for the animal may be important to the owner when deciding how aggressively to pursue diagnostic and therapeutic alternatives. Diseases that affect the vascular and the nervous systems are particularly prone to ocular manifestations. Hence, animals with systemic disease should undergo a complete eye examination, including ophthalmoscopy.

The Dog

CONGENITAL DISEASES

ALBINISM AND PARTIAL ALBINISM

Partial albinism in the dog is associated with multiple ocular anomalies as well as with unilateral or bilateral inner ear defects that result in deafness. The condition has been described in several breeds with merling genes; the merling gene is inherited through an incompletely dominant mechanism. In general, the severity of the lesions correlates with merling on the basis of the amount of white in the coat of the homozygous individual. Affected Australian Shepherds have microphthalmia of varying degrees, scleral staphylomas, choroidal colobomas, choroidal hypoplasia, retinal dysplasia, retinal detachments, retinal fibrosis, cataracts, lenticular colobomas, pupillary membranes, iridal colobomas, dyscorias, corectopia, goniodysgenesis, and corneal epithelial dysplasia.

459

The embryogenesis of these defects stems from a primary abnormality of the pigment epithelium in the retina or the outer layer of the optic cup. Other breeds with this syndrome and homozygous merling include the Collie, Great Dane, and Longhaired Dachshund. The Dalmatian is not a merled breed, but it does have an association between blue irides and deafness from cochleosaccular degeneration that is suggestive of a further association with pigmentation.

EHLERS-DANLOS SYNDROME

Ehlers-Danlos syndrome (i.e., cutaneous asthenia) has been reported in the dog. It is a congenital, inherited syndrome involving collagen, and it is characterized by skin that is fragile and easily torn. Some affected animals have excessive joint laxity as well. One reported dog with the complete syndrome had ocular lesions of bilateral lens luxation, cataracts, corneal edema, thin sclera, and lax lids. The lenses in this dog were subluxated dorsally and were colobomatous ventrally; they also had a diffuse cortical cataract.

DWARFISM AND OCULAR DEFECTS

Syndromes involving short appendages with a normal axial skeleton (i.e., short-limbed dwarfism) and ocular lesions are inherited in the Samoyed and the Labrador Retriever. In the Labrador Retriever, skeletal changes consist of the following:

1. The front legs are more affected than the back,
2. The radius and ulna are shorter and more bowed than normal,
3. The elbows may have un-united anconeal and coronoid processes, and
4. Delayed development of epiphysis and hip dysplasia occur (Fig. 17-1).

FIGURE 17-1. *Short-limbed dwarfism in a Labrador Retriever.*

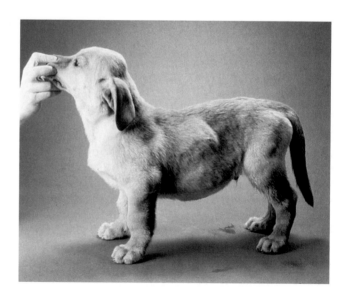

In the Labrador Retriever, this syndrome is an incomplete, dominant trait for the ocular lesions and is recessive for the skeletal lesions. Ocular lesions in this breed vary from mild to blinding, and they usually occur among the field-trial strains. In general, those animals manifesting skeletal dysplasia have more severe ocular lesions, but the relevant litter may have a spectrum of lesions ranging from mild to severe. **Heterozygous animals may (or may not) have retinal lesions, and whether two genetic forms of dysplasia exist in the Labrador Retriever has not been not resolved. Heterozygous individuals usually manifest with focal or geographic retinal dysplasia, which is typically observed as hyperreflective areas with pigment clumping dorsal to the optic disc.** Animals with focal lesions may exhibit a loss of central vision (e.g., failing to mark downed birds or stationary handlers). Milder degrees of manifestation may involve smaller, branching retinal folds and be located in other fundic regions. Severely affected animals may be presented as puppies with retinal detachments, or such detachments may occur during the first 2 to 3 years of life. **Homozygous dogs inconsistently exhibit a variety of ocular lesions, including those of axial myopia, superficial corneal opacities, varying degrees of cataract formation, prominent hyaloid artery remnants, tapetal hypoplasia, and changes in the color and size of the optic nerve.**

The Samoyed syndrome of short-limbed dwarfism is postulated to be an autosomal, simple recessive trait. The ocular lesions consist of **focal cortical cataracts, retinal detachments, multifocal retinal dysplasia, prominent hyaloid remnants, and red tapetal fractures or fissures.** Retinal detachment usually occurs during the first 6 months of life, and it may occur in retinas having no obvious lesions of dysplasia.

CONGENITAL HYDROCEPHALUS

Congenital hydrocephalus may produce enlargement of the calvarium, which may then impinge on the orbit from the dorsolateral aspect. In turn, this pushes the eyes in a ventrolateral direction and produces a "sunset" appearance to the corneas. Rarely, hydrocephalus may produce papilledema.

AMBLYOPIA AND QUADRIPLEGIA

A syndrome of decreased vision with nystagmus, ataxia, and tremors has been described in the Irish Setter and the Kerry Blue Terrier. The ocular fundus is normal on examination, but most affected animals are unable to stand at birth. Instead, walking movements are made that propel them in a "seal-like" manner when prone. **Vision is difficult to evaluate in a very young animal, but those affected lack fixation as well as menace and dazzle responses. Even so, the pupillary light reflexes are normal. As mentioned, the ocular fundus is normal as well, though electroretinographic (ERG) findings have not been reported.** Central nervous system (CNS) lesions include degeneration and necrosis of the cerebellar cortex, with severe loss of Purkinje cells. The condition is inherited as a postnatally lethal, autosomal recessive gene.

INFECTIOUS DISEASES

VIRAL

Viral diseases in the dog that involve include ocular manifestations include canine distemper, infectious canine hepatitis, canine herpesvirus infection, and papillomavirus.

Canine Distemper

Canine distemper is caused by a single-stranded, RNA paramyxovirus that infects a wide variety of various Canidae, Procyonidae, Ursidae, Mustelidae, and Hyaenidae. Clinical signs of distemper will vary with the strain of the virus, immunity of the host, and age of the host. **Acute signs of distemper usually are associated with a bilateral conjunctivitis that progresses from serous to mucopurulent in nature. The distemper virus itself may produce an inflammatory reaction in the lacrimal gland, which is characterized by mononuclear and neutrophilic inflammatory infiltration as well as by marked, degenerative changes in the glandular tissue. Corneal ulceration is often quite profound, with multiple descemetocele formations or corneal perforations in one or both eyes. Sicca usually resolves in 4 to 8 weeks, however, if the animal recovers from the systemic infection.**

Distemper often produces a multifocal, nongranulomatous chorioretinitis, but this is usually an incidental finding. Dogs with neurologic forms of distemper may have a 41% overall prevalence of chorioretinal lesions; in contrast, dogs with chronic leukoencephalopathy syndromes have an 83% overall prevalence of chorioretinal lesions. Typically, these lesions are multifocal, and they may occur more frequently in the peripheral to the midperipheral nontapetal fundus (Fig. 17-2). Acute lesions must be differentiated from scars, however, because the latter will not correlate well with the acute systemic signs. Active lesions in the nontapetal region are white, somewhat fluffy, and have mildly indistinct borders; later, they progress to white, flat, and have sharp-bordered scars. In the tapetal region, the acute lesions are subtle, with loss of tapetal detail, and they may have a mild, overlying haziness. With time, these lesions develop into hyperreflective lesions with sharp borders and varying degrees of pigment clumping.

The most dramatic clinical ocular problem associated with distemper is optic neuritis, which is characterized by an acute onset of bilateral blindness and mydriasis. If the inflammation extends rostrally to the optic papilla, ophthalmoscopic signs of peripapillary hemorrhages and edema, retinal vascular congestion, and elevation of the papilla are observed. If the neuritis remains retrobulbar, the diagnosis is established on the basis of exclusion (i.e., blind eyes with dilated pupils and normal retinal function as tested by ERG). Distemper-associated blindness also may occur with inflammation of the optic tracts, lateral geniculate, optic radiation, or occipital cortex (e.g., central or cortical blindness).

Ocular signs are suggestive of—but are not definitive for—distemper. Acute lesions of chorioretinitis usually correlate well with concur-

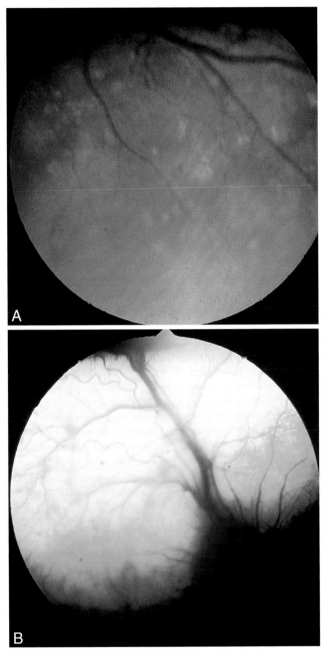

FIGURE 17-2. *Distemper-induced chorioretinitis.* **A.** *Multifocal, white lesions deep to the retinal vessels. Most lesions are active, as evidenced by hazy borders, and do not displace the vessels.* **B.** *Multifocal, gray, hazy lesions in the tapetal fundus that do not displace the retinal vessels.*

rent systemic disease, but chorioretinal scars may not. The finding of distemper inclusions or positive immunofluorescence on conjunctival scrapings may be helpful diagnostically early in the course of systemic disease (5–21 days postinoculation), but a negative finding is inconclusive. **Treatment is mainly symptomatic. Conjunctivitis and decreased tear production are treated with topical antibiotics and lubricants, and if other signs of distemper are absent, syndromes of acute optic neuritis are treated with systemic anti-inflammatory dosages of glucocorticoids.**

Infectious Canine Hepatitis

The ocular lesions of infectious canine hepatitis have mostly become an historical footnote since Rubarth first described them in 1947. Canine adenovirus-1 (CAV-1) is the causative agent, and it produces clinical disease in the dog, fox, and in Ursidae. **It also produces the ocular lesions of anterior uveitis and corneal edema, and it has been estimated to produce ocular lesions in approximately 20% of dogs during the recovery phase of a natural infection.** More troubling, however, have been the modified live strains of CAV-1 used during vaccine production that could also produce ocular lesions, with an estimated prevalence of 0.4% or less. **The universal use of canine adenovirus-2 (CAV-2) for immunization against infectious canine hepatitis has all but eliminated this complication of vaccination.** The ocular lesions manifest approximately 7 to 21 days after viral inoculation. The virus invades the eye earlier (4–8 days postinoculation), however, and may produce a mild, subclinical anterior uveitis.

Canine Herpesvirus Infection

Infection with the canine herpesvirus in adult dogs may produce only a transient conjunctivitis and vaginitis with a duration of 4 to 5 days. Canine herpesvirus is almost exclusively a disease of the neonate, however, in which it usually is fatal. Puppies dying of herpesvirus infection have a bilateral panuveitis with keratitis, synechiae, cataracts, retinal necrosis and disorganization, retinal atrophy and dysplasia, and optic neuritis as well as atrophy. Because of the high fatality rate, the clinical implication of these lesions is unknown.

Papillomavirus

Papillomas involving the canine eye and adnexa have been associated with two different DNA viruses. The oral papillomas, which usually occur in young animals, result from infection with a canine oral papilloma (COP) virus, and the solitary skin lesions that occur in older animals result from infection with a cutaneous papilloma-producing virus. **In addition to the oral papillomas, the COP virus may produce lesions on the eyelids, conjunctiva, and cornea. Lesions are characteristically pedunculated and have a cauliflowerlike surface. Not all ocular papillomas result from the COP virus, but lesions in dogs younger than 2 years of age or with multiple lesions probably do.** Most viral papillomas spontaneously regress; the ocular forms may not. **Excision should involve minimal handling of the lesion, wide excision (if possible), and perhaps, cryotherapy at the base of the lesion.**

RICKETTSIAL INFECTIONS

Canine ehrlichiosis is a tickborne disease produced by *Ehrlichia canis*, *E. platys*, and *E. equii*. *Ehrlichia canis* is the most important agent, however, and is transmitted by the brown dog tick (*Rhipicephalus sanguineus*). The disease is divided into the acute (1–3 weeks), subclinical (average, 11 weeks), and chronic stages. **Ocular signs may occur during all stages, but animals usually are not presented for diagnosis until the chronic stage. The prevalence of ocular lesions has been reported as ranging from 10 to 15%; when present, such lesions can produce devastating functional results.** The ocular lesions themselves result from a platelet deficiency or, more commonly, a vasculitis (or both). **Massive orbital and ocular hemorrhages may develop, but more commonly, a uveitis with hemorrhages occurs. Retinal hemorrhages are common as well, and retinal detachments may be observed, either resulting from massive subretinal hemorrhage or from exudates. Optic neuritis with engorged retinal vessels and papillary hemorrhages also may occur.**

Ehrlichia platys, **which is the agent of infectious cyclic thrombocytopenia, has a more restricted geographic distribution (i.e., the southern United States). It has been described as producing uveitis in a dog, but the syndrome was mild and improved rapidly.** *Rickettsia rickettsii,* which is the agent of Rocky Mountain spotted fever, produces ocular lesions that are similar to (albeit much milder than) those produced by *E. canis.* The vector and reservoir are the ticks *Dermacentor andersoni, D. variabilis,* and *Amblyomma americanum.* **Signs of conjunctivitis, chemosis, retinal vasculitis, mild anterior uveitis, and petechiae of the conjunctiva, iris, and retina are common.**

Serologic testing for antibody titer is the most readily available method with which to diagnosis both ehrlichiosis and Rocky Mountain spotted fever. If either disease is suspected, trial therapy with tetracyclines is warranted until the test results are available, because response to therapy is usually rapid and also is used to establish a presumptive diagnosis. The inflammatory lesion of the anterior ocular segment should be treated with topical or subconjunctival glucocorticoids in addition to systemic antibiotics. The ocular lesions of Rocky Mountain spotted fever usually resolve quickly with therapy, but the sequelae of glaucoma, retinal detachments, and severe ocular hemorrhages in dogs with ehrlichiosis may be blinding.

BACTERIAL

Any sporadic bacteremia may result in seeding of the uveal tract and create various degrees of inflammation. Bacteremia from endocarditis, salmonellosis, pyorrhea, and local abscessation sometimes also may result in various degrees of focal chorioretinal lesions of hemorrhage or exudates (or both), which often go unnoted.

Canine Brucellosis

Brucella canis is a Gram-negative coccobacillus that is usually associated with abortions, infertility, and vaginal discharge in females and with testicular and epididymal problems in males. Transmission is either venereal or via absorption of contaminated tissues, urine, or discharges through the mucous membranes. *Brucella canis* has been isolated from the eye, and it has been recognized as a cause of uveitis in both experimental and naturally occurring disease.

Dogs usually are presented with rather advanced ocular lesions of nongranulomatous uveitis/endophthalmitis. Ocular hemorrhage associated with the inflammation is common in the anterior chamber or the vitreous, and extensive synechiae typically are present. The usual screening diagnostic method is the rapid slide agglutination test. Negative results are considered to be accurate, but false-positive results are common. Therefore, a positive slide agglutination test should be followed by more specific tests (e.g., the tube agglutination test). A titer of 1:200 or greater is very suggestive of active infection. Before treatment is recommended, however, the zoonotic potential and difficulty in clearing the organism from the animal should be carefully explained to the owner. A variety of systemic antibiotic regimens have been employed, but relapses are common. In one report, a treatment regimen of oral tetracycline HCl, 30 mg/kg given twice a day for 1 month, and intramuscular streptomycin, 20 mg/kg once a day for the first 2 weeks, resulted in an apparent cure rate of 94%. The anterior uveitis is treated with topical corticosteroids and atropine. If the condition is blinding and painful, enucleation is recommended.

Borreliosis

Lyme disease (i.e., borreliosis) is a tickborne spirochetal disease that is produced by *Borrelia burgdorferi*. It is transmitted primarily by ticks of the *Ixodes* sp., but *Amblyomma americanum* has also been associated with outbreaks. The primary reservoir for *B. burgdorferi* is the white-footed mouse. In the dog, *B. burgdorferi* may produce ocular lesions. In a retrospective review of 132 seropositive dogs, five had the primary complaint of ocular lesions that included conjunctivitis, anterior uveitis, corneal edema, retinal petechiae, chorioretinitis, and retinal detachment.

Vaccination and tick control, both in the environment and on the animal, are important to prevent infection. A variety of systemic antibiotics (e.g., the tetracyclines, doxycycline, minocycline, penicillin, ampicillin, ceftriaxone, and cefotaxime) have been reported to be effective. The duration of therapy is usually 10 to 14 days. Topical chloromycetin, atropine, and corticosteroids are indicated for anterior uveal inflammation.

MYCOTIC

Dermatophytosis (i.e., cutaneous infections with fungi) usually result from *Microsporum canis, M. gypseum, Trichophyton mentagrophytes,* or some combination of these organisms. Because dermatophytes cause facial dermatitis, they frequently involve the eyelids and typically produce a dry, crusty, periocular alopecia. The diagnosis is established on the basis of direct microscopic examination of scrapings, Wood's light examination, or more frequently, direct fungal culturing with use of dermatophyte test medium. If necessary, therapy is oral griseofulvin for 4 to 6 weeks and environmental decontamination. When treating facial dermatophytes with most of the current antifungal shampoos, the material should not be allowed to contact the eyes.

Blastomycosis

North American blastomycosis is produced by *Blastomyces dermatitidis*. It is endemic to various river valleys in the United States, Canada, Europe, Mexico, Latin America, and Africa. Sporting dogs and hounds are at increased risk, presumably because of their greater outdoor exposure. After inhalation, *Blastomyces* sp. becomes established in the lung. Then, it disseminates via the lymphatics or hematogenous routes to the preferred sites of the skin, eyes, bones, lymph nodes, brain, and testicles.

Ocular signs have been reported in as many as 48% of dogs with blastomycoses, and they have been the only sign of infection in 1.5 to 3.0% of diagnosed dogs. Approximately 50% of the ocular lesions are bilateral. Regarding prognosis, the ocular lesions have been divided into anterior segment lesions (5–30%), anterior and posterior segment lesions (endophthalmitis, 26–72%), and posterior segment lesions (22–43%). **Granulomatous chorioretinitis with systemic signs, which might include weight loss, cough, fever, skin lesions, or lameness in an endemic area, is suggestive of blastomycosis. Examination of tissue aspirates (including ocular centesis) usually demonstrates the organism.** If the yeast cannot be seen on tissue imprints, aspirates, or biopsy specimens, however, a positive serologic examination using the agar-gel immunodiffusion test in combination with compatible thoracic radiographs is also indicative of blastomycosis.

Therapy can become prohibitively expensive for many owners, because most affected dogs are large breeds, therapy may be very chronic, and imidazole medications are very expensive. Approximately 80% of dogs can be treated effectively, however, with the degree of pulmonary involvement being the main determinant of success. Reported overall therapeutic success rates for the eyes are 42% with oral itraconazole, 5 mg/kg twice a day for 60 days, and 40% with a protocol of amphotericin B, 0.5 to 1.0 mg/kg intravenously every 48 hours for a cumulative dose of 4 to 6 mg/kg, or ketoconazole, 10 to 20 mg/kg every 24 hours for 30 to 90 days.

Coccidioides

Coccidioides immitis is a biphasic fungus that can be found during the mycelial phase among the soil of the Lower Sonoran life zone, which comprises the southwestern United States, Mexico, and Central America. Signs of other organ system involvement occur approximately 4 months after the primary pulmonary infection. Preferred tissues for dissemination are the bones, skin, eyes, visceral organs, testicles, CNS, and heart. **The incidence of ocular lesions with coccidioidomycosis is unknown, but in one study, 42% of patients with ocular lesions had no systemic clinical signs. Keratitis occurred in 49% of the animals reported, anterior uveitis in 43%, and glaucoma in 31%.**

A granulomatous uveitis, either unilateral or bilateral, in an endemic area is suggestive of coccidioidomycosis. Vitreal centesis will demonstrate the organism at cytology in most cases, but culture is discouraged because of the highly contagious nature of the mycelial

phase. Serologic examination with precipitin and complement fixation tests can be performed if the organism is not found in tissue specimens. The precipitin test becomes negative after 4 to 5 weeks, so many patients with the ocular lesions will have a negative precipitin test result. The complement fixation test remains elevated for months, however, and a titer of greater than 1:16 is indicative of disseminated disease. **Treatment is similar to that for other systemic mycoses (i.e., extended azole therapy; see Appendix F).**

Histoplasmosis

Histoplasmosis is produced by a dimorphic fungus *Histoplasma capsulatum*. Though quite widespread among North and South America, the endemic areas include the Ohio, Missouri, and Mississippi river valleys. The dog is the most prone of all domestic animals to develop clinical disease, yet ocular lesions appear to be rare. Most of these infections probably are subclinical respiratory infections. **The choroid appears to be the target organ, undergoing a pyogranulomatous reaction that either extends into the subretinal space and produces focal lesions or that coalesces and results in retinal detachments.** A presumptive clinical diagnosis can be established on the basis of typical respiratory or gastrointestinal signs that have been nonresponsive to antibiotics in an endemic area. **Granulomatous chorioretinitis is similar in clinical appearance to other systemic mycoses. Cytologic and biopsy results may establish the diagnosis with use of the agar-gel immunodiffusion test, which is 80% sensitive and almost 100% specific.** Dogs with ocular lesions have not been reported to respond to antifungal therapy.

Cryptococcosis

Cryptococcosis results from *Cryptococcus neoformans*. In the dog, cryptococcosis is usually a disseminated disease, with the most consistent localization occurring in the CNS and the eye. **The ocular lesions generally involve a granulomatous to pyogranulomatous reaction of the choroid that extends subretinally to detach the retina (Fig. 17-3). The anterior segment may have a mild to modest inflammatory reaction as well. The latex agglutination test for *C. neoformans* is an antigen test against a capsular antigen. Treatment is long-term imidazole therapy (see Appendix F), but the prognosis is guarded in most dogs because of the CNS involvement.** Therapy should be monitored on the basis of both clinical improvement and the *C. neoformans* titers and should be continued until these titers have dropped to 1:10 or less.

Disseminated Opportunistic Fungal Diseases

Disseminated opportunistic fungal diseases usually occur in the female German Shepherd and may be associated with a variety of common saprophytic fungi. Agents that have been isolated with this syndrome include *Geotrichum candidum, Candida albicans, Aspergillus terreus, A. fumigatus, A. flavus, A. niger, A. nidulans, Penicillium* sp., *Paecilomyces*

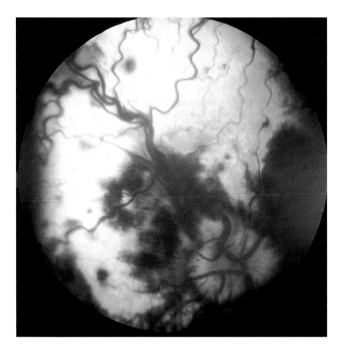

FIGURE 17-3. *A Labrador Retriever with tetraparesis and cryptococcus in the cerebrospinal fluid. Optic neuritis and multiple retinal hemorrhages are present, and a granuloma adjacent to the optic disc is obscured by a hemorrhage. Vasculitis is evident as well, with multiple hemorrhages, perivascular infiltrate around the smaller vessels, and marked hyperemia.*

sp., *Chrysosporium* sp., and *Pseudallescheria boydii*. Predisposing immune suppression of individuals is not obvious, and the most common signs relate to discospondylitis (e.g., vertebral pain, paresis, paralysis). **Ocular lesions of chronic anterior and posterior uveitis may occur as well. Urine and vitreous centesis may establish the diagnosis through cytologic and culture results. Treatment is long-term imidazole therapy (see Appendix F).**

PROTOZOAL DISEASES

Toxoplasmosis

Toxoplasmosis is produced by *Toxoplasma gondii*, which is an obligate and common intracellular protozoal parasite with a worldwide distribution. A wide variety of warm-blooded animals are susceptible, but the definitive hosts are Felidae. **In both experimental and natural canine infections with *T. gondii*, the ocular lesions, listed here in order of decreasing frequency, have been mononuclear anterior uveitis, retinitis, choroiditis, extraocular myositis, scleritis, and optic neuritis. Episcleritis in the dog also may be the presenting—and the only—clinical sign in dogs with elevated and rising toxoplasmal titers.** Systemic disease in a dog with *T. gondii* is relatively rare, but when it does occur, it usually is associated with other diseases (e.g., distemper) or with other systemic, debilitating states. **The diagnosis of toxoplasmosis usually is established on the basis of serologic tests using an enzyme-linked immunosorbent assay (ELISA) for *T. gondii*–specific immunoglobulin (Ig) M and IgG.** Paired serum samples obtained at 2- to 3-week intervals are preferred for determining rising titers or seroconversion from IgM to IgG titers.

Toxoplasmosis may be a self-limiting disease that does not require therapy. If systemic signs or active intraocular inflammation are present, however, systemic therapy usually is advised. Oral clindamycin, 25 mg/kg every 12 hours for 21 to 30 days, and topical corticosteroids as well as atropine are recommended for surface and anterior uveal inflammation. Clindamycin and oral corticosteroids are recommended for posterior uveal inflammation.

Neosporosis

Neospora caninum is a protozoal parasite that is morphologically similar to *Toxoplasma gondii*. Currently, the only identified mode of transmission is the transplacental route; consequently, in the dog, reports have involved neonatal infections. The most typical sign is an ascending limb paralysis. Puppies either die or are euthanized because of neurologic signs, but ocular lesions are also present in most cases. These ocular lesions mainly involve a retinitis with extension into the choroid (i.e., retinochoroiditis), though a mild anterior uveitis and extraocular myositis may occur as well. An indirect fluorescent antibody test and peroxidase-antiperoxidase test can distinguish *N. caninum*. Therapy is similar to that for toxoplasmosis.

Leishmaniasis

Leishmania sp. are diphasic protozoa that infect a wide range of vertebrates, including humans. The disease syndromes are divided into Old World and New World leishmaniases. *Leishmania donovani infantum* is responsible for Old World leishmaniasis, which is endemic to the Mediterranean region, Africa, and Asia, and the dog is a reservoir for *L. donovani infantum*. New World leishmaniasis is produced by *L. donovani chagasi* and may be found in Central and South America as well as in some regions of the United States. The leishmanoid life cycle includes two hosts: a vertebrate, and an insect (i.e., sand flies). Approximately 90% of infected dogs ultimately develop clinical disease, usually before 5 years of age. The incubation period ranges from a few months to between 3 and 4 years. The disseminated disease produces emaciation with muscular weakness, chronic renal failure, and chronic, nonpruritic skin lesions. The lesions begin on the head, thereby producing a blepharitis that is characterized by scaliness and loss of hair and that begins at the medial canthus. A vesicular-bullous blepharitis similar to pemphigus complex also may develop, and this results in ulcerative/erosive lesions. Focal granulomatous blepharitis is a typical lid reaction as well. **Ocular lesions consist of simple or granulomatous conjunctivitis, scleritis, superficial or deep keratitis, anterior uveitis, and secondary glaucoma. Most cases reported in North America have involved dogs imported from endemic areas, but reports involving a closed research colony of English Foxhounds in Ohio and Oklahoma are indicative that once introduced, this infection can be transmitted in the United States. The diagnosis is established on identifying the organism, which is round to oval in shape and 2.5 to 5.0 by 1.5 to 2.0 μm in size, in the bone marrow, lymph node aspirates, or skin biopsy specimens.** Available serologic examination use ELISA and indirect fluorescent antibody testing.

Therapy with intravenous pentavalent antimonial compounds every 48 hours for 20 to 30 treatments produces remission of the clinical signs, but the relapse rate is high (75%). Therapy with allopurinol, 15 mg/kg per day for the life of the dog, has produced promising results.

Hepatozoonosis

Hepatozoonosis is produced by a protozoan *Hapatozoon canis*, and it has a worldwide distribution. In the United States, this condition usually is reported among states bordering the Gulf Coast. The organism is transmitted by *Ripicephalus sanguineus* that were, in turn, infected by feeding on an infected host. The role of this organism in disease production has been questioned, however, because it also may be present in clinically normal dogs. The clinical picture is one of a chronic, febrile disease with generalized emaciation and variable appetite. **Ophthalmic signs may include chronic and mucopurulent ocular discharge, KCS, retinal scars, papilledema, and active uveitis.** Additional systemic signs of joint and back pain, paresis and ataxia, and generalized weakness are also common. **A definitive diagnosis is established on the basis of identifying the schizonts (i.e., cysts) in muscle biopsy specimens.** Outside the United States, gametes are frequently observed in the cytoplasm of peripheral leukocytes and in the bone marrow.

Dogs may respond within 2 to 3 days of anticoccidial therapy with toltrazuril (not available in the United States) at 5 mg/kg every 12 hours for 5 days. Unfortunately, relapse with death is common. Remissions average 6 months and, if treated, respond to therapy.

Trypanosomiasis

Trypanosoma venezuelense has produced blepharitis, conjunctivitis, keratitis, and endophthalmitis in a dog, and the organism was present in the eye as well as in the blood. *Trypanosoma brucei* infections in the dog frequently produce corneal opacification, blepharitis, conjunctivitis, and keratitis. Aqueous centesis may demonstrate the trypanosomes, and use of suramin, pentamidine, and berenil have been advocated as therapy.

PROTOTHECOSIS

Protothecosis is a rare disease in the dog that results from a colorless algae that is a ubiquitous saprophyte having a wide geographic distribution and being found in soil, water, and some vegetable matter. Three species have been recognized, but only *Prototheca wickerhamii* and *P. zophii* are known to be pathogens. *Prototheca zophii* is usually isolated from disseminated cases, whereas *P. wickerhamii* produces a cutaneous syndrome. Most ocular syndromes are associated with systemic signs, but in some cases, these systemic signs are occult. The tissues most commonly affected include the eyes, digestive tract, kidney, heart, and brain. **Ocular lesions include a granulomatous, posterior uveitis or panuveitis that often is bilateral and blinding. Exudative retinal detachments are the**

usual cause of blindness. A definitive diagnosis usually is established on the basis of finding the organism in ocular aspirates, tissue exudates, excretions (i.e., urine sediment), or biopsy specimens. Because colitis is one of the more common systemic signs, any dog with a history of hemorrhagic diarrhea and ocular lesions should be considered a candidate for prototothecosis. The organism can be cultured on Sabouraud's dextrose media and speciated by sugar and alcohol assimilation, electron microscopy, and indirect fluorescent antibodies. **The most commonly attempted therapy has been amphotericin B, an imidazole antifungal drug, or both (see Appendix F). To date, however, no efficacious therapy has been reported.**

METAZOAN PARASITES

Dirofilariasis

Dirofilaria immitis is the most commonly reported intraocular parasite among dogs in North America. Aberrant migration of fourth-stage larvae from the subconjunctival space and into the eye, with subsequent development to immature adults or fifth-stage larvae, is postulated. Approximately half of these dogs do not have microfilaremia, however, or are occult. **The German Shepherd was overrepresented in one series, in which all ocular involvement was unilateral. The worm was in the anterior chamber in 20 of the 21 cases, but it also may be found in the vitreous (Fig. 17-4). Anterior uveitis was consistent in the series, and pain was exacerbated by examination with a light, which stimulated movement of the parasite.**

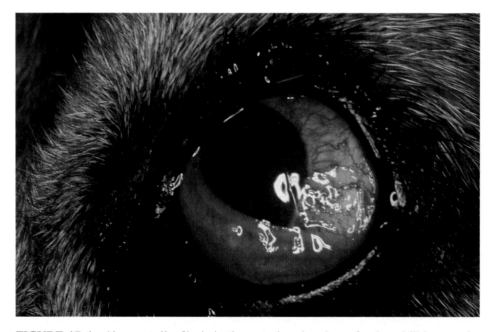

FIGURE 17-4. *Aberrant dirofilaria in the anterior chamber of a dog. Mild corneal edema and anterior uveitis are present as well.*

Corneal edema may be severe and hinder deep examination. The uveitis and corneal edema are postulated to be associated with mechanical trauma from the worm, toxic metabolic byproducts from the worm, or an immune reaction to the worm.

Therapy involves removal of the worm through a limbal incision, which has been successful in 90% of the patients reported to date. Vision has been maintained in 89% of cases, but vision usually has been lost when glaucoma is a complication. The most common complication has been residual corneal edema, which has persisted in 24% of cases. **The uveitis is treated with topical corticosteroids and atropine.**

Other Parasitic Diseases

Toxocara canis, which is the extremely common round worm or ascarid of the dog, is thought to be responsible for the migrating larvae that occasionally may be aberrant in the eye of both humans and the dog. **Aberrant migration of *T. canis* to the canine eye may produce small (i.e., one-fourth to one-sixth of a disc diameter), solitary, focal chorioretinal granulomas.** *Angiostrongylus vasorum* is a nematode that inhabits the pulmonary arteries and right heart of dogs and wild carnivores in parts of Europe, Great Britain, and Uganda, and severe granulomatous uveitis and secondary glaucoma have been observed with chronic involvement. Infection also may manifest in acute cases as a free nematode in the anterior chamber. Therapy for infection with *A. vasorum* may be either levamisole, 10 mg/kg for 3 days, or subcutaneous ivermectin, 200 mg/kg. Periocular onchocerciasis has been described in dogs from the western United States, which were presented with periocular granulomas attached to the sclera and involving the palpebral conjunctiva and third eyelid.

The term *ophthalmomyiasis interna* refers to the intraocular migration of fly *(Diptera* sp.) larvae in the dog. The syndrome is quite characteristic, but which type of fly larvae is present generally is not determined. The point of entry is unknown but is postulated to be across the conjunctival surfaces. Affected animals may be presented during the acute stages if an anterior uveitis is produced, but the syndrome usually is noted as an incidental finding during the chronic stages. **The characteristic ophthalmoscopic lesions are wandering, curvilinear tracts that frequently intersect and are associated with both retinal and preretinal hemorrhages during the acute stage.** If the larva is observed, it typically is photosensitive and moves away from a strong light.

Visualization of the larvae in either the anterior or the posterior compartment of the eye may occur. More commonly, however, the finding is of typical wandering tracts in the fundus. Only acute cases warrant therapy, and topical or systemic steroids are indicated depending on the location of the lesion (or lesions).

DEMODICOSIS

The *Demodex canis* mite is considered to be a normal finding in the skin of the dog, but for unknown reasons, these mites sometimes multiply to produce either local or generalized demodicosis. Localized demodicosis typically develops in young dogs (age, 3 months to 1 year), starting preferentially around the eyes, lips, and forelegs. Lesions are typically circumscribed, dry, scaly, and hairless. Skin scrapings are the main method of establishing the diagnosis, and the mites typically are easy to find. **All forms of blepharitis should indicate the need for skin scrapings, and demodicosis should be an important factor in the differential diagnosis of blepharitis affecting young dogs.** Local demodicosis heals in 6 to 8 weeks, with or without therapy. Lesions that increase in size or number can be treated with topical antiparasitic preparations.

METABOLIC DISEASES

DIABETES MELLITUS

The most consistent and earliest ocular manifestation in the diabetic dog is blinding cataracts. Diabetic cataract formation varies, however, with the species, the individual dog, the dog's age, and both the duration and severity of hyperglycemia. The young dog is very susceptible to diabetic cataract formation. Such cataracts are present at the initial examination of almost 60% of spontaneous canine diabetics as well. The increase in the blood glucose level produces diffusion of increased amounts of sugar into the lens. When the supply of sugar increases, it becomes shunted to the sorbitol pathway, which normally supplies only 5% of the glucose metabolism. Aldose reductase is the first enzyme in this pathway, and it forms polyols (i.e., sorbitol with glucose, dulcitol with galactose) that do not diffuse through the cell membranes and, thus, accumulate in the lens. This results in an osmotic gradient that draws water into the lens, which in turn results in swelling and opacification. Sorbitol is slowly metabolized to fructose, which can slowly diffuse across cellular membranes, whereas dulcitol is not further metabolized, thereby resulting in more rapid changes.

   Initially, cataractous changes are observed as vacuoles in the equatorial cortex that extend into the anterior and the posterior cortex (Fig. 17-5). The cortical sutures may be accentuated as well. This process then progresses to complete cortical opacification, and the sutures are often either fractured or widened because of water imbibition. Cataracts from a variety of causes may progress rapidly, but diabetes should be considered as the cause when a dog is presented with bilateral cataracts having a history of rapid progression. Early diabetic retinopathy, which is characterized by microaneurysms, has been demonstrated in both spontaneous and experimentally induced diabetes as well as in the galactosemic canine model. Diabetic retinopathy takes approximately 3 to 5 years to develop, and almost invariably, cataracts will develop during this period and obscure the retinopathy. **The success rate of cataract surgery among diabetic dogs is approximately the same as that for nondiabetic cataracts.**

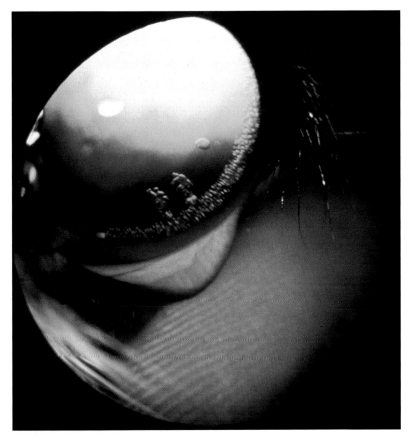

FIGURE 17-5. *Early diabetic cataract in a dog, with vacuoles extending from the lens equator.*

HYPOCALCEMIA

Hypocalcemia in the dog has been associated with focal punctate to linear opacities in the anterior and the posterior lens cortex. These opacities may occur at different levels in the cortex, and they may reflect different episodes of hypocalcemia. Possible causes of hypocalcemia include severe dietary imbalance of calcium and phosphorus, hypoparathyroidism, postparturient hypocalcemia, and chronic renal failure. Treatment involves correction of the underlying disease, if possible, and calcium supplementation with vitamin D_2, vitamin D_3, or dihydrotachysterol. New focal cataracts may manifest for a period after correction, however, and the existing opacities will remain.

HYPERADRENOCORTICISM

Hyperadrenocorticism occurred with ocular lesions of progressive corneal ulcerations, nonhealing ulcerations, corneal calcification, cataracts, lipemia retinalis, and lesions associated with systemic hypertension.

Hyperlipidemia may produce lipemia retinalis or lipids in the aqueous. In one series of cushingoid dogs, an association with KCS was observed as well.

HYPOTHYROIDISM

Hypothyroidism can be associated clinically with a variety of ocular lesions; as many as 20% of dogs with hypothyroidism have also been reported to have KCS. The association has been thought to be one of multiglandular, immune-mediated inflammation. Because hypothyroidism results in vascular disease characterized by atherosclerosis, the association with retinal lesions of hypertension and arteriosclerosis is neither surprising nor consistent. Hypertensive retinal changes of retinal hemorrhages and, less frequently, bullous retinal detachments also may be observed. Hyperlipidemia with hypothyroidism may manifest with lipemia retinalis, corneal lipid degeneration, and lipids in the aqueous humor. Corneal lipid deposits with hypothyroidism may take various forms as well, from diffuse and rapidly developing opacities at all levels of the cornea to the characteristic, peripheral arcus lesion adjacent to the limbus. The diagnosis of hypothyroidism is established on the basis of comparing resting T_4 levels with those occurring after administration of thyrotrophin-stimulating hormone.

INBORN ERRORS OF METABOLISM (LYSOSOMAL STORAGE DISEASES)

Inborn errors of metabolism are relatively rare diseases. The lysosomal storage diseases result from a deficiency in a specific degradative enzyme (i.e., acid hydrolases), which allows the enzyme substrate to accumulate in the cells. Because this excess material is a normal component, the histopathologic changes result from distortion of the cells rather than from an actual toxic effect (Table 17-1).

BLOOD/VASCULAR DISORDERS

HYPERTENSION

Hypertension-induced retinopathy can occur in the dog, but it is observed more commonly in the cat. Hypertension now is recognized as being a common complication of renal disease (60–80% of cases), hyperadrenocorticism (59–86%), pheochromocytoma (>50%), primary aldosteronism, hypothyroidism, and hyperthyroidism. Although apparently rare, primary hypertension has also been documented in the dog. Renal disease appears to be the usual underlying cause, and 60 to 80% of dogs with

TABLE 17-1

INBORN ERRORS OF METABOLISM IN THE DOG, CAT, AND FOOD ANIMALS

Disease	Breeds Affected
Dog	
Gangliosidoses	
Fucosidosis	English Springer Spaniel
Mucopolysaccharidosis	Plott Hound
Globoid cell leukodystrophy	Cairn Terrier
Ceroid lipofuscinosis	English Setter, Australian Blue Heeler, Chihuahua, Border Collie, Saluki, Tibetan Terrier, Dachshund, Dalmation, Miniature Schnauzer, American Cocker Spaniel
Tyrosinemia	
Cat	
GM$_1$-gangliosidosis	Domestic Shorthair, Siamese, Korat
GM$_2$-gangliosidosis	Domestic Shorthair, Korat
α-Mannosidosis	Persian, Domestic Shorthair
Mucopolysaccharidosis I	Domestic Shorthair
Mucopolysaccharidosis IV	Siamese
Food Animals	
Gangliosidoses	Cattle
Mannosidosis	Angus cattle, Nubian goats
α-Mannosidosis	Aberdeen Angus, Murray Gray cattle
Globoid cell leukodystrophy (Krabbe's disease)	Sheep
Ceroid lipofuscinoses	Devon cattle, Hampshire sheep

renal disease are hypertensive. **Ocular lesions reported to be associated with canine hypertension have been tortuous retinal vessels, variable-sized retinal and preretinal hemorrhages, papilledema, variable degrees of retinal detachment, and tapetal reflectivity changes (Fig. 17-6).** Hemorrhage may occur in the anterior segment and the vitreous, and uveitis as well as glaucoma may be complications. **Repeated indirect measurements of systolic blood pressure greater than 160 to 180 mm Hg in a relatively relaxed patient are indicative of hypertension.**

The primary condition should be managed, if possible, and dietary salt should be restricted (0.1–0.4% dry wt basis) and antihypertensive therapy administered. **The drug (or drugs) of choice are unresolved**

FIGURE 17-6. *Multiple retinal hemorrhages and possible papilledema associated with hypertension in a dog.*

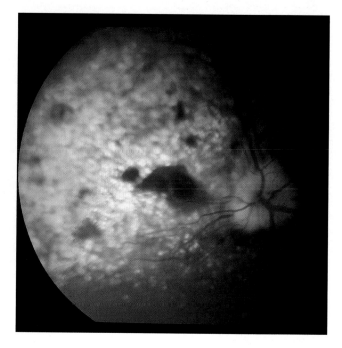

in the dog, but in a research model of hypertension, a combination of angiotensin-converting enzyme inhibitors and calcium channel blockers worked best.

HYPERLIPIDEMIA

Hyperlipidemia is an elevated serum level of cholesterol or triglycerides (or both). Because the latter are transported in the blood by various proteins, the term *hyperlipoproteinemia* is often used. Hyperlipidemia or hyperlipoproteinemia may produce ocular lesions depending on the quantity and the class of the lipoprotein with the elevated level. The usual causes for secondary hyperlipidemia include pancreatitis, hypothyroidism, diabetes mellitus, hyperadrenocorticism, and renal as well as hepatic disease. **Visible lipemia in the dog is produced by elevations of triglyceride levels and can be detected in the ocular vessels of the conjunctiva and retina as pink, engorged vessels. It most easily is observed in the retinal vessels over the non-tapetal region. Hyperlipidemia also may manifest with lipids in the anterior chamber.** A prerequisite for gaining access to the anterior chamber by the large, lipid-laden molecules is alteration of the blood-aqueous barrier, presumably resulting from pre-existing uveitis. **Hyperlipidemia characterized by elevated cholesterol levels may result in corneal lipidosis with varying patterns. A rapid, rather diffuse, and bilateral stromal syndrome has been observed to be associated with elevated cholesterol levels in hypothyroid dogs.** Evidence of ocular lesions from lipemia retinalis and aqueous lipids should prompt the taking of a good dietary and medical history as well as a clinical workup to determine the cause of the hyperlipidemia. All owners of patients with lipid keratopathy should be asked about the dietary level of fat, because diet is an important modifier.

POLYCYTHEMIA

Absolute polycythemia may be a primary or secondary condition. Secondary polycythemia is more common, however, and results from increased levels of erythropoietin or an erythropoietinlike substance. It can also result from cyanotic heart disease and pulmonary disease, but renal neoplasia (e.g., adenocarcinoma) should be considered as well. **Polycythemia may manifest as dark, ruddy-colored conjunctival and retinal blood vessels that are dilated and tortuous. Left untreated, retinal detachment and ocular hemorrhage may eventually occur.**

ANEMIA

Severe anemia often manifests in the retinal vasculature as pale vessels, varying degrees of retinal hemorrhage, and subtle changes in the tapetal reflectivity. Hemorrhages are more likely to be observed, however, and are more dramatic if they are accompanied by thrombocytopenia, but hemorrhages routinely are observed when the hematocrit approaches 5 to 7%. Small intraretinal hemorrhages are typical and may reabsorb quickly with correction of the anemia, though retinal pigmentary disturbances may be a residual change.

THROMBOCYTOPENIA

Thrombocytopenia and thromboasthenia, from any origin, is a rather frequent cause of ocular and periocular hemorrhage. The presence of bleeding signs at a given platelet level vary between individuals, but platelet counts generally are less than 50,000 cells/mL when ocular petechiae form. **Petechiae in the ocular fundus often are present without visible petechiae in the skin or other mucous membranes. The most common causes of thrombocytopenia include infectious diseases, immune-mediated causes, and drug-induced reactions. Therapy is directed at correcting the underlying cause.**

ICTERUS

The sclera is the classic location for the detection of icterus or jaundice. The yellow hue of icterus may be detected in the intraocular structures as well.

HYPERVISCOSITY SYNDROME

Hyperviscosity syndrome is associated with elevated levels of large molecules (e.g., IgM or polymerized IgA) in the bloodstream, but it is uncommonly associated with elevated levels of IgG. The underlying cause usually is a malignancy (e.g., lymphoma, chronic lymphocytic leukemia, plasmacytoma, multiple myeloma), but infectious diseases (e.g., ehrlichiosis) also may produce the syndrome. **The ocular lesions most frequently noted include dilated and tortuous retinal vessels, which may develop kinking or "boxcarring," papilledema, retinal hemorrhages,**

intraretinal cysts, and bullous retinal detachments. Anterior segment complications such as glaucoma and anterior uveitis may develop as well. The diagnosis of hyperviscosity syndrome is established on the basis of demonstrating the hyperproteinemia with electrophoresis and determining the serum viscosity. A detailed medical workup is necessary to determine the cause of the hyperproteinemia, because specific antineoplastic therapy directed at the underlying cause is indicated.

INTRAVENOUS FLUID OVERLOAD

Bullous retinal detachments have been associated with isotonic fluid administered to patients having varying degrees of renal compromise. This syndrome begins with multiple, small, subretinal bullae forming in both eyes. The small bullae then coalesce to form larger detachments, and eventually, they progress to total retinal detachments that are associated with a clear, subretinal fluid. Retinal hemorrhages are absent, however, and affected animals have normal blood pressure. Correction of the underlying renal problem or decreasing the fluid intake will cause the fluid to be reabsorbed and the retinas to reattach, even though retinal folds may persist. Therapy should concentrate on decreasing fluid administration or regaining renal compensation (or both).

IMMUNE-MEDIATED CONDITIONS

VOGT-KOYANAGI-HARADA–LIKE SYNDROME

Vogt-Koyanagi-Harada–like or uveodermal syndrome affects many breeds of dog, including the Akita, Siberian Husky, Chow Chow, Golden Retriever, Samoyed, Irish Setter, Shetland Sheepdog, Saint Bernard, Old English Sheepdog, and Australian Shepherd. The mean age of the patients is approximately 3 years, and ocular lesions usually precede the dermatologic lesions. Often, the patients are presented for sudden blindness. Ocular lesions vary from bilateral anterior uveitis to severe panuveitis. Bullous retinal detachments also may occur, and secondary glaucomas as well as cataracts are common. The iris and retinal pigment epithelium develop progressive depigmentation. As the depigmentation progresses, the tapetal fundus becomes hyperreflective, and retinal vascular attenuation as well as optic nerve atrophy may develop. Dermal and hair depigmentation develop, either gradually or rapidly, and may be ulcerative in nature. The lesions usually are restricted to the face, involving the eyelids, nasal planum, and lips, but the scrotum and footpads are other possible areas of dermal involvement.

Skin biopsy specimens are most useful for establishing the diagnosis on the basis of lichenoid dermatitis, histiocytes, and small mononuclear cell as well as giant cell infiltration. The prognosis is guarded, and therapy should be considered to be lifelong. If therapy is stopped or tapered, relapses are frequent, and because of the immunosuppressive therapy, periodic rechecks as well as blood and liver evaluations are neces-

sary. Initial therapy involves immunosuppressive doses of oral prednisolone, 0.5 to 1.0 mg/kg daily, and azathioprine, 1 to 2 mg/kg daily.
Maintenance therapy may require use of one or both drugs at a
markedly reduced dose. Topical corticosteroids may be used for lesions of the anterior segment.

MASTICATORY MYOPATHY

In the dog, inflammatory and atrophic syndromes involving the muscles of
mastication (i.e., temporalis, masseter, and pterygoid muscles) are thought
to be immune mediated. The syndrome affects relatively young dogs (average age, 3.1 years) and predominantly large breeds. Signs include tris-
mus, pain on muscle palpation, muscle swelling, or later, muscle atrophy.
Whether the atrophic syndrome is an extension of the acute syndrome with
muscular swelling, however, is unclear. **Ocular signs generally are present in 45% of cases and consist of exophthalmos, conjunctival injection, enophthalmos, and rarely, blindness from optic nerve atrophy. In
addition, ocular signs are usually (but not invariably) bilateral.**

Clinical signs, elevated levels of serum creatinine kinase, electromyog-
raphy, and muscle biopsy with immunocytochemistry for antibodies
against type 2M fibers are diagnostic. **Immunosuppressive doses of prednisolone, 0.5 to 1.0 mg/kg orally for a minimum of 1 month before ta-
pering, are recommended at any stage of the disease.**

KERATOCONJUNCTIVITIS SICCA

**Keratoconjunctivitis sicca (KCS) in the dog has several causes, but one
of the common underlying causes appears to be a multiglandular, inflammatory destruction that is probably immune mediated.** Evidence of
immune-mediated glandular inflammation is provided by the presence of
circulating autoantibodies (i.e., rheumatoid factor [RF], anti-nuclear antibody [ANA]) in a significant number of affected animals (34% and 40%,
respectively), breed specificity, glandular pathology, and the presence of
various other diseases (in 40% of KCS patents) that may have an immune-
mediated component. The salivary and thyroid are two glands that frequently are involved (in 20% of cases each) with the lacrimal glands. **Recommended treatment is topical cyclosporin A as needed.**

FACIAL DERMATOSES

Both allergic and autoimmune diseases often produce a facial dermatitis
that involves the eyelids and the conjunctiva. Such disorders include pemphigus vulgaris, pemphigus vegetans, pemphigus foliaceus, pemphigus
erythematosus, and bullous pemphigoid. The pemphigus complex is characterized by autoantibodies against intercellular substances. In most cases,
facial lesions involve the mucocutaneous regions, and they are characterized by pustules and vesicles that eventually rupture, thereby leaving erosions and ulcers, crusting, scaling, and hypopigmentation. Discoid lupus
erythematosus is associated with facial dermatitis, which is predominantly
nasal, as well as with oral ulcers.

JUVENILE PYODERMA/JUVENILE CELLULITIS

A syndrome of acute pyoderma, which usually is restricted to the head, in puppies younger than 3 months of age is relatively common. One or more puppies in a litter may be involved. Pustules form acutely and then fistulate and drain, thereby creating a moist, crusty lesion. Though the lesions appear to be induced by bacteria, they are actually sterile and cannot be transmitted. A bacterial hypersensitivity has been postulated to explain the response to corticosteroids and the explosive course. **Systemic, broad-spectrum antibiotics as well as immunosuppressive doses of systemic corticosteroids are indicated.** Some clinicians prefer to use antibiotics for a few days before initiating corticosteroids. Nursing care, which consists of gentle cleansing or soaking of the lesions, also may be attempted.

NUTRITIONAL DISORDERS

MILK-REPLACEMENT FORMULAS

Cataract formation has been recognized in puppies and a variety of other species fed commercial or homemade orphan milk formulas. In one report, levels of arginine were deficient in the canine and the feline formulas, and supplementation prevented cataracts in wolf cubs, puppies, and kittens. Various attempts to correct commercial formulas, however, have still resulted in cataract formation. The lens changes begin as vacuolar changes separating the anterior and the posterior cortex from the nucleus and outlining the sutures. By 5 weeks, the opacity remains, appearing as a white, posterior subcapsular opacity. **With growth, this opacity occupies the fetal nucleus and appears as a spheroidal or ring-shaped fetal nuclear opacity.**

VITAMIN E DEFICIENCY

The antioxidant action of vitamin E limits the peroxidation of lipids and the production of free radicals, which are very damaging to cellular constituents. Phospholipids are a significant structural component of the photoreceptors, and normal shedding and phagocytosis by the retinal pigment epithelium produces a peroxidized lipoprotein or lipofuscin from the lysosomes in the cell. Lipofuscin is a yellow-brown, autofluorescent pigment. In the dog, vitamin E deficiency causes muscular and testicular degeneration, reproductive problems, hemolytic anemia, as well as weak and dying puppies. **Ocular lesions occur only with prolonged vitamin E deficiency, however, and they consist of cataracts, decreased vision to blindness, and retinal degeneration.** The retinal degeneration is first noted at ophthalmoscopy as a fine stippling in the central deep retina. The mottling then increases in intensity, with brown accumulations and night blindness later developing. After 6 months on a vitamin E–deficient diet, the tapetal fundus develops central hyperreflectivity, and retinal vascular attenuation is noted. After 8 to 12 months of deficiency, discrete, yellow-brown, multifocal accumulations are noted in the tapetal fundus, as are tapetal hyperreflectivity and attenuated retinal vessels with focal constrictions. **Clinical reports of vitamin E deficiency and retinal pigment epitheliopathy or central retinal degeneration closely parallel those involving experimental models. Therapy is directed at dietary correction and vitamin E supplementation.**

ZINC-RESPONSIVE DERMATOSIS

Zinc deficiency has been implicated in dogs with dermatitis that is characterized by dry, scaly skin and change in hair coloration. Canine zinc deficiency has also been described as producing ocular signs of mucopurulent exudation, blepharitis, and keratitis.

SYSTEMIC AND CENTRAL NERVOUS SYSTEM NEOPLASIA

LYMPHOSARCOMA

Lymphosarcoma is the most common secondary neoplasia of the canine eye and is usually bilateral. In one large, prospective study, 37% of cases had ocular lesions. Of these, 49% were anterior uveitis, 9% posterior uveitis, 14% panuveitis, 23% retinal hemorrhages only, and 6% adnexal diseases (Fig. 17-7). Combined lesions of one or more categories accounted for 57% of the ocular lesions, and some form of uveitis accounted for 71%. Most animals with ocular lesions were seen during the advanced stages of lymphoma (i.e., stage V), and 78% of the cases with leukemia involved ocular disease. Orbital involvement produces marked bilateral

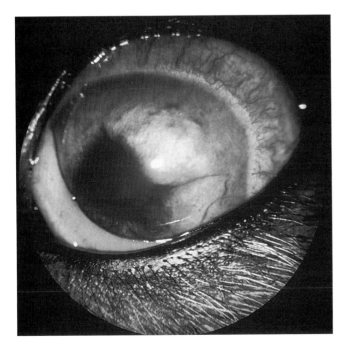

FIGURE 17-7. *Secondary glaucoma in a dog with ocular lymphosarcoma. Note the iris bombé. This condition was bilateral, and marked lymphadenopathy was present.*

exophthalmos, chemosis, and exposure keratitis. Rarely, lymphoma will be diagnosed on the basis of a diffusely enlarged third eyelid with no obvious accompanying systemic lesions.

Lymphadenopathy combined with endogenous bilateral uveitis or hemorrhages should undergo fine-needle aspirations of enlarged organs or lymph nodes to confirm the diagnosis of lymphosarcoma. **For details regarding current therapeutic options, the reader should consult the appropriate internal medicine texts for lymphosarcoma protocols.**

SYSTEMIC HISTIOCYTOSIS

The Bernese Mountain Dog experiences a syndrome of systemic histiocytosis that is characterized by a multisystemic, perivascular infiltration of histiocytes. The systemic signs vary, but they include anorexia, depression, weight loss, cutaneous nodules, and nasal infiltration. **Ocular lesions may include eyelid masses, episcleral masses, exophthalmos, anterior and posterior uveitis, retinal detachment, glaucoma, and corneal edema. The course of the disease may wax and wane but, eventually, progressive and unresponsive to immunosuppressive therapy.**

INTRACRANIAL NEOPLASIA AND INFLAMMATIONS

Intracranial neoplasia or granulomatous disease, whether primary or secondary, often produces ocular/orbital signs. Brain tumors frequently produce visual deficits and papilledema in association with neurologic signs. Because of the great variation in myelination of the canine papilla, however, early papilledema is difficult to detect unless it is asymmetrical or has a definite rim of edema. Intracranial tumors also may produce blindness, which may be acute in nature.

Granulomatous meningoencephalitis in the dog is a syndrome with both neoplastic and inflammatory characteristics. The cause is unknown, but viral infection has been postulated. The condition is characterized by multifocal signs that are responsive, at least temporarily, to systemic corticosteroids. **The disease process may involve the optic nerves, thus producing a syndrome of acute blindness, papilledema, retinal and peripapillary hemorrhages, and occasionally, extension into the globe, which in turn produces retinal detachments and retinal infiltrates.** A definitive diagnosis is difficult to establish, but multifocal CNS deficits, increased cerebrospinal fluid protein levels, pleocytosis with mononuclear cells, and response to corticosteroids are suggestive. **Most animals die within 3 months of their initial presentation, though aggressive therapy has produced long remissions in some cases.**

TUMOR METASTASES TO THE EYE AND ORBIT

Though relatively rare, a variety of carcinomas and sarcomas have been described as metastasizing to the eye and the orbit. Bilateral ocular involvement may occur as well, because most tumors spread via a hematogenous route. The usual site is the uveal tract and, specifically, the ciliary body. The tumors may be masked by hemorrhage, inflammation, and glaucoma; thus, neoplasia, whether primary or secondary, should be included in the differential diagnosis of undetermined spontaneous hemorrhage or secondary glaucoma. Ocular metastasis usually is a late occurrence, so the systemic history or physical examination generally will be significant.

SYSTEMIC TOXICITIES

Ocular toxicity may result from several drugs that are used clinically. Toxicity from systemic trimethoprim-sulfadiazine is probably the most common and significant in the dog, and the most common effect is decreased tear production and resultant KCS (Table 17-2).

SUDDEN ACQUIRED RETINAL DEGENERATION SYNDROME

Sudden acquired retinal degeneration syndrome (SARDS) has been recognized among dogs in the United States for two decades now. The syndrome involves systemic signs and altered laboratory test results in 40 to 60% of patients. The cause of SARDS is unknown, despite the syndrome being relatively common. Animals characteristically are presented with acute blindness and a normal to near-normal ocular fundus. After several weeks to months, however, more advanced retinal vascular attenuation and tapetal hyperreflectivity become apparent. Because of the acute onset, most dogs are quite disoriented. In most patients, vision loss occurs during the course of 1 to 2 weeks, and nyctalopia may be observed. The mean age of affliction is 8.5 to 10.0 years. The syndrome occurs predominantly in neutered females, in both purebred and mixed breeds, and with a predisposition for Dachshunds. A seasonal incidence has been reported as well, with 46% of cases occurring in December and January. Many patients also have polyuria, polydipsia (28–36%), and polyphagia (39%), and a history of weight gain (57%). Laboratory values are variable, but lymphopenia (30%), lymphopenia with neutrophilia (21%), and abnormal biochemical profiles (68%) may be present as well. Elevated levels of alkaline phosphatase (30–40% of cases) and cholesterol (42%) are the most common biochemical changes. In one report, adrenocorticotropic hormone stimulation or a low-dose dexamethasone suppression test was abnormal in six of 10 patients. Overall, 12 to 17% of patients have adrenal profile changes that are compatible with those of Cushing's syndrome; however, these changes may be adaptations to other diseases as well.

The ERG response is extinguished in dogs with SARDS. Levels of excitotoxins (e.g., glutamate) are elevated in the vitreous of affected animals, but the significance of this is unknown.

To date, no therapy has stopped the progression or reversed the blindness. Once past the initial adjustment to an acute blindness, however, most animals still make acceptable pets.

TABLE 17-2

OCULAR TOXICITIES IN THE DOG

Drug	*Ocular Manifestations*
Trimethoprim-sulfadiazine	Given systemically, KCS developed in 4–15% of dogs; more than 63% of animals on the drug have decreased STT readings. The decrease in tear production may occur in a few days after sulfa therapy is initiated, and 50% will develop it within 30 days.
Phenazopyridine	An urinary analgesic. Within 7–10 days after doses of 25 mg/kg in the dog, the STT decreased below 10 mm/min, and signs of KCS developed. Lacrimal glands develop a grossly visible, brown-black discoloration within 48 hours of administration.
Hypolipidemic compounds	Compounds of the hydroxymethylglutaryl–coenzyme A reductase inhibitor group may produce cataracts in the dog. Cataracts begin as posterior subcapsular equatorial opacities.
Ivermectin	Observed after gross overdosing, usually when large-animal anthelmintic preparations are used. The Collie may develop toxicosis with as little as 220 μg/kg. Depending on the dose, CNS signs such as muscle fasciculations, ataxia, and stupor may be present. Blindness may occur without marked CNS signs, and this is usually accompanied by pupillary dilation. Ophthalmoscopic findings are papilledema and retinal edema with folds. Residual pigment disruption may be visible in the nontapetal fundus with recovery. Vision loss is temporary, with recovery in 2–10 days.
Disophenol	An old, injectable anthelmintic used for ancylostomiasis during the 1970s. Experimentally, cataracts could be routinely produced with three times (30 mg/kg) the recommended parenteral dose. The onset of cataracts is within 24–36 hours, typically with a vacuolar lesion beginning at the equator, then progressing axially, both anteriorly and posteriorly, in the superficial cortex. In most cases, resolution occurs within 3–7 days.
Tocainide	An oral, antiarrhythmic agent. In Doberman Pinschers with cardiomyopathies receiving at recommended doses for more than 2 months, a bilateral, progressive, irreversible corneal edema developed in some animals.
Coumarin poisoning	Signs manifest with ocular or orbital hemorrhages. The source is usually rodenticides.
Ionizing radiation	Complication rates between 76–84%. Approximately 45–59% are sight-threatening or chronic in nature. Conjunctivitis (35% of cases); signs of keratoconjunctivitis, KCS, and ulcerative keratitis are more common (64–78%); anterior uveitis (8–10%); cataract formation delayed for 1.0–9.6 months (11–26%); and multifocal retinal hemorrhages delayed from 1–6 months and present in 19% of patients. Additional late-onset lesions are noted at histopathology, but not clinically, include retinal atrophy and tapetal atrophy.

continued

TABLE 17-2	
OCULAR TOXICITIES IN THE DOG—*continued*	
Drug	*Ocular Manifestations*
Electricity	Electric shocks and lightning strikes may produce cataracts that manifest months later. Cataracts are more likely to be produced by electric shocks to the head.

CNS, central nervous system; *KCS,* keratoconjunctivitis sicca; *STT,* Schirmer tear test.

The Cat

DERMATOLOGIC CONDITIONS

DEMODICOSIS

Feline demodicosis results from two species of mites: *Demodex cati,* and a species of Demodex that has not yet been named. Lesions usually affect the eyelids, periocular area, head, and neck. Such lesions are variably pruritic, and they are characterized by alopecia, erythema, and scaling. The diagnosis is established on the basis of lesion scrapings and identification of the mite. **Treatment with lime-sulfur solutions or mild parasiticides may be used, but these agents should not be allowed to contact the eye.**

The causative agent of feline scabies is *Notoedres cati,* but cats also **may be infected with the mite that causes canine scabies, *Sarcoptes scabiei* var *canis.*** Typically, lesions begin around the medial edge of the ear pinna and then progress to involve the upper ear, face, eyelids, and neck. Intense pruritus is characteristic, and the diagnosis is suggested by the location of the lesions and the intense pruritus. The diagnosis is confirmed on the basis of the results from lesion scrapings. **Treatment should include clipping all hair and applying a 3% lime-sulfur solution every seventh day until the lesions have resolved.** All other cats on the premises must be treated as well.

Ringworm is a mycotic skin infection and, in the cat, may be caused by one of several species of *Microsporum* or *Trichophyton*. The most common species affecting the cat is *M. canis*. Lesions are characterized by alopecia, with or without scales, and most commonly affect the head, pinnae, and paws; however, they also may involve the eyelids. The diagnosis is best established on the basis of fungal culture of the affected hair and scales. **Treatment includes clipping the hair in the affected region, which is followed by topical therapy with antifungal agents that continues for 2 weeks beyond clinical resolution.**

Several immune-mediated skin diseases may affect the eyelids of the cat, usually with other accompanying head lesions and with variable lesions on the rest of the body. These diseases include pemphigus foliaceous, pemphigus erythematosus, pemphigus vulgaris, food hypersensitivity, and feline atopy. Biopsy is necessary to establish the diagnosis of pemphigus complex diseases. Food hypersensitivity may be diagnosed on the basis of food elimination trials, whereas atopy may be best diagnosed on the basis of skin testing. Treatment is aimed at the underlying disease process but often includes topical or systemic anti-inflammatory therapy as well.

OPHTHALMOMYIASIS

The term *ophthalmomyiasis interna* refers to the presence of dipteran fly larvae within the eye. These larvae may gain access to the eye via a hematogenous route or via direct migration through the ocular tunics. Retinal lesions consisting of curvilinear tracts are characteristic of parasitic migration, but no report has identified the actual larval species that is associated with these retinal tracts. Migration of *Cuterebra* sp. larvae in the subcutaneous tissues of the cat is common, and the eyelids or conjunctiva may be affected as well. Removal of the larvae is indicated.

NEURO-OPHTHALMIC DISEASES

INTRACRANIAL PARASITE MIGRATION

Intracranial migration of *Cuterebra* sp. larvae has been documented in the cat, with both multifocal neurologic signs and blindness being reported. Anisocoria and unilateral blindness also were reported in a cat with progressive neurologic signs and cerebral coenurosis caused by *Taenia serialis*.

ISCHEMIC ENCEPHALOPATHY

Ischemic encephalopathy occurs when the arterial supply to part of the brain is disrupted. Most often, a portion of one side of the cerebrum supplied by the middle cerebral artery is involved, thereby resulting in necrosis. The cause is unknown in most cases. Acute visual deficits may accompany other neurologic signs (e.g., behavior change, seizures, ataxia, motor deficits) and usually are cortical in origin. Occasionally, the optic chiasm may be involved, thus resulting in dilated and nonresponsive pupils.

HEPATIC ENCEPHALOPATHY

Hepatic encephalopathy most frequently occurs in cats with portosystemic shunts, but it also may occur in cats with acute or chronic liver failure from many causes. Clinical signs may include cortical blindness, anorexia, vomiting, ptyalism, depression, disorientation, aggressive or maniacal behavior, aimless walking, circling, head pressing, weakness, collapse, seizures, and coma. **Therapy is aimed at correcting the underlying cause of the liver disease, if possible, and general supportive care as well as minimization of the clinical signs are indicated.**

HYPOXIA

Hypoxia most commonly occurs during use of anesthetics, and it may relate to apnea, cardiopulmonary failure, improper intubation, overdose of anesthetic agent, failure of anesthetic equipment, or paralysis in the respiratory muscles. **Clinical signs of cerebral hypoxia include blindness, stupor or coma, paralysis with decerebrate rigidity, seizures, and deafness.** Pupillary light responses, however, generally are normal. These signs may be either partially or wholly reversible after a period of days to months, because both astrocytes and macrophages proliferate and remove necrotic debris. **Immediate treatment should include supplemental oxygen at a level of 40 to 60%, either in an oxygen cage or by nasal insufflation. Glucocorticoids have not proved to be effective treatment of the cytotoxic edema also seen with hypoxia.**

DYSAUTONOMIA

Feline dysautonomia (i.e., Key-Gaskell syndrome) was first reported in England in 1982. **Since then, the disease, which produces widespread dysfunction of the autonomic nervous system, has been reported in many cats throughout Europe, but only a few cases have been documented in the United States.** The cause of dysautonomia has not been determined. **Reported ophthalmic signs most consistently include mydriasis that is unresponsive to light, decreased tear production, and protruding nictitating membranes. Vision is unaffected, and photophobia is variable.** Systemic signs include general malaise, dehydration, anorexia, vomiting or regurgitation, urinary bladder distention, and constipation. Pharmacologic testing with ocular autonomic stimulants can aid in establishing the diagnosis of feline dysautonomia. Affected eyes respond to dilute concentrations of drugs that will not affect a normal eye: 0.1% pilocarpine produces miosis; 1:10,000 epinephrine induces retraction of a prolapsed nictitating membrane; and 0.06% echothiophate iodide causes miosis in a normal cat but has no effect on a dysautonomic pupil. **The prognosis for cats with dysautonomia ranged from guarded to poor, though some cats have been maintained for long periods of time on supportive therapy or even recovered after a prolonged period.**

INTRACRANIAL NEOPLASIA

Blindness has been associated with intracranial neoplasia (i.e., pituitary carcinoma and meningiomas) in the cat. Other signs include mydriasis, aniscoria, and positional nystagmus.

INFECTIOUS DISEASES

Systemic infectious disease may lead to a variety of ocular manifestations, ranging from ocular surface disease to intraocular disease, with or without accompanying systemic signs.

FELINE HERPESVIRUS-1

Infection with feline herpesvirus type 1 (FHV-1) is common, and the virus itself is widespread among cat populations. **Primary FHV-1 disease is characterized by malaise, fever, sneezing or coughing, and nasal as well as ocular discharge.** The virus is spread from cat to cat either by direct contact or by aerosolization of the virus, which infects the epithelial surfaces of the respiratory tract and conjunctiva and, to a lesser degree, the corneal epithelium, thereby causing necrosis of these tissues as the virus replicates and invades the adjacent cells. **Several eye diseases have been reported in association with FHV-1 (Table 17-3). Diagnostic tests are summarized in Chapter 12, and recommended treatments are summarized in Table 17-4.**

TABLE 17-3

OPHTHALMIC DISEASES ASSOCIATED WITH FELINE HERPESVIRUS-1 IN THE CAT

Condition	Clinical Signs
Neonatal ophthalmia	Kittens younger than 10–14 days and before normal eyelids opening.
Primary conjunctivitis	Hyperemia, blepharospasm, chemosis, and ocular discharge.
Recurrent conjunctivitis	Adults, usually 1–2 years or older; after stress.
Keratoconjunctivitis sicca	Persistent mucopurulent exudates; low Schirmer tear test values. Superficial keratitis with vascularization.
Corneal ulceration	Dendritic or geographic corneal ulcer; stromal keratitis (deep corneal vascularization, edema, and cellular infiltrates).
Corneal sequestration	Focal area of degeneration, with a brown-to-black discoloration; variable corneal vascularization and pain.
Symblepharon	Adherence of bulbar/palpebral conjunctiva to cornea.

TABLE 17-4	

TREATMENT OF FELINE HERPESVIRUS-1–RELATED OPHTHALMIC DISEASES IN THE CAT

Condition	Recommended Therapy
Primary infection	Respiratory tract: systemic, broad-spectrum antibiotics; subcutaneous fluids; cleansing of nasal and ocular discharge. Conjunctivitis: broad-spectrum, topical ophthalmic antibiotic.
Recurrent conjunctivitis	Topical broad-spectrum antibiotics; other drugs under evaluation include recombinant interferon (natural oral human interferon at a dose of 5 and 25 IU) and oral lysine (100 mg of lysine, given once or twice daily; watch for gastric upset).
Corneal ulcerations	Debridement and an ophthalmic antiviral (trifluridine, idoxuridine, or vidarabine)
Corneal sequestra	Surgically removed by keratectomy, and placement of a conjunctival or corneoconjunctival graft.
Keratoconjunctivitis sicca	Topical 0.2% cyclosporin A ointment in addition to antiviral therapy.

CHLAMYDIA PSITTACI

Chlamydia psittaci, which is an obligate intracellular bacterium, is a common pathogen in the cat that primarily causes conjunctivitis. **The acute phase of infection with *C. psittaci* results in conjunctival hyperemia, chemosis, serous ocular discharge, and blepharospasm.** Mild nasal discharge and sneezing also may occur. Conjunctivitis often initially is unilateral, but it then progresses to involve the second eye during the next few days. If untreated, infection with *C. psittaci* can produce chronic conjunctivitis. Asymptomatic carrier states can exist as well, and these may be significant in spreading the organism within the population. The diagnosis is established on the basis of identifying the characteristic inclusion body within the conjunctival epithelial cell cytoplasm or a positive fluorescent antibody (FA) test using a conjunctival scraping. **Chlamydial organisms are sensitive to tetracyclines and to erythromycin.** Topical administration of tetracycline four times daily to both eyes for 1 to 2 weeks after resolution of conjunctivitis is sufficient treatment in many cats. Oral administration of tetracycline or doxycycline may be necessary to treat refractory infections, however, and also may be advisable to clear the gastrointestinal tract of latent infection. Vaccination with a live chlamydial vaccine provides the best clinical protection.

CALICIVIRUS

Feline calicivirus, which is a picornavirus, is primarily a pathogen of the respiratory tract in the cat but also may cause oral ulcers and polyarthritis.

MYCOPLASMA SP.

Mycoplasma sp. are the smallest free-living organisms, and they are classified as being prokaryotes. *Mycoplasma felis, M. gatae,* and *M. arginini* have all been isolated from both sick and healthy cats. **The role of** *Mycoplasma* **sp. as a cause of conjunctivitis in the cat has been controversial, because the organism has been isolated from the eyes of normal cats as well as from those of cats with conjunctivitis.** The diagnosis of mycoplasmosis can be established on the basis of culturing the organism using special media or finding the characteristic, small, coccoid inclusions within the cytoplasm of the epithelial cells. *Mycoplasma* **sp. are sensitive to many routinely used ophthalmic antibiotics.**

UVEITIS ASSOCIATED WITH INFECTIOUS DISEASES

Anterior uveitis is a common disorder in the cat, and it may relate to a variety of underlying mechanisms. Whether unilateral or bilateral, uveitis may be the only presenting clinical sign even if the cat is infected with a systemic pathogenic agent. Many cats with uveitis do not exhibit ocular pain, which may allow the uveitis to advance without being detected and, thereby, lead to the development of glaucoma in many instances. The cause of many cases of feline uveitis remains idiopathic despite extensive testing. Infectious agents associated with uveitis in the cat include *Toxoplasma gondii* (Fig. 17-8) feline immunodeficiency virus, feline coronavirus (i.e., feline infectious peritonitis; Fig. 17-9), feline leukemia virus (FeLV), the various causes of the systemic mycoses (i.e., *Cryptococcus neoformans, Histoplasma capsulatum, Blastomyces dermatitidis, Coccidioides immitis,* and *Candida albicans*), *Mycobacterium bovis,* and occasionally, *M. tuberculosis* as well as, rarely, *M. avium*). (For more details regarding therapy, see Chapter 12 and consult the third edition, pp. 1018–1025 and 1456–1462.)

PANLEUKOPENIA VIRUS

Kittens infected with panleukopenia virus, either during gestation or shortly after birth, develop cerebellar hypoplasia and retinal dysplasia. The cerebellar disease becomes apparent at approximately 3 to 4 weeks of age (i.e., when kittens begin to walk). Hypermetria and ataxia are apparent as well.

METASTATIC NEOPLASIA

The most frequent feline systemic neoplasia with ocular metastases is lymphosarcoma, yet surprisingly few reports have appeared in the literature.

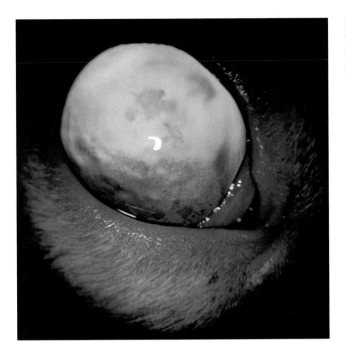

FIGURE 17-8. *Anterior uveitis with keratic precipitates in a cat with positive serum antibody titers for* Toxoplasma gondii.

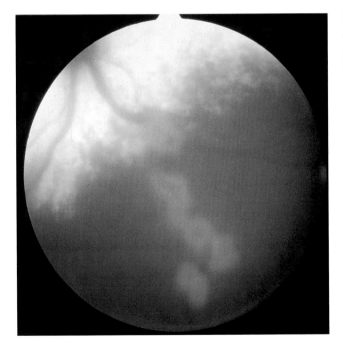

FIGURE 17-9. *Chorioretinitis in a young cat with feline infectious peritonitis. Note the inflammatory infiltrate sheathing the retinal vessels.*

The uveal tract has been involved in all eyes, and nodular iris lesions have been the most common manifestation, being present in 35 of the 50 eyes reported (Fig. 17-10). Seventeen of these cats were tested for FeLV, and seven were positive. Survival times ranged from 0 days to 31 months, with a mean survival time of 14 months. Aggressive treatment of cats with ocular

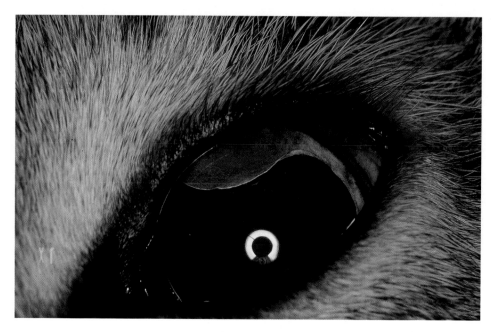

FIGURE 17-10. *Early intraocular lymphosarcoma in a 2-year-old cat. Note the raised infiltrate of cells in the dorsolateral iris.*

lymphosarcoma using topical corticosteroids (e.g., 1% prednisolone acetate) as well as using systemic therapy with corticosteroids or other chemotherapeutic protocols is indicated.

Other metastatic tumors include adenocarcinomas (from lung, mammary tissue, and uterus), soft-tissue fibrosarcoma, and squamous cell carcinoma.

NUTRITIONAL DISEASES

Several eye diseases have been associated with nutritional disorders in cats, and these include taurine-deficiency retinopathy (see Chapter 12), thiamine deficiency, and nutritional cataracts in kittens. Thiamine deficiency may occur in cats that eat large amounts of raw fish, which contains thiaminases, or in cats that eat processed commercial foods in which thiamine has been destroyed by heat processing but not adequately replaced. In addition, cats with severe gastrointestinal disease may not absorb sufficient amounts of thiamine. **The clinical signs of thiamine deficiency include initial inappetence and occasional vomiting, which are followed by pupillary dilatation without visual deficits, ataxia, and ventroflexion of the head and neck.** The final—and irreversible—stage involves progression of the signs to a semicomatose state that is characterized by crying, opisthotonos, and extensor rigidity. Normal blood thiamine levels in the cat are approximately 32 mg/dL. **Before development of a comatose state, cats will respond favorably to parenterally administered**

preparations of vitamin B complex containing 50 to 75 mg of thiamine per dose every 8 hours.

Cataracts have been reported in growing kittens fed a commercial milk-replacer diet, and the low serum arginine concentration in these kittens was thought to relate to the diet and, possibly, to the cataract formation.

INHERITED DISEASES

Chediak-Higashi syndrome is an autosomal recessive disorder of the cat and other species. **In the cat, the syndrome has been reported only in the Persian breed.** The disease is characterized by giant cytoplasmic granules within lysosomes, melanocytes, and neutrophils. Systemic manifestations of the syndrome include cutaneous hypopigmentation, increased susceptibility to infections, and bleeding tendencies; ocular manifestations include photophobia, pale irises, and fundus hypopigmentation. Cataracts have been noted in some cats with Chediak-Higashi syndrome, as has spontaneous nystagmus.

The lysosomal storage diseases include a group of inherited disorders in which a specific lysosomal enzyme is lacking, thereby causing a buildup of the substrate (Table 17-1). **Systemic signs are variable, but the most consistent ocular manifestation is corneal opacification or cloudiness secondary to vacuoles.**

DISORDERS OF THE VASCULAR SYSTEM

ELEVATED BLOOD PRESSURE

Systemic hypertension is a relatively common disease among aged cats, and it has most consistently been associated with chronic renal failure and hyperthyroidism. The ocular manifestations of systemic hypertension can be severe and even lead to blindness. Reported ocular abnormalities have included retinal hemorrhages, retinal detachments, retinal edema, retinoschisis, retinal degeneration, hyphema, and secondary glaucoma. Cats with diseases such as chronic renal failure and hyperthyroidism should be screened for systemic hypertension. In many cats, hypertensive retinopathy is a slow, insidious process in which vision may be spared if the retinopathy is identified and controlled before severe ocular disease can develop.

Measurement of the blood pressure in the cat is most easily accomplished in a clinical setting through indirect measurement using an oscillometric or ultrasonic detection device. Reported hypertensive values for cats are 160/100 mm Hg or greater, and one group reported that the mean blood pressure in normal cats is 118/84 mm Hg. Treatment of hypertensive retinopathy is aimed primarily at controlling the underlying disease processes as well as treating the systemic hypertension. Antihypertensive agents used in the cat include β-blockers, such as propranolol or atenolol; diuretics, such as spironolactone/thiazide, furosemide, and hydrochlorothiazide; and angiotensin-converting enzyme inhibitors, such as captopril. **The calcium channel blocker amlodipine was recently used successfully in cats at an oral dose of 0.625 mg, and it has the advantage of being administered only once daily.**

LIPEMIA RETINALIS

The term *lipemia retinalis* describes excess lipid within the retinal vessels, thus giving them a pale appearance. Hyperlipidemia can occur in the cat for several reasons, including postprandial hyperlipidemia, diabetes mellitus, administration of exogenous corticosteroids or megestrol acetate, nephrotic syndrome, lipoprotein lipase deficiency, and idiopathic hyperchylomicronemia.

ANEMIC RETINOPATHY

Retinal hemorrhages may occur in cats with anemia. Cats with anemia and hemoglobin values of less than 5 g/dL are apt to have retinal hemorrhages. Causes of anemia include infection with *Hemobartonella felis*, thrombocytopenia, autoimmune hemolytic anemia, aplastic anemia, lymphosarcoma, FeLV, and bleeding duodenal ulcer.

HYPERVISCOSITY SYNDROMES

Hyperviscosity syndromes involve an increase in plasma protein levels such that the blood becomes more viscous than normal. Most frequently, this has been associated with multiple myeloma, in which a certain class of Ig is produced to excess. The clinical signs are variable but often include listlessness, pale mucous membranes, neurologic signs, and lameness. Ocular manifestations are common and include retinal hemorrhages, dilated and tortuous retinal vessels, retinal detachment, perivascular effusion, papilledema, and retinal degeneration. Treatment is aimed at the underlying disease process, if possible. Reducing the serum viscosity using plasmapheresis sometimes is helpful as well.

DRUG TOXICITIES

Griseofulvin is teratogenic in the cat. Reported ocular anomalies include cyclopia, anophthalmia, absence of optic nerves, and rudimentary optic tracts. Acute renal failure secondary to **ethylene glycol intoxication** has produced bilateral retinal detachments and edema. Cats treated with **long-term megestrol acetate** for dermatologic disease may develop diabetes mellitus and diabetic retinopathy.

The Horse

DERMATOLOGIC CONDITIONS

A number of parasites cause skin disease that may involve the face and eyelids in the horse. These parasites include *Demodex equi* and *D. caballi, Sarcoptes scabei,* chiggers (i.e., harvest mites) and straw-itch mites, lice, *Microsporum* or *Trichophyton* sp. (i.e., ringworm), *Onchocerca cervicalis, O. gutturosa,* and *O. reticulata.* The diagnosis usually is established on the basis of skin scrapings or biopsy findings, and specific treatment is then administered. (For more details, the reader should consult the third edition, pp. 1473–1475.)

Pemphigus foliaceus is the most commonly reported immune-mediated skin disease in the horse. There are no breed or sex predilections in this species, but Appaloosas may be predisposed. Lesions are characterized initially by vesicles and pustules and then by crusts, scales, oozing, and annular erosions. The head is a common site of involvement, with the skin of the eyelids frequently being affected. The diagnosis is established on the basis of skin biopsy findings, with samples being preserved in Michel's media.

SYSTEMIC DISEASES

A number of systemic diseases and toxicities have been associated with ophthalmic signs in the horse. Often, the clinical ophthalmic signs are not diagnostic in themselves, but when combined with other signs may aid in diagnosing the specific disorder (Table 17-5). Other diseases that have been reported either infrequently or rarely include cryptococcosis, histoplasmosis, aspergillosis, and toxoplasmosis. (For more details, the reader should consult the third edition, pp. 1479–1486.)

OPTIC NERVE DEGENERATION

Optic nerve atrophy may occur after head trauma in the horse. Immediately after trauma such as a fall, rearing and striking of the poll, or other blunt injury to the head or poll, horses are noted to be blind. They simultaneously also may act dazed and have epistaxis. The pupillary light responses are slow or absent, and the fundic examination may be normal. Alternatively, hemorrhages of the optic disc and peripapillary edema may occur. With chronicity, the optic discs become pale, the retinal vessels attenuated, and the peripapillary pigment disrupted (Fig. 17-11).

Medical therapy usually has not been successful in preventing blindness. Because optic nerve damage secondary to swelling or contusion necrosis is treatable, however, the horse should be given high-dose intravenous

TABLE 17-5

SYSTEMIC DISEASES AND TOXICITIES WITH OPHTHALMIC SIGNS IN THE HORSE

Disease	Clinical/Ophthalmic Signs
Equine protozoal myeloencephalitis	Ataxia, tetraparesis, head tilt, facial paralysis, circling nystagmus, and blindness (with or without pupillary light abnormalities), and Horner's syndrome.
Leukoencephalomalacia (toxin produced by corn fungus, *Fusarium moniliforme*)	Depression, ataxia, recumbency, blindness (with or without abnormal pupillary light response), head pressing, circling, seizures, or frantic running behavior.
Eastern, Western, and Venezuelan equine encephalomyelitis	Aggression, head pressing, blindness, fever, stuporous state, paralyzed tongue and pharynx, nystagmus, strabismus, and pupillary dilatation.
Meningitis	Fever, neck pain and stiffness, hyperesthesia, anorexia, and diarrhea. Ophthalmic signs may include optic neuritis, blindness, nystagmus, anisocoria, strabismus, and ptosis.
Thiamine deficiency	Ataxia, blindness, bradycardia, heart block, muscle fasciculations, weight loss, diarrhea, and hypothermia of the extremities.
Horner's syndrome	Ptosis, miosis, enophthalmos, and protrusion of the nictitating membrane. Sweating and increased skin temperature on the denervated side of the face.
Tetanus (*Clostridium tetani*)	Sawhorse stance to the legs, retraction of the ears and lips, elevation of the tail, rapid retraction of the globe, hyperesthesia, third-eyelid prolapse.
Botulism	Toxin from *Clostridium botulinum*, weakness, dysphagia, drooling and inability to retract the tongue, ptosis, and mydriasis (with slow pupillary light responses).
Equine viral arteritis	Fever, depression, coughing, nasal and ocular discharge, and abortion. Ophthalmic signs include periorbital and peripheral edema, conjunctivitis, corneal opacity, and photophobia.
Equine infectious anemia	Cyclical anemia, thrombocytopenia, fever, and ventral edema. Ophthalmic signs are infrequent: intraocular and conjunctival hemorrhages.
African horse sickness	Peracute or pulmonary form; subacute, edematous or cardiac form; acute or mixed form; and fever form. Ophthalmic signs are mainly vascular congestion of the conjunctiva and subcutaneous edema affecting eyelids and the supraorbital fossa.
Equine herpesvirus-2	Mainly respiratory disease. Ophthalmic abnormalities include excessive tearing, mucopurulent discharge, chemosis, conjunctival hyperemia, linear and punctate keratopathy, corneal irregularity, and corneal edema as well as vascularization.

continued

TABLE 17-5	
SYSTEMIC DISEASES AND TOXICITIES WITH OPHTHALMIC SIGNS IN THE HORSE—*continued*	
Disease	***Clinical/Ophthalmic Signs***
Adenoviral infection	In immunodeficient Arabian foals. Fever, pneumonia, and leukopenia. Thick, yellow discharge from the eyes and nares that adheres to the eyelids, muzzle, and forelegs. Dyspnea, cough, and diarrhea.
Equine influenza	Harsh, dry, and nonproductive cough; fever; lethargy; and anorexia. Ophthalmic signs include conjunctival hyperemia and excessive tearing.
Streptococcus equi (strangles)	Purulent pharyngitis and lymphadenitis of the upper respiratory tract. Initial serous and later mucopurulent ocular discharge, panophthalmitis, and chorioretinitis.
Rhodococcus equi	Bronchopneumonia in foals; also uveitis.
Brucellosis (*Brucella abortus*)	Fistulous withers; uveitis.
Leptospira sp.	Initial pyrexia, renal disease, and liver dysfunction are often undetected. *Leptospira interrogans* serovar *pomona* most frequently associated with uveitis in the horse, but serovars *icterohaemorrhagiae, grippotyphosa, canicola,* and *hardjo* are also reported.
Lyme disease	Caused by *Borrelia burgdorferi*. Arthritis and lameness, encephalitis, limb edema, dermatitis, abortion, and foal mortality and panuveitis.
Salmonellosis	Infectious diarrhea among adult horses; iridocyclitis and hypopyon usually in bacteremic animals.
Babesiosis (piroplasmosis)	Fever, hemolytic anemia, jaundice, hemoglobinuria, and death. Swelling of the eyelids, icterus of the conjunctiva and sclera, conjunctival petechial, and ecchymotic hemorrhages.

dexamethasone as soon as possible after head trauma. **Resolution of peripapillary edema and reduced vision has occurred in one horse treated with both dexamethasone and phenylbutazone.**

OPTIC NEURITIS

Optic neuritis has been reported infrequently in the horse. Suppurative optic neuritis associated with endocarditis and *Actinobacillus equuli* as well as granulomatous optic neuritis thought to be secondary to parasitic migration have been reported. Optic nerve degenerations secondary to extensive blood loss, orbital cellulitis, parasitism and anemia, guttural pouch mycosis, intra-arterial injection of phenylbutazone, pituitary mass, and associated

FIGURE 17-11. *Traumatic optic nerve degeneration and peripapillary pigment disruption in a horse. (Courtesy of C. Martin.)*

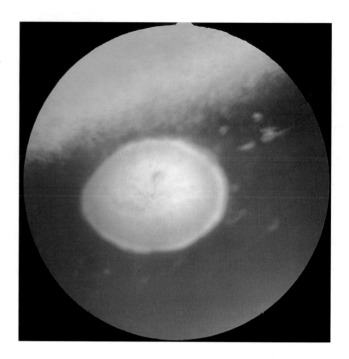

with carotid arterial occlusion for guttural pouch mycosis have also been reported. Extensive blood loss in the horse is thought to lead to ischemic optic neuropathy, whereas occlusion of both the internal and the external carotid arteries with guttural pouch mycosis and epistaxis may lead to an immediate loss of the blood supply to the optic nerve and retina.

PARASITIC DISEASES

Numerous parasites can infect the horse. Some may affect the equine eye as well, either through aberrant migration or by localization near or in the eye itself as part of their normal life cycle.

Onchocerciasis

Onchocerca cervicalis **is one of the most important parasites that affect the equine eye.** The adult nematode lives in the nuchal ligament of the horse, and their microfilariae migrate through the subcutaneous tissues until they are ingested by a biting midge (*Culicoides* sp.). In the midge, they develop to the infectious stage in approximately 25 days and are then transmitted to the horse by the bite of the midge. In the horse, they next develop into adults. The adult worm appears to cause no disease in the horse, but the migrating microfilariae may cause both dermatologic and ocular disease. The prevalence of *O. cervicalis* microfilariae among horses in the United States was at one time high, but it has been reduced by periodic worming with systemic ivermectin. Ocular manifestations of onchocerciasis include anterior and posterior uveitis, peripapillary chorioretinitis, keratitis, keratoconjunctivitis, and lateral conjunctival vitiligo. The diagnosis of onchocerciasis is best established on the basis of biopsy results that show infected tissue. Systemic ivermectin, 0.2 mg/kg, has a high rate of efficacy in killing microfilariae; however, horses can become reinfected with *O. cervicalis* during insect seasons. In addition, there is no treatment regarding the adult nematode; thus, microfilariae will continue to be produced. Systemic nonsteroidal anti-inflammatory agents as well as topical or subconjunctival corticosteroids should be used.

Setaria and *Dirofilaria* Infestations

***Setaria digitata* and *S. equina* occasionally invade the equine eye.** Normally, these nematodes are found living free within the abdominal cavity, and their migration into the eye and anterior chamber is aberrant. **Severe intraocular inflammation may occur secondary to the presence of the parasite.** Successful surgical removal of *S. digitata* from the anterior chamber of a horse has been reported. ***Dirofilaria immitis* also has been removed from the anterior chamber of a horse.**

Habronemiasis

Habronemiasis results from the aberrant migration by larvae of the spirurid nematodes *Habronema muscae, H. microstoma,* and *Draschia megastoma*. The adult parasites reside in the equine stomach, and stable flies (*Stomoxys calcitrans*) serve as the intermediate hosts. The L3 larvae may be deposited on wounds or near the eye, and larval migration through the tissue incites a granulomatous inflammatory response. **Lesions may affect the conjunctiva, typically near the medial canthus, or the periocular area, and they have a raised, irregular, yellow (i.e., "sulphur granules") appearance.** The tissue tends to bleed easily, and pruritus as well as self-trauma often are evident. The diagnosis may be established on the basis of the characteristic appearance of the lesions during fly season and by the histopathologic results (i.e., granulomatous inflammatory infiltrate with eosinophils and mast cells along with collagenolysis, but the larvae are variable). **Treatment with systemic ivermectin, 0.2 mg/kg, is effective at killing the larvae.**

Hydatid Disease

Hydatid cyst disease (*Echinococcus granulosus*) affects the horse in many countries, but reports of it affecting the equine eye have been few. Cysts have been reported in the orbit, however.

METASTATIC NEOPLASIA

Lymphosarcoma is the most common systemic neoplastic disease that affects the equine eye. **Ocular manifestations of equine lymphosarcoma include eyelid swelling, nictitating membrane masses, uveitis, chemosis and conjunctivitis, corneoscleral masses, and orbital lymphosarcoma.**

PLANT TOXICITY

Numerous plants may be toxic to the horse and produce visual abnormalities. Many plants also have teratogenic effects in the horse, especially if they are eaten during the first trimester of pregnancy. Pregnant mares may produce foals with a centrally placed, single eye if they eat *Veratrum eschscholtzii* during early pregnancy, much as ewes will produce such lambs if they eat *Veratrum californicum* on day 14 of gestation. (For more details, the reader should consult the third edition, pp. 1487–1488.)

Food Animals

Many systemic diseases in food animals have ophthalmic manifestations. Often, specific ophthalmic tissues are affected by specific diseases, thereby facilitating their detection. A thorough examination of the ocular fundus can be easily performed in food animals and may provide diagnostic information regarding many systemic diseases.

CONGENITAL DISORDERS

CHEDIAK-HIGASHI SYNDROME

Chediak-Higashi syndrome has been described in cattle, cats, minks, and mice. Affected animals have a partial oculocutaneous albinism, susceptibility to infection, tendency for prolonged bleeding, and enlarged cytoplasmic granules in most cells. Ocular manifestations of Chediak-Higashi syndrome include photophobia, light or pale irides, and fundic hypopigmentation. In cattle, the corpora nigra are absent.

HYDROCEPHALUS, MICROPHTHALMIA, AND RETINAL DYSPLASIA

In Shorthorn calves, a syndrome of microphthalmia, cataracts, retinal detachments, retinal dysplasia, optic nerve hypoplasia, persistent pupillary membranes, and vitreous hemorrhage has been associated with hydrocephalus. The cause has not been determined, but it has been postulated to be genetic.

BOVINE VIRAL DIARRHEA–INDUCED OCULAR ABNORMALITIES

Bovine viral diarrhea results from a pestivirus with a worldwide distribution that infects cattle, sheep, goats, and wild ruminants. In cattle, in utero infection with the virus between 76 and 150 days of gestation may result in congenital defects of the eye and brain. Central nervous system lesions include microencephaly, cerebellar hypoplasia, hydranencephaly, and hydrocephalus. **The ocular lesions of cataracts, retinal degeneration and dysplasia, optic nerve gliosis, optic neuritis, and microphthalmia have been described with experimentally induced disease as well.** At ophthalmoscopy, the tapetal coloration is altered, and pigment clumping is visible. Cataracts and optic nerve lesions may not be present in spontaneous cases, however, and may relate to the time of infection.

INFECTIOUS DISEASES

Several systemic diseases may affect the ophthalmic tissues. These ocular changes may collectively assist in establishing the diagnosis of the specific infection (Table 17-6).

INBORN ERRORS OF METABOLISM (LYSOSOMAL STORAGE DISEASES)

Inborn errors of metabolism are relatively rare among food animals (Table 17-1). The lysosomal storage diseases result from a deficiency in a specific degradative enzyme (i.e., acid hydrolases), which in turn allows the enzyme substrate to accumulate in the cells. In most cases, the eyes have histopathologic lesions, though clinical ophthalmic lesions may not be visible.

NUTRITIONAL DISEASES

Vitamin A deficiency has been studied extensively among cattle, both in spontaneous and experimentally induced cases. In young, growing animals, vitamin A deficiency produces clinical signs when the levels fall to less than 20 mg of vitamin A per 1 dL of plasma and less than 2 mg/g of liver. A lag period of from 3 to 12 months may be necessary before the effects of vitamin A deficiency are noted, and the effects themselves depend on the age at onset, degree of deficiency, and amount of liver stores. **Animals younger than 6 months of age are more susceptible and more likely to have blindness as a presenting sign because of sphenoid bone overgrowth constricting the optic nerve. Blindness, with or without convulsions, is the first outward sign to be noted in most cases among young, growing animals.** At critical examination of animals, night blindness may be noted. Blindness is accompanied by dilated, fixed pupils, and at ophthalmoscopy, papilledema will be present. **Papilledema occurs well before blindness in both adult- and young-onset deficiency and presumably results from increased cerebrospinal fluid pressure.**

TABLE 17-6

OPHTHALMIC MANIFESTATIONS OF INFECTIOUS DISEASES IN FOOD ANIMALS

Disease	Systemic and Ophthalmic Signs	Diagnosis
Bovine rhinotracheitis	Rhinotracheitis, conjunctivitis/keratitis, infectious pustular vulvovaginitis, and abortion. Raised, red-to-white plaques of lymphocyte follicles; nonulcerative keratitis; and anterior uveitis.	Viral isolation, fluorescent antibody testing
Malignant catarrhal fever	Head-and-eye variation; corneal edema; anterior uveitis; and panophthalmitis.	Histopathology
Bluetongue	Cattle: severe conjunctivitis accompanied by mucosal lesions, laminitis, and edema of the lips. Sheep: deformed lambs, brain deformities, and choroiditis and retinitis with retinal necrosis and retinal dysplasia.	Histopathology
Scrapie	Sheep and goats; multifocal, round tapetal lesions; focal retinal detachments resulting from subretinal accumulations of lipid.	Histopathology
Blue eye disease	Central nervous system disorders, reproductive failure, corneal edema, blindness, with dilated pupils and nystagmus. Conjunctivitis.	Virus isolation and hemagglutination-inhibition tests
Hog cholera	Anterior uveitis, focal choroiditis, retinitis, and optic neuritis develop with time.	
Pseudorabies	Acute blindness, depression, head pressing, and death.	
Chlamydia psittaci serotype 2	Cattle: polyarthritis, polyserositis, keratoconjunctivitis, pneumonia, and encephalomyelitis. Lambs and kids: polyarthritis; conjunctivitis, petechial hemorrhages, epiphora and mucopurulent exudation, and conjunctival lymphoid follicular proliferation. Peripheral corneal edema and neovascularization.	Cytology; culture
Thromboembolic meningoencephalitis	Peracute to chronic septicemia of yearling cattle. Blindness, strabismus, and nystagmus; retinal hemorrhages and focal exudates associated with endarterioles; focal retinal detachments and modest papilledema.	Histopathology (fibrinopurulent meningitis and multifocal hemorrhagic necrosis of the brain)

continued

TABLE 17-6		
OPHTHALMIC MANIFESTATIONS OF INFECTIOUS DISEASES IN FOOD ANIMALS—*continued*		
Disease	*Systemic and Ophthalmic Signs*	*Diagnosis*
Tuberculosis	Anterior and posterior uveitis, subretinal exudation and retinal detachment, and endophthalmitis.	Cytology and culture
Listeriosis	Involvement of the brainstem with facial nerve paralysis.	Culture
Neonatal septicemias	Polyarthritis, umbilical infections, and diarrheal signs may sporadically involve the eye. Anterior and posterior uveitis; endophthalmitis.	*Streptococcus* sp., *Escherichia coli, Cornybacterium pyogenes, Salmonella* sp., and *Pasteurella* sp. are usually cultured

Causes of blindness vary with the age of onset for the deficiency. Blindness may result from retinal degeneration at all ages, however, or from constriction and ischemic necrosis of the optic nerve at the optic foramen in growing animals. Eventually, optic nerve atrophy develops as well. Additional changes in the fundus are papillary and peripapillary hemorrhages as well as disruption of the pigment in the nontapetal region. Retinal degeneration primarily occurs in the nontapetal region.

In general, severe deficiency is accompanied by unthriftiness, diarrhea, poor growth, decreased appetite, and pneumonia.

The clinical signs, history, and ophthalmoscopic signs are very suggestive of hypovitaminosis A. If vitamin supplementation has not been instituted, plasma blood levels for vitamin A of less than 20 mg/dL will confirm the diagnosis. Vision will not be restored in calves that are day blind, but animals with vision and papilledema as well as older animals may benefit from parenteral administration of vitamin A, 440 IU/kg.

Vitamin A deficiency in pregnant sows causes a high incidence of varying degrees of microphthalmos and blindness in piglets. In extreme cases, anophthalmia is present as well.

NEOPLASIA

Cattle sometimes experience a syndrome of orbital involvement with lymphosarcoma that results in a progressive, bilateral or unilateral exophthalmos (Fig. 17-12). The resultant exposure keratitis may be severe, but

FIGURE 17-12. *Bilateral exophthalmos in a cow with severe exposure keratitis resulting from orbital lymphosarcoma. (Courtesy of W. Rebhun.)*

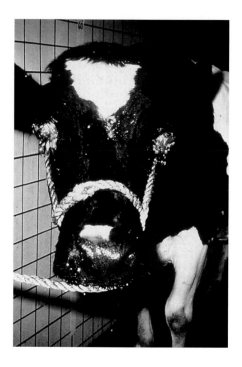

intraocular involvement is rare. Systemic involvement of the peripheral or the visceral lymph nodes, however, usually is present. A syndrome of bilateral conjunctival involvement without obvious orbital involvement also has been observed.

TOXIC PLANTS AND DRUGS

Food animals are subject to the adverse effects of poisonous plants, which are encountered not infrequently in their environment, and the clinical effects resulting from some of these plants primarily involve the visual system (Table 17-7). (For more information, the reader should consult the third edition, pp. 1501–1502.)

TABLE 17-7

OPHTHALMIC MANIFESTATIONS OF TOXIC PLANTS AND DRUGS IN FOOD ANIMALS

Plant	Clinical Signs
Male fern poisoning	*Dryopteris filix mas* consumption by cattle causes lethargy, constipation, and blindness. Acutely blind cattle: dilated pupils, papilledema, and retinal and preretinal hemorrhages.
Bracken fern poisoning	Ingestion of *Pteridium aquilinum* in chronic, low-level amounts causes bright blindness among sheep and cattle (England and Wales). Retinal degeneration with blindness, including retinal vascular attenuation, tapetal hyperreflectivity, and optic nerve atrophy.
Helichrysum argyrosphaerum	Blindness, paresis, and paralysis in sheep and cattle.
Coumarin poisoning	Sweet-clover poisoning in cattle, sheep, pigs, and horses. Hemorrhages are either limited or predominantly located in the eye and orbit.
Veratrum poisoning	Cyclopia in lambs may be produced by ingestion of *Veratrum californicum* or skunk cabbage in pregnant ewes on day 14 of gestation. The teratogen cyclopamine is found in the green leaves, stems, and especially, the roots. The incidence of anomalies may be as high as 25%.
Locoweed poisoning	Ingestion of locoweed by cattle and sheep may produce ocular signs of blindness and a "dull" eye.
Phenothiazine toxicity	Cattle on a low plane of nutrition may develop diffuse corneal edema via exposure to sunlight within 24 hours after receiving phenothiazine as a dewormer. Ulceration may develop secondary to the edema, and recovery may occur in 1 week (if the animal is restricted indoors) or be prolonged for 2–3 months (if the animal is kept in the pasture).
Hygromycin B	Pigs receiving this aminoglycoside antibiotic, fed at 13.2 gm per 1000 kg of feed for 14 months on continuous feed, or pigs with elevated levels of hygromycin B (10–11 months), develop cataracts. The opacities begin as axial, posterior subcapsular opacities and then progress to complete cortical cataracts.
Arsanilic acid	Used in swine as a growth stimulant and a therapy for swine dysentery. Arsanilic acid poisoning has occurred from long-term administration, errors in feed formulation, or when water has been restricted. Clinical signs of blindness and pupillary dilation occur with toxicity, and additional signs of ataxia, torticollis, and paralysis may develop as well.

Suggested Readings

Suggested readings include selected references from within the past 10 years, and occasional older references that are vital to our veterinary ophthalmic foundation of knowledge.

CHAPTER 1: Ophthalmic Examination and Diagnostic Procedures

Bauer GA, Spiess BM, Lutz H. Exfoliative cytology of conjunctiva and cornea in domestic animals: a comparison of four collecting techniques. Vet Comp Ophthalmol 1996;6:181–186.

Collins BK, Gross ME, Moore CP, Branson KR. Physiological, pharmacological, and practical considerations for anesthesia of domestic animals with eye diseases. J Am Vet Med Assoc 1995;207:220–230.

Cooley PL. Normal equine ocular anatomy and eye examination. Vet Clin North Am Eq Pract 1992;8:427–449.

Dziezyc J, Millichamp NJ, Smith WB. Comparison of applanation tonometers in dogs and horses. J Am Vet Med Assoc 1992;201:430–433.

Feenstra RPG, Tseng CG. What is actually stained by rose Bengal? Arch Ophthalmol 1992;110:984–993.

Gelatt KN. Diagnostic procedures in comparative ophthalmology, 2nd ed. Elkland: Am Anim Hosp Assoc, 1974.

Gelatt KN, Cure TH, Guffy MM, Jessen C. Dacryocystorhinography in the dog and cat. J Small Anim Pract 1972;13:381–397.

Hazel SJ, Thrall MA, Severin GA, Lauerman LH, Lavach JD. Laboratory evaluation of aqueous humor in the healthy dog, cat, horse, and cow. Am J Vet Res 1985;46:657–659.

Hirsh SG, Kaswan RL. A comparative study of Schirmer tear test strips in dogs. Vet Comp Ophthalmol 1995;5:215–217.

Latimer CA, Wyman M, Diesem CD, Burt JK. Radiographic and gross anatomy of the nasolacrimal duct of the horse. Am J Vet Res 1984;45:451–458.

Miller PE, Pickett JP. Comparison of the human and canine Schiotz tonometry conversion tables in clinically normal dogs. J Am Vet Med Assoc 1992;201:1021–1025.

Murphy CJ, Howland JC. Optics of comparative ophthalmoscopy. In: Proceedings of the Sixteenth Annual Scientific Program of the College of Veterinary Ophthalmologists, 1985;16:132–157.

Priehs DR, Gum GG, Whitley RD, Moore LE. Evaluation of three applanation tonometers in dogs. Am J Vet Res 1990;51:1547–1550.

Stiles J, Buyukmichi NC, Farver TB. Tonometry of normal eyes in raptors. Am J Vet Res 1994;55:477–479.

Whitley RD, Moore CP. Ocular diagnostic and therapeutic techniques in food animals. Vet Clin North Am Large Anim Pract 1984;6:553–575.

Wilkie DA. Ophthalmic procedures and surgery in the standing horse. Vet Clin North Am Eq Pract 1991;7:535–547.

Wyman M, Gilger B, Mueller P, Norris K. Clinical evaluation of a new Schirmer tear test in the dog. Vet Comp Ophthalmol 1995;5:211–214.

CHAPTER 2: Diseases and Surgery of the Canine Orbit

Brightman A, Magrane WG, Huff RW, Helper LC. Intraocular prosthesis in the dog. J Am Anim Hosp Assoc 1977;13:481–485.

Carpenter JL, Schmidt GM, Moore FM, Albert DM, Abrams KL, Elner VM. Canine bilateral extraocular polymyositis. Vet Pathol 1989;26:510–512.

Gilger BC, Hamilton HL, Wilkie DA, van der Woerdt A, McLaughlin SA. Traumatic ocular proptoses in dogs and cats—84 cases (1980–1993). J Am Vet Med Assoc 1995;206:1186–1190.

Kern TJ. Orbital neoplasia in 23 dogs. J Am Vet Med Assoc 1985;186:489–491.

Martin C. Augenkrankheiten bei Hund und Katze. Hannover, Germany: M & H Schaper, 1995.

Millichamp N, Spencer CP. Orbital varix in a dog. J Am Anim Hosp Assoc 1991;27:56–60.

O'Brien MG, et al. Total and partial orbitectomy for the treatment of periorbital tumors in 24 dogs and 6 cats: a retrospective study. Vet Surg 1996;25:471–479.

Ruehli M, Spiess BM. Retrobulbar space-occupying lesions in dogs and cats: clinical signs and diagnostic work-up. Tierarztl Prax 1995;23:306–312.

Ruehli MB, Spiess BM. Treatment of orbital abscesses and phlegmon in dogs and cats. Tierarztl Prax 1995;23:398–401.

Shelton GD, Cardinet GHD, Bandman E. Canine masticatory muscle disorders: a study of 29 cases. Muscle Nerve 1987;10:753–766.

Slatter DH, Abdelbaki Y. Lateral orbitotomy by zygomatic arch resection in the dog. J Am Vet Med Assoc 1979;175:1179–1182.

Spiess B, Williams MM. Protruding eye. In: Binnington A, Cockshutt JR, eds. Decision making in small animal soft tissue surgery. Toronto: BC Decker, 1988:164–165.

Spiess BM, Ruhli MB, Bauer GA. Therapy of orbital neoplasms in small animals. Tierarztl Prax 1995;23:509–514.

Walde I, Hittmair K, Henninger W, Czedik-Eysenberg T. Retrobulbar dermoid cyst in a dachshund. Vet Comp Ophthalmol 1997;7:239–244.

CHAPTER 3: Diseases and Surgery of the Canine Eyelids

Bedford PGC. Surgical correction of facial droop in the English Cocker Spaniel. J Small Anim Pract 1990;31:255–258.

Bedford PGC. Technique of lateral canthoplasty for the correction of macropalpebral fissure in the dog. J Small Anim Pract 1998;39:117–121.

Bigelbach A. A combined tarsorrhaphy-canthoplasty technique for the repair of entropion and ectropion. Vet Comp Ophthalmol 1996;6:220.

Johnson BW, Gerding PA, McLaughlin SA, Helper LC, Szajerski ME, Cormany KA. Non-surgical correction of entropion in Shar Pei puppies. Vet Med 1988;83:482.

Munger RJ, Carter JD. A further modification of the Khunt-Szymanowski procedure for correction of atonic entropion in dogs. J Am Anim Hosp Assoc 1984;20:651.

Robertson BF, Roberts SM. Latent canthus entropion in the dog. Part I: comparative anatomic studies. Vet Comp Ophthalmol 1995;5:151.

Robertson BF, Roberts SM. Lateral canthus entropion in the dog. 2: surgical correction. Results and follow-up from 21 cases (1991–1994). Vet Comp Ophthalmol 1995;5:162.

Stades FC. A new method for surgical correction of upper eyelid trichiasis-entropion. Operation method. J Am Anim Hosp Assoc 1987;23:603.

Stades FC, Boeve MH. Surgical correction of upper eyelid trichiasis-entropion: results and follow-up in 55 eyes. J Am Anim Hosp Assoc 1987;23:607.

Stades FC, Boeve MH, van der Woerdt A. Palpebral fissure length in the dog and cat. Prog Vet Comp Ophthalmol 1992;2:155.

Wheeler CA, Severin GA. Cryosurgical epilation for the treatment of distichiasis in the dog and cat. J Am Anim Hosp Assoc 1984;20:877.

CHAPTER 4: Diseases and Surgery of the Canine Tear and Nasolacrimal Systems

Berger S, Scagliotti R, Lund EM. A quantitative study of the effects of Tribrissen on canine tear production. J Am Anim Hosp Assoc 1995;31:236–241.

Kaswan RL, Salisbury MA. A new perspective on canine keratoconjunctivitis sicca. Treatment with ophthalmic cyclosporine. Vet Clin North Am Small Anim Pract 1990; 20:583–613.

Kern TJ, Erb HN, Schaedler JM, Dougherty EP. Scanning electron microscopy of experimental keratoconjunctivitis sicca in dogs: cornea and bulbar conjunctiva. Vet Pathol 1988;25:468–474.

Moore CP, Collier LL. Ocular surface disease associated with loss of conjunctival goblet cells in dogs. J Am Anim Hosp Assoc 1990;26:458–465.

Moore CP, Frappier B. Density and distribution of canine third eyelid excretory ducts: effects of two surgical techniques. Vet Comp Ophthalmol 1996;4:258–264.

Morgan RV, Abrams KL. Topical administration of cyclosporine for treatment of keratoconjunctivitis sicca in dogs. J Am Vet Med Assoc 1991;199:1043–1046.

Morgan RV, Duddy JM, McClug K. Prolapse of the gland of the third eyelid in dogs. A retrospective study of 89 cases (1980–1990). J Am Anim Hosp Assoc 1993;29:56–60.

Salisbury MA, et al. Topical application of cyclosporine in the management of keratoconjunctivitis sicca in dogs. J Am Anim Hosp Assoc 1990;26:269–274.

CHAPTER 5: Diseases and Surgery of the Canine Conjunctiva

Collins BK, Collier LL, Miller MA, Linton LL. Biologic behavior and histologic characteristics of canine conjunctival melanoma. Prog Vet Comp Ophthalmol 1993;3: 135–140.

Davidson MG, Breitschwerdt EB, Nasisse MP, Roberts SM. Ocular manifestations of Rocky Mountain spotted fever in dogs. J Am Vet Med Assoc 1989;194:777–781.

Eichenbaum JD, Lavach JD, Severin GA, Paulsen ME. Immunology of the ocular surface. Comp Cont Educ Pract Vet 1987;9:1101–1109.

Gelatt KN, Gelatt JP. Surgical procedures of the conjunctiva. In: Handbook of small animal ophthalmic surgery. Vol 1: extraocular procedures. Oxford: Pergamon, 1994: 165–188.

Gerding PA, McLaughlin SA, Troop MW. Pathogenic bacteria and fungi associated with external ocular diseases in dogs: 131 cases (1981–1986). J Am Vet Med Assoc 1988;193:242–244.

Hakanson NE, Merideth RE. Conjunctival pedicle grafting in the treatment of corneal ulcers in the dog and cat. J Am Anim Hosp Assoc 1987;23:641–648.

Moore CP, Collier LL. Ocular surface disease associated with loss of conjunctival goblet cells in dogs. J Am Anim Hosp Assoc 1990;26:458–466.

Moore CP, Wilsman NJ, Nordheim EV, Majors LJ, Collier LL. Density and distribution of canine conjunctival goblet cells. Invest Ophthalmol Vis Sci 1987;28:1925–1932.

Peiffer RL Jr, Gelatt KN, Gwin RM. Tarsoconjunctival pedicle grafts for deep corneal ulceration in the dog and cat. J Am Anim Hosp Assoc 1977;13:387–391.

Ramsey DT, Ketring KL, Glaze MB, Render JA. Ligneous conjunctivitis in four Doberman Pinschers. J Am Anim Hosp Assoc 1996;32:439–447.

Scagliotti RH. Tarsoconjunctival island graft for the treatment of deep corneal ulcers, descemetocels, and perforations in 35 dogs and 6 cats. Semin Vet Med Surg Small Anim 1988;3:69–76.

Scherlie PH, Smedes SL, Feltz T, Dougherty SA, Riis RC. Ocular manifestation of systemic histiocytosis in a dog. J Am Vet Med Assoc 1992;201:1229–1232.

Wagner J, Nasisse MP, Davidson MG. A retrospective study of conjunctival flaps in 67 dogs and 17 horses, 1987–1991 (abstract). Vet Pathol 1992;29:476.

Wheeler CA, Blanchard GL, Davidson HJ. Cryosurgery for treatment of recurrent proliferative keratoconjunctivitis in five dogs. J Am Vet Med Assoc 1989;195:354–357.

CHAPTER 6: Diseases and Surgery of the Canine Nictitating Membrane

Collins BK, Collier LL, Miller MA, Linton LL. Biologic behavior and histologic characteristics of canine conjunctival melanoma. Prog Vet Comp Ophthalmol 1993;3: 135–140.

Crispin S. Treating the everted membrana nictitans. In: Boden E, ed. Canine practice. London: Bailliere Tindall, 1991:33–36.

Dugan SJ, Ketring KL, Severin GA, Render JA. Variant nodular granulomatous episclerokeratitis in four dogs. J Am Anim Hosp Assoc 1993;29:403–409.

Gelatt KN, Gelatt JP. Handbook of small animal ophthalmic surgery. Vol 1: extraocular procedures. Tarrytown, NY: Pergamon, 1994:158–159.

Kaswan RL, Martin CL. Surgical correction of third eyelid prolapse in dogs. J Am Vet Med Assoc 1985;186:83.

Moore CP. Imbrication technique for replacement of prolapsed third eyelid gland. In: Bojrab MJ, ed. Current techniques in small animal surgery. Philadelphia: Lea & Febiger, 1990:126–128.

Morgan RV, Duddy JM, McClurg K. Prolapse of the gland of the third eyelid in dogs: a retrospective study of 89 cases (1980–1990). J Am Anim Hosp Assoc 1993;29: 56–60.

Read RA. Treatment of canine nictitans plasmacytic conjunctivitis with 0.2 percent cyclosporine ointment. J Small Anim Pract 1995;36:50–56.

Stanley RG, Kaswan RL. Modification of the orbital rim anchorage method for surgical replacement of the gland of the third eyelid in dogs. J Am Vet Med Assoc 1994;205:1412–1414.

Wilcock B, Peiffer RJ. Adenocarcinoma of the gland of the third eyelid in seven dogs. J Am Vet Med Assoc 1988;193:1549–1550.

CHAPTER 7: Diseases and Surgery of the Canine Cornea and Sclera

Champagne ES, Munger RJ. Multiple punctate keratotomy for the treatment of recurrent epithelial erosions in dogs. J Am Anim Hosp Assoc 1992;28:213–216.

Crispin SM. Crystalline corneal dystrophy in the dog. Histochemical and ultrastructural study. Cornea 1988;7:149–161.

Crispin SM. Ocular manifestations of hyperlipoproteinemia. J Small Anim Pract 1993;34:500–506.

Eichenbaum JD, Lavach JD, Gould DH, Severin GA, Paulsen ME, Jones RL. Immunohistochemical staining patterns of canine eyes affected with chronic superficial keratitis. Am J Vet Res 1986;47:1952–1955.

Gelatt KN, Samuelson DA. Recurrent corneal erosions and epithelial dystrophy in the Boxer dog. J Am Anim Hosp Assoc 1982;18:453–460.

Gilger BC, Whitley RD, McLaughlin SA, Wright JC, Drane JW. Canine corneal thickness measured by ultrasonic pachymetry. Am J Vet Res 1991;52:1570–1572.

Gratzek AT, Calvert CA, Martin CL, Kaswan RL. Corneal edema in dogs treated with tocainide. Prog Vet Comp Ophthalmol 1996;3:47.

Gwin RM, Lerner I, Warren K, Gum G. Decrease in canine corneal endothelial cell density and corneal thickness as a function of age. Invest Ophthalmol Vis Sci 1982;22:267–271.

Hacker DV. Frozen corneal grafts in dogs and cats: a report of 19 cases. J Am Anim Hosp Assoc 1991;27:387–398.

Kirschner SE. Persistent corneal ulcers. What to do when ulcers won't heal. Vet Clin North Am Small Anim Pract 1990;20:627–642.

Marlar AB, Miller PE, Canton DD, Scagliotti R, Murphy CJ. Canine keratomycosis: a report of eight cases and literature review. J Am Animal Hosp Assoc 1994;30: 331–340.

Morgan R, Abrams K. A comparison of six different therapies for persistent corneal erosions in dogs and cats. Vet Comp Ophthalmol 1994;4:38–43.

Sullivan TC, Nasisse MP, Davidson MG, Glover TL. Photocoagulation of limbal melanoma in dogs and cats: 15 cases (1989–1993). J Am Vet Med Assoc 1996;208: 891–894.

Williams DL, Hoey AJ, Smitherman PJ. The use of topical cyclosporine and dexamethasone in the treatment of canine chronic superficial keratitis: a comparison of therapeutic effects. Vet Rec 1995;137:635–639.

CHAPTER 8: The Canine Glaucomas

Barnett KC, Mason IK. Primary glaucoma in the Great Dane. Trans Am Coll Vet Ophthalmol 1993;24:112.

Bentley E, Nasisse MP, Glover T, Nelms S. Implantation of filtering devices in dogs with glaucoma: preliminary results in 13 eyes. Vet Comp Ophthalmol 1996,6:243–246.

Bjerkås E, Peiffer RL, Ekesten B. Primary glaucoma in the Norwegian Elkhound. Trans Am Coll Vet Ophthalmol 1994;25:74.

Brooks D, Strubbe D, Kubilis P, Mackay EO, Samuelson DA, Gelatt KN. Histomorphometry of the optic nerves of normal dogs and dogs with hereditary glaucoma. Exp Eye Res 1995; 60:71–89.

Brooks DE, Garcia GA, Dreyer EB, Zurakowski D, Franco-Bourland RE. Vitreous body glutamate concentration in dogs with glaucoma. Am J Vet Res 1997;58:864–867.

Brooks DE, Samuelson DA, Gelatt KN, Smith PJ. Morphologic changes in the lamina cribrosa of Beagles with primary open-angle glaucoma. Am J Vet Res 1989; 50:936–941.

Cook C, Davidson M, Brinkmann M, Priehs D, Abrams K, Nasisse M. Diode laser transscleral cyclophotocoagulation for the treatment of glaucoma in dogs: results of six and twelve months follow-up. Vet Comp Ophthalmol 1997;7:148–154.

Corcoran KA, Koch SA, Peiffer RL. Primary glaucoma in the Chow Chow. Vet Comp Ophthalmol 1994;4:193–197.

Ekesten B. Correlation of intraocular distances to the iridocorneal angle in Samoyeds with special reference to angle-closure glaucoma. Prog Vet Comp Ophthalmol 1993;3:67–73.

Ekesten B, Narfström K. Age-related changes in intraocular pressure and iridocorneal angle in Samoyeds. Prog Vet Comp Ophthalmol 1992;2:37–40.

Ekesten B, Narfström K. Correlation of morphologic features of the iridocorneal angle to intraocular pressure in Samoyed. Am J Vet Res 1991;52:1875–1878.

Garcia GA, Brooks DE, Gelatt KN, Kubilis PS, Gil F, Whitley RD. Evaluation of valved and nonvalved gonioimplants in 83 eyes of 65 dogs with glaucoma. Anim Eye Res 1998;17:9–16.

Gelatt KN, Brooks DE, Miller TR, Smith PJ, Sapienza JS, Pellicane CP. Issues in ophthalmic therapy: the development of anterior chamber shunts for the clinical management of the canine glaucomas. Prog Vet Comp Ophthalmol 1992;2: 59–64.

Gelatt KN, Gum GG, Mackay EO, Gelatt KJ. Estimations of aqueous humor outflow facility by pneumatonography in normal, genetic carrier and glaucomatous Beagles. Vet Comp Ophthalmol 1996;6:148–151.

Gum GG, Metzger KJ, Gelatt KN. The tonographic effects of pilocarpine and pilocarpine-epinephrine in normal Beagles and Beagles with inherited glaucoma. J Small Anim Pract 1993;34:112–116.

Håkanson NW. Extraorbital diversion of aqueous in the treatment of glaucoma in the dog: a pilot study including two recipient sites. Vet Comp Ophthalmol 1996;6:82–90.

Miller PE, Poulsen GL, Nork TM, Galbreath EJ, Dubielzig RR. Photoreceptor cell death by apoptosis in spontaneous acute glaucoma in dogs. Invest Ophthalmol Vis Sci (Abstract) 1997;38:163.

Read RA, Wood JL, Laklani KH. Pectinate ligament dysplasia and glaucoma in Flat Coated Retrievers. I. Objectives, technique, and results of survey. Vet Ophthalmol 1998;1:85–90.

Samuelson DA, Gum GG, Gelatt KN. Ultrastructural changes in the aqueous outflow apparatus of Beagles with inherited glaucoma. Invest Ophthalmol Vis Sci 1989; 30:550–561.

Smith PJ, Brooks DE, Lazarus JA, Kubilis PS, Gelatt KN. Ocular hypertension following cataract surgery in dogs: 139 cases (1992–1993). J Am Vet Med Assoc 1996; 209:105–111.

Smith RIE, Peiffer RL, Wilcock BP. Some aspects of the pathology of canine glaucoma. Vet Comp Ophthalmol 1993;3:16–28.

Tinsley DM, Betts DM. Clinical experience with a glaucoma drainage device in dogs. Vet Comp Ophthalmol 1994;4:77–84.

CHAPTER 9: Diseases and Surgery of the Canine Anterior Uvea

Collins BK, et al. Familial cataracts and concurrent ocular anomalies in Chow Chows. J Am Vet Med Assoc 1992;200:1485–1491.

Crispin SM. Uveitis in the dog and cat. J Small Anim Pract 1988;29:429–436.

Dubielzig RR. Ocular neoplasia in small animals. Vet Clin North Am Small Anim Pract 1990;20:837–848.

Gerding PA, Essex-Sorlie D, Vasaune S, Yack R. Use of tissue plasminogen activator for intraocular fibrinolysis in dogs. Am J Vet Res 1992;53:890–894.

Hakanson N, Forrester SD. Uveitis in the dog and cat. Vet Clin North Am 1990; 20:715–734.

Krohne SG, et al. Prevalence of ocular involvement in dogs with multicentric lymphosarcoma: prospective evaluation of 94 cases. Vet Comp Ophthalmol 1994;4: 127–134.

Millichamp NJ, Dziezyc J. Mediators of ocular inflammation. Prog Comp Vet Ophthalmol 1991;1:41–58.

Swanson JF. Ocular manifestations of systemic disease in the dog and cat: recent developments. Vet Clin North Am 1990;20:849–867.

Van der Woerdt A, Nasisse MP, Davidson MG. Lens-induced uveitis in dogs: 151 cases (1985–1990). J Am Vet Med Assoc 1992;201:921–926.

Ward DA. Comparative efficacy of topically applied flurbiprofen, diclofenac, tolmetin, and suprofen for the treatment of experimentally induced blood-aqueous barrier disruption in dogs. Am J Vet Res 1996;57:875–878.

Ward DA, et al. Comparison of the blood-aqueous barrier stabilizing effects of steroidal and nonsteroidal anti-inflammatory agents in the dog. Prog Vet Comp Ophthalmol 1992;2:117–124.

Wilcock BP, Peiffer RL. Morphology and behavior of primary ocular melanomas in 91 dogs. Vet Pathol 1986;23:418–424.

Wilcock BP, Peiffer RL. The pathology of lens-induced uveitis in dogs. Vet Pathol 1987;24:549–553.

Wilkie DA. Control of ocular inflammation. Vet Clin North Am 1990;20:693–713.

CHAPTER 10: Diseases and Surgery of the Canine Lens

Bagley LH, Lavach JD. Comparison of postoperative phacoemulsification results in dogs with and without diabetes mellitus: 153 cases (1991–1992). J Am Vet Med Assoc 1994;205:115–1169.

Bjerkas E, Bergsjo T. Hereditary cataract in the Rottweiler dog. Prog Vet Comp Ophthalmol 1991;1:7–10.

Boevé M, Stades F, van der Linde-Sipman J, Vrensen G. Persistent hyperplastic tunica vasculosa lentis and primary vitreous (PHTVL/PHPV) in the dog: a comparative review. Prog Vet Comp Ophthalmol 1993;2:163–172.

Boevé M, van der Linde-Sipman J, Stades F. Early morphogenesis of persistent hyperplastic tunica vasculosa lentis and primary vitreous. The dog as an otogenetic model. Invest Ophthalmol Vis Sci 1988;29:1076–1086.

Collins B, Collier L, Johnson G, Shibuya H, Moore C, DaSilva-Curiel J. Familial cataracts and concurrent ocular anomalies in Chow Chows. J Am Vet Med Assoc 1992;200:1485–1491.

Da Costa P, Merideth R, Sigler R. Cataracts in dogs after long-term ketoconazole therapy. Vet Comp Ophthalmol 1996;6:176–180.

Davidson MG, Nasisse MP, Jamieson VE, English RV, Olivero DK. Phacoemulsification and intraocular lens implantation: a study of surgical results in 158 dogs. Prog Vet Comp Ophthalmol 1991;1:233–238.

Davidson MG, Nasisse MP, Rusnak IM, Corbett WT, English RV. Success rates of unilateral vs. bilateral cataract extraction in dogs. Vet Surg 1990;19:232–236.

Gaiddon J, Rosolen S, Crozafon P, Steru D. A new technique for lens extraction in surgery on dogs: endocapsular phaco-emulsification. Eur J Implant Refract Surg 1988;6:30–35.

Gaiddon J, Rosolen SG, Lallemnet PE, LeGargassojn JF. New intraocular lens (IOL) for dogs: the foldable cani 15S. Preliminary results of surgical technique. Invest Ophthalmol Vis Science (Abstract) 1997;38(Suppl):179.

Jamieson V, Davidson M, Nasisse M, English R. Ocular complications following cobalt-60 radiotherapy of neoplasma in the canine head region. J Am Anim Hosp Assoc 1991;27:51–55.

Miller PE, Stanz KM, Dubielzig RR, Murphy CJ. Mechanisms of acute intraocular pressure increases after phacoemulsification lens extraction in dogs. Am J Vet Res 1997;58:1159–1165.

Miller TR, Whitley RD, Meek LA, Garcia GA, Wilson MC, Rawls BH. Phacofragmentation and aspiration for cataract extraction in dogs: 56 cases (1980–1984). J Am Vet Med Assoc 1987;190:1577–1580.

Nasisse MP, Davidson MG, Jamieson VE, English RV, Olivero DK. Phacoemulsification and intraocular lens implantation in dogs: a study of technique in 158 dogs. Prog Vet Comp Ophthalmol 1990;1:225–232.

Neumann W. Chirurgische Behandlung der Katarakt beim Kleintier (1. Mitteilung). Kleintierpraxis 1991;36:17–28.

Smith PJ, Brooks DE, Lazarus JA, Kubilis PS, Gelatt KN. Ocular hypertension following cataract surgery in dogs: 139 cases (1992–1993). J Am Vet Med Assoc 1996; 209:105–111.

Van der Woerdt A, Nasisse M, Davidson M. Lens-induced uveitis in dogs: 151 cases (1985–1990). J Am Vet Med Assoc 1992;20:921–926.

Van der Woerdt A, Wilkie D, Myer C. Ultrasonographic abnormalities in the eyes of dogs with cataracts: 147 cases (1986–1992). J Am Vet Med Assoc 1993;203:838–841.

CHAPTER 11: Diseases and Surgery of the Canine Posterior Segment

Acland GM, Blanton SH, Hershfield B, Aguirre G. XLPRA: a canine retinal degeneration inherited as an X-linked trait. Am J Med Genet 1994;52:27–33.

Anderson RE, Maude MB, Alvarez RA, Acland GM, Aguirre GD. Plasma lipid abnormalities in the Miniature Poodle with progressive rod-cone degeneration. Exp Eye Res 1991;52:349–355.

Bjerkås E. Collie eye anomaly in the rough collie in Norway. J Small Anim Pract 1991;32:82–92.

Bloom JD, Hamor RE, Gerding PA Jr. Ocular blastomycosis in dogs: 73 cases, 108 eyes, 1985–1993. J Am Vet Med Assoc 1996;209:1271–1274.

Boevé MH, Stades FC, van der Linde-Sipman JS, Vrensen GFJM. Persistent hyperplastic tunica vasculosa lentis and primary vitreous in the dog: a comparative review. Vet Comp Ophthalmol 1992;2:163–172.

Boevé MH, van der Linde-Sipman JS, Stades FC. Early morphogenesis of persistent hyperplastic tunica vasculosa lentis and primary vitreous. The dog as an ontogenetical model. Invest Ophthalmol Vis Sci 1988;29:1076–1086.

Breitschwerdt EB, et al. Efficacy of chloramphenicol, enrofloxacin, and tetracycline for treatment of experimental Rocky Mountain spotted fever in dogs. Antimicrob Agents Chemother 1991;35:2375–2381.

Brooks DE, Legendre AM, Gum GG, Laratta LJ, Abrams KL, Morgan RV. The treatment of canine ocular blastomycosis with systemically administered itraconazole. Prog Vet Comp Ophthalmol 1991;1:263–268.

Carrig CB, Sponenberg DP, Schmidt GM, Tvedten HW. Inheritance of associated ocular and skeletal dysplasia in Labrador Retrievers. J Am Vet Med Assoc 1988;193:1269–1272.

Clements PJM, Gregory CY, Peterson-Jones SM, Sargan DR, Bhattacharya SS. Confirmation of the rod cGMP phosphodiesterase beta subunit (PDEb) nonsense mutation in affected rcd1 Irish Setters in the U.K. and development of a diagnostic test. Curr Eye Res 1993;12:861–866.

Curtis R, Barnett KC. Progressive retinal atrophy in Miniature Longhaired Dachshund dogs. Br Vet J 1993;149:71–85.

Davidson EM, et al. Vascular permeability and coagulation during Rickettsia rickettsii infection in dogs. Am J Vet Res 1990;51:165–170.

Håkansson N, Narfström K. Progressive retinal atrophy in Papillon dogs in Sweden. A clinical survey. Vet Comp Ophthalmol 1995;5:83–87.

Hendrix DV, Nasisse MP, Cowen P, Davidson MG. Clinical signs, concurrent diseases, and risk factors associated with retinal detachment in dogs. Prog Vet Comp Ophthalmol 1993;3:87–91.

Huss BT, Collier LL, Collins BK, Pittman LL Jr, Aronson E, Rottinghaus AA. Polyarthropathy and chorioretinitis with retinal detachment in a dog with systemic histoplasmosis. J Am Anim Hosp Assoc 1994;30:217–224.

McLellan GJ, Richelle M, Elks R, Lybaert P, Bedford PGC. Vitamin E deficiency in canine retinal epithelial dystrophy (RPED) results of the oral vitamin E tolerance test in clinically normal dogs and in RPED affected cocker spaniels. WSAVA Congress, Birmingham, UK, 1997.

Miller PE, Murphy CJ. Vision in dogs. J Am Vet Med Assoc 1995,207:1623–1634.

O'Toole D, Roberts S, Nunamaker C. Sudden acquired retinal degeneration ("silent retina syndrome") in two dogs. Vet Rec 1992;130:157–161.

Parshall C, Wyman M, Nitroy S, Acland G, Aguirre G. Photoreceptor dysplasia: an inherited progressive retinal trophy of miniature schnauzer dogs. Prog Vet Comp Ophthalmol 1991;1:187–203.

Paulsen ME, Severin GA, LeCouteur RA, Young S. Primary optic nerve meningioma in a dog. J Am Anim Hosp Assoc 1989;25:147–152.

Ray K, Baldwin V, Acland G, Aguirre G. Molecular diagnostic tests for ascertainment of genotype at the rod cone dysplasia 1 (rcd1) locus in Irish setters. Curr Eye Res 1995;14:243–247.

Schmid V, Murisier N. Color doppler imaging of the orbit in the dog. Vet Comp Ophthalmol 1996;6:35–44.

Vainisi S, Peyman G, Wolf D, West S. Treatment of serous retinal detachments associated with optic disk pits in dogs. J Am Vet Med Assoc 1989;195:1233–1236.

Vainisi SJ, Packo K, Schmidt GM. Retinal detachments in the Shih Tzu. Proceedings 25th Am Coll Vet Opthalmol 1990;25:115.

Vainisi SJ, Packo KH. Management of giant retinal tears in dogs. J Am Vet Med Assoc 1995;206:491–495.

Venter IJ, van der Lugt JJ, van Rensburg IBJ, Petrick SW. Multiple congenital eye anomalies in Bloodhound puppies. Vet Comp Ophthalmol 1996;6:9–13.

CHAPTER 12: Feline Ophthalmology

Anderson RE, Maude MB, Nilsson SEG, Narstrom K. Plasma lipid abnormalities in the Abyssinian cat with a hereditary rod-cone degeneration. Exp Eye Res 1991;53:415–417.

Brightman AH, Ogilvie GK, Tompkins M. Ocular disease in FeLV-positive cats: 11 cases (1981–1986). J Am Anim Hosp Assoc 1991;198:1049–1051.

Brown MH, Brightman AH, Butine MD, Moore TL. The phenol red thread tear test in healthy cats. Vet Comp Ophthalmol 1997;7:249–252.

Corcoran KA, Peiffer RL, Koch SA. Histopathologic features of feline ocular lymphosarcoma: 49 cases (1978–1992). Vet Comp Ophthalmol 1995;5:35–41.

Davidson MG, Nasisse MP, English RV, Wilcock BP, Jamieson V. Feline anterior uveitis: a study of 53 cases. J Am Anim Hosp Assoc 1991;27:77–83.

Dubielzig RR, Hawkins KL, Toy KA, Rosebury WS, Mazur M, Jasper TG. Morphological features of feline ocular sarcomas in 10 cats: light microscopy, ultrastructure, and immunohistochemistry. Vet Comp Ophthalmol 1994;4:7–12.

Duncan DE, Peiffer RL. Morphology and prognostic indicators of anterior melanomas in cats. Prog Vet Comp Ophthalmol 1991;1:25–32.

Espinola MB, Lilenbaum W. Prevalence of bacteria in the conjunctival sac and on the eyelid margin of clinically normal cats. J Small Animal Pract 1996;37:364–366.

Gilger BC, et al. Orbital neoplasms in cats: 21 cases (1974–1990). J Am Vet Med Assoc 1992;201:1083–1086.

Gilger BC, Hamilton HL, Wilkie DA, van der Woerdt A, McLaughlin SA, Whitley RD. Traumatic ocular proptoses in dogs and cats: 84 cases (1980–1993). J Am Anim Hosp Assoc 1995;206:1186–1190.

Glover TL, Nasisse MP, Davidson MG. Acute bullous keratopathy in the cat. Vet Comp Ophthalmol 1994;4:66–70.

Gunn-Moore DA, Jenkins PA, Lucke VM. Feline tuberculosis: a literature review and discussion of 19 cases and an unusual mycobacterial variant. Vet Rec 1996;138:53–58.

Henik RA. Diagnosis and treatment of feline hypertension. Comp Cont Educ Pract Vet 1997;19:163–179.

Henik RA, Synder PS, Volk LM. Treatment of systemic hypertension in cats by amlodipine besylate. J Am Anim Hosp Assoc 1997;33:226–234.

Johnson BW. Congenitally abnormal visual pathways of Siamese cats. Comp Cont Educ Pract Vet 1991;13:374–377.

Kerlin RL, Dubielzig RR. Lipogranulomatous conjunctivitis in cats. Vet Comp Ophthalmol 1997;7:177–179.

Kline KL, Joseph RJ, Averill DR. Feline infectious peritonitis with neurologic involvement: clinical and pathological findings in 24 cats. J Am Anim Hosp Assoc 1994;30:111–118.

Lappin MR, Burney DP, Dow SW, Potter TA. Polymerase chain reaction for the detection of *Toxoplasma gondii* in aqueous humor of cats. Am J Vet Res 1996;57:1589–1593.

Martin CL, Stiles J, Willis M. Feline colobomatous syndrome. Vet Comp Ophthalmol 1997;7:39–43.

McLaughlin SA, Whitley RD, Gilger BC, Wright JC. Eyelid neoplasia in cats: a review of demographic data (1979–1989). J Am Anim Hosp Assoc 1993;29:63–67.

Morgan RV. Feline corneal sequestration: a retrospective study of 42 cases (1987–1991). J Am An Hosp Assoc 1994;30:24–28.

Morgan RV, Abrams KL, Kern TJ. Feline eosinophilic keratitis: a retrospective study of 54 cases (1989–1994). Prog Vet Comp Ophthalmol 1996;6:131–134.

Nasisse MP, Guy JS, Stevens JB, English EV, Davidson MG. Clinical and laboratory findings in chronic conjunctivitis in cats: 91 cases (1983–1991). J Am Vet Med Assoc 1993;203:834–837.

Nasisse MP, Weigler BJ. The diagnosis of ocular feline herpesvirus infection. Vet Comp Ophthalmol 1997;7:44–51.

Nuyttens J, Simoens P. Protrusion of the third eyelid in cats. Vlaams Diergeneeskundig Tijdschrift 1994;63:80–86.

Olivero DK, Riis RC, Dutton AG, Murphy CJ, Nasisse MP, Davidson MG. Feline lens displacement: a retrospective analysis of 345 cases. Prog Vet Comp Ophthalmol 1991;1:239–244.

Peiffer RL, Wilcock BP. Histopathological study of uveitis in cats: 139 cases (1978–1988). J Am Vet Med Assoc 1991;198:135–138.

Pentlarge VW. Eosinophilic conjunctivitis in five cats. J Am Anim Hosp Assoc 1991;27:21–28.

Prasse KW, Winston SM. Cytology and histopathology of feline eosinophilic keratitis. Vet Comp Ophthalmol 1996;6:74–81.

Ramsey DT, et al. Ophthalmic manifestations and complications of dental disease in dogs and cats. J Am Anim Hosp Assoc 1996;32:215–224.

Remillard RL, Pickett JP, Thatcher CD, Davenport LJ. Comparison of kittens fed queen's milk with those fed milk replacers. Am J Vet Res 1993;54:901–907.

Stiles J. Treatment of cats with ocular disease attributable to herpesvirus infection: 17 cases (1983–1993). J Am Vet Med Assoc 1995;207:599–603.

Stiles J, McDermott M, Willis M, Roberts W, Greene C. Comparison of nested polymerase chain reaction, virus isolation, and fluorescent antibody testing for identifying feline herpesvirus in cats with conjunctivitis. Am J Vet Res 1997;58:804–807.

Weigler BJ, Babinaeu CA, Sherry B, Nasisse M. A polymerase chain reaction for studies involving the epidemiology and pathogenesis of feline herpesvirus type 1. Vet Rec 1997;140:335–338.

Wilcock B, Peiffer RL, Davidson MG. The causes of glaucoma in cats. Vet Pathol 1990;27:35–40.

CHAPTER 13: Equine Ophthalmology

Andrew SE, Brooks DE, Smith PJ, Gelatt KN, Chmielewski NT, Whittaker C. Equine ulcerative keratomycosis: visual outcome and ocular survival in 39 cases (1987–1996). Eq Vet J 1998;30:109–116.

Ball MA, Rebhun WC, Gaarder JE, Patten V. Evaluation of itraconazole-dimethyl sulfoxide ointment for treatment of keratomycosis in nine horses. J Am Vet Med Assoc 1997;211:199–203.

Brooks DE. Ocular emergencies and trauma. In: Auer JA, ed. Equine surgery. Philadelphia: WB Saunders, 1992:666–672.

Brooks DE, et al. Histomorphometry of the optic nerves of normal horses and horses with glaucoma. Vet Comp Ophthalmol 1995;5:193–210.

Brooks DE, Andrew SE, Dillavou CL, Ellis G, Kubilis PS. Antifungal susceptibility patterns of fungi isolated from cases of ulcerative keratomycosis in Florida horses. Am J Vet Res 1998;59:138–142.

Chmielewski NT, et al. Visual outcome and ocular survival following iris prolapse in the horse: a review of 32 cases. Eq Vet J 1997;29:31–39.

Dugan SJ, Curtis CR, Roberts SM, Severin GA. Epidemiologic study of ocular/adnexal squamous cell carcinoma in horses. J Am Vet Med Assoc 1991;198: 251–256.

Dwyer AE, Crockett RS, Kalsow CM. Association of leptospiral seroreactivity and breed with uveitis and blindness in horses: 372 cases (1986–1993). J Am Vet Med Assoc 1995;207:1327–1331.

Dziezyc J, Millichamp NJ, Keller CB. Use of phacofragmentation for cataract removal in horses: 12 cases (1985–1989). J Am Vet Med Assoc 1991;198:1774–1778.

Gelatt KN. Congenital and acquired ophthalmic diseases in the foal. Anim Eye Res 1993;1–2:15–27.

Gilger BC, Davidson MG, Nadelstein B, Nasisse M. Neodymium:yttrium-aluminum-garnet laser treatment of cystic granula iridica in horses: eight cases (1988–1996). J Am Vet Med Assoc 1997;211:341–343.

Grahn B, Wolfer J, Keller C, Wilcock B. Equine keratomycosis: clinical and laboratory findings in 23 cases. Prog Vet Comp Ophthalmol 1993;3:2–7.

Hallenda RM, Grahn BH, Sorden SD, Collier LL. Congenital equine glaucoma: clinical and light microscopic findings in two cases. Vet Comp Ophthalmol 1997;7:105–116.

Hardy J, Robertson JT, Wilkie DA. Ischemic optic neuropathy and blindness after arterial occlusion for treatment of guttural pouch mycosis in two horses. J Am Vet Med Assoc 1990;196:1631–1634.

Hendrix DVH, et al. Corneal stromal abscesses in the horse: a review of 24 cases. Eq Vet J 1995;27:440–447.

Joyce JR, Martin JE, Storts RW, Skow L. Iridial hypoplasia (aniridia) accompanied by limbic dermoids and cataracts in a group of related quarterhorses. Eq Vet J Suppl 1990;2:26–28.

Kalsow CM, Dwyer AE, Smith AW, Nifong TP. Pinealitis accompanying equine recurrent uveitis. Br J Ophthalmol 1993;77:46–48.

Kellner SJ. Glaucoma in the horse (in German). Pferdeheilkunde 1994;10:107–113.

Kellner SJ. Glaucoma in the horse. Part 2 (in German). Pferdeheilkunde 1994;10: 261–266.

King TC, Priehs DR, Gum GG, Miller TR. Therapeutic management of ocular squamous cell carcinoma in the horse: 43 cases (1979–1989). Eq Vet J 1991;23: 449–452.

Lavach JD. The eyelids. In: Handbook of Equine Ophthalmology, Fort Collins: Gidding Studio Publishing, 1987:63–97.

Madigan JE, Kortz G, Murphy C, Rodger L. Photic headshaking in the horse: 7 cases. Eq Vet J 1995;27:306–311.

Matthews AG, Crispin SM, Parker J. The equine fundus. II: normal anatomical variants and colobomata. Eq Vet J Suppl 1990;10:50–54.

Mätz-Rensing, Drommer W, Kaup FJ, Gerhards H. Retinal detachment in horses. Eq Vet J 1996;28:111–116.

Miller TR, Brooks DE, Smith PJ, Sapienza JS. Equine glaucoma: clinical findings and response to treatment in 14 horses. Vet Comp Ophthalmol 1995;5:170–182.

Moore CP, Collins BK, Fales WH. Antibacterial susceptibility patterns for microbial isolates associated with infectious keratitis in horses: 63 cases (1986–1994). J Am Vet Med Assoc 1995;207:928–933.

Morgan RV, Daniel GB, Donnell RL. Magnetic resonance imaging of the normal eye and orbit of the horse. Prog Vet Comp Ophthalmol 1993;3:127–134.

Munroe G. Congenital ocular disease. In: Robinson NE, ed. Current therapy in equine medicine, 4th ed. Philadelphia: WB Saunders, 1997:355–359.

Rehhun WC. Retinal and optic nerve diseases. Vet Clin North Am 1992;8:587–608.

Roberts SM. Equine vision and optics. Vet Clin North Am Eq Pract 1992;8:451–457.

Schoster JV. The assembly and placement of ocular lavage systems in horses. Vet Med 1992;87:460–471.

Sweeney CR, Irby NL. Topical treatment of *Pseudomonas* sp.–infected corneal ulcers in horses: 70 cases (1977–1994). J Am Vet Med Assoc 1996;209:954–957.

Théon AP, Pascoe JR, Crlson GP, Krag DN. Intratumoral chemotherapy with cisplatin in oily emulsion in horses. J Am Vet Med Assoc 1993;202:261–267.

Werry H, Gerhards H. The surgical therapy of equine recurrent uveitis. Tierarztl Prax 1992;20:178–186.

Wheeler CA, Collier LL. Bilateral colobomas involving the optic discs in a quarterhorse. Eq Vet J Suppl 1990;10:39–41.

Whitley RD, Meek LA, Millichamp NJ, McRae EE, Priehs DR. Cataract surgery in the horse: a review of six cases. Eq Vet J Suppl 1990;10:85–90.

Whittaker CJG, et al. Therapeutic penetrating keratoplasty for deep corneal stromal abscesses in eight horses. Vet Comp Ophthalmol 1997;7:19–28.

Wilcock BP, Brooks DE, Latimer CA. Glaucoma in horses. Vet Pathol 1991;28:74–78.

CHAPTER 14: Food Animal Ophthalmology

Allen LJ, George LW, Willits NH. Effect of penicillin or penicillin and dexamethasone in cattle with infectious bovine keratoconjunctivitis. J Am Vet Med Assoc 1995;206:1200–1203.

Anderson DE, Badzioch M. Association between solar radiation and ocular squamous cell carcinoma in cattle. Am J Vet Res 1991;52:784–788.

Bailey CM, Hanks DR, Hanks MA. Circumocular pigmentation and incidence of ocular squamous cell tumors in *Bos taurus* and *Bos indicus* x *Bos taurus* cattle. J Am Vet Med Assoc 1990;196:1605–1608.

Brown MH, et al. Infectious bovine keratoconjunctivitis—a review. J Vet Intern Med 1996;12:259–266.

Dagnall GJ. The role of *Branhamella ovis*, *Mycoplasma conjunctivae* and *Chlamydia psittaci* in conjunctivitis of sheep. Br Vet J 1994;150:65–71.

Davidson HJ, Blanchard GL, Coe PH. Idiopathic uveitis in a herd of Holstein cows. Prog Vet Comp Ophthalmol 1992;2:113–116.

Den Otter W, et al. Ocular squamous cell carcinoma in Simmental cattle in Zimbabwe. Am J Vet Res 1995;56:1440–1441.

Distl O, Scheider A. An uncommon eye defect in Highland cattle: divergent unilateral strabismus. Dtsch Tierarztliche Wochenschr 1994;101:202–203.

Distl O, Wenninger A, Krausslich H. Inheritance of convergent strabismus with exophthalmos in cattle. Dtsch Tierarztliche Wochenschr 1991;98:354–356.

Hosie BD, Greig A. Role of oxytetracycline dihydrate in the treatment of mycoplasma associated ovine keratoconjunctivitis in lambs. Br Vet J 1995;151:83–88.

Kagonyera GM, George LM, Munn R. Light and electron microscopic changes in corneas of healthy and immunomodulated calves infected with *Moraxella bovis*. Am J Vet Res 1988;49:386–395.

Leipold HW. Congenital ocular defects in food producing animals. Vet Clin North Am Large Anim Pract 1984;6:577–595.

Lepper AW, et al. The protective efficacy of cloned *Moraxella bovis* pili in monovalent and multivalent vaccine formulations against experimentally induced infectious keratoconjunctivitis. Vet Microbiol 1995;45:129–138.

Lepper AW, et al. The protective efficacy of pili from different strains of *Moraxella bovis* within the same serogroup against infectious bovine keratoconjunctivitis. Vet Microbiol 1992;32:177–187.

Mertel L, et al. Clinical and pathologic study of a cow with chronic glaucoma. Vet Comp Ophthalmol 1996;6:18–26.

Moritomo Y, et al. Congenital anophthalmia with caudal vertebral anomalies in Japanese Brown Cattle. J Vet Med Sci 1995;57:693–696.

Odorfer G. Occurrence and frequency of eye diseases among cattle in Austria. Wien Tierarztliche Monatsschr 1995;82:170.

O'Toole D, et al. Selenium induced "blind staggers" and related myths. A commentary on the extent of historical livestock losses attributed to selenosis on Western U.S. rangelands. Vet Pathol 1996;33:104–116.

Ruehl WW, et al. Infection rates, disease frequency, pilin gene rearrangement, and pilin expression in calves innoculated with *Moraxella bovis* pilin–specific isogenic variants. Am J Vet Res 1993;54:248–253.

Ruehl WW, et al. Q-pili enhance the attachment of *Moraxella bovis* to bovine corneas in vitro. Mol Microbiol 1993;7:285–288.

Walker B, et al. Excision of neoplasms of the bovine lower eyelid by H-blepharoplasty. Vet Surg 1991;20:133–139.

Ward JL, Rebhun WC. Chronic frontal sinusitis in dairy cattle: 12 cases (1978–1989). J Am Vet Med Assoc 1992;201:326–328.

Wilsmore AJ, Dagnall GJ, Woodland RM. Experimental conjunctival infection of lambs with a strain of *Chlamydia psittaci* isolated from the eyes of a sheep naturally affected with keratoconjunctivitis. Vet Rec 1990;127:229–231.

CHAPTER 15: Exotic Animal Ophthalmology

Bauck L. Ophthalmic conditions in pet rabbits and rodents. Comp Cont Educ Pract Vet 1989;11:258–268.

Bellhorn R. Laboratory animal ophthalmology. In: Gelatt KN, ed. Veterinary ophthalmology. 2nd ed. Philadelphia: Lea & Febiger, 1991:656–679.

Besch-Williford DL. Biology and medicine of the ferret. Vet Clin North Am 1987;17: 1155–1183.

Brooks DE. Avian cataracts. In: Murphy CJ, Paul-Murphy J, eds. Seminars in avian and exotic pet medicine—ophthalmology. Philadelphia: WB Saunders, 1997:131–137.

Brooks DE, McCracken MD, Collins BR. Heterotopic bone formation in the ciliary body of an aged guinea pig. Lab Anim Sci 1991;40:88–90.

Burling K, Murphy CJ, Curiel JS, Koblick P, Bellhorn RW. Anatomy of the rabbit nasolacrimal duct and its clinical implications. Prog Vet Comp Ophthalmol 1991,1:33–40.

Buyukmihci NC, Murphy CJ, Schulz T. Developmental ocular disease of raptors. J Wildl Dis 1988;24:207.

Davidson MG. Ocular consequences of trauma in raptors. In: Murphy CJ, Paul-Murphy J, eds. Seminars in avian exotic pet medicine—ophthalmology. Philadelphia: WB Saunders, 1997:121–130.

Dupont C, Carrier M, Gauvin J. Bilateral precorneal membranous occlusion in a dwarf rabbit. J Small Exotic Anim Med 1995;3:41–44.

Fox JG, Pearson RC, Gorham JR. Viral and chlamydial diseases. In: Fox JG, ed. Biology and diseases of the ferret. Philadelphia: Lea & Febiger, 1988:217–234.

Harkness JE, Ridgway MD. Chromodacryorrhoea in laboratory rats (*Rattus norvegicus*): etiologic considerations. Lab Anim Sci 1980;30:841–844.

Kempster RC, et al. Ocular response of the koala (*Phascolarctos cinereus*) to infection with *Chlamydia psittaci*. Vet Comp Ophthalmol 1996;6:14–17.

Kern TJ. Rabbit and rodent ophthalmology. Semin Avian Exotic Pet Med 1997;6: 138–145.

Kern TJ, et al. Disorders of the third eyelid in birds: 17 cases. J Avian Med Surg 1996;10: 12–18.

Knepper PA, McLane DG, Goossens W, Van Der Hoek T, Higbee RG: Ultrastructural alterations in the aqueous outflow pathway of adult buphthalmic rabbits. Exp Eye Res 1991;52:523–533.

McCalla TL, et al. Lymphoma with orbital involvement in two ferrets. Vet Comp Ophthalmol 1997;7:36–38.

Meagher M, Quinn WJ, Stackhouse L. Chlamydial-caused infectious keratoconjunctivitis in bighorn sheep of Yellowstone National Park. J Wildl Dis 1992;28: 171–176.

Mikaelian I, Paillet I, Williams D. Comparative use of various mydriatic drugs in kestrels (*Falco tinnunculus*). Am J Vet Res 1994;55:270.

Miller PE. Ferret ophthalmology. Semin Avian Exotic Pet Med—Ophthalmology 1997;6:146–151.

Miller PE, Dubielzig RR. Autosomal dominant microphthalmia, cataract and retinal dysplasia in a laboratory colony of ferrets. Invest Ophthalmol Vis Sci (Abstract) 1995;36:S64.

Miller PE, Marlar AB, Dubiezig RR. Cataracts in a laboratory colony of ferrets. Lab Anim Sci 1993;43:562–568.

Millichamp NJ. Management of ocular disease in exotic species. In: Murphy CJ, Paul-Murphy J, eds. Seminars in avian and exotic pet medicine—ophthalmology. Philadelphia: WB Saunders, 1997:152–159.

Millichamp NJ, Jacobson ER, Dziezyc J. Conjunctivoralostomy for treatment of an occluded lacrimal duct in a blood python. J Am Vet Med Assoc 1986; 189:1136.

Moore CP, Dubielzig R, Glaza SM. Anterior corneal dystrophy of American Dutch belted rabbits: biomicroscopic and histopathological findings. Vet Pathol 1987; 24:28–33.

Murphy CJ, et al. Enucleation in birds of prey. J Am Vet Med Assoc 1983;183:1234.

Nielsen JN, Carlton WW. Colobomatous microphthalmos in a New Zealand White rabbit, arising from a colony with suspected vitamin E deficiency. Lab Anim Sci 1995;45:320–322.

Petersen-Jones SM, Carrington SD. Pasteurella dacryocystitis in rabbits. Vet Rec 1988;122:514–515.

Ramer JC, et al. Effects of mydriatic agents in cockatoos, African gray parrots, and Blue-fronted Amazon parrots. J Am Vet Med Assoc 1996;208:227.

Rubin LF. Ocular abnormalities in rats and mice: a survey of commonly occurring conditions. Anim Eye Res 1986;5:15–30.

Saunders LZ. Ophthalmic pathology in rats and mice. In: Cotchin E, Roe FJC, eds. Pathology of laboratory rats and mice. Oxford: Blackwell Scientific Publications, 1967:349–371.

Shibuya K, Tajima M, Yamate J. Spontaneously occurring corneal lesions in nine strains of mice. Anim Eye Res 1993;12:29–36.

Wilcock BP, Dukes TW. The eye. In: Ferguson HW, ed. Systemic pathology of fish. Ames, IA: Iowa State University Press, 1989:168.

Williams DL. Ophthalmology. In: Mader DR, ed. Reptile medicine and surgery. Philadelphia: WB Saunders, 1996:175–184.

Williams DL, Whitaker BR. The amphibian eye—a clinical review. J Zool Wildl Med 1994;25:18–28.

Wolfer J, Grahn B, Wilcock B, Percy D. Phacoclastic uveitis in the rabbit. Prog Vet Comp Ophthalmol 1993;3:92–97.

CHAPTER 16: Comparative Neuro-Ophthalmology

Barrett PM, Scagliotti RH, Merideth RE, Jackson PA, Alarcon FA. Absolute corneal sensitivity and corneal trigeminal nerve anatomy in normal dogs. Prog Vet Comp Ophthalmol 1991;1:245–254.

Collins BK, O'Brien D. Autonomic dysfunction of the eye. Semin Vet Med Surg Small Anim 1990;5:24–36.

DeLahunta A, Cummings JF. Neuro-ophthalmologic lesions as a cause visual deficits in dogs and horses. J Am Vet Med Assoc 1967;150:944–1011.

Fischer CA. Retinal and retinochoroidal lesions in early neuropathic canine distemper. J Am Vet Med Assoc 1971;158:740–752.

Green SL, Cochrane SM, Smith-Maxie L. Horner's syndrome in ten horses. Can Vet J 1992;33:330–333.

Hacker DV. "Crocodile tears" syndrome in a domestic cat: case report. J Am Anim Hosp Assoc 1990;26:245–246.

Kern TJ, Aromando MC, Erb HN. Horner's syndrome in dogs and cats: 100 cases (1975–1985). J Am Vet Med Assoc 1989;195:369–373.

Kern TJ, Erb HN. Facial neuropathy in dogs and cats: 95 cases (1975–1985). J Am Vet Med Assoc 1987;191:1604–1609.

Little CB, Hilbert BJ, McGill CA. A retrospective study of head fractures in 21 horses. Aust Vet J 1985;62:89–91.

Madigan JE, Kortz G, Murphy C, Rodger L. Photic headshaking in the horses: 7 cases. Eq Vet J 1995;27:306–311.

Martin CL, Kaswan R, Chapman W. Four cases of traumatic optic nerve blindness in the horse. Eq Vet J 1986;18:133–137.

Miller PE, Murphy CJ. Vision in dogs. J Am Vet Med Assoc 1995;207:1623–1634.

Palmer AC, Malinowski W, Barnett KC. Clinical signs including papilledema associated with brain tumors in twenty-one dogs. J Small Anim Pract 1974;15:359–386.

Parker AJ, Cusick PK, Park RD, Small E. Hemifacial spasms in a dog. Vet Rec 1973;93:514–516.

Roberts SR, Vainisi SJ. Hemifacial spasm in dogs. J Am Vet Med Assoc 1967; 150:381–385.

Simoens P, Lauwers H, DeMuelenare C, Muylle C, Steenhaut M. Horner's syndrome in the horse: a clinical, experimental and morphological study. Eq Vet J Suppl 1990;10:62–65.

Thibos LN, Levick WR, Morstyn R. Ocular pigmentation in white and Siamese cats. Invest Ophthalmol Vis Sci 1980;19:475–486.

CHAPTER 17: Ocular Manifestations of Systemic Diseases

The Dog

Appel MJ. Lyme disease in dogs and cats. Comp Cont Educ Pract Vet 1990;12: 617–664.

Blogg JR, Sykes JE. Sudden blindness associated with protothecosis in a dog. Aust Vet J 1995;72:147–149.

Brooks DE, Legendre AM, Gum GG, Laratta LJ, Abrams KL, Morgan RV. The treatment of canine ocular blastomycosis with systemically administered itraconazole. Prog Vet Comp Ophthalmol 1991;1:263–268.

Carastro SM, Dugan SJ, Paul AJ. Intraocular dirofilariasis in dogs. Comp Cont Educ Pract Vet 1992;14:209–212.

Collier LL, Collins KB. Excision and cryosurgical ablation of severe periocular papillomatosis in a dog. J Am Vet Med Assoc 1994;204:881–885.

Crispin SM. Ocular manifestations of hyperlipoproteinaemia. J Small Anim Pract 1993;34:500–506.

Davidson MG, et al. Acute blindness associated with intracranial tumors in dogs and cats: eight cases (1984–1989). J Am Vet Med Assoc 1991;199:755–758.

Davidson MG, Geoly F, Gilger BC, Whitley W, McLellan GL, Walker EJ. Vitamin E deficiency retinopathy in a group of North Carolina hunting dogs. Prog Sci Meet ACVO 1996;27:39–40.

Diehl KJ, Roberts SM. Keratoconjunctivitis sicca in dogs associated with sulfon-amide therapy: 16 cases (1980–1990). Prog Vet Comp Ophthalmol 1991;1:276–282.

Gelatt KN, Chrisman CL, Samuelson DA, Shell LG. Ocular and systemic aspergillo-sis in a dog. J Am Anim Hosp Assoc 1991;27:427–431.

Gilmour MA, Morgan RV, Moore FM. Masticatory myopathy in the dog: a retro-spective study of 18 cases. J Am Anim Hosp Assoc 1992;28:300–306.

Gratzek AT, Calvert CA, Martin CL, Kaswan RL. Corneal edema in dogs treated with tocainide. Prog Vet Comp Ophthalmol 1993;3:47–51.

Greibrokk T. Hereditary deafness in the dalmatian: relationship to eye and coat color. J Am Anim Hosp Assoc 1994;30:170–176.

Hendrix DVH, Gelatt KN, Smith PJ: Ophthalmic disease as the presenting complaint in five dogs with multiple myeloma. J Am Anim Hosp Assoc 1998;34:121–128.

Hopkins KD, Marcella KL, Strecker AE. Ivermectin toxicosis in a dog. J Am Vet Med Assoc 1990;197:93–94.

Huss BT, Collier LL, Collins BK, Pittman LL, Aronson E. Polyarthropathy and chorioretinitis with retinal detachment in a dog with systemic histoplasmosis. J Am Anim Hosp Assoc 1994;30:217–224.

Jacobs GJ, Medleau L, Brown J, Calvert C. Cryptococcal infection in cats: factors in-fluencing treatment outcome and results of sequential serum antigen titers in 35 cats. J Vet Intern Med 1997;11:1–4.

Jamieson VE, Davidson MG, Nasisse MP, English RV. Ocular complications follow-ing cobalt-60 radiotherapy of neoplasms in the canine head region. J Am Anim Hosp Assoc 1991;27:51–55.

Jolly RD, Palmer DN. The neuronal ceroid-lipofuscinoses (Batten disease): compar-ative aspects. Neuropathol Appl Neurobiol 1995;21:50–60.

Keller CB, Lamarre J. Inherited lysosomal storage disease in an English Springer Spaniel. J Am Vet Med Assoc 1992;200:194–195.

King MC, Grose RM, Startup G. Angiostrongylus vasorum in the anterior chamber of a dog's eye. J Small Animal Pract 1994;35:326–328.

Kontos VJ, Koutinas AF. Old world canine leishmaniasis. Comp Cont Edu Pract Vet 1993;15:949–960.

Krohne SG, Henderson NM, Richardson RC, Vestre WA. Prevalence of ocular in-volvement in dogs with multicentric lymphoma: prospective evaluation of 94 cases. Vet Comp Ophthalmol 1994;4:127–134.

Lester SJ, Kenyon JM. Use of allopurinol to treat visceral leishmaniosis in a dog. J Am Vet Med Assoc 1996;209:615–617.

Martin CL. Glaskorper und Augenhintergrund. In: Augenkrankheiten bei Hund und Katze. Hannover, Germany: M & H Schaper, 1995:333–402.

Mattson A, Roberts SM. Clinical features suggesting hyperadrenocorticisim associ-ated with sudden acquired retinal degeneration syndrome in a dog. J Am Anim Hosp Assoc 1992;28:199–202.

Nell B, Angerer M, Walde I. Fetthaltiges Kammerwasser und Uveitis als Okulare Manifestation einer Hyperlipidamie Infolge Primarer Hypothyreose bei Einem Hund. Wien Tierarztl Mschr 1995;82:122–129.

Perry AW, Hertling R, Kennedy MJ. Angiostrongylosis with disseminated larval infection associated with signs of ocular and nervous disease in an imported dog. Can Vet J 1991;32:430–431.

Rudmann DG, Coolman BR, Perez CM, Glickman LT. Evaluation of risk factors for blastomycosis in dogs: 857 cases (1980–1990). J Am Vet Med Assoc 1992:201: 1754–1759.

Sansom J, Barnett KC, Blunden AS, Smith KC, Turner S, Waters L. Canine conjunctival papilloma: a review of five cases. J Small Anim Pract 1996;37:84–86.

Smith RI, Sutton RH, Jolly RD, Smith KR. A retinal degeneration associated with ceroid-lipofuscinosis in adult Miniature Schnauzers. Vet Comp Ophthalmol 1996;6: 187–191.

Swanson JF. Ocular manifestations of systemic disease in the dog and cat. Vet Clin North Am Small Anim Pract 1990;20:849–867.

Theisen SK, Podell M, Schneider T, Wilkie DA, Fenner WR. A retrospective study of cavernous sinus syndrome in 4 dogs and 8 cats. J Vet Intern Med 1996;10:65–71.

Thomas W, Sorjonen D, Steiss J. A retrospective evaluation of 38 cases of canine distemper encephalomyelitis. J Am Anim Hosp Assoc 1993;29:129–133.

Van der Woerdt A, Nasisse MP, Davidson MG. Sudden acquired retinal degeneration in the dog: clinical and laboratory findings in 36 cases. Prog Vet Comp Ophthalmol 1991;1:11–18.

The Cat

Alroy J, et al. Clinical, neurophysiological, biochemical and morphological features of eyes in Persian cats with mannosidosis. Virchows Arch B Cell Pathol Incl Mol Pathol 1991;60:173–180.

Breider MA, et al. Blastomycosis in cats: five cases (1979–1986). J Am Vet Med Assoc 1988;193:570–572.

Brightman AH, Ogilvie GK, Tompkins M. Ocular disease in FeLV-positive cats: 11 cases (1981–1986). J Am Vet Med Assoc 1991;198:1049–1051.

Chavkin MJ, et al. Seroepidemilogic and clinical observations of 93 cases of uveitis in cats. Prog Vet Comp Ophthalmol 1992;2:29–36.

Collins BK, Nasisse MP, Moore CP. In vitro efficacy of L-lysine against feline herpesvirus type-1. Proc Am Coll Vet Ophthalmol (Abstract) 1995;26:141.

Davidson MG, et al. Acute blindness associated with intracranial tumors in dogs and cats: eight cases (1984–1989). J Am Vet Med Assoc 1991;199:755–758.

Davidson MG, et al. Feline anterior uveitis: a study of 53 cases. J Am Anim Hosp Assoc 1991;27:77–83.

Davidson MG, English RV, Tompkins MB. Feline immunodeficiency virus predisposes cats to acute generalized toxoplasmosis. Am J Pathol 1993;143:1486–1497.

English RV, et al. Intraocular disease associated with feline immunodeficiency virus infection in cats. J Am Vet Med Assoc 1990;196:1116–1119.

Forrester SD, Greco DS, Relford RL. Serum hyperviscosity syndrome associated with multiple myeloma in two cats. J Am Vet Med Assoc 1992;200:79–82.

Greek JS. Feline pemphigus foliaceous: a retrospective study of 23 cases. Proc Am Acad Vet Dermatol 1993;9:27–28.

Gunn-Moore DA, et al. Prevalence of *Chlamydia psittaci* antibodies in healthy pet cats in Britain. Vet Rec 1995;136:366–367.

Gwin RM, et al. Ophthalmomyiasis interna posterior in two cats and a dog. J Am Anim Hosp Assoc 1984;20:481–486.

Haesebrouck F, et al. Incidence and significance of isolation of *Mycoplasma felis* from conjunctival swabs of cats. Vet Microbiol 1991;26:95–101.

Helton KA, Nesbitt GH, Caciolo PL. Griseofulvin toxicity in cats: literature review and a report of seven cases. J Am Anim Hosp Assoc 1986;22:453–458.

Henik RA, Snyder PS, Volk LM. Treatment of systemic hypertension in cats with amlodipine besylate. J Am Anim Hosp Assoc 1997;33:226–334.

Hill SL, Lappin MR, Carman J, et al. Comparison of methods for estimation of *Toxoplasma gondii*–specific antibody production in the aqueous humor of cats. Am J Vet Res 1995;56:1181–1187.

Holland CT. Horner's syndrome and ipsilateral laryngeal hemiplegia in three cats. J Small Anim Pract 1996;37:442–446.

Huss BT, et al. Fatal cerebral coenurosis in a cat. J Am Vet Med Assoc 1994; 205:69–71.

Lappin MR, et al. Detection of *Toxoplasma gondii*–specific IgA in the aqueous humor of cats. Am J Vet Res 1995;56:774–778.

Lappin MR, et al. Serologic prevalence of selected infectious diseases in cats with uveitis. J Am Vet Med Assoc 1992;201:1005–1009.

Leon A, Levick WR, Sarossy MG. Lesion topography and new histological features in feline taurine deficiency retinopathy. Exp Eye Res 1995;61:731–741.

Lewis DT, Foil CS, Hosgood G. Epidemiology and clinical features of dermatophytosis in dogs and cats at Louisiana State University: 1981–1990. Vet Dermatol 1991;2:53–58.

Medleau L, Greene CE, Rakich PM. Evaluation of ketoconazole and itraconazole for treatment of disseminated cryptococcosis in cats. Am J Vet Res 1990;51:1454–1458.

Muir P, et al. A clinical and microbiological study of cats with protruding nictitating membranes and diarrhoea: isolation of a novel virus. Vet Rec 1990;127:324–330.

Nasisse MP, et al. Immunologic, histologic, and virologic features of herpesvirus-induced stromal keratitis in cats. Am J Vet Res 1995;56:51–55.

Sansom J, et al. Ocular disease associated with hypertension in 16 cats. J Small Anim Pract 1994;35:604–611.

Shell LG. Feline ischemic encephalopathy (cerebral infarct). Fel Pract 1996;24:32–33.

Stiles J, et al. Comparison of nested polymerase chain reaction, virus isolation and fluorescent antibody testing for identifying feline herpesvirus in cats with conjunctivitis. Am J Vet Res 1997;58:804–807.

Stiles J, et al. Use of nested polymerase chain reaction to identify feline herpesvirus in ocular tissue from clinically normal cats and cats with corneal sequestra or conjunctivitis. Am J Vet Res 1997;58:338–342.

Stiles J, Polzin DJ, Bistner SI. The prevalence of retinopathy in cats with systemic hypertension and chronic renal failure or hyperthyroidism. J Am Anim Hosp Assoc 1994;30:564–572.

Stiles J, Prade R, Greene C. Detection of *Toxoplasma gondii* in feline and canine biological samples by use of the polymerase chain reaction. Am J Vet Res 1996;57: 264–267.

Symonds HW, et al. A cluster of cases of feline dysautonomia (Key-Gaskell syndrome) in a closed colony of cats. Vet Rec 1995;136:353–355.

The Horse

Alexander CS, Keller H. Etiology and occurrence of periodic eye inflammation of horses in the area of Berlin. Tierarztl Prax 1990;18:623 627.

Collinson PN, et al. Isolation of equine herpesvirus type 2 (equine gammaherpesvirus 2) from foals with keratoconjunctivitis. J Am Vet Med Assoc 1994;205: 329–331.

Dwyer AE, Crockett RS, Kalsow CM. Association of leptospiral seroreactivity and breed with uveitis and blindness in horses: 372 cases (1986–1993). J Am Vet Med Assoc 1995;207:1327–1331.

Fenger CK, et al. Epizootic of equine protozoal myeloencephalitis on a farm. J Am Vet Med Assoc 1997;210:923–927.

Glaze MB, et al. A case of equine adnexal lymphosarcoma. Eq Vet J Suppl 1990; 10:83–84.

Green SL, Cochrane SM, Smith-Maxie L. Horner's syndrome in ten horses. Can Vet J 1992;33:330–333.

Hardy J, Robertson JT, Wilkie DA. Ischemic optic neuropathy and blindness after arterial occlusion for treatment of guttural pouch mycosis in two horses. J Am Vet Med Assoc 1990;196:1631–1634.

Matz K, et al. Bilateral blindness after injury in a riding horse. Tierarztl Prax 1993; 21:225–232.

Parker JL, White KK. Lyme borreliosis in cattle and horses: a review of the literature. Cornell Vet 1992;82:253–274.

Rebhun WC, Del Piero F. Ocular lesions in horses with lymphosarcoma: 21 cases (1977–1997). J Am Vet Med Assoc 1998;212:852–854.

Reppas GP, et al. Trauma-induced blindness in two horses. Aust Vet J 1995;72: 270–272.

Shanks G, et al. An outbreak of acute leukoencephalomalacia associated with fumonsin intoxication in three horses. Aust Eq Vet 1995;13:17–18.

Simoens P, et al. Horner's syndrome in the horse: a clinical, experimental and morphological study. Eq Vet J Suppl 1990;10:62–65.

Timoney JF. Strangles. Vet Clin North Am Eq Pract 1993;9:365–374.

Timoney PJ, McCollum WH. The epidemiology of equine viral arteritis. Vet Clin North Am Eq Pract 1993;9:295–309.

Wilson WD. Equine influenza. Vet Clin North Am Eq Pract 1993;9:257–282.

Food Animals

Rakich PM, Latimer KS, Mispagel ME, Steffens WL. Clinical and histologic characterization of cutaneous reactions to stings of the imported fire ant (*Solenopsis invicta*) in dogs. Vet Pathol 1993;30:555–559.

Van der Lugt JJ, Olivier J, Jordaan P. Status spongiosis, optic neuropathy, and retinal degeneration in Helichrysum argyrosphaerum poisoning in sheep and a goat. Vet Pathol 1996;33:495–502.

Appendices

APPENDIX A

ADRENERGICS

Adrenergics:
 Topical: Causes conjunctival vasoconstriction; lowers IOP a few mm Hg; additive effects with the parasympatholytic mydriatics. Used in Horner's syndrome to determine the site of sympathetic denervation. Occasionally causes irritation.

  Epinephrine (1–2%), 1 to 2 times daily.
  Dipivalyl epinephrine (0.1%), 1 to 2 times daily.

 Systemic (IV):
  1:1,000 to 1:10,000 in irrigating solution (usually lactated Ringer's solution) during anterior segment surgery for mydriasis and to assist in blood clotting. Use caution with halothane anesthesia.

β-Blockers (β-antagonists): Lowers IOP in cats and dogs by several mm Hg and is usually combined with other topical antiglaucoma drugs to decrease IOP to normal levels. Timolol in cats produces miosis. Generally instilled 2 to 3 times daily. Use caution in very small dogs and cats with cardiovascular and pulmonary diseases.

  Timolol (0.25–0.5%), β_1- and β_2-receptor antagonist.
  Betaxolol (0.5%), β_1-receptor antagonist.
  Levobunolol (0.5%), β_1- and β_2-receptor antagonist.
  Metipranolol (0.6%), nonselective β-antagonist.

α-Agonists:
  Apraclonidne (0.5%), α_2-agonist. In dogs, causes mydriasis, variable decline in IOP, and variable decrease in heart rate. In cats, causes miosis, vomiting, decreased IOP and decreased heart rate, and is not recommended for clinical use.

IOP, intraocular pressure.

APPENDIX B

ARTIFICIAL TEAR SUBSTITUTES

Product	Viscosity Agents/ Concentration(s)[a]	Preservative	Source
Polyvinyl alcohol solutions			
AKWA Tears	PVA 1.40%	BAC, EDTA	Akorn
Artificial Tears	PVA 1.40%	BAC, EDTA	Generic (many)
Dry Eyes	PVA 1.40%	BAC, EDTA	Bausch & Lomb
Liquifilm Forte	PVA 3%	Thimerosal, EDTA	Allergan
Liquifilm Tears	PVA 1.40%	Chlorobutanol	Allergan
Ocu-tears PF	PVA 0.10%	None	Ocumed
Cellulose-based solutions			
Cellufresh	CMC 0.50%	None	Allergan
Celluvlsc	CMC 1%	None	Allergan
Comfort Tears	HEC	BAC, EDTA	Barnes-Hinds
Isopto Alkaline	HPMC 1%	BAC, EDTA	Alcon
Isopto Tears Plain	HPMC 0.50%	BAC, EDTA	Alcon
Murocel	MC 1%	Methylparaben, propylparaben	Bausch & Lomb
Refresh plus	CMC 0.50%	None	Allergan
TearGard	HPMC 0.50%	Sorbic acid, EDTA	Med Tech
Tearisol	HPMC 0.50%	BAC, EDTA	Iolab
Polymer combinations			
Adsorbotear	HEC 0.40%, povidone 1.67%, adsorbobase	Thimerosal, EDTA	Alcon
Aqua Site	PEG-400 0.20%, DEX 0.10%	EDTA	Ciba
Bion Tears	DEX 0.10%, HPMC 0.30%	None	Alcon
Hypotears	PVA 1%, HEC, DEX	BAC, EDTA	Iolab
Hypotears PF	PVA 1%, HEC, DEX 3.30%	EDTA	Iolab
Lacril	HPMC 0.50%, GEL 0.01%, PSB	Chlorobutanol	Allergan
Lubrifair Solution	DEX-70, HPMC	None	Pharmafair
Lubri Tears	HPMC 0.50%, DEX 0.10%	BAC, EDTA	Bausch & Lomb
Murine Eye Lubricant	PVA 1.40%, Povidone 0.60%	BAC, EDTA	Ross
Moisture Drops	HPMC 0.50%, DEX 0.10%, povidone 0.10%, glycerin 0.20%	BAC, EDTA	Bausch & Lomb
Nature's Tears	HPMC 0.40%, DEX	BAC, EDTA	Rugby

Product	Viscosity Agents/ Concentration(s)[a]	Preservative	Source
Polymer combinations—cont'd			
Refresh	PVA 1.40%, povidone 0.60%	None	Allergan
Tears Naturale	HPMC 0.30%, DEX 0.10%	BAC, EDTA	Alcon
Tears Naturale II	HPMC 0.30%, DEX-70 0.10%	POLYQUAD, EDTA	Alcon
Tears Naturale Free	HPMC 0.30%, DEX 0.10%	None	Alcon
Tears Plus	PVA 1.40%, povidone 0.60%	Chlorobutanol	Allergan
Tears Renewed	HPMC 0.30%, DEX-70 0.10%	BAC, EDTA	Akorn
Vasoclastic products			
Hylashield	Hylan 0.15%	None	I-Med
Hylashield Nite	Hylan 0.40%	None	I-Med
Glycerin products			
Dry Eye Therapy	Glycerin 0.30%	None	Bausch & Lomb
Eye-Lube-A	Glycerin 0.25%	BAC, EDTA	Optoptics
Ointments			
AKWA Tears Ointment	White petrolatum, MO	None	Akorn
Dry Eyes	White petrolatum, MO	None	Bausch & Lomb
Duolube	White petrolatum 80%, MO 20%	None	Bausch & Lomb
Duratears Naturale	White petrolatum, lanolin, MO	None	Alcon
Hypo Tears	White petrolatum 85%, lanolin, MO 15%	None	Iolab
Lacri-Lube	White petrolatum 55%, lanolin, MO 41.50%	Chlorobutanol	Allergan
Lacri-Lube NP	White petrolatum 55%, lanolin, MO 42.50%	None	Allergan
Lacri-Lube S.O.P.	White petrolatum 55%, MO 41.50%, 2% nonionic lanolin derivatives	Chlorobutanol	Allergan
Lipotears	White petrolatum, MO	None	Coopervision
Lubri Tears	White petrolatum, lanolin, MO	Chlorobutanol	Bausch & Lomb
Ocutube	White petrolatum	Methylparaben	Ocumed
Paralube	White petrolatum, lanolin 2%, MO	None	Fourgera

Product	Viscosity Agents/ Concentration(s)[a]	Preservative	Source
Ointments—cont'd			
Refresh PM	White petrolatum 56.80%, lanolin, MO 41.50%	None	Allergan

BAC, benzalkonium chloride; *CMC*, carboxymethyl cellulose; *DEX*, dextran; *EDTA*, ethylenediaminetetraacetic acid; *GEL*, gelatin; *HEC*, hydroxyethyl cellulose; *HPMC*, hydroxypropyl methylcellulose; *MC*, methylcellulose; *MO*, mineral oil; *PEG*, polyethylene glycol; *POLYQUAD*, polyquaternium-1; *PSB*, polysorbate 80; *PVA*, polyvinyl alcohol.

[a]Percentage compositions are given when available.

TOPICAL AND LOCAL ANESTHETICS

Topical:

Administer 1 to 2 drops per eye. Repeat instillations are not recommended.

Produce surface anesthesia of the conjunctiva and cornea within 10–20 seconds and for a duration of 15–20 minutes. Multiple drops may increase duration but not depth within the eye tissues. Less effective in inflamed eyes, probably because of edema.

May cause local irritation, corneal epithelial toxicity, and reduce tear production by as much as 50%. Generally avoid before bacterial culturing of the cornea and conjunctiva. Use only for diagnostics.

Tetracaine (0.5%) is more irritating (usually conjunctival hyperemia) than proparacaine (0.5%).

Local/injectable:

Used for auricuopalpebral (1 mL [small animals] to 5 mL [horse and cow]) and retrobulbar nerve blocks (20–30 mL for horse and cow).

Addition of 1:200,000 epinephrine prolongs the anesthetic's action. Addition of hyaluronidase (15000 IU/100 mL) increases local tissue infiltration by the local anesthetic.

Lidocaine. Mepivacaine. Bupivacaine (longer acting).

APPENDIX D

ANTIBIOTICS

Frequently Used Topical Antibiotics

Chloramphenicol (avoid in food animals)
Fusidic acid
Gentamycin
Neomycin-Polymyxin B-Gramicidin combinations
Neomycin-Polymyxin B-Bacitracin
Terramycin (often used in cats for *Chlamydia* sp. and *Mycoplasma* sp.)
Tobramycin

Availability may vary by country.

Administered 2–12 times daily depending on the ophthalmic disease.

Selection on Initial Antibiotics by Smear Morphology

Gram Stain	Suggested Antibiotics
G$^+$ cocci	Topical 5% cefazolin, 5% vancomycin, or 0.3% ciprofloxacin. Subconjunctival cefazolin or cephaloridine (100 mg).
G$^+$ rods	Topical 1.4% gentamicin or 1.4% tobramycin. Subconjunctival gentamicin (20–40 mg).
G$^-$ cocci	Topical penicillin G (100,000 U/mL) or 0.3% ciprofloxacin.
G$^-$ rods	Topical 1.4% gentamicin, 1.4% tobramycin, 0.3% ciprofloxacin, or 0.4% carbenicillin. Subconjunctival gentamicin or tobramycin (20–40 mg).

Concentrated or Fortified Antibiotics for Topical Ophthalmic Use

	Concentration		
Antibiotic[a]	Commercial Eye Solutions	Formulated Eye Solutions	Shelf Life
Amikacin	N/A[b]	10 mg/mL	30 days
Carbenicillin	N/A	4–8 mg/mL	3 days
Cefazolin	N/A	50 mg/mL	4 days
Gentamicin	3 mg/mL	14 mg/mL	30 days
Penicillin G	N/A	100,000 U/mL	4 days
Tobramycin	3 mg/mL	14 mg/mL	30 days
Vancomycin	N/A	50 mg/mL	4 days

[a]Used primarily for infected corneal ulcerations.

[b]Drug not available in an ophthalmic formulation.

Suggested Dosages of Subconjunctival Antibiotics

Antibiotic	Dosage (mg)
Amikacin	25–125
Ampicillin	50–100
Carbenicillin	100
Cephaloridine	100
Cephalotin	100
Cefazolin	100
Gentamicin	20–40
Lincomycin	50–150
Tobramycin	20–40
Vancomycin	25

Inject only once or twice into the dorsal bulbar subconjunctival tissues. Limit volume of the injection to 0.25–0.5 ml/site.

APPENDIX E

ANTIVIRALS

Drug[a]	Trade Name (Manufacturer)	Vehicle	Mechanism of Action	Recommended Dosage
Topical Drugs:				
Idoxuridine (0.1%)	Stoxil (Smith, Kline & French)	Ointment	Competes with thymidine for incorporation into viral DNA, producing a defective genome	Ointment, 5 times daily
	Herplex (Allergan)	Solution		Every 2 hours
Adenine arabinoside (3.0%)	Vira-A (Parke-Davis)	Ointment	Inhibits viral DNA polymerase	5 times daily
Trifluorothymidine (1.0%)	Viroptic (Burroughs Wellcome Co) Trifluridine (Schein)	Solution	Competes for incorporation into viral DNA to inhibit viral mRNA	Hourly the first day, then reducing to 5 times daily
Systemic Drugs:				
Acyclovir	Zovirax (Glaxo Wellcome)	Capsules (200/400 mg)	Interferes with viral DNA polymerase and inhibits replication	200 mg orally 2–3 times daily for 14 days. Watch for toxic effects

[a]Drug availability may vary by country.

ANTIFUNGALS

Agent	Dose	Spectrum (sp.)
Topical:[a]		
Natamycin	Topical: 5% suspension	*Fusarium* *Candida* *Aspergillus* *Cephalosporium* *Penicillium*
Miconazole	Topical: 1% (IV) solution Subconjunctival injection, 5–10 mg	*Candida* *Aspergillus* *Fusarium* *Mucor* *Penicillium*
Nystatin	Topical: ointment (100,000 mg)	*Aspergillus* *Candida*
Ketaconazole	Topical: 2% solution	*Candida*
Amphotericin B	Topical: 2.5–10.0 mg/mL in 5% dextrose solution Subconjunctival: 750 mg/mL in dextrose every other day	*Candida* *Blastomyces* *Coccidioides* *Histoplasma*
Flucytosine	Topical: 1% solution	*Candida* *Cryptococcus*

Systemic:

Horse
Generally administered for 4–6 weeks and very expensive.
Ketoconazole, 30 mg/kg orally once or twice a day.
Fluconazole, 4 mg/kg orally once a day.
Thiabendazole, 44 mg/kg orally once a day.
Itraconazole, 3 mg/kg orally twice a day.

Dog
Generally administered for several months; recurrences are not infrequent.
Amphotericin B, 0.5–1.0 mg/kg IV every 48 hours for a cumulative dose of
4–6 mg/kg.
Ketaconazole, 10–20 mg/kg every 24 hours for 60–90 days.

[a]Topical antifungals agents generally are fungiostatic and administered 6–8 times daily for several weeks.

APPENDIX G

CARBONIC ANHYDRASE INHIBITORS

Recommended Dosage (mg/kg)[a]	*Effects on Intraocular Pressure (hours)*			
	Mean Onset	*Maximum*	*Decrease*	*Duration*
Systemic (single-dose studies)[b]				
Acetazolamide 10	1	7	19	8+
Dichlophenamide				
5	1	8	15	8+
10	1	3	24	8
Ethoxzolamide				
5	1	5	17	8
7.5	1	2	20	8+
Methazolamide				
5	1	6	28	8+
7.5	1	7	29	8+
Topical (2–3 times daily)[c]				
Dorzolamide (2%)				
Brinzolamide (1%)				

[a]Recommended clinical doses for the dog: acetazolamide, 10 mg/kg 2–3 times daily; dichlorphenamide, 2–5 mg/kg 2–3 times daily; methazolamide, 2.5–5 mg/kg 2–3 times daily; ethoxzolamide, 4.0–7.5 mg/kg 2–3 times daily.

[b]Cats seem not to tolerate the long-term systemic carbonic anhydrase inhibitors. In the cat, dichlorphenamide (0.5–2.0 mg/kg) reduces intraocular pressure for 4+ hours and acetazolamide (10–25 mg/kg) for 5+ hours.

[c]In the dog and cat, topical carbonic anhydrase inhibitors are administered 2–3 times daily. Controlled studies are limited, but three administrations daily seem to be most effective.

CORTICOSTEROIDS

Topical Corticosteroids

Eyelid/nasolacrimal/conjunctival diseases: 2.5% hydrocortisone and 0.25–0.5% prednisolone recommended. Use often as antibiotic/corticosteroid combinations. Administer 2–4 times daily.

Cornea/iris/ciliary body diseases: Stronger steroids and those with good corneal penetration generally are recommended: 1% prednisolone, 0.1% dexamethasone, and 0.1% betamethasone. Administer 4–6 times daily.

Retina/choroid/optic nerve diseases: Systemic route most important. Prednisolone is usually used:

Dog: 0.5–1.0 mg/kg orally once daily (anti-inflammatory dose), 2.2 mg/kg orally once daily (immunosuppressant).

Cat: 0.5–2.0 mg/kg orally once daily (anti-inflammatory), 2.2–6.6 mg/kg orally once daily (immunosuppressant).

Horse: 0.5–1.0 mg/kg orally or IM once daily.

Depot Glucocorticoids for Subconjunctival Administration

Drug[a]	Dosage (mg/eye)			
	Cats	Small & Medium Dogs	Large Dogs	Horses
Methylprednisolone acetate	4	4–8	8–12	40
Triamcinolone acetonide	4	4–8	8–12	40
Betamethasone sodium phosphate plus acetate	0.75	0.75–1.5	2	15
Dexamethasone acetate	0.75	0.75–1.5	2	15

[a]Generally used for severe or refractory anterior uveitis, anterior episcleritis, and scleritis. Only one injection is recommended, either weekly or biweekly.

APPENDIX I

NONSTEROIDAL ANTI-INFLAMMATORY DRUGS

Route/Agent	Indications/Use
Topical:	
0.03% Flurbiprofen	To prevent synthesis of prostaglandins and
0.1% Diclofenac	breakdown of the blood-aqueous barrier. To pre-
1.0% Indomethacin	vent and maintain miosis after anterior chamber
0.5% Ketorolacromethamine	entry during paracentesis and intraocular surgery.
1.0% Suprofen	Can slow or prevent corneal vascularization.
Systemic:	
Flunixin megumine	Dog only: 0.2 mg/kg IV immediately before cataract surgery.
	Horse: 0.25–1.0 mg/kg orally twice a day.
Carprofen	Dog only: 0.5 mg/kg orally twice a day.
Phenylbutazone	Horse only: 1 g IV or orally twice a day.
Aspirin	Horse only: 25 mg/kg orally twice a day.

APPENDIX J

HYPEROSMOTICS

Topical: To decrease corneal edema temporarily; often irritating. Usually administered 2–4 times daily or to effect.

2–5% NaCl ointment
2–5% NaCl solution
40% Glucose solution
100% Anhydrous glycerin ointment

Systemic: To lower intraocular pressure and reduce the size of the vitreous body.[a] Usually administered only once or twice.

Mannitol: 1–2 g/kg IV over 10–20 minutes. In the dog, the intraocular pressure begins to decrease 0.5 hours after administration and lasts for at least 5.5 hours. Considerable diuresis may result. Use caution or avoid in older patients with cardiovascular diseases.

Glycerin: 1–2 g/kg PO. In the dog, the intraocular pressure begins to decline 1.0 hours after ingestion and remains low for 10 hours. Frequently vomiting after administration (solution's taste, temperature, and dose are important). Avoid use in diabetic patients, because it will increase blood glucose levels. Limited diuresis.

[a]Less effect on intraocular pressure and vitreous body with osmotic agents in inflamed eyes because of the altered blood-aqueous barrier.

APPENDIX K

MIOTICS

Miotic[a]	Miosis			Intraocular Pressure		
	Time of Onset	Duration	Minimum Pupil Size	Time of Onset	Duration	Mean Decrease[c]
Dog						
Pilocarpine solution 1%[b]	45 minutes	>6 hours	1.5 mm	3 hours	>6 hours	5–10 mm Hg
Pilocarpine solution 2%[b]	30 minutes	>6 hours	1.0 mm	1 hour	>6 hours	5–15 mm Hg
Pilocarpine solution 4%[b]	30 minutes	>6 hours	1.0 mm	45 minutes	>6 hours	5–15 mm Hg
Pilocarpine gel 4%	30 minutes	16 hours	2.0–5.0 mm	1 hour	24 hours	4–8 mm Hg
Pilocarpine 2% & epinephrine 1%	1 hour	>8 hours	2.0 mm	1 hour	>8 hours	18–22 mm Hg
Pilocarpine 4% & epinephrine 1%	45 minutes	>8 hours	1.5 mm	1 hour	>8 hours	18–22 mm Hg
Carbachol solution 1.5%	15 minutes	>8 hours	1.5 mm	45 minutes	>8 hours	2–4 mm Hg
Carbachol solution 3%	15 minutes	>8 hours	1.0–1.5 mm	15 minutes	>8 hours	5–7 mm Hg
Demecarium bromide 0.125%	1 hour	49–55 hours	0.5 mm	1 hour	49–51 hours	9–13 mm Hg
Demecarium bromide 0.25%	1 hour	53–77 hours	0.5 mm	1 hour	55 hours	10–20 mm Hg
Echothiophate iodide 0.125%	1 hour	49–51 hours	0.5 mm	1 hour	25–49 hours	10–13 mm Hg
Echothiophate iodide 0.25%	1 hour	53–55 hours	0.5 mm	1 hour	51–53 hours	10–13 mm Hg
Cats						
Pilocarpine solution 2%	30 minutes	>12 hours	4.5 mm	2 hours	>12 hours	2–3 mm Hg

[a]Availability of these drugs may vary by country. Clinical dose of these drugs also may vary and is based on the extent to which the intraocular pressure is lowered, but for topical pilocarpine and carbachol, it is usually 2–3 times daily and for demecarium and echothiophate usually 1–2 times daily.

[b]Causes irritation (i.e., conjunctival hyperemia, blepharospasm, tearing, mild aqueous flare) that appears related to the pH of the commercial solutions.

[c]Mean intraocular pressure decreases in glaucomatous dogs.

APPENDIX L

MYDRIATICS

The Dog

Drug[a]	Time to Maximum Dilation (hours)	Duration (hours)	Extent of Dilation
Parasympatholytics:			
1% Atropine[b]	1.0	96–120	Maximal
4% Atropine[b]	0.75	96–120	Maximal
0.25% Scopolamine[c]	0.75	96–120	Maximal
1% Cyclopentolate	0.75	60	Maximal
1% Tropicamide[d]	0.5	12	Maximal
2% Homatropine	0.75	48	Moderate
5% Homatropine	0.75	48	Moderate
Sympathomimetics:			
10% Phenylephrine[e]	2.0	12–18	Maximal
0.1% Epinephrine	—	—	None
1% Epinephrine	1.0	9	Maximal
2% Epinephrine	0.75	6	Moderate

[a]Generally administered 2–4 times daily, but are best used to effect (onset and duration of mydriasis) to reduce the possibility of adverse effects.

[b]Because of its bitter taste, topical atropine may induce salivation in puppies and smaller adult dogs (usually occurs very soon after administration). Topical atropine also may reduce the rate of tear formation by 50% in normal dogs and can induce temporary keratoconjunctivitis sicca in dogs with marginal tear production. Hence, measurement of tear formation by the Schirmer tear test during topical atropine therapy is recommended. A substitute drug is 1% tropicamide.

[c]Scopolamine (0.25%) combined with 10% phenylephrine is a very strong mydriatic combination and is used to breakdown recent (usually < 1 week of duration) posterior synechiae.

[d]Tropicamide (1%) is the recommended mydriatic for the routine eye examination because of its rapid onset and short duration of mydriasis. Its bitter taste can cause occasionally salivation in puppies. Incomplete or slow onset of mydriasis after 1% tropicamide often suggests anterior uveitis or iridocyclitis.

[e]Phenylephrine (10%) is a very weak mydriatic in the dog, but it is additive in promoting mydriasis with many other parasympatholytic mydriatics in inflamed eyes. The 2.5% solution also is used in the determination of sympathetic denervation in Horner's syndrome.

The Cat

Drug[a]	Time to Maximum Dilation (hours)	Duration (hours)	Extent of Dilation
Parasympatholytics:			
1% Atropine[b]	1.0	60	Maximal
4% Atropine	0.5	144	Maximal
1% Cyclopentolate	0.5	66	Maximal
2% Cyclopentolate	0.5	108	Maximal
0.5% Tropicamide	0.75	8–9	Maximal
1% Tropicamide[c]	0.75	8–9	Maximal
2% Homatropine	0.75	7	Moderate
Sympathomimetics:			
10% Phenylephrine[d]	—	—	None
2% Epinephrine[d]	—	—	None
Parasympatholytic/sympathomimetic combinations:			
1% Atropine/10% phenylephrine	1.0	120	Maximal
1% Cyclopentolate/10% phenylephrine	0.5	108	Maximal
2% Homatropine/10% phenylephrine	1.0	24	Moderate

[a]Mydriatics (mainly 1% atropine ointment) are administered 2–4 times daily in cats with anterior uveitis. Once pupillary dilation occurs, the frequency of atropine may be reduced to once daily or once every other day.

The different colors of the feline iris probably affect the onset and duration of mydriatics. Blue irides may be more sensitive, with a more rapid onset and shorter duration, because of the drug's affinity to melanin.

[b]Ophthalmic solutions of atropine commonly induce salivation in cats because of its bitter taste and its passage down the nasolacrimal system and contact with the cat's tongue. Hence, 1% atropine ointment is usually recommended.

[c]Tropicamide (1%) is recommended for mydriasis during the routine ophthalmic examination. Slow or incomplete mydriasis is suggestive of anterior uveitis or iridocyclitis.

[d]Both phenylephrine (2.5% and 10%) and epinephrine (1–2%) are weak mydriatics in cats but are additive to the parasympatholytic mydriatics. They also are used in the diagnosis of Horner's syndrome and for bilateral nictitating membrane protrusions in young cats.

The Cow

Drug[a]	Time to Maximum Dilation (hours)	Duration (hours)	Extent of Dilation
Parasympatholytics:			
1% Atropine[b]	0.75	24	Moderate
3% Atropine	2	168	Maximal
0.25% Scopolamine	2	144	Maximal
1% Cyclopentolate	12	48	Moderate
2% Cyclopentolate	12	96	Maximal
0.5% Tropicamide	3	3	Moderate
1% Tropicamide[c]	3	8	Moderate
2% Homatropine	2	48	Moderate
Sympathomimetics:			
10% Phenylephrine[d]	—	—	None
Parasympatholytic/sympathomimetic combinations:			
1% Atropine/10% phenylephrine	2	24	Moderate

[a]Mydriatics (usually 1% atropine solution or ointment) are administered 2–4 times daily or to effect (maintain mydriasis).

[b]Atropine (1%) is the preferred mydriatic for anterior uveitis in cattle because of its costs and availability.

[c]Tropicamide (1%) is recommended for mydriasis during the routine ophthalmic examination in cattle because of its short onset and brief duration of action.

[d]Phenylephrine (10%) is a very weak mydriatic in cattle but is additive to the parasympatholytic agents. It also is used in the diagnosis of Horner's syndrome.

The Horse

Drug[a]	Time to Maximum Dilation (hours)	Duration (hours)	Extent of Dilation
Parasympatholytics:			
1% Atropine[b]	10	132	Maximal
3% Atropine	12	264	Maximal
0.25% Scopolamine[c]	4	108	Maximal
1% Cyclopentolate	12	96	Maximal
2% Cyclopentolate	12	120	Maximal
0.5% Tropicamide	1	5	Maximal
1% Tropicamide[d]	5	12	Maximal
2% Homatropine	3	8	Moderate
Sympathomimetics:			
10% Phenylephrine	—	—	None
Parasympatholytic/sympathomimetic combinations:			
1% Atropine/10% phenylephrine	8	84	Maximal

[a]Mydriatics are used frequently in horses because of anterior uveitis or iridocyclitis. They usually are administered 2–4 times daily but are best used to effect (to maintain mydriasis).

[b]Of the domestic species, the horse appears to be most sensitive to topical mydriatics, especially 1% atropine (they may reduce gut motility and even colic). Hence, daily monitoring of fecal output, gut sounds, and mydriasis of the opposite or fellow eye for pupillary dilation (for systemic absorption) is recommended. Gastrointestinal problems can necessitate cessation of topical atropine administration. Topical atropine in foals may produce acute salivation because of its bitter taste, passage down the nasolacrimal system, and contact with the foal's tongue.

[c]Scopolamine (0.25%) combined with phenylephrine (10%) is a very strong mydriatic combination for the horse. It may be instilled hourly for 4–6 times to attempt to break down the posterior synechiae (<1 to 2 weeks of duration). Generally, this intense treatment period is attempted only once, and monitoring of the gastrointestinal tract function is a must.

[d]Tropicamide (1%) is recommended for the routine ophthalmic examination because of its rapid onset and short duration of mydriasis.

The Bird

Agent[a]	Recommendations
D-Tubocurarine	Topical instillation of solution of 3 mg of tubocurarine powder per 1 mL of NaCl solution with 0.025% benzalkonium chloride 3–4 times over 20 minutes.
Vecuronium bromide	Produces mydriasis in kestrels, 4 mg/mL given as 2 drops every 15 minutes for 3 instillations to only one eye (concern about systemic absorption if both eyes are dilated).
Ketamine and xylazine	Short-acting, IM anesthetic combination produces variable mydriasis. Ketamine, 10–15 mg/kg, and xylazine, 1–2 mg/kg.

[a]Birds have striated iridal muscles that control pupil size; paralysis of these muscles by neuroparalytic drugs produces mydriasis.

The serious complications of these drugs are variable effects on the systemic musculature (e.g., eyelid paralysis, limb and neck paralysis, breathing problems). Dilation of both eyes has a greater chance of inducing side effects than unilateral instillation and less systemic drug absorption. For more details, the reader should consult the third edition, pp. 1286–1287.

APPENDIX M

OTHER OPHTHALMIC DRUGS

Drug	*Indications/Use*

Stains:

Fluorescein: Solution and impregnated paper strip. Use for corneal ulcers; naso-lacrimal patency. Used to measure tear film breakup times. A 10% solution (IV) for fluorescein angiography and blood-aqueous barrier studies.

Rose Bengal: Solution and impregnated paper strip. Used to identify damaged corneal and conjunctival epithelium. In cats, used for feline herpesvirus microul-cers; in dogs, used for early keratoconjunctivitis sicca.

Viscoelastics:

Highly viscous fluids injected during intraocular surgery to physically separate tissues; facilitate sliding of intraocular lens; inflate the anterior chamber for phacoemulsification, anterior and posterior capsulorhexis, and during repair of full-thickness corneal lacerations with iris prolapse. Agents include sodium hyaluronate, sodium chondroitin sulfate combined with sodium hyaluronate, and hydroxypropylmethylcellulose.

Antifibrin formation:

Use heparin, 1–2 IU/mL in irrigating solution (usually lactated Ringer's solution), to inhibit fibrin formation in the anterior chamber during intraocular surgery.

Fibrinolysis:

Tissue-plasminogen activator, 25–40 μg. When injected, causes fibrinolysis in the anterior chamber. Fibrin must be recent ($\leq$10–14 days). Use for hypopyon, hyphema, and early postoperative fibrin stands. Do not use if clotting is very recent; rebleeds may occur.

Tissue (butylcyanoacrylate) glue:

Used to treat corneal ulcerations. For success use, carefully debride all nonvi-able corneal tissue, stabilize the eye and dry the ulcer site with cotton swabs and/or a hair dryer, carefully spread a very thin layer of glue using a 30-g hypo-dermic needle (do not apply a thick layer), and let the glue completely dry to prevent accidental contact with the eyelids. Dried glue will slough sponta-neously in 7–14 days.

Ethylenediaminetetraacetate:

Used to chelate calcium. Probably does not penetrate the intact corneal epithe-lium. Use as 0.1–1.0% solution or ointment.

Antifibrotics:

Chemotherapeutic drugs used intra- and postoperatively after glaucoma surg-eries to prevent closure of filtering tissues and stents. Include 0.2–0.4 mg of mit-omycin (applied by surgical sponges directly to the surgical site) and 5-fluo-rouracil injections (total dose of 20–40 mg by subconjunctival injection).

INHERITED EYE DISEASES IN THE DOG

Breed	Microphthalmia	Eyelid Defects[a]	Keratoconjunctivitis Sicca/Dry Eye	Nictitans Defects[b]	Chronic Superficial Keratitis/Pannus	Corneal Dystrophy[c]	Uveodermatologic Syndrome	Glaucoma	Cataract	Lens Luxation	Persistent Lenticular Vascular Membranes[d]	Vitreous Degeneration	Choroidal Hypoplasia, ± Coloboma, ± Retinal Detachment	Retinal Dysplasia[e]	Retinal Degeneration[f]	Optic Nerve Defects[g]	RPE Dystrophy (CPRA)[h]
Afghan Hound						✓			✓								
Airedale Terrier						✓					✓			✓	✓		
Akita	✓	✓					✓	✓	✓		✓				✓		
Alaskan Malamute																	
American Staffordshire Terrier		✓							✓	✓	✓						
Australian Cattle Dog[i]																	
Australian Shepherd	✓	✓				✓			✓				✓		✓	✓	
Basenji									✓		✓					✓	
Basset Griffon Vendeen, Petite											✓			✓			

	Microphthalmia	Eyelid Defects[a]	Keratoconjunctivitis Sicca/Dry Eye	Nictitans Defects[b]	Chronic Superficial Keratitis/Pannus	Corneal Dystrophy[c]	Uveodermatologic Syndrome	Glaucoma	Cataract	Lens Luxation	Persistent Lenticular Vascular Membranes[d]	Vitreous Degeneration	Choroidal Hypoplasia, ±Coloboma, ±Retinal Detachment	Retinal Dysplasia[e]	Retinal Degeneration[f]	Optic Nerve Defects[g]	RPE Dystrophy (CPRA)[h]
Basset Hound		✓						✓									
Beagle[j]	✓			✓		✓			✓						✓		
Bearded Collie						✓			✓		✓			✓			
Bedlington Terrier[k]	✓	✓							✓					✓			
Belgian Malinois														✓			
Belgian Sheepdog					✓				✓		✓				✓	✓	
Belgian Tervuren					✓				✓		✓					✓	
Bernese Mountain Dog		✓															
Bichon Frise						✓			✓								
Bloodhound		✓		✓							✓						
Border Collie									✓	✓			✓		✓		✓
Borzoi															✓		
Boston Terrier		✓				✓		✓	✓								

Bouvier Des Flandres

Boxer

Briard*ˡ*

Brittany

Brussels Griffon

Bulldog (English)

Bullmastiff

Cairn Terrier

Cardigan Welsh Corgi

Cavalier King Charles Spaniel

Chesapeake Bay Retriever

Chihuahua

Chinese Shar Pei

Chow Chow

Clumber Spaniel

Cocker Spaniel (American)

Collie

Curly-Coated Retriever

Dachshund

Dalmatian*ⁱ*

Doberman Pinscher

English Cocker Spaniel

English Springer Spaniel

Breed	Microphthalmia	Eyelid Defects[a]	Keratoconjunctivitis Sicca/Dry Eye	Nictitans Defects[b]	Chronic Superficial Keratitis/Pannus	Corneal Dystrophy[c]	Uveodermatologic Syndrome	Glaucoma	Cataract	Lens Luxation	Persistent Lenticular Vascular Membranes[d]	Vitreous Degeneration	Choroidal Hypoplasia, ±Coloboma, ±Retinal Detachment	Retinal Dysplasia[e]	Retinal Degeneration[f]	Optic Nerve Defects[g]	RPE Dystrophy (CPRA)[h]
English Toy Spaniel		✓							✓								
Field Spaniel		✓												✓			
Flat-Coated Retriever		✓															
German Shepherd		✓			✓	✓			✓					✓	✓	✓	
German Shorthaired Pointer		✓		✓					✓		✓				✓		
Golden Retriever[m]		✓				✓		✓	✓		✓	✓		✓	✓		✓
Gordon Setter		✓							✓		✓			✓	✓		
Great Dane	✓			✓				✓	✓						✓		
Greyhound					✓										✓		
Havanese		✓							✓								
Irish Setter		✓		✓					✓		✓	✓					
Irish Wolfhound									✓		✓				✓		
Italian Greyhound						✓			✓			✓			✓	✓	

Jack Russell Terrier

Japanese Chin

Labrador Retriever

Lakeland Terrier

Lhasa Apso

Lowchen

Mastiff

Miniature Bull Terrier

Miniature Pinscher

Miniature Schnauzer

Newfoundland

Norbottenspets

Norwegian Elkhound

Nova Scotia Duck Tolling Retriever

Old English Sheepdog

Papillon

Pekingese

Pembroke Welsh Corgi

Poodle (all)

Portuguese Water Dog

Pug

Rottweiler

Saint Bernard

Breed	Microphthalmia	Eyelid Defects[a]	Keratoconjunctivitis Sicca/Dry Eye	Nictitans Defects[b]	Chronic Superficial Keratitis/Pannus	Corneal Dystrophy[c]	Uveodermatologic Syndrome	Glaucoma	Cataract	Lens Luxation	Persistent Lenticular Vascular Membranes[d]	Vitreous Degeneration	Choroidal Hypoplasia, ±Coloboma, ±Retinal Detachment	Retinal Dysplasia[e]	Retinal Degeneration[f]	Optic Nerve Defects[g]	RPE Dystrophy (CPRA)[h]
Samoyed		✓				✓		✓	✓		✓			✓	✓		
Scottish Terrier									✓		✓						
Sealyham Terrier										✓				✓			
Shetland Sheepdog		✓				✓			✓		✓		✓		✓	✓	
Shih Tzu			✓						✓								
Siberian Husky		✓				✓	✓		✓			✓			✓		
Smooth Fox Terrier		✓						✓	✓	✓					✓		
Soft-Coated Wheaten Terrier	✓							✓						✓			
Staffordshire Bull Terrier (English)		✓							✓		✓						
Standard Schnauzer			✓						✓		✓						
Tibetan Spaniel		✓							✓						✓		
Tibetan Terrier									✓		✓				✓		
Vizsla		✓				✓			✓	✓							

Weimaraner

Welsh Springer Spaniel

West Highland White Terrier

Whippet

Wire Fox Terrier

Yorkshire Terrier

[a]Includes: Ciliated Caruncle, Distichiasis, Ectopic Cilia, Ectropion, Macroblepharon, & Entropion

[b]Includes: Eversion/Prolapse of 3rd Eyelid Gland

[c]Includes: Corneal Dystrophy—Endothelial, Endothelial Erosion, Stromal, & Posterior Polymorphous

[d]Includes: Persistent Pupillary Membranes, Persistent Hyaloid Artery, Persistent Hyperplastic Primary Vitreous (PHPV) & Persistent Hyperplastic Tunica Vasculosa Lentis (PHTVL)

[e]Includes: Retinal Dysplasia: Folds, Geographic, & Detachments

[f]Includes: Retinal Atrophy—Generalized & Rod/Cone Dysplasia Type 2 (rcd2), Retinal Degeneration, Day Blindness

[g]Includes: Optic Nerve—Coloboma & Hypoplasia

[h]Includes: Retinal Pigment Epithelial Dystrophy or Central Progressive Retinal Atrophy.

[i]Australian Shepherd & Dalmatian specific disorder—Ceroid Lipofuscinosis

[j]Beagle specific disorder—Tapetal Degeneration

[k]Bedlington Terrier specific disorder—Imperforate Lacrimal Punctum

[l]Briard specific disorder—Congenital Stationary Night Blindness

[m]Golden Retriever specific disorders—Iris Cysts, Pigmentary Uveitis

APPENDIX O

INHERITED EYE DISEASES IN THE CAT

Breed	Ophthalmic Disease
Abyssinian	Early onset progressive retinal atrophy, late-onset progressive retinal atrophy.
Birman	Dermoids, cataracts.
Burmese	Dermoids, congenital nictitans gland enlargement.
Himalayan	Epiphora, cataracts.
Korat	GM_1- and GM_2-gangliosidosis.
Persian	Multiple ocular anomalies, epiphora, entropion, iridal heterochromia, cataracts, retinal atrophy, α-mannosidase.
Shorthair	Multiple ocular anomalies, dermoids, cataracts, GM_1- and GM_2-gangliosidosis, α-mannosidosis, mucopolysaccharidosis I.
Siamese	Esotropia, nystagmus, iridal heterochromia, glaucoma, GM_1-gangliosidosis, mucopolysaccharidosis VI.

INHERITED EYE DISEASES IN THE HORSE

Appaloosa
Congenital stationary night blindness
Congenital cataracts
Glaucoma
Equine recurrent uveitis
Optic disc colobomas

Arabian
Congenital cataracts

Belgian
Aniridia and secondary cataracts

Morgan
Cataracts (nuclear, bilateral, symmetrical, and nonprogressive)

Quarter horse
Congenital cataracts
Entropion

Thoroughbred
Congenital cataracts
Microphthalmia associated with multiple ocular defects
Retinal dysplasia associated with retinal detachments in some cases
Entropion

Color-dilute breeds
Iridal hypoplasia (photophobia)

Standardbred
Retinal detachments
Congenital stationary night blindness

Paso Fino
Congenital stationary night blindness
Glaucoma

American Saddlebred
Cataracts

Warm bloods
Glaucoma

Rocky Mountain horse
Anterior segment dysgenesis

INHERITED EYE DISEASES IN FOOD ANIMALS

Cattle:

Aberdeen Angus	Osteopetrosis, mannosidosis.
Ayrshire	Heterochromia irides, porphyria, nystagmus.
Beef Master	Neuronal lipodystrophy.
Brown Swiss	Supernumerary lacrimal drainage openings, multiple ocular anomalies.
Charolais	Posterior segment/optic disc colobomata.
Devon	Ceroid lipofuscinosis.
Guernsey	Heterochromia irides, multiple ocular anomalies, nystagmus.
Hereford	Iridal heterochromia, optic disc coloboma with incomplete albinism, dermoids, cataracts, retinal dysplasia and hydrocephalus, Chediak-Higashi syndrome, squamous cell carcinoma.
Holstein-Friesian	Cataracts, gangliosidosis, heterochromia irides, nystagmus, corneal edema, porphyria, glaucoma.
Jersey	Strabismus, cataracts, multiple ocular anomalies, nystagmus.
Shorthorn	Corneal edema, strabismus, exophthalmia, cataracts, retinal dysplasia and hydrocephalus, porphyria, glycogen storage disease type II.

Sheep:

Many breeds	Entropion, upper eyelid coloboma.
Corriedale	Glucocerebroside storage disease type II, glycogen storage diseases type II.
South Hampshire	Ceroid lipofuscinosis.
New Zealand Romney	Cataracts.

Swine:

Breeds with white hair	Heterochromia irides.
Sinclair miniature	Cutaneous melanomas/uveitis.
Yorkshire	Cerebrospinal lipodystrophy, glucocerebroside storage disease.

Glossary

Common Ophthalmic Roots

blepharo lid

cor pupil

cyclo ciliary body

dacryo tears

hyal vitreous

hyp anterior chamber

irido iris

kerato cornea

ophthalmo globe or eye

papilla optic disc

phako/phaco lens

Common Words

Ablation Removal of the globe or part of the eye (as destruction of the ciliary body).

Ablepharon Partial or complete congenital absence of the eyelids.

Accommodation Changes in the shape (and power) of the lens for seeing near objects. Limited in the domestic species.

Amaurosis Total loss of vision.

Amblyopia Reduced or partial loss of sight without detectable lesions in the eye and the optic nerve.

Aniridia Iris is absent clinically; some remnants may be demonstrated at histopathology.

Anisocoria Unequal pupils.

561

Ankyloblepharon   Adhesion of the eyelids to each other. Physiologic in kittens and puppies during the first 10 to 14 days of life.

Anophthalmia   Congenital absence of the globes. Usually a severe hypoplasia of the globe (i.e., microphthalmia)

Aphakia   Absence of the lens.

Aphakic Crescent   Area of the pupil not covered by a luxated or a displaced lens.

Aqueous Flare   Aqueous humor with increased levels of proteins. Best demonstrated using a focal light beam projected across the anterior chamber or a commercial laser flaremeter.

Asteroid Hyalosis   Calcium lipid bodies/opacities suspended in the vitreous.

Bergmeister's Papilla   Remnants of the posterior hyaloid artery that appear as a small, white projection from the center of the surface of the optic disc.

Bernard-Horner Syndrome   Ptosis, miosis, enophthalmos, and protrusion of the nictitating membrane (also regional sweating in the horse). Commonly called *Horner's syndrome*.

Biomicroscopy   Microscopic examination of the various ocular structures.

Blepharitis   Inflammation of the eyelids. May be diffuse or focal.

Blepharospasm   Contractions of the orbicularis oculi muscles.

Blepharostenosis (Blepharophimosis)   Inability to open the palpebral fissure to a normal extent; a palpebral fissure that is smaller than normal.

Buphthalmos   Enlargement of the globe. Also called *hydrophthalmia* or *megaloglobus*.

Canaliculus   Connects the lacrimal punctum to the nasolacrimal sac.

Canthotomy   Incision of the lateral or the medial canthus.

Caruncle   Small mass often covered with hair at the medial canthus in front of the nictitating membrane.

Cataract   Opacity of the lens and its capsules.

Chalazion   Chronic and often granulomatous inflammation of the tarsal or the meibomian glands.

Chemosis   Edema of the conjunctiva.

Choroid   Posterior uvea; consists of pigmented cells, blood vessels, and in some animal species, a special layer in the dorsal fundus, the tapetum lucidum (*T. cellulosum* [in carnivores] or *T. fibrosum* [in herbivores]).

Choroiditis   Inflammation of the choroid.

Ciliary Body   Part of the anterior uvea and the primary source of aqueous humor.

Ciliary Flush   Hyperemia of the bulbar conjunctiva; usually associated with intraocular inflammations.

Cilium/Cilia   Another name for eyelashes.

Coloboma   A defect of the eye. Commonly divided into typical (i.e., 6-o'clock position) and atypical (i.e., all other positions) types.

Conjunctiva   Mucous membrane connecting the eyelid margin to the limbus of the globe. Divided into the palpebral, fornix (or cul-de-sac), and bulbar conjunctiva.

Conjunctivorhinostomy   Surgically created fistula between the medial conjunctival fornix and the nasal cavity as an alternate drainage route for tears.

Conjunctivobuccostomy   Surgically created fistula for the passage of tears from the ventral conjunctival fornix to the mouth.

Consensual Pupillary Reflex   Constriction of the pupil when the opposite eye (i.e., the retina) is stimulated. Sometimes called the *indirect pupillary response*.

Corectasia   Dilation of the pupil

Corectopia   An off-center pupil.

Coreoplasty   Construction of a new pupil.

Corneal Dystrophy   Bilateral, inherited corneal disease that is usually characterized by the deposition of materials, usually lipid substances. Must be distinguished from the unilateral corneal degeneration, which occurs secondary to other corneal diseases. Can also involve the corneal epithelium and endothelium.

Corpora Nigrum/Nigra   Pigmented, irregular mass on the dorsal and, occasionally, the ventral pupillary margin of the iris in herbivores. Also, more recently called *granula iridica*.

Cul-de-Sac   Junction of the palpebral and the bulbar conjunctiva; also called the *fornix*.

Cryoextraction   Removal of the lens using ultracold devices.

Cyclitis   Inflammation of the ciliary body.

Cyclocryothermy   Application of an ultracold probe on the sclera to destroy the ciliary body epithelium and reduce the formation of aqueous humor.

Cyclodialysis   Surgical fistula from the anterior chamber beneath the iris and the ciliary body to exit thorough the sclera.

Cycloplegia   Usually drug-induced paralysis of the ciliary body, along with the resultant loss of accommodation.

Dacryoadenitis   Inflammation of the lacrimal gland.

Dacryocystitis   Inflammation of the nasolacrimal sac.

Dacryocystorhinography   Radiopaque studies of the nasolacrimal apparatus.

Dermoid   Congenital mass involving the eyelids, conjunctiva, nictitating membrane, or cornea and consisting of normal skin and its components. Sometimes also called a *choristoma*.

Descemetocele   A deep corneal ulcer characterized by the exposure and possible protrusion of the Descemet's membrane. Does not stain with topical fluorescein.

Dialysis   Retinal tear at the ora ciliaris retinae, with separation of the neurosensory retina from the retinal pigment epithelium.

Diathermy   Application of heat to various parts of the eye (especially the ciliary body).

Diopter (D)   Refracting power of a lens focused at 1 m (i.e., 1 D = 1/1 m).

Discission   Incision of a structure, usually the anterior capsule of the lens.

Distichiasis   Presence of abnormal eyelashes (cilia).

Dyscoria   An irregular pupil.

Ectasia   Protrusion of the cornea or sclera.

Ectopic Lentis   Luxation or displacement of the lens.

Ectropion   Outward folding of the eyelid and its margin.

Electroretinography   Recording of retinal electrical potentials generated by a rapid change in illumination. Divided into flash and pattern types.

Emmetropia   Normal eye in refraction; the image focused on the retina with the eye at rest.

Endophthalmitis   Inflammation of the globe involving the inner structures.

Enophthalmos   Recession of the globe in the orbit.

Entropion   Infolding of the eyelid and its margin.

Enucleation   Surgical removal of the globe.

Epilation   Manual removal by forceps of cilia (eyelashes).

Epiphora   Overflow of tears onto the medial canthus or the eyelid margin. May signal overproduction, inadequate drainage, or both.

Equine Recurrent Uveitis   Recurrent (or chronic) iridocyclochoroiditis in the horse.

Esotropia   Convergent strabismus.

Evisceration   Removal of the structures of the eye, leaving only the sclera or the cornea and sclera.

Exenteration   Removal of all the contents from the orbit.

Exophthalmos   Protrusion of the globe; eyelids can usually still function and cover the cornea.

External Hordeolum (Stye)   Inflammation and frequent abscessation of the glands of Zeis and Moll.

Exotropia   Divergent strabismus.

"Flare"   An increase in the protein levels of the aqueous humor with a positive Tyndell phenomenon.

Fluorescein (Resorcinol-Phthalein)   Water-soluble compound that yields a bright green fluorescence. Used for the detection of corneal ulcers, chorioretinal circulation time, integrity of the blood-aqueous barrier, and patency of the nasolacrimal apparatus.

Glands of Moll   Apocrine (sweat) glands near the eyelid margin. When inflamed, a stye (or external hordeolum) is observed.

Glands of Zeiss   Sebaceous glands of the eyelid margins. When inflamed, a stye (or external hordeolum) is observed.

Glaucoma   Abnormal increase in the intraocular pressure and optic neuropathy.

Gonioscopy   Examination of the anterior chamber angle (iridocorneal angle and sclerociliary cleft) using a special contact lens.

Granula Iridica   Pigmented mass on the edge of the upper and the lower pupil in herbivores.

Haws   Lay term for the nictitating membrane.

Hemeralopia   Day blindness.

Heterochromia Iridis   Two or more colors in an iris or between two irides in one individual.

Hordeolum (External)   Inflammation of the glands of Moll and Zeiss. Also called a *stye*.

Hordeolum (Internal)   Inflammation of the meibomian gland; an abscess or granuloma. Also called a *chalazion*.

Horner's Syndrome   Sympathetic denervation of the eye and the orbit. Clinical signs include miosis, nictitating membrane protrusion, enophthalmos, ptosis, and in some animal species, regional vascular hyperemia and sweating.

Hyaloid   Vitreous.

Hydrophthalmos   Congential globe enlargement. A dated term; currently, *buphthalmos* is preferred.

Hyperopia   Farsightedness. Objects can be seen distinctly when at a distance. The image is not in focus at the level of the retina; instead, the image is in focus behind the retina.

Hyphema   Hemorrhage in the anterior chamber.

Hypopyon   Pus in the anterior chamber.

Hypotony   Abnormally low intraocular pressure (usually < 5 mm Hg).

Iridectomy   Excision of the iris. Divided into basal, peripheral, and sphincterectomy.

Iridencleisis   A surgical procedure used to treat glaucoma that consists of a pillar of iris positioned through a scleral incision (creating a "wick").

Iridocorneal Angle   The angle created by the iris and cornea. In nonprimate mammals, the angle is composed of the basal iris, ciliary body (i.e., ciliary cleft), and sclera. Also called the *anterior chamber angle* or *filtration angle*.

Iridocyclitis   Inflammation of iris and the ciliary body. Also called *anterior uveitis*.

Iridodonesis   Tremulousness of the iris, usually associated with lens instability, an intraocular lens, or a small lens. Observed with lens luxation, aphakia, hypermature cataracts, and cataract resorption.

Iridoplegia   Pupillary dilation and paralysis of the iridal sphincter muscles.

Iridotomy   Incision of the iris.

Iris Bombé   Focal or generalized bulging of the iris that indicates impaired pupillary passage of the aqueous humor. Associated with focal or annular posterior synechiae.

Iritis   Inflammation of the iris.

Keratectomy   Excision (usually superficial) of the cornea.

Keratitis   Inflammation of the cornea.

Keratocentesis   Puncture of the cornea and removal of portions of the aqueous humor.

Keratoconus (Anterior)   Conical anterior protrusion of the center of the cornea.

Keratoglobus   An enlarged cornea, usually with buphthalmos.

Keratoplasty   Corneal grafts. Divided into lamellar (i.e., superficial) and complete (i.e., full thickness).

Krause's glands   Accessory lacrimal glands of the upper and the lower conjunctiva fornix.

Lacrimation   Used clinically as a term to imply excessive rates of tear formation.

Lagophthalmos   Inability to close the palpebral fissure; mainly the inability of the upper eyelid to close.

Lenticular   Relating to the lens.

Lenticulodenesis   Instability of the lens associated with zonulary loss.

Leukoma   A dense corneal scar.

Limbus   The transitional zone between the cornea and the sclera. Also called the *blue zone*.

Luxation   Dislocation of a structure. In ophthalmology, term is used for the globe (i.e., proptosis) and for dislocation of the lens.

Manometry   Direct measurement of the intraocular pressure using a needle inserted into the anterior chamber or the vitreous body.

Megalocornea   An enlarged cornea, usually with buphthalmos.

Microcornea   A small or hypoplastic cornea.

Microphakia   An abnormally small lens.

Microphthalmia   An abnormally small eye.

Miosis   Contraction of the pupil.

Miotic   A drug that produces constriction of the pupil. Two types are available: direct (i.e., parasympathomimetic), and indirect (i.e., anticholinesterase).

Mittendorf's dot   Hyaloid vascular remnant at posterior pole of the lens.

Morgagnian Cataract   Type of hypermature cataract with a liquified cortex and a solid nucleus.

Motility   Movement of the globe.

Mydriatic   A drug that produces dilation of the pupil. Two types are available: parasympatholytic, and sympathomimetic.

Myopia   Nearsightedness. Objects are seen distinctly when close. The image is not in focus at the level of the retina; instead, it is in focus in front of the retina.

Nevus   A focal, pigmented area in the iris, choroid, and so on.

Nyctalopia   Night blindness

Nystagmus   Oscillation of the globe.

OD   Oculus dextor; the right eye.

Ophthalmia Neonatorum   Conjunctivitis in the neonate with physiologic ankyloblepharon; occurs in kittens and puppies.

Ophthalmoplegia   Paralysis of the extraocular muscles. Divided into internal (with mydriasis) and external types.

Ophthalmoscopy   Examination of the ocular fundus using an ophthalmoscope. Both direct and indirect methods are available.

OS   Oculus sinister; the left eye.

OU   Oculi unitas; both eyes.

Pannus   Invasion of the cornea, with subepithelial neovascularization and pigmentation.

Panophthalmitis   Inflammation involving all layers of the globe.

Papilla   Another term for the optic nerve head or optic disc.

Papilledema   Edema of the optic disc or papilla.

Papillitis   Inflammation of the optic disc or papilla.

Periodic Ophthalmia   An older term for equine recurrent uveitis.

Peripheral Anterior Synechia   Inflammatory attachments of the basal iris and the peripheral posterior cornea.

Persistent Pupillary Membrane   Congenital remnants of the prenatal pupillary vascular membrane that extend from the collarette region of the iris to the cornea, lens, or other areas of the iris.

Phacodonesis   Instability of the lens, usually secondary to the loss of zonulary attachments.

Photophobia   Increased sensitivity to light.

Photopic   Conditions under light or bright illumination, as with photopic vision or electroretinography.

Phthisis bulbus   Atrophy of the globe with low intraocular pressure; usually associated with trauma and inflammation.

Polycoria   Two or more pupils in an eye. Divided into false (i.e., no sphincter muscle) and true (i.e., with sphincter muscle) types. Must be differentiated from iris atrophy.

Proptosis   Forward displacement of the globe out of the orbit.

Provocative Tests   Procedures to demonstrate the tendency toward glaucoma in an eye. Such tests include use of corticosteroids, water, mydriatics, and a dark room.

Pterygium   Invasion of the cornea by the bulbar conjunctiva. Has not been documented in animals.

Ptosis   Drooping of the upper eyelid.

Pupil   Opening in the central iris.

Rose Bengal   Topical ophthalmic stain used to outline dead and degenerating corneal as well as conjunctival cells.

Rubeosis Iridis   Neovascularization of the iris, with frequent involvement of the anterior chamber angle, pupil, anterior surface of the lens, and ciliary body processes.

Sclerotomy   Incision of the sclera.

Scleritis   Inflamation of the sclera.

Scotopic   Dark conditions, as with vision or electroretinography.

Spherophakia   Round or spherical lens.

Sicca   Dryness.

Squint   Strabismus.

Staphyloma   Protrusion of the cornea or sclera lined with uveal tissue. May be congenital, traumatic, or surgical.

Strabismus   When the visual axes of the eyes are not parallel. Common types are *S. convergens* (i.e., internal squint) and *S. divergens* (i.e., external squint). Also called *heterotropia*.

Striate Keratopathy   Irregular, linear lines in the cornea, usually associated with glaucoma (i.e., breaks), and phthisis bulbi (i.e., folds), and changes in the Descemet's membrane.

Stye   Inflammations of the glands of Moll and Zeiss.

Subluxation Partial lens displacement; associated with partial loss of the lens zonules.

Symblepharon Adhesion of one or both eyelids to the conjunctiva, the cornea, or both.

Synechia Adhesion of the iris to the cornea (i.e., anterior synechia), of the iris to the lens (i.e., posterior synechia), and in the iridocorneal angle (i.e., peripheral anterior synechia).

Syneresis Liquefaction of the vitreous.

Synchysis Scintillans Liquified vitreous with cholesterol crystals.

Tapetum Lucidum A special reflective layer within the dorsal choroid that provides additional reflection of light, thereby permitting double retinal stimulation of the retina. Divided into *T. cellulosum* (in carnivores) and *T. fibrosum* (in herbivores).

Tarsorrhaphy Temporary (using sutures) or permanent apposition of part (i.e., partial tarsorrhaphy) or all (i.e., complete tarsorrhaphy) of the eyelids.

Tear film breakup Development of dry spots (measured in seconds) in the tear film, as observed at biomicroscopy with the preocular film stained using fluorescein.

Tenon's Capsule Fascia bulbus.

Tonography Continuous measurement of the intraocular pressure to estimate pressure-sensitive aqueous humor outflow (in μL/ mm Hg per minute).

Tonometry Measurement of the intraocular pressure. Divided into indentation and applanation types.

Transillumination Passage of light through the tissues. May facilitate the differentiation of solid from hollow tissue masses.

Trichiasis Contact of hair with the eye, as in entropion or nasal fold trichiasis.

Uvea The iris, ciliary body and choroid.

Uvea (Anterior) The iris and ciliary body.

Uvea (Posterior) The choroid.

Uveitis Inflammation of the uveal tract.

Uveitis (Anterior) Inflammation of the iris and the ciliary body.

Uveitis (Posterior) Inflammation of the choroid.

Panuveitis Inflammation of the iris, ciliary body, and choroid.

Vibrissae Large, tachile hair about the eyelids and face of large animals.

Wolfring Accessory lacrimal gland of the dorsal palpebral conjunctiva.

Xerophthalmia Dryness of the cornea and conjunctiva. Also called *keratoconjunctivitis sicca* or *xerosis*.

Zonules Suspensory ligaments connecting the lens periphery (i.e., equator) to the ciliary body.

Zonulolysis Enzymatic (i.e., α-chymotrypsin) or surgical transection of the lens zonules.

Index

Page numbers in *italics* denote figures; those followed by a "t" denote tables; those followed by a "b" denote boxes.

569